T0145389

Lecture Notes on Data Engineering and Communications Technologies

Volume 127

The aim of the book series is to present cutting edge engineering approaches to data technologies and communications. It will publish latest advances on the engineering task of building and deploying distributed, scalable and reliable data infrastructures and communication systems.

The series will have a prominent applied focus on data technologies and communications with aim to promote the bridging from fundamental research on data science and networking to data engineering and communications that lead to industry products, business knowledge and standardisation.

Indexed by SCOPUS, INSPEC, EI Compendex.

All books published in the series are submitted for consideration in Web of Science.

More information about this series at https://link.springer.com/bookseries/15362

Faisal Saeed · Fathey Mohammed ·
Fuad Ghaleb
Editors

Advances on Intelligent Informatics and Computing

Health Informatics, Intelligent Systems, Data Science and Smart Computing

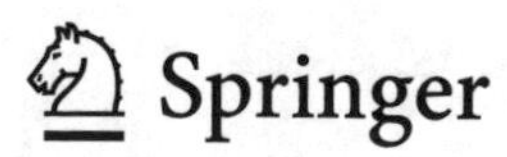

Editors
Faisal Saeed
Birmingham City University
Birmingham, UK

Fathey Mohammed
School of Computing
Universiti Utara Malaysia (UUM)
Sintok, Kedah, Malaysia

Fuad Ghaleb
Department of Computer Science,
School of Computing
Universiti Teknologi Malaysia
Skudai, Malaysia

ISSN 2367-4512 ISSN 2367-4520 (electronic)
Lecture Notes on Data Engineering and Communications Technologies
ISBN 978-3-030-98740-4 ISBN 978-3-030-98741-1 (eBook)
https://doi.org/10.1007/978-3-030-98741-1

This Springer imprint is published by the registered company Springer Nature Switzerland AG
The registered company address is: Gewerbestrasse 11, 6330 Cham, Switzerland

Preface

We are pleased to welcome all of you to the 6th International Conference of Reliable Information and Communication Technology 2021 (IRICT 2021) that is held online on December 22–23, 2021. RICT 2021 is organized by the Yemeni Scientists Research Group (YSRG), in collaboration with Behavioral Informatics Research Group (INFOBEE) in Universiti Teknologi Malaysia (Malaysia) and College of Engineering, IT and Environment at Charles Darwin University (Australia). IRICT 2021 is a forum for the presentation of technological advances in the field of information and communication technology. The main theme of the conference is "Advances on Intelligent Informatics and Computing".

The conference book includes 66 papers that discuss several research topics such as health informatics, artificial intelligence, soft computing, data science, big data analytics, Internet of Things (IoT), intelligent communication systems, cybersecurity, and information system. These papers were presented in three parallel sessions during the two days.

We would like to express our appreciations to all authors and the keynote speakers for sharing their expertise with us. And, we would like to thank the organizing committee for their great efforts in managing the conference. In addition, we would like to thank the technical committee for reviewing all the submitted papers.

Finally, we thank all the participants of IRICT 2021 and hope to see you all again in the next conference.

Organization

IRICT 2021 Organizing Committee

International Advisory Board

Abdul Samad Haji Ismail	Universiti Teknologi Malaysia, Malaysia
Ahmed Yassin Al-Dubai	Edinburgh Napier University, UK
Ali Bastawissy	Cairo University, Egypt
Ali Selamat	Universiti Teknologi Malaysia, Malaysia
Ayoub AL-Hamadi	Otto-von-Guericke University Magdeburg, Germany
Eldon Y. Li	National Chengchi University (NCCU), Taiwan
Kamal Zuhairi Zamil	Universiti Malaysia Pahang, Malaysia
Kamarulnizam Abu Bakar	Universiti Teknologi Malaysia, Malaysia
Mohamed M S Nasser	Qatar University, Qatar
Srikanta Patnaik	SOA University, Bhubaneswar, India

Conference General Chair

Faisal Saeed (President)	Yemeni Scientists Research Group (YSRG)

Program Committee Chair

Fathey Mohammed	Universiti Utara Malaysia (UUM), Malaysia

General Secretary

Nadhmi Gazem	Taibah University, Kingdom of Saudi Arabia

Technical Committee Chair

Faisal Saeed	Taibah University, Kingdom of Saudi Arabia
Tawfik Al-Hadhrami	Nottingham Trent University, UK
Mamoun Alazab	Charles Darwin University, Australia

Publications Committee

Fathey Mohammed	Universiti Utara Malaysia
Fuad A. Ghaleb	University Teknologi Malaysia, Malaysia
Abdulaziz Al-Nahari	Unitar, International University, Malaysia

Publicity Committee

Wahid Al-Twaiti (Chair)	Universiti Tun Hussein Onn Malaysia
Maged Nasser	Universiti Teknologi Malaysia
Mohammed Omar Awadh Al-Shatari	Universiti Teknologi Petronas
Ali Ahmed Ali Salem	Universiti Tun Hussein Onn Malaysia

IT & Multimedia Committee

Sameer Hasan Albakri (Chair)	Sana'a University, Yemen
Mohammed Alsarem	Taibah University, KSA
Amer Alsaket	Sitecore, Malaysia

Treasure Registration Committee Chair

Abdullah Aysh Dahawi	Universiti Teknologi Malaysia

International Technical Committee

Abdelhamid Emara
Abdelrahman Elsharif Karrar
Abdulmajid Aldaba
Abdulrahman A Alsewari
Abdulrahman Alqarafi
Abdulwahab Almazroi
Adel Ammar
Ahmad Alzu'Bi
Ahmed Awad
Ahmed Rakha
Aisyah Ibrahim
Akram Osman
Alaa Alomoush
Ali Nasser
Ammar Alqadasi
Amr Tolba
Ashraf Osman
Bakr Salim Ba-Quttayyan
Bouchaib Cherradi
Badiea Abdulkarem Mohammed Al-Shaibani
Ghassan Aldharhani
Heider Wahsheh
Hiba Zuhair

Fadi Herzallah
Faisal Saeed
Fathey Mohammed
Funminiyi Olajide
Hakeem Flayyih
Hany Harb
Hussien Abualrejal
Ibrahim Fadhel
Ibrahim Mahgoub
Jawad Alkhateeb
Kamal Alhendawi
Kamal Karkonasasi
Khairul Shafee Kalid
Khalil Almekhlafi
Lamia Berriche
Maged Rfeqallah
Maha Idriss
Manal A.Areqi
Masud Hasan
Mohamamed A. Al-Sharafi
Mohamed Abdel Fattah
Mohamed Elhamahmy
Mohammed A. Hajar
Mohammed Al Sarem
Mohammed Azrag
Mounira Kezadri Hamiaz
Nadhmi Gazem
Nejood Hashim Al-Walidi
Noor Suhana Sulaiman
Nouf Alharbi
Osama Sayaydeh
Othman Asiry
Qasim Alajmi
Rashiq Marie
Rayan Alanazi
Safa Ben Atitallah
Salisu Garba
Siwar Rekik
Tariq Saeed
Tawfik Al-Hadhrami
Wadii Boulila
Waleed Abdulmaged Hammood
Waseem Alromimah
Yogan Jaya Kumar
Yousef Fazea
Yousif Aftan Abdullah
Zahid Khan
Zeyad Ghaleb Al-Mekhlafi

Contents

Data Science

Cyber Security

Information Systems

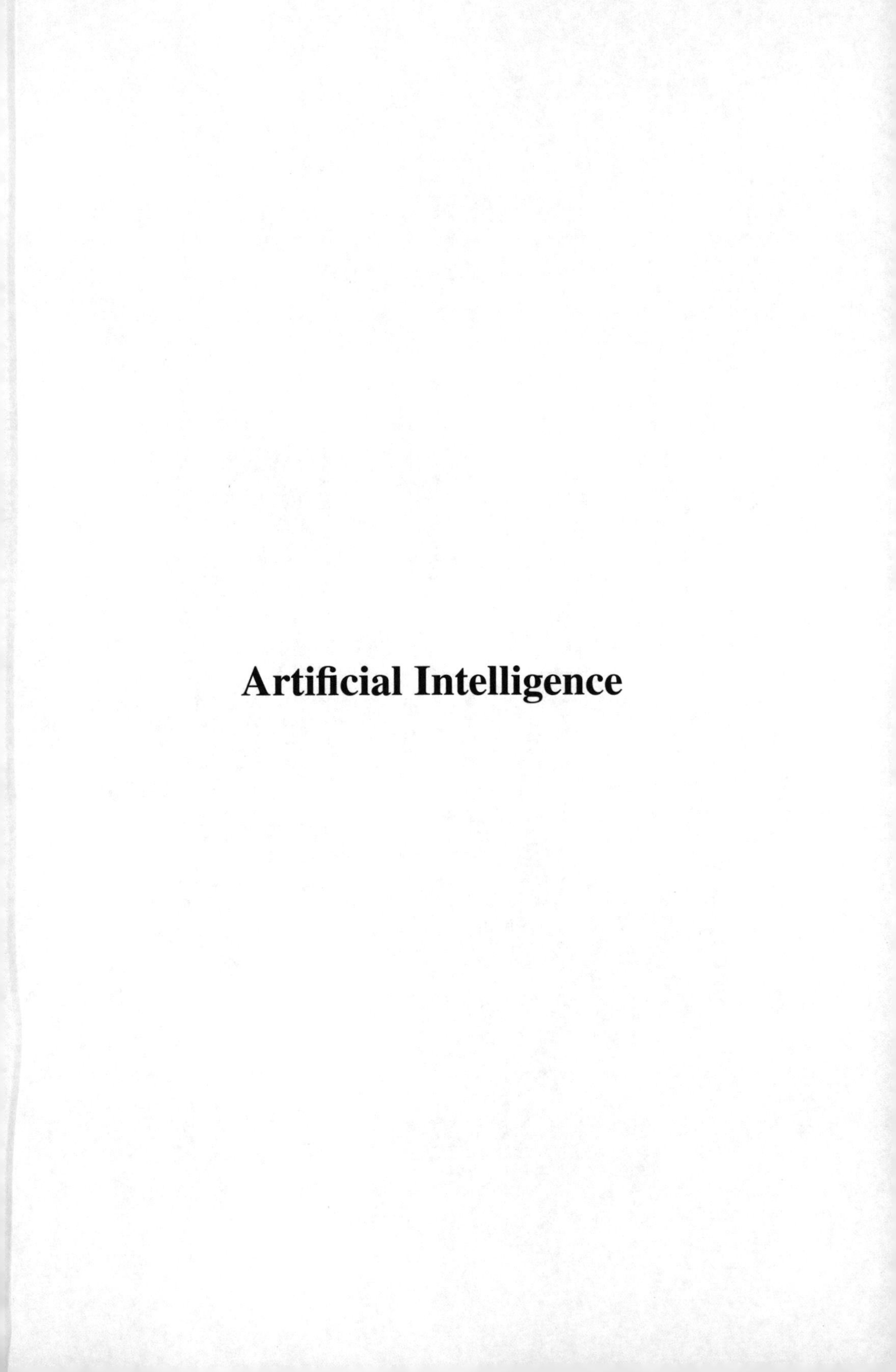

Artificial Intelligence

Automatic Saudi Arabian License Plate Detection and Recognition Using Deep Convolutional Neural Networks

Maha Driss[1,2](✉), Iman Almomani[1], Rahaf Al-Suhaimi[3], and Hanan Al-Harbi[3]

[1] Security Engineering Lab, CS Department, CCIS, Prince Sultan University, Riyadh, Saudi Arabia
maha.idriss@riadi.rnu.tn

[2] RIADI Laboratory, National School of Computer Sciences, University of Manouba, Tunis, Tunisia

[3] IS Department, CCSE, Taibah University, Medina, Saudi Arabia

Abstract. Automatic License Plate (LP) detection and recognition algorithms have become a necessity for intelligent transportation systems due to their efficiency in multiple applications such as parking control and traffic management. Vehicle LP detection and recognition is the process of identifying and locating the LP from the vehicle and then extracting and recognizing the characters from this plate. Several academic studies have addressed the problem of LP detection and recognition and have proposed implementations with different performance indicators' values. However, many of the current studies' solutions are still not robust and efficient in complex real-world situations. In this paper, an automatic LP detection and recognition approach is proposed for the context of Saudi Arabia using Deep Learning (DL) techniques. The core of the proposed approach is to develop a sequence of Faster Region-based Convolutional Neural Networks (Faster-RCNN) and Convolutional Neural Networks (CNN). The Faster-RCNN model is used for LP detection, whereas CNN is applied for characters' recognition from LPs. The obtained experimental results prove the robustness and effectiveness of the proposed approach. We obtained a precision of 92% for LP detection and an accuracy of 98% for LP recognition.

Keywords: License plate · Detection · Recognition · Faster-RCNN · CNN · Saudi Arabia

1 Introduction

Automatic License Plate (LP) detection and recognition have become an interesting research field since it contributes significantly to the enhancement of smart cities' applications such as traffic flow control, stolen and criminals' vehicles detection, enforcement of traffic laws, and management of parking lots, etc. This topic has been largely studied and is still receiving significant attention from researchers and the industry. In the literature, several research works have been proposed [1]. Traditional methods based

F. Saeed et al. (Eds.): IRICT 2021, LNDECT 127, pp. 3–15, 2022.
https://doi.org/10.1007/978-3-030-98741-1_1

on image pre-processing techniques such as object localization, character extraction, and pattern recognition did not provide good results, especially with different image acquisition conditions. With the technological progress made on the graphics processing unit, running high-performance computing algorithms becomes possible, and several Machine Learning (ML) and Deep Learning (DL) models are increasingly used in image classification applications and provide impressive results [2–5]. In the last decade, many research studies have been conducted using DL-based methods to propose more robust and efficient systems for LP detection and recognition.

In this paper, an efficient approach for LP detection and recognition in the context of Saudi Arabia is proposed. The proposed approach is based on three steps: 1) license plate detection, 2) image pre-processing, and 3) character segmentation and recognition.

The main contributions of the proposed work are summarized as follows:

- To the best of the authors' knowledge, this paper constitutes the first study that investigates the problem of LP detection and recognition for the context of Saudi Arabia using DL techniques;
- The proposed approach is based on two DL models; the Faster-RCNN model for LP detection and CNN for characters' recognition from LPs;
- A new dataset is created consisting of 1150 real-world Saudi Arabian cars. The car images were collected under various lighting and weather conditions. Besides, the images cover different types of cars and vehicles such as pickup trucks, vans, hatchbacks, buses, ambulances, and sports coupes cars, etc.
- Experiments that were conducted on the collected dataset showed that the proposed approach achieved a precision of 92% for LP detection and an accuracy of 98% for LP recognition.

This paper is organized as follows. Section 2 presents related works for LP detection and recognition. Section 3 details the proposed approach. Implementations and experiments are illustrated in Sect. 4. Finally, Sect. 5 concludes the paper and provides potential future work.

2 Related Works

In the literature, a limited number of works were conducted to ensure detection and recognition for Saudi Arabian LPs. Most of these works used image processing and analysis techniques [6, 7]. Other works used simple neural networks to ensure either LP detection or recognition [8, 9]. Our focus in this work is to examine research studies that have been conducted to resolve both the detection and recognition problems of LP using DL techniques.

In [10], Hendry and Chen used You Only Look Once (YOLO) to detect LP for Taiwan's car, which contains six digits. They modified the original YOLO to detect a single class by using a sliding window. Experiments that were made under different conditions such as rainy background, darkness, and dimness showed that the proposed system achieved good performance results in terms of detection and recognition accuracy, average model loss, and average speed. Kessentini et al. [11] proposed a real-time

LP recognition system based on two DL stages. The first stage aimed to detect LP using full raw images by applying the YOLOv2 CNN model. The second stage recognized LPs captured on cropped images. In this paper, two fully annotated datasets were considered and experiments carried out showed that the proposed system achieved acceptable rates in terms of LP recognition accuracy. The authors in [12] developed a DL-based system for automatic recognition of Brazilian LP. Montazzolli et al. used two YOLO CNN networks to detect LP and to recognize characters within cropped LPs. The authors introduced a method to annotate car bounding boxes. The results of experiments applied on a Brazilian public dataset showed good performance of this approach in terms of character segmentation and recognition accuracy. In [13], Omar et al. proposed using semantic segmentation to split images into regions that were fed into two CNN models for both Arabic number recognition and city determination. Omar et al. have conducted their experiments using a new LP dataset composed of images taken in the northern region of Iraq. Experiments showed that the proposed approach achieved acceptable results in terms of recognition recall, precision, and F-measure scores. Laroca et al. [14] presented an automatic LP recognition system based on a YOLO object detector. The authors trained their model using images from different datasets. To improve training accuracy, more than 38,000 bounding boxes were labeled. Obtained results showed that the proposed approach achieved good performance results for LP recognition across eight public datasets.

In this work, our purpose is to take advantage of the previous experiences to propose enhancements of the deployed DL models to detect and efficiently recognize Saudi Arabian LPs.

3 Proposed Approach

This paper proposes a new approach for the automatic detection and recognition of license plates. This approach consists of 3 successive phases as shown in Fig. 1.

3.1 License Plate Detection Phase

For this phase, the input is an image of a car, and the output encloses the detected LP. This phase is automated by applying the region-based object detector Faster-RCNN model, which delimits the LP by surrounding it with a bounding box. Faster-RCNN is the modified version of Fast-RCNN. The main difference between these two DL models is that Fast-RCNN applies the selective search for generating Regions of Interest (RoI). In contrast, Faster-RCNN applies the Region Proposal Network (RPN), which takes image feature maps as input and produces a set of object proposals, each with an objectness score as output. Our choice of Faster-RCNN is justified by its effectiveness in detecting objects from images or videos, which has been proven in different applications [15, 16]. To detect LPs from car images, the network flow of the Faster-RCNN model consists of 4 successive steps as shown by Fig. 2:

1) A car image is taken as input and then transmitted to the convolutional layers, which return the feature maps for this image;

2) RPN is applied to the feature maps. It returns the object proposals along with their objectness score;
3) An RoI pooling layer is applied to these proposals to bring down all the proposals to the same size;
4) Finally, the proposals are passed to a fully connected layer, which has a multiclass classification layer and a regression layer at its top that allow classification and return the bounding boxes for detected objects.

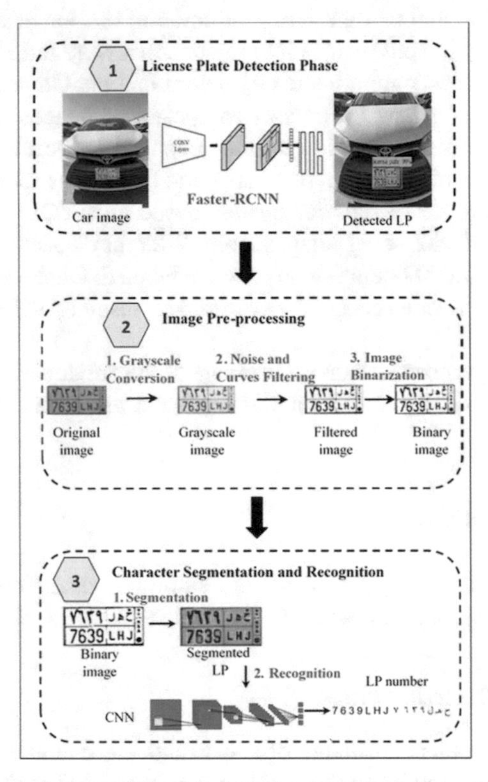

Fig. 1. The proposed approach for LP detection and recognition using DL networks.

3.2 Image Pre-processing Phase

The preprocessing phase aims to transform the raw data into clean data by reducing the noise in the image before it is fed to the DL networks. Preprocessing is essential to get a better result when performing the recognition of LP. Because real-world data is often inconsistent, incomplete, and contains noise caused by multiple factors such as lighting, weather, and camera position, preprocessing of data is a proven method for solving such problems. In this phase, an RGB image is converted into a grey-level image and then into a binary image. Filters that were used to remove the noise are:

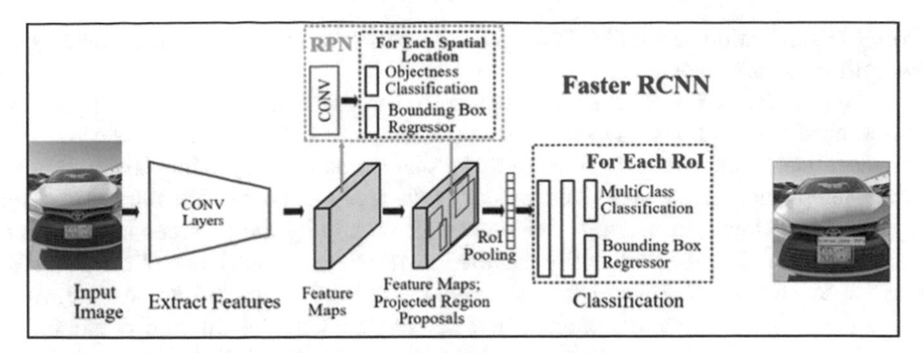

Fig. 2. Network flow of Faster-RCNN-based LP detection

- ***RGB to grayscale conversion***: the captured input image is in RGB format. The first step of preprocessing consists of converting the RGB image into a grayscale image. The RGB image is 24 bit, and processing it is time-consuming. Therefore, we need to convert the color image into a grayscale image to reduce the number of colors;
- ***Noise and curve filtering***: the input image contains different types of noise that reduce the efficiency of detecting thc LPs. This filter aims to remove noise and distortions from the input image. The noise can happen during camera capturing and can also result from the weather and illumination conditions. The noise and curves filtering is performed by applying the Gaussian blur filter;
- ***Image binarization***: by using this filter, the grayscale image is converted into a binary image (black and white image). This transformation is useful to reduce computational complexity.

3.3 Character Segmentation and Recognition Phase

After the preprocessing phase, a segmentation of the license plate characters is necessary before identifying the characters. This step aims to localize the characters to facilitate their recognition. In addition, it allows extracting any black object from the white background of the binary image. For this phase, we choose to apply the horizontal and vertical projection profile method for character segmentation. This method uses horizontal and vertical projection histograms. First, the horizontal histogram is used to find relevant regions that contain characters of the LP. Then, the vertical histogram is applied to find out a series of valley points separating characters. Finally, the image is segmented at the resulting valley points.

After the segmentation, the last step is character recognition. There are several techniques for character recognition, such as syntactic, statistical, and neural networks-based techniques. Our proposed approach is performed using the CNN DL model. CNN classifies the LP characters into several classes. For training, classes were divided into English digits class (0 to 9), upper case letters class (A to Z), and non-letters class. The Saudi Arabian LPs use two different languages, which are English and Arabic. In our approach, we choose to recognize only the English numbers and letters, then we propose to apply a character matching method to match each English character with its corresponding Arabic character, and this for the purpose to reduce the computational complexity resulting from the application of the CNN model for the recognition of characters belonging to two different languages.

CNN receives 28 × 28 grey and segmented images as input, and it has 11 layers, including 6 convolutional layers, 3 pooling layers, and 2 fully connected layers. The convolutional layers extract features from the source image. The pooling layers allow to down-sample the feature size of the output of the previous layers. The fully connected layers are employed to flatten the characteristics found by the previous layers into a vector and calculate the probability that the image belongs to each one of the potential classes. Since only 17 Arabic letters are used in the Saudi Arabian LPs, so we have to recognize 27 types of mappings characters (17 English letters + 10 English numbers). As a final result, the output of the recognition step is a string of all characters extracted from the LP (both English and Arabic characters) as shown by Fig. 3.

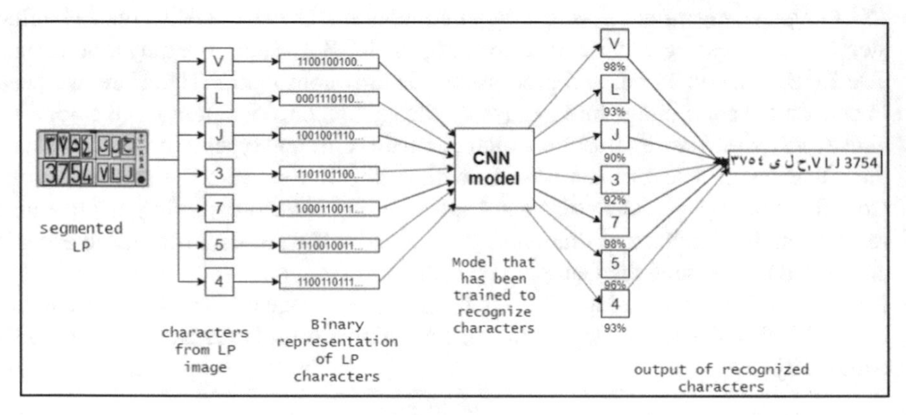

Fig. 3. The working process of the CNN-based character recognition.

4 Implementation and Experiments

The LP detection and recognition experiments were carried out using a PC with the following configuration properties: an x64-based processor; an Intel Core i7-8565U CPU @ 1.80 GHz 1.99 GHz; and a 32 GB RAM running on Windows 10 with NVIDIA GeForce MX. The deep convolutional neural networks were implemented using python 3.7 on Jupyter notebook [17]. In addition, we have utilized the Keras library [18] and TensorFlow [19] backend. To speed up the computation runtime, we used the Nvidia GeForce MX 250 GPU with CUDA and cuDNN libraries.

4.1 Dataset Collection and Labeling

For the experimentation of the proposed approach, we created our own dataset consisting of 1150 real-world Saudi Arabian cars. The car images were collected under various lighting and weather conditions. Besides, the images cover different types of cars and vehicles such as pickup trucks, crossovers, vans, hatchbacks, buses, ambulances, and sports cars, etc. We used 80% of this dataset for deep convolutional neural networks' training and 20% for testing. Figure 4 presents examples of the different types of Saudi Arabian LPs that were considered in our dataset. Figure 5 shows some training and testing sample images.

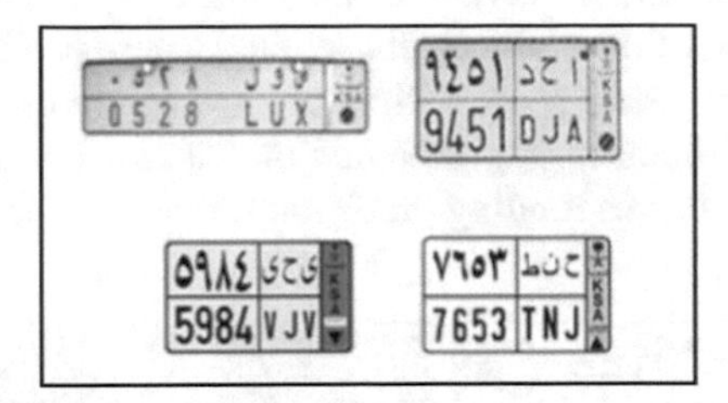

Fig. 4. Examples of different types of LPs that are considered in the constructed dataset.

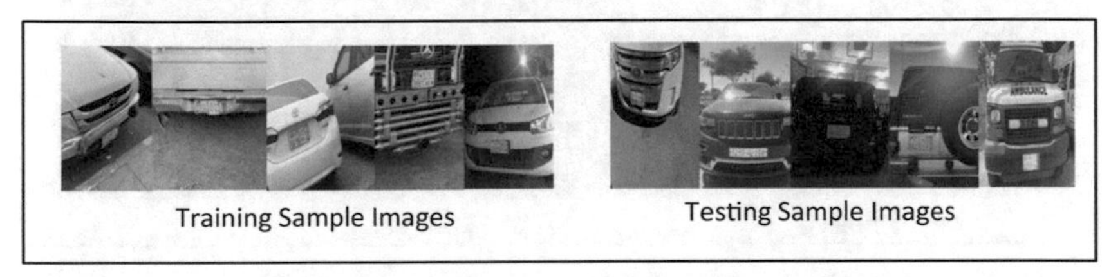

Fig. 5. Sample images used in the training and testing of the proposed deep CNNs.

To automatically label our dataset, the labelImg tool [20] is used. It allows localizing the LP region in each vehicle image. The obtained result is a boundary box drawn around the LP accompanied by the generation of a textual description of the identified region. LabelImg allows also to describe the identified region with an XML file that contains label information regarding the LP object, which are mainly: the name and the path of the image, the name, the width, the height, the depth, and the coordinates of the LP object.

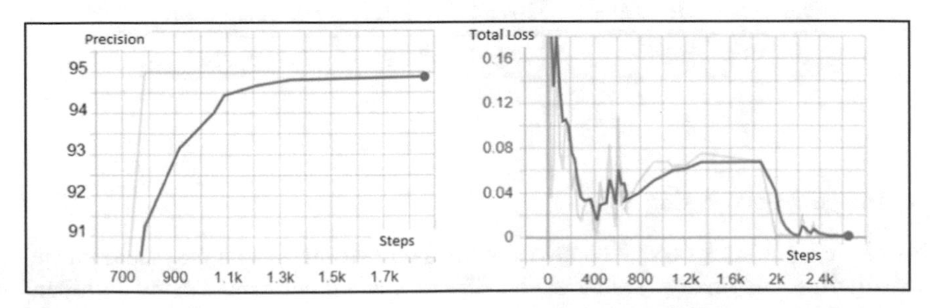

Fig. 6. Training precision (left) and total loss (right) of Faster-RCNN with InceptionV2 for LP detection.

4.2 Faster-RCNN-Based LP Detection

For LP detection, we used the training images' set to train the Faster-RCNN using the Inception-V2 model. The training is performed by using Tensorflow. This model is trained over 20 epochs. Figure 6 shows the precision and the total loss versus the number of steps of the whole training of Faster-RCNN using InceptionV2.

After the completion of the training phase, the Faster-RCNN model is tested using the images from the testing set. Figure 7 illustrates the results obtained by testing Faster-RCNN on two different images. The obtained outputs are bounding boxes identifying the location of LPs with corresponding precision scores.

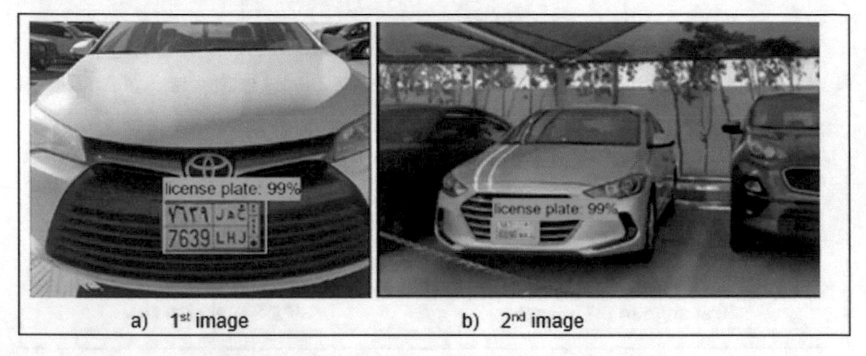

Fig. 7. Faster-RCNN testing for LP detection.

We validated the Faster-RCNN model by computing these performance metrics: loss, precision, recall, IoU (Intersection over Union), and response time. These metrics are detailed in [21]. As shown in Table 1, Faster-RCNN provides high performance results.0.0018 of loss, 92% of precision and recall, 0.98 of IoU, and 1.56–5.82s of response time.

Table 1. FASTER-RCNN testing performance for LP detection

Loss	Precision	Recall	IoU	Response time
0.0018	92%	92%	0.98	1.56–5.82s

4.3 Image Preprocessing

This phase includes 3 steps: 1) conversion of the RGB image to a grayscale image, 2) noise filtering, and finally 3) binarization. The first step is performed using the OpenCV library [22], the second step is implemented using the Gaussian blur filter, which applies a low-pass filter to images, and finally, the last step is achieved by applying the Otsu thresholding algorithm. Figure 8 shows the preprocessing results obtained for 2 different LP images.

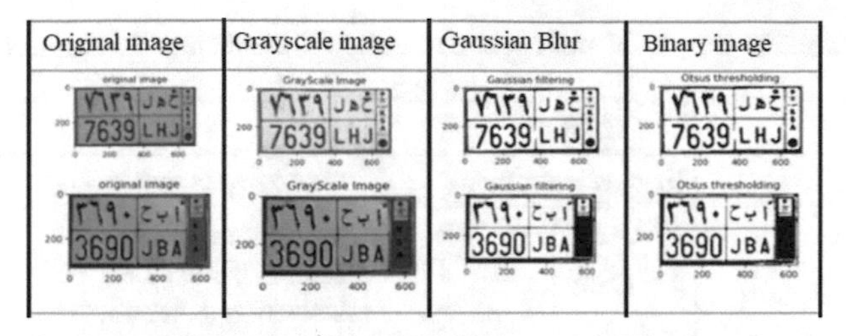

Fig. 8. Steps and results of the preprocessing phase.

4.4 LP Segmentation and Recognition

English characters' dataset preparation and creation is the first step in the LP segmentation and recognition phase. The collected dataset is composed of 27 classes of English characters. For each class, we have between 30 to 90 28×28 JPG images. The total number of images forming the collected characters' English dataset is 2174. These images are labeled to be prepared for the DL training and testing. Since the Saudi Arabian LP use only 17 Arabic letters, we propose correspondence between English characters and Arabic characters as illustrated by Fig. 9.

Arabic letters	ا	ب	ح	د	ر	س	ص	ط	ع	ق	ك	ل	م	ن	هـ	و	ى
English letters	A	B	J	D	R	S	X	T	E	G	K	L	Z	N	H	U	V
Arabic numbers	٠	١	٢	٣	٤	٥	٦	٧	٨	٩							
English numbers	0	1	2	3	4	5	6	7	8	9							

Fig. 9. Arabic characters and their corresponding characters in English.

After the preprocessing phase, LP images are segmented. The segmentation starts by finding contours for each black character identified in the white background of the LP. Each contour is a NumPy array of (x,y) coordinates of boundary points that delimit the identified character. Segmentation consists of drawing the characters' contours to split the LP image into disjoint characters. As we are interested in the recognition of English characters, Fig. 10 shows the result of the segmentation on the second part of the LP.

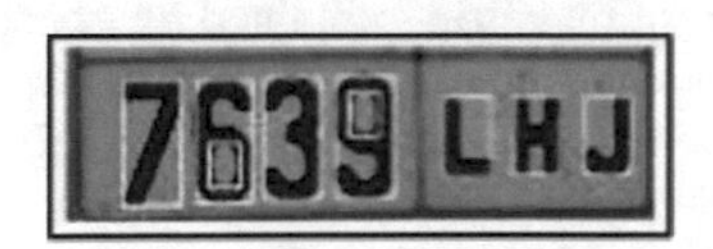

Fig. 10. Segmentation of the English characters of an LP image.

For LP characters' recognition, we propose to use a CNN model. The architecture of the considered CNN is detailed in Table 2.

After training the considered CNN model, the recognition testing is performed by following these steps:

Table 2. The CNN architecture used for LP characters' recognition.

Layer	Description	Values
Input layer	Images input layer	28 × 28 grey and segmented images
Hidden block 1	1st Conv2D 2nd Conv2D	32 feature maps Kernel size = (2,2) Activation = "ReLu"
	MaxPool2D	Pool size = (2,2) Strides = (2,2)
Hidden block 2	3rd Conv2D 4th Conv2D	32 feature maps Kernel size = (2,2) Activation = "ReLu"
	MaxPool2D	Pool size = (2,2) Strides = (2,2)
Hidden block 3	5th Conv2D 6th Conv2D	32 feature maps Kernel size = (2,2) Activation = "ReLu"
	MaxPool2D	Pool size = (2,2) Strides = (2,2)
Classification layer	2 FC layer	1st layer units = 33280 2nd layer units = 18468 Activation = "ReLu"
	SoftMax	27 classes

1) CNN takes as input segmented characters/non-characters identified in the LP separately;
2) The segmented characters/non-characters are converted to the binary format;
3) CNN takes each segmented character/non-character and compares it with the different classes that it has learned during the training phase;
4) CNN recognizes English letters and numbers and returns each identified character with its corresponding precision score.

The LP number is the resulting string obtained by concatenating the different recognized characters while respecting the order of their appearance in the LP. The Arabic part of the LP is finally added by using character mapping. The final output is presented in Fig. 11.

We validated the proposed CNN model by computing the following performance metrics for the testing phase: loss, accuracy, and response time. As shown by Table 3, the proposed CNN model achieves 0.0544 of loss rate, 98% of accuracy, and 0066s as response time for the recognition of LPs.

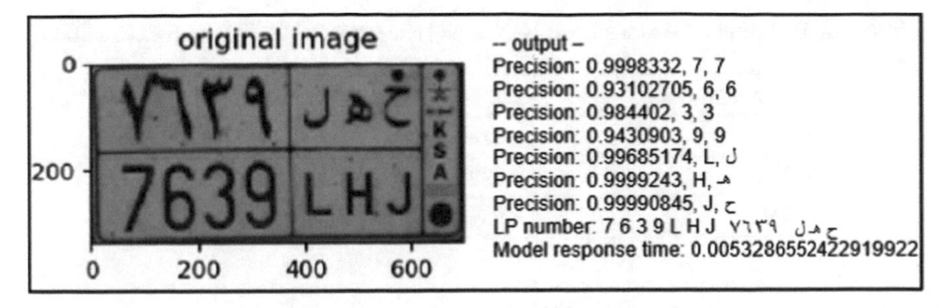

Fig. 11. Recognition output.

Table 3. CNN testing performance for LP recognition

Loss	Accuracy	Response time
0.0544	98%	0.0066s

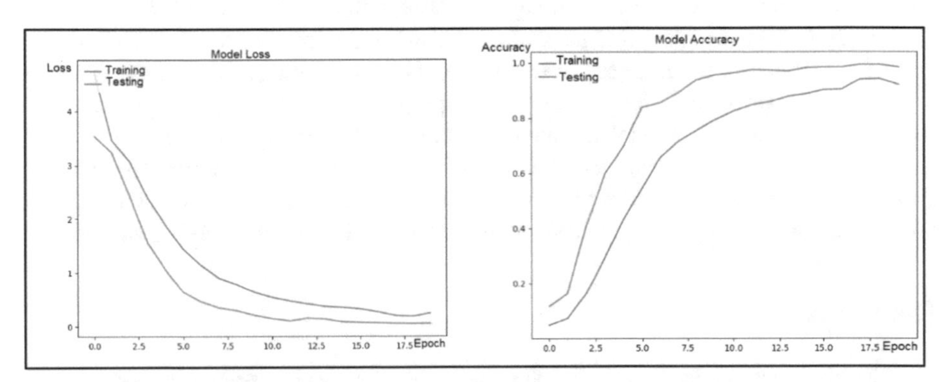

Fig. 12. Training and testing loss (left) and accuracy (right) of the proposed CNN model for LP recognition.

In addition, as illustrated by Fig. 12, the CNN recognition model provides high performance in terms of loss rate and accuracy in both training and testing phases.

To validate the choice of the CNN model, we trained our collected dataset with the Multilayer Perceptron (MLP) model and the K-Nearest Neighbors (K-NN) classifier. The testing results provided in Table 4 show that the CNN model got the highest accuracy and the lowest loss. MLP is composed of fully connected layers that include too many parameters, which will be resulting in redundancies and inefficiencies, unlike CNN, which has layers of convolution and pooling, fewer parameters than MLP, weights that are smaller and shared. Concerning KNN, it stores the whole training data, which requires high memory and makes the recognition process slower. CNN was less wasteful, easier to train, and more effective too.

Table 4. Performance Results MLP, K-NN, and our proposed CNN for LP Recognition

Model/algorithm	Loss	Accuracy
MLP	3.4735	91%
K-NN	0.1822	93%
CNN	**0.0544**	**98%**

5 Conclusion and Future Work

This paper proposes an efficient approach for LP detection and recognition using deep convolutional neural networks. The presented work applies Faster-RCNN using Inception V2 to ensure LP detection from vehicles' images. A CNN model is proposed, trained, and tested to ensure LP recognition. The LP detection and recognition process goes through three successive phases: detection phase, image pre-processing phase, and character segmentation and recognition phase. Our experiments of the proposed DL models were implemented on real images' dataset including 1150 Saudi Arabian vehicles' images. The vehicles' images were collected under various lighting and weather conditions. Besides, the images cover different types of vehicles. The obtained experimental results prove the effectiveness of the proposed approach showing precision of 92% of the Faster-CNN model and an accuracy of 98% of the CNN model.

As future work, we intend to improve the proposed models to ensure LP detection and recognition from real-time videos and for other countries. Also, we will work on collecting more vehicles images that are captured under more challenging conditions.

References

1. Shashirangana, J., Padmasiri, H., Meedeniya, D., Perera, C.: Automated license plate recognition: a survey on methods and techniques. IEEE Access **9**, 11203–11225 (2020)
2. Boulila, W., Sellami, M., Driss, M., Al-Sarem, M., Safaei, M., Ghaleb, F.: RS-DCNN: a novel distributed convolutional-neural-networks based-approach for big remote-sensing image classification. Comput. Electron. Agric. **182**, 106014 (2021)
3. Ben Atitallah, S., Driss, M., Boulila, W., Ben Ghézala, H.: Randomly initialized convolutional neural network for the recognition of COVID-19 using X-ray images. Int. J. Imaging Syst. Technol. **32**, 55–73 (2021)
4. Ur Rehman, M., Shafique, A., Khalid, S., Driss, M., Rubaiee, S.: Future forecasting of COVID-19: a supervised learning approach. Sensors **10**, 3322 (2021)
5. Alkhelaiwi, M., Boulila, W., Ahmad, J., Koubaa, A., Driss, M.: An efficient approach based on privacy-preserving deep learning for satellite image classification. Remote Sens. **13**(11), 2221 (2021)
6. Almustafa, K.: On the automatic recognition of Saudi license plate. Int. J. Appl. Inf. Syst. (IJAIS) **5**, 34–44 (2013)
7. Basalamah, S.: Saudi license plate recognition. Int. J. Comput. Electr. Eng. **5**(1), 1 (2013)
8. Sarfraz, M., Ahmed, M.J.: An approach to license plate recognition system using neural network. In: Exploring Critical Approaches Evolutionary Computation, pp. 20–36. IGI Global (2019)

9. Alzubaidi, L., Latif, G., Alghazo, J.: Affordable and portable realtime saudi license plate recognition using SoC. In: 2nd International Conference on New Trends in Computing Sciences (ICTCS), pp. 1–5. IEEE (2019)
10. Chen, R.: Automatic license plate recognition via sliding-window darknet-YOLO deep learning. Image Vis. Comput. **87**, 47–56 (2019)
11. Kessentini, Y., Besbes, M., Ammar, S., Chabbouh, A.: A two-stage deep neural network for multi-norm license plate detection and recognition. Expert Syst. Appl. **136**, 159–170 (2019)
12. Silva, S., Jung, C.: Real-time license plate detection and recognition using deep convolutional neural networks. J. Vis. Commun. Image Representation **71**, 102773 (2020)
13. Omar, N., Sengur, A., Al-Ali, S.: Cascaded deep learning-based efficient approach for license plate detection and recognition. Expert Syst. Appl. **149**, 113280 (2020)
14. Laroca, R., Zanlorensi, L., Gonçalves, G., Todt, E., Schwartz, W., Menotti, D.: An efficient and layout-independent automatic license plate recognition system based on the YOLO detector. IET Intell. Transp. Syst. **15**(4), 483–503 (2021)
15. Omar, N., Mohsin Abdulazeez, A., Sengur, A., Saeed Al-Ali, S.G.: Fused faster RCNNs for efficient detection of the license plates. Indones. J. Electr. Eng. Comput. Sci., **19**(2), 874 (2020)
16. Yin, S., Li, H., Teng, L.: Airport detection based on improved faster RCNN in large scale remote sensing images. Sensing Imaging **21**(1), 1–13 (2020). https://doi.org/10.1007/s11220-020-00314-2
17. Jupyter Notebook. https://jupyter.org/. Accessed 20 Oct 2021
18. Keras: the Python deep learning API. https://keras.io/. Accessed 20 Oct 2021
19. TensorFlow. https://www.tensorflow.org/. Accessed 20 Oct 2021
20. labelImg. https://pypi.org/project/labelImg/1.4.0/. Accessed 20 Oct 2021
21. Ben Atitallah, S., Driss, M., Boulila, W., Koubaa, A., Ben Ghézala, H.: Fusion of convolutional neural networks based on Dempster–Shafer theory for automatic pneumonia detection from chest X-ray images. Int. J. Imaging Syst. Technol. **32**, 658–672 (2021)
22. OpenCV. https://opencv.org/. Accessed 20 Oct 2021

Ship Detection Approach Using Machine Learning Algorithms

Abdirahman Osman Hashi[1(✉)], Ibrahim Hassan Hussein[1], Octavio Ernesto Romo Rodriguez[2], Abdullahi Ahmed Abdirahman[1], and Mohamed Abdirahman Elmi[1]

[1] Faculty of Computing, SIMAD University, Mogadishu, Somalia
Wadani12727@gmail.com, {aaayare,m.abdirahman}@simad.edu.so
[2] Department of Computer Science, Faculty of Informatics, Istanbul Teknik Üniversitesi, 34469 Maslak, İstanbul, Turkey

Abstract. The control of territorial waters is critical, since water occupies more than 70% of earth surface. Due to that fact, maritime security and safety is essential, in order to reduce illegal operations including piracy, illegal fishing and transportation of illicit goods. With the rapid development of artificial intelligence, ship detection research has increased as well. Several researchers have addressed this issue by proposing a variety of solutions such as VGG and Dense Net. Nevertheless, these proposed solutions have not provided enough accuracy in term of ship detection. Therefore, the primary objective of this work is to propose a robust model that can detect ships by applying artificial intelligence and machine learning models, those are Random Forest, Decision Tree, Naive Bayes and CNN. The result achieved in this experiment will tackle the forementioned problems and conduct research on how ships could be detected. Based on the result, Random Forest outperforms other models in terms of accuracy, scoring 97.20% for RGB and 98.90% for HSV, in comparison with Decision Tree and Naive Bayes those are scored 96.82% for RGB and 97.18% for HSV and 92.43 for RGB and 96.30% for HSV respectively. Meanwhile, CNN scored 90.45% for RGB and 98.45% for HSV. Overall, Random Forest is the best model so far, achieving a good result in terms of RGB and HSV 97.20% and 98.90% respectively. The significance of the proposed method for the field of artificial intelligence is to introduce a novel method to detect Ships.

Keywords: Deep learning · Naive Bayes · Random forest · Artificial intelligence · Convolutional neural network

1 Introduction

The precise and concurrent identification of moving ships has become an important part of marine video surveillance, resulting in increased traffic safety and security. With the fast advancement of artificial intelligence, intelligent methods to improve ship identification outcomes in marine applications are becoming possible. The visual picture quality is often reduced in real-world imaging settings owing to poor weather conditions, such

F. Saeed et al. (Eds.): IRICT 2021, LNDECT 127, pp. 16–25, 2022.
https://doi.org/10.1007/978-3-030-98741-1_2

as rain, haze, and low light, among others. The apparent degradation has the potential to jeopardize the safety and security of maritime traffic. Furthermore, since it enables for accurate and real-time identification of moving ships, high-quality images has become an essential component in maritime video surveillance. As a result, a great deal of effort has gone into improving low-visibility enhancement and ship recognition in a variety of imaging scenarios [1].

As a consequence of many international cooperation efforts, the frequency of cases of maritime piracy has recently reduced. The Ministry of Defense proposed 3,200 million JPY for anti-piracy operations off the coast of Somalia in Japan's FY2017 national budget. A important marine route between Japan and Europe must pass through this area through the Suez Canal. The Japanese Maritime Self-Defense Force has sent a fleet to protect Japanese ships [2]. This works well, but it would have been much better if Somalis had been able to identify ships using ship detection models.

Machine learning has opened new opportunities for better picture categorization and detection in recent years. It has started Machine learning methods to learn picture characteristics automatically and discover possible object characters and distribution rules across the object that are not defined by human cognition [3]. Three criteria should be fulfilled by a competent ship detecting technique. The first is robustness; the detecting technique should be resistant to changes in light, clouds, and waves. The second need is generality; the detection technique must be capable of detecting both in-shore and offshore ships. Last but not least, computational efficiency: the detecting technique should be computationally efficient. This is particularly important when working with large-scale remote sensing pictures [4]. Recent years, numerous researchers such as [5, 6] and [7] have proposed different solutions for ship detection. However, these proposed solutions were not provided enough accuracy in term of ship detection. Hence, the primary key objective of this paper is to intend by proposing robust model that can detect ships in the sea by applying four machine learning models, those are CNN, Random forest, Decision Tree and Naive Bayes.

This paper is organized with five sections. The upcoming section discusses the related work of ship detection methods that other researchers have proposed before. Section three explains the proposed methodology for ship detection that uses four machine learning algorithms. The next section illustrates the experiment result and dataset description that is applied for the proposed model. And the final section presents the conclusion and future work recommendations.

2 Background and Related Work

Due to the increasing need for applications in the scope of maritime security and safety, marine monitoring research has increased recently. With the objective of maritime border control, fight against piracy, observing ocean pollution, and related missions, several organizations and government agencies must guarantee the safety of ships and the overall security of maritime operations. The oceans and seas occupy about 71% of the earth's surface, as a result of that, water transportation has played a significant role in global economies throughout history [8]. However, the sea is fraught with threats ranging from piracy to the potential of mishaps. Furthermore, numerous illegal operations, including illegal fishing and the transportation of illicit goods might take place, especially in the Indian Ocean. There are resources such as satellites that can be used to keep track of these enormous seas. However, sophisticated image processing techniques are required for the identification and the following categorization of ships and maritime transportation-vehicles traversing the seas using satellite images. In conjunction with monitoring the seas for the intention of ships guard, prevention of illegal fishing and illicit goods transportation, countries must also control their shores and nearby waterbodies in search of military threats, including enemy ships and submarines from a defensive standpoint [7].

Through history; Airbus, previously known as the European-Aeronautic-Defense Space-Company, has offered a wide range of maritime surveillance services with effective solutions and intense monitoring of marine areas with fine fidelity [8]. Airbus supplied researchers with data in order for them to create an automatized prediction model that could track the activity of ships, correctly identify every ship in all the satellite pictures given, therefore preventing illegal maritime operations [9]. Given the increment of maritime traffic, there is a greater chance of illicit operations occurring in the water, such as piracy and illegal goods transportation. Airbus had the aim to develop a comprehensive maritime surveillance system to constantly check ship traffic and prevent criminal operations including piracy, illegal fishing, and the transport of illicit goods. Furthermore, a system like that would safeguard the maritime environment, since it would help prevent accidents that could result in pollution [5].

On account of the benefits that automated surveillance of the seas or oceans areas could result in, ship location is an imperative application when we talk about area of computer vision or in specific an image processing field. The benefits of creating a model that can locate and examine ships in an autonomous way range from stopping piracy, illegal fishing, illicit transportation of goods. As a result of recent technological advancements, the interest in Neural-Network research for detecting and classificating specific items in pictures has increased. Ship detection is one of these applications that may provide significant benefits to the parties involved but yet not implemented in Somalia which is currently dealing with the forementioned problems [3].

On the other hand, to predict the object's minimal circumscribed rectangle and minimize the redundant detection area, a method based on rotation anchor approach was developed [10]. For identifying ships, the experiment's dataset relies on remote sensing photos from Google Earth. The RDFPN performed better in ship identification in complicated pictures, particularly in identifying densely packed ships, according to the findings. The authors used K-Nearest Neighbors, Random Forest, Naive Bayes in another approach for ship identification using satellite imagery [11]. Deep Learning techniques were also put to the test, with researchers using pre-trained network designs as a comparison network. When the Deep Learning technique was compared to conventional methods, the Random-Forest model had the highest accuracy in the category of classical methods, scoring 93% of accuracy in detection. In contrast, the methods in the category of Deep Learning obtained 94% of accuracy in detection [12].

Since last decade most researchers were always working on ways to enhance current algorithms, which is something that typically happens as the quantity of datasets grows. Between the input and output layers of a typical deep learning classifier, there are many layers of CNN that allow for sophisticated non-linear information processing [13]. Chua et al. [14] compared three traditional machine learning algorithms: histogram of oriented gradient (HOG), exemplar-SVM, and latent-SVM [15] to determine their particular benefits, and discovered that exemplar SVM is excellent for specificity measurement. Chen et al. [15] proposed a detection technique that uses a fully convolutional neural network (FCNN) segmentation method and then identifies the item using bounding box regressions, with the class labelled by a CNN classifier.

3 Proposed Methodology

It is well know that the research methodology presents the sequence of the follows and the structure overview of the proposed model, this proposed model consists of four models: CNN, Random forest, Decision Tree and Naive Bayes. As already mention we are trying to find which algorithms can give us the best accuracy of ship detection and we are dealing with images that airbus ship detection provides. It is also a notable to mention that we used Yolovov3 as it is one of the most advanced of object detection.

Hence, to do the pre-processing, the images in this research are first subjected to a block section. Following this phase, the color and texture characteristics are retrieved from the picture blocks to be utilized as training data. A hybrid feature vector is created by combining these characteristics. Then, using the previously extracted feature vectors, the Naive Bayes, Decision Tree, and Random Forest classifiers are trained, this method has been done other researchers too. The categorization of ship blocks and non-ship blocks on the blocks of test images was done as the last step after the classifiers had been trained. There are three main steps that have done before applying the models. Here are the steps:

1. Block division
2. Feature Extraction
3. Color Feature

For the block division, in comparison to pixel-based detection, the block-based method offers more meaningful and comprehensive detection. It offers more homogenous information based on the image's color and texture richness, as well as the ability to create vectors quickly. This research used 64×64 pixel blocks throughout the pre-processing stage, but there are other researchers that have applied 16×16 and 32×32 pixel blocks. The second step is to apply a binary mask in order to label images if they are from a ship or not.

As it is important to choose the appropriate features in order to achieve the right classification, it is also important to do a feature selection based on the image blocks by creating a feature vector from the extracted features in the data. Similar to that, the color feature is also important as it gives information about the visual perception of pixels. This proposed method considers two different color spaces: HSV (Hue-Saturation-Value) and RGB (Red-GreenBlue) (Fig. 1).

From this figure, we can see that after the pre-processing stage, there are numerous steps to follow before applying the model, such as block division, feature extraction, and color features that will play an important role in extracting the appropriated images. After that, we trained CNN, Random forest, Decision Tree and Naive bayes.

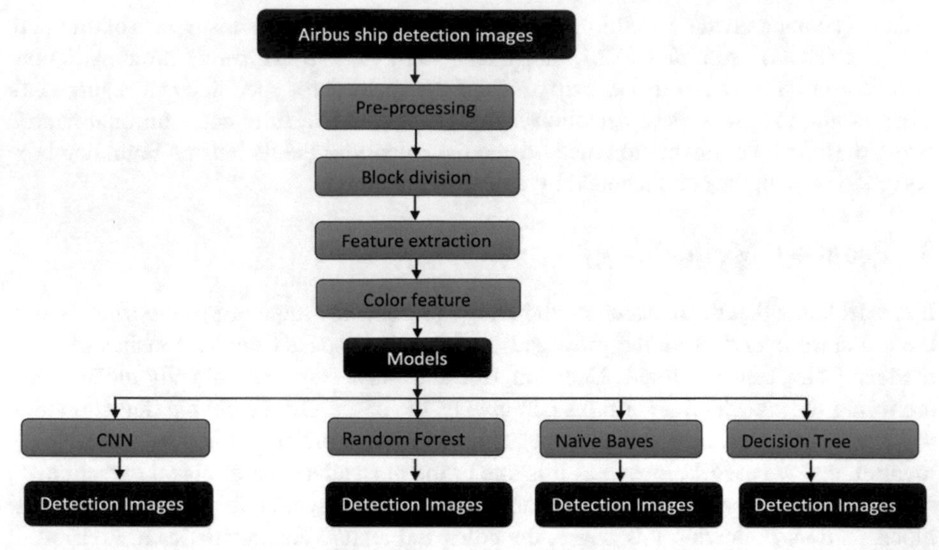

Fig. 1. Proposed methodology

It is well know that Convolutional Neural Networks (CNN) have achieved significant success in the perception and detection of the image as it consists of one or more layers and these layers are the input layer, sub-sampling, and fully connected layer. The upcoming figure demonstrates how CNN is applied to image detection by applying the sub-sampling layer followed by the convolution layer, and then again by doing sub-sampling later and finally producing a fully connected MLP (Fig. 2).

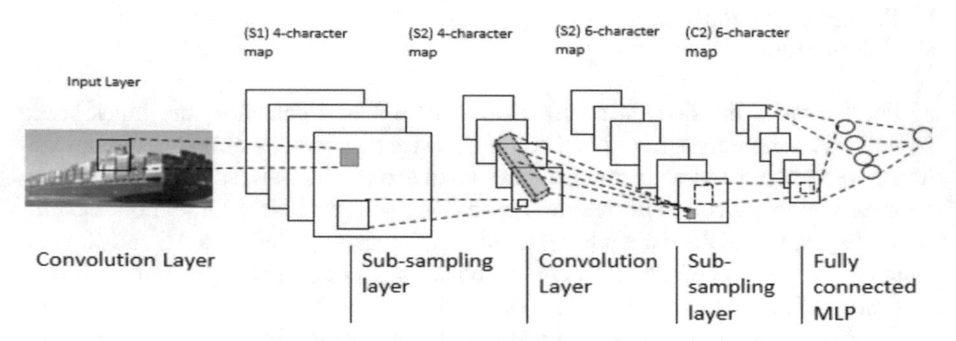

Fig. 2. CNN to Fully connected MLP

On the other hand, the second model we trained is the Random Forest, which is one of the most popular machine learning models. RF is a decision tree-based community learning algorithm that solves supervised learning tasks such as classification. It has a low noise tolerance and does not oversleep. It has much better performance categorization outcomes than the NB and DT approaches. It integrates several decision trees by generating stronger models in order to get a more accurate and stable estimate. During the training phase, the method uses a random data sample to build a model of several decision trees based on various data subsets. The unpredictability of the random forest model is a benefit, since it makes it more resilient than a single decision tree and eliminates the issue of conventional data being too compatible and comparable.

It is also applied to the Decision Tree (DT) algorithm, which is the second technique that delivers the most effective outcomes among machine learning algorithms. It may be used for regression and classification. A knot, branch, and leaf make up a decision tree. The root is at the top, the branch is the route from the root to the other nodes, and the leaf is the final outcome of these branches. This algorithm asks a series of questions to the data to be trained, and the outcomes are determined based on the responses. The information gain and information gain rate methods are computed while constructing a decision tree, depending on the criteria or attribute value of the branch in the tree.

The last model we applied is the Naive Bayes (NB) algorithm, which is a machine learning method that is regulated. It's a straightforward probability model for multiple classifications based on the premise of feature independence. NB implies that each feature contributes to the possibilities given to a class in its own right.

4 Results and Discussion

4.1 Dataset

The Kaggle platform [16] was used to generate a dataset of ship pictures from satellite photos for this study. The satellite pictures show the earth's surface, including farmland, buildings, roads, and other features. PlanetScope complete views of the San Francisco Bay and San Pedro Bay regions of California were used to create these pictures. It contains 4000 RGB pictures with a resolution of 80 × 80 pixels for two issue classes: "ship" and "non-ship."

Table 1. Total number of samples

Class	Numbers of imges in each sample
Ships	1000
Non-Ships	3000

The pictures for the ship class must show the whole look of a single ship. It comes in a variety of sizes and orientations, as well as some ambient sounds. A non-ship class is made up of one or more of the following three elements: 1) random samples of various land cover characteristics such as buildings, water, vegetation, bare soil, and so on; 2) a partial picture of a ship; and 3) noises produced by bright pixels or strong linear features (Table 1).

4.2 Results

Following the steps that are mentioned after preprocessing in the methodology, we have obtained a hybrid vector by extracting color from each image's contents based on the block size. After that, the results were evaluated based on the block sizes while keeping in mind the successful classification. As we are dealing with each block size, we created different vectors that have different sizes based on block size and then apply the color space. As mentioned before, in this study it used 64×64 block sizes, and after we divided them into 64×64 block sizes, we found 40752 images.

By using Yolovov3 as mentioned in the methodology, we have created the bounding box and bounding area to make it more clear by feeding it into our models, so that the classification will be more accurate. Here is the picture that demonstrates the division of each picture into bounding boxes and bounding areas (Fig. 3).

	ImageId	Ship	Boundingbox	BoundingboxArea
0	000194a2d.jpg	1	[0.625, 0.38671875, 0.026041666666666668, 0.02...	440.0
1	000194a2d.jpg	1	[0.09830729166666667, 0.4967447916666667, 0.01...	153.0
2	000194a2d.jpg	1	[0.3665364583333333, 0.23372395833333334, 0.01...	517.0
3	000194a2d.jpg	1	[0.09765625, 0.5032552083333334, 0.00130208333...	6.0
4	000194a2d.jpg	1	[0.4557291666666667, 0.244140625, 0.0247395833...	722.0

Fig. 3. Image bounding box

We can see from this figure that each image has a bounding box and a bounding box area, which is a vector based on the block size for each image. Hence, it is easy to fit the model or to apply it with a blanched bounding box. Before applying any model, here is the dataset images which we meant to detect the ships from inside the images.

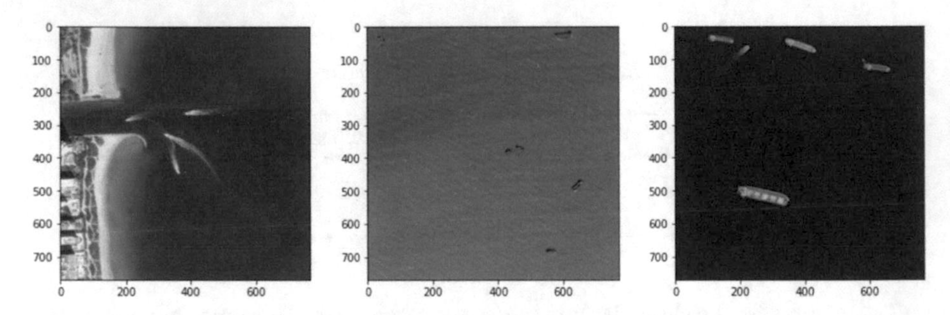

Fig. 4. Image of undetected images

From Fig. 4, we can see that there are certain ships in each image. However, after applying the models, we detected the ships in each image. Here is the detected result after applying the models.

Figure 5 illustrates how each image is block sized and then detected the ship by putting a red rectangle box which clearly shows that the model has performed and segmented the image accurately. Although there are other images where there is no ship in the image, the trained model returned without block sizing it and putting the rectangle boundary box around it.

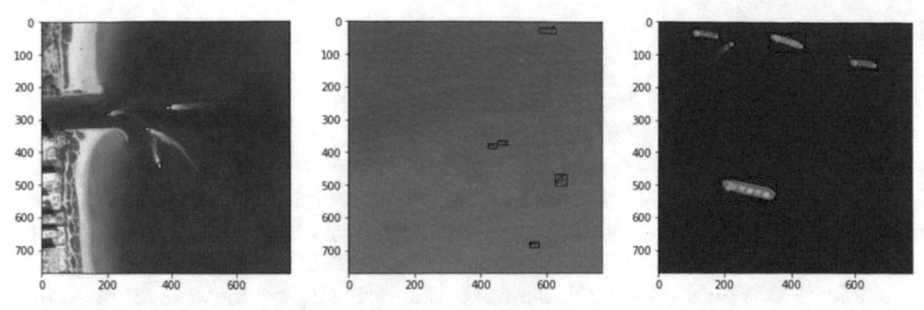

Fig. 5. Detected ship results

In terms of classification performance of the Random Forest, Decision Tree, and Naive Bayes, we applied only based on the forementioned color features that are RGB and HSV. Here is the accuracy of the classification performance (Table 2).

Table 2. Accuracy of the classification performance

Color space	Models			
Color features	Random forest	Decision tree	Naive Bayes	CNN
RGB	97.20	96.82	92.43	90.45
HSV	98.90	97.18	96.30	98.45

It can be seen from this table that Random Forest has achieved the highest accuracy compared to the decision tree, Naive Bayes, and CNN, yet the decision tree has also outperformed compared with Naive Bayes. However, the decision tree has also achieved a good accuracy performance, close enough to the Random Forest and better than CNN and Naive Bayes. Though our benchmark author [12] has also implemented these models, nevertheless, our implemented Random Forest has overall outperformed compared even with other author [12] results. However, the decision tree accuracy of the other author has scored 98.75, which is close enough to the Random Forest but still lower accuracy than the HSV that we obtained for this model. It is also worth noting that other researchers' Naive Bayes outperformed our implemented model, scoring 95.03, 98.72, RGB, and HSV, respectively. However, our model's Naive Bayes has achieved 92.43, 96.30 RGB and HSV respectively.

Due to the complexity and number of convolutional layers, our CNN model has achieved slightly lower performance compared with other Random Forests. CNN has achieved 98.45 compared to Random Forest, which has scored 98.90 in the HSV. Overall, Random Forest is the best model so far that has achieved a good result in terms of RGB and HSV, 97.20 and 98.90 respectively.

5 Conclusions

This work addresses the issue of detecting ships using artificial intelligence. We proposed a more accurate ship detection approach using four machine learning models. Those are Random Forest, Decision Tree, Naive Bayes, and CNN. Before applying the model, it was observed that doing block size and color highlighting played an essential role for feature extraction. Based on the results, Random Forest outperformed other models in terms of accuracy, as it scored 97.20% for RGB and 98.90% for HSV. Although other models have also performed well, their accuracy was slightly lower than the Random Forest technique.

For future work, it is important to classify the detected ships into categories based on the ship's operation. This will require the implementation of more complex features such as classifying objects according to their shapes and sizes.

Acknowledgments. It is imperative to acknowledge the support given by SIMAD Research Center in order to make this research a success. In addition to that, the authors of this paper are honored to thank SIMAD University for making this research possible by granting the Research University Grant.

References

1. Liu, R.W., Yuan, W., Chen, X., Lu, Y.: An enhanced CNN-enabled learning method for promoting ship detection in maritime surveillance system. Ocean Eng. **235**, 109435 (2021)
2. Watanabe, K., Takashima, K., Mitsumura, K., Utsunomiya, K., Takasaki, S.: Experimental study on the application of UAV drone to prevent maritime pirates attacks. TransNav Int. J. Marine Navigation Saf. Sea Transp **11**(4), 705–710 (2017)
3. Nie, G.H., Zhang, P., Niu, X., Dou, Y., Xia, F.: Ship detection using transfer learned single shot multi box detector. In: ITM Web of Conferences, vol. 12, p. 01006). EDP Sciences (2017)
4. Zhang, T., Zhang, X., Shi, J., Wei, S.: HyperLi-Net: a hyper-light deep learning network for high-accurate and high-speed ship detection from synthetic aperture radar imagery. ISPRS J. Photogramm. Remote. Sens. **167**, 123–153 (2020)
5. Zhou, L., Suyuan, W., Cui, Z., Fang, J., Yang, X., Ding, W.: Lira-YOLO: a lightweight model for ship detection in radar images. J. Syst. Eng. Electron. **31**(5), 950–956 (2020)
6. Li, J., Qu, C., Shao, J.: Ship detection in SAR images based on an improved faster R-CNN. In: 2017 SAR in Big Data Era: Models, Methods and Applications (BIGSARDATA), pp. 1–6. IEEE, November 2017
7. Petrescu, R.V., Aversa, R., Akash, B., Corchado, J., Apicella, A., Petrescu, F.I.: Home at airbus. J. Aircraft Spacecraft Technol. **1**(2), 97–118 (2017)
8. Corbane, C., Pecoul, E., Demagistri, L., Petit, M.: Fully automated procedure for ship detection using optical satellite imagery. In: Remote Sensing of Inland, Coastal, and Oceanic Waters, vol. 7150, p. 71500R, December 2008
9. Yang, X., et al.: Automatic ship detection in remote sensing images from google earth of complex scenes based on multi-scale rotation dense feature pyramid networks. Remote Sens. **10**(1), 132 (2018)
10. Chen, Y., Zheng, J., Zhou, Z.: Airbus Ship Detection-Traditional vs Convolutional Neural Network Approach, Stanford

11. Dolapci, B., Özcan, C.: Automatic ship detection and classification using machine learning from remote sensing images on apache spark. J. Intell. Syst. Theory Appl. **4**(2), 94–102 (2021)
12. Wang, Y., Wang, C., Zhang, H., Dong, Y., Wei, S.: A SAR dataset of ship detection for deep learning. Remote Sens. **11**(765), 6–11 (2019)
13. Ma, M., Chen, J., Liu, W., Yang, W.: Ship classification and detection based on CNN using GF-3 SAR images. Remote Sens. **2043**(10), 2–22 (2018)
14. Li, H., Chen, L., Li, F., Huang, M.: Ship detection and tracking method for satellite video based on multiscale saliency and surrounding contrast analysis. Remote Sens. **13**(2), 6–10 (2019)
15. Kaggle. Dataset for Airbus Ship Detection Challenge (2018). https://www.kaggle.com/c/airbus-shipdetection/data

A New Deep Learning System for Wild Plants Classification and Species Identification: Using Leaves and Fruits

Nehad M. Abdulrahman Ibrahim[1(✉)], Dalia Goda Gabr[2], and Abdel-Hamid M. Emara[3,4]

[1] Department of Computer Science, College of Computer Science and Information Technology, Imam Abdulrahman Bin Faisal University, Dammam, Saudi Arabia
nmaibrahim@iau.edu.sa

[2] Botany and Microbiology Department, Faculty of Science (Girls Branch), AL Azhar University, Cairo, Egypt
daliaGabr.el20@azhar.edu.eg

[3] Department of Computers and Systems Engineering, Faculty of Engineering, Al-Azhar University, Cairo 11884, Egypt

[4] College of Computer Science and Engineering, Taibah University, Medina 41477, Saudi Arabia

Abstract. Many studies are based on the study of plant classification and their identification using its leaves, and there are many studies to identify plants using its fruits. Most of these studies are based on the leaves of the plant in general as well as the fruits in general as well. In this research, we present a new tool using artificial intelligence to classify and identify wild plants through the leaves of these plants, or by using their fruits, or by using both leaves and fruits together. This tool has proven an excellent result compared to similar tools in the same field. More than one AI model was applied to three datasets, lower plants dataset (LPDS), upper plant dataset (UPDS), and fruit plant dataset (FPDS). The aim of this study is to use machine learning methods to serve in the plant taxonomy and identification. The wild plant's dataset was gathered in its natural habitat in Egypt. The developed convolution neural network model (AlexNet CNN), the Random Forest (RF), and the support vector machine (SVM) techniques were contrasted in the species classifications. The highest degree of accuracy achieved was 98.2% by using the developed CNN model.

Keywords: Plant taxonomy · Deep learning · Support vector machine · Random forest

1 Introduction

Botanists, especially plant taxonomists, after collecting plant samples from the fields, the first step before starting work on plant samples is to identify plants in terms of family, genus and species. Taxonomists use flora books and also comparisons with herbarium

F. Saeed et al. (Eds.): IRICT 2021, LNDECT 127, pp. 26–37, 2022.
https://doi.org/10.1007/978-3-030-98741-1_3

samples to obtain an accurate and correct identification of plant samples and this process is delicate and a little cumbersome. Recently, some programming scientists have implemented a set of applications and websites to identify plants using artificial intelligence algorithms to facilitate this process for scientists and those interested in botany as, PlantNet, PlantDetect Lite, Plant D, PlantSnap Pro and Picture This. Botanists used morphology, anatomy, genomic analysis, and photochemistry to identify and classify plants, among other methods. The first is through the plant's morphological characteristics, especially the flower. When the flowering stage is unavailable, the fruit characters are useful for species identification and separation [1]. In recent years, Deep Learning has demonstrated the highest machine learning efficiency, and its image rating has skyrocketed. Several linear and non-linear layers make up a standard deep learning system. The term "deep" refers to the multiple layers of deep stacking. Deep learning approaches' progress is largely dependent on the development of devices that can manage large amounts of data and network architecture. Convolutional neural networks CNN, in particular, have recently achieved the highest image classification success and are commonly used in modern deep learning techniques [2]. To identify and classify plants, recent studies of image recognition and taxonomy approaches have been used. These techniques used texture and color-based features to perform classification. Aspect ratio, kurtosis, skewness, energy, correlation, sum variance, entropy, and compactness are some of these characteristics. The computing power is disproportionate. The major drawback of these traditional methods is the lengthy computation time needed for handcrafted feature extraction. All conventional approaches have been replaced by machine learning techniques in recent years. The convolution layers are concerned with the digital filtering techniques, that are used to highlight or extract the most noticeable features. The pooling mainly concerned lowering the volume of the feature maps received from the convolution layer, decreasing the overfitting of the maps in the network layers, and reducing the computations.

Most of the implemented applications depend on datasets for cultivated plants, not wild plants. One of the main objectives of the current study is to work on the wild plant's dataset, this research aims to create a system to help the scientists to identified plant specimens using only images. This system can be considered a kernel of an electronic herbarium for wild plants.

2 Review of Related Literatures

In this section, we will list the recent studies related to plants image classification based on the leaf and the fruits.

Using the large and deep learning method, a model that integrates a linear and a deep learning models to solve fine-grained plant image classification challenge [2].

The CNNs had five convolutional layers at the time, but ensemble systems outperformed them in terms of true deep learning. Another method used handcrafted visual features and qualified SVM classifiers for various view styles [3]. Using the ImageNet model and dataset released in [3], a new model to classify plant images using the convolution neural network architecture [4]. The study [5] present three models, Alexnet, DLeaf, and AyurLeaf; the AyurLeaf CNN model is evaluated and compared to AlexNet, Leaf, and fine-tuned AlexNet versions using two classifiers, CNN and SVM with accuracy 96.76%. Plant taxonomy is the study of how various species of plants are categorized.

In comparison to other transfer learning strategies, the study found that transfer learning improves the performance of deep learning models, especially models that apply deep features and use fine-tuning to provide better performance [6], the research applies deep learning features SVM and LDA to four publicly accessible plant datasets using two deep learning models, Alexnet and VGG16 (Flavia, Swedish Leaf, UCI Leaf, and Plantvillage). The study [7] present the extension work to [8] with an adaptive algorithm that relies on a deep adaptive Residual Neural Network to deal with the identification of multiple plant diseases in real-world acquisition environments, where numerous modifications have been proposed for early disease detection using a Residual Neural Network, including several enhancements to the augmentation scheme and tile cropping. The study [9] presents D-Leaf, a modern CNN-based approach that was proposed. After pre-processing the leaf images, the three pretrained Convolutional Neural Network (CNN) models: pre-trained AlexNet, fine-tuned AlexNet, and D-Leaf. Support Vector Machine (SVM), Artificial Neural Network (ANN), K-Nearest-Neighbour (K-NN), Nave-Bayes (NB), and CNN are five machine learning methods which used to extract and identify the features. The accuracy of these techniques is 90–98% on three publicly available datasets: MalayaKew, Flavia, and Swedish Leaf Dataset. [10] present the three neural network architectures, Inception v3, ResNet50, and DenseNet201 to improve the performance of plant species classification, used a variety of augmentation operations to increase the dataset diversity further, using dataset holds 256.288 samples and the noisy set 1.432.162. These samples are for 10.000 different plants, as well as a robust Orchid family plant database built for algorithm evaluation. The study [11] present a pre-trained AlexNet was fine-tuned, which resulted in the 4th place. The study [12] providing a detailed empirical guide showing that residual networks are easier to refine and can achieve precision by increasing depth substantially, also test performed on the residual nets with a depth of 152 layers in the ImageNet dataset, but with lower complexity, on the ImageNet test range, an ensemble of these residual nets achieves a 3.57% error. The model was pre-trained with ImageNet and fine-tuned with the PlantCLEF database, using an Inception Convolutional Neural Network (CNN) model-based network. They merged the outputs of five CNNs, which were fine-tuned with randomly selected sections of the database. The optimization of hyperparameters, on the other hand, was not completed [13]. The study [14] design A multi-input convolutional neural network for large scale flower grading and achieves 89.6 after data augmentation. The study [15] presents a method for extracting distinctive invariant features from images that can be used to perform reliable matching between different views of an object or scene. The study [16] propose model that use different training epochs, batch sizes and dropouts. Compared with popular transfer learning approaches, the proposed model achieves better performance when using the validation data. After an extensive simulation, the proposed model achieves 96.46% classification accuracy. The study [17] present overview on the plant species recognition methods and features extraction using leaf image. The study [18] provide a data article for a dataset that holds samples of images of healthy citrus fruits and leaves. The study [19] the pre-processing, feature extraction, and categorization into one of the species. Several morphological parameters such as centroid, major axis length, minor axis length, solidity, perimeter, and orientation are retrieved from digital pictures of various leaf categories with an accuracy rate of 95.85%

In the study [20], builds an unique multiscale convolutional neural network with attention (AMSCNN) model for plant species detection, with a maximum accuracy of 95.28%.

3 Description of the Implemented Techniques

Taxonomy and family classification of plants are difficult to decipher. There have been several studies on the classification and recognition of plant images. We used a matrix of multiple models with multiple plant parts in this study. On the lower leaf, upper leaf, and fruit images, CNN developed model, Random Forest with parameter optimization, and SVM are used. Deep Learning has shown the best outcomes of machine learning. Convolutional neural networks (CNN) have recently achieved the greatest success in image recognition and are commonly used in most advanced deep learning techniques. Most recent studies have focused on using deep learning to classify images.

Support Vector Machine: The main objective of the SVM is to find the hyperplane that can separate the data most efficiently and most accurately. In both classification and regression, the support vector machine (SVM) is used.

In a linear SVM, the given data set is represented as a p-dimensional vector that can be separated by a maximum of p-1 planes. These planes divide the data space or define the boundaries between data classes in classification and regression problems [21].

Deep Learning: VGGNet, LeNet, GoogLeNet, and AlexNet are the most common CNN architectures used in current state-of-the-art Deep Learning research to solve various Computer Vision problems such as Image Classification, Object Recognition. AlexNet is a CNN model that has been pre-trained using images from the ImageNet dataset. It can distinguish 1000 different animals. There are five convolutional layers, three completely linked layers, and a softmax classification layer in this model [22]. Mathematical formula for a convolution layer:

$$Conv(I,K)x,y = \sum_{i=1}^{nH}\sum_{j=1}^{nW}\sum_{k=1}^{nC}(Ki,j,kIx+i-1,y+j-1,k)$$

where: I: image, K: filter, nH: the size of the Height, nW: the size of the Width, nC: the number of Channels.

Random Forest: Random Forest is a powerful and scalable that classify as the supervised learning of the machine learning algorithms that creates a "forest" by growing and combining more than one of the decision trees that are compiled to enhance the prediction. It can be used to solve problems involving classification and regression.

4 Empirical Studies

4.1 Description of Dataset

- Reviewed all images of (lower leaf, upper leaf, and fruit) and ensured that the image is clear.
- Ensured that all images are uniform in length.
- Distortion cleaning.
- Standardized the image features.

4.2 Dataset Analysis

The dataset is 51 original images for 17 species belonging to two families, is not useful in the training of the CNN model. We use the augmentation to increase the dataset to 3954 images for 51 species belong to two different families. The image dimensions are 224 ×224, divided into 3164 for training and 790 images for testing, as shown in Table 1. Eight for the first family (Apiaceae), and nine images from the second family (Brassicaceae) as shown in Fig. 1, and Fig. 2 respectively. In our work we used different four plants species in identification testing, which does not train by our system.

Table 1. Plant dataset information.

Family name	No. of plants	Fruit images	Lower leaf images	Upper leaf images	Total
Apiaceae	8	608	608	608	1824
Brassicaceae	9	710	710	710	2130
Total	17	1318	1318	1318	3954

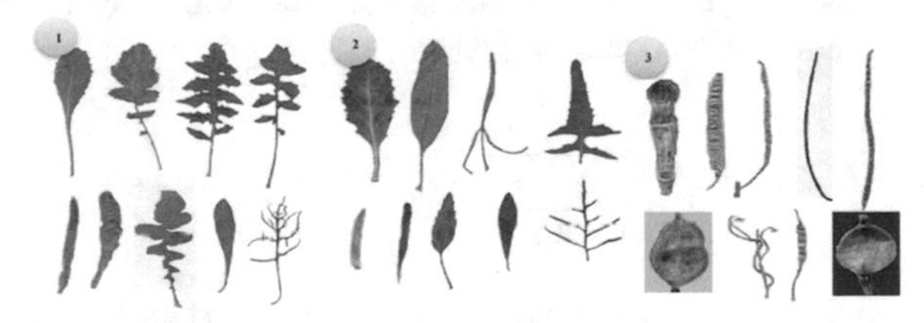

Fig. 1. The image of family Apiaceae used for the dataset (1- Lower leaf, 2- Upper leaf, and 3- fruit).

One of the contributions in the current study is preparing this dataset, because the current study is the first machine learning and AI experiments applied on this dataset. The dataset consists of three parts; the first is lower leaf images, the second is upper leaf images and the third is the fruits images. All images related to two plant families as shown in Table 1.

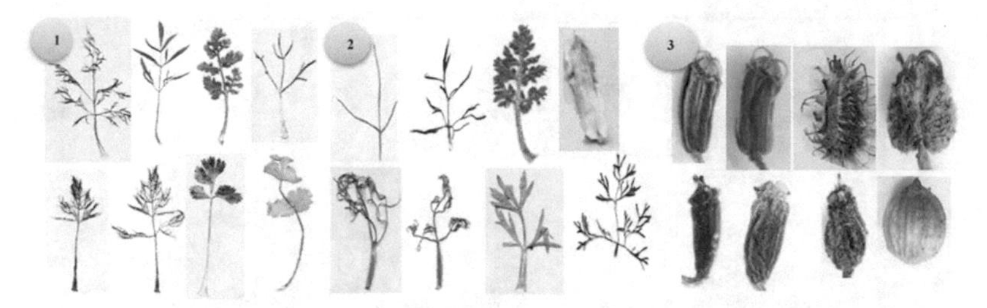

Fig. 2. The image of family Brassicaceae used for the dataset (1- Lower leaf, 2- Up*per leaf, and 3- fruit).*

4.3 Feature's Extraction

Features are parts or patterns of an object in an image that help to identify it. The HOG (Histogram of Oriented Gradients) descriptor is one of commonly used global explored in the object detection group. It is based on the idea of counting the number of times a gradient orientation appears in a particular localized region of an image [23]. We extract the Histogram of Oriented Gradients (HOG) for the plant's images, and compute a HOG by using python package (SKIMAGE) that working on:

- Global image normalization
- Computing the gradient image
- Computing gradient histograms
- Normalizing across blocks
- Flattening into a feature vector
- Combine color and hog features.

HOG descriptors are not tied to a specific machine learning algorithm.

In the current study we have developed the features extraction process based on the CNN model.

5 Proposed Models and Results

More than one AI model was applied to three datasets, lower plants dataset (LPDS), upper plant dataset (UPDS), and fruit plant dataset (FPDS). The AlexNet CNN (Convolution Neural Network) model developed and implemented to extract the fruit and the leaves features, classify each plant to its family, and use the trained model to identify the plant and to classify it to the belongs family. The current study propose the system for family classification and species identification based on the developed CNN model as shown in Fig. 3:

- Developed CNN
- SVM (Support Vector Machine)
- Random Forest.

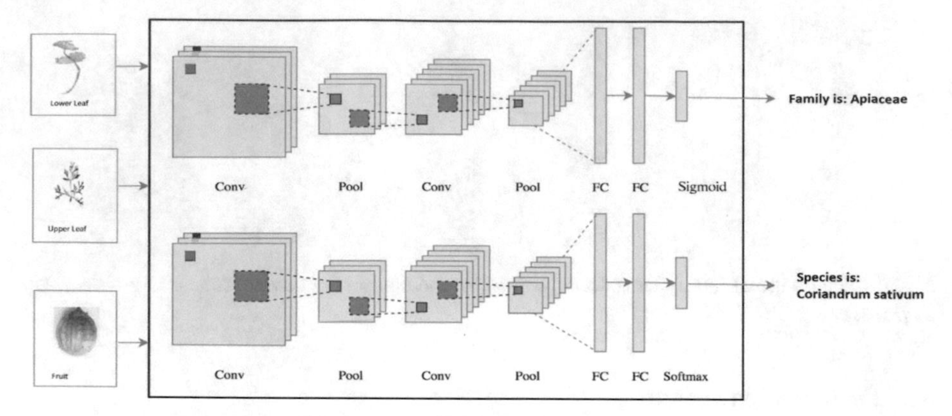

Fig. 3. Proposed System Architecture based on developed CNN.

5.1 Families Classification (Binary Classification)

In this section we implemented different deep learning models of binary classification to classify the plants into two families (Apiaceae and Brassicaceae) with validation on these models.

First Experiment Description. The dataset described in Table 1 is the input for the first developed CNN model, the model architecture consists of 11 layers. In this experiment the three datasets (LPDS, UPDS, and FPDS) applied and the accuracy is near to 99% as shown in Fig. 4, also the loss is near to zero. This result is individual for each dataset type standalone the result is binary and classify two families based on supervising training, as shown in Fig. 4, the accuracy of fruit and lower leaf are better than the accuracy of upper leaf and the best result with the fruit.

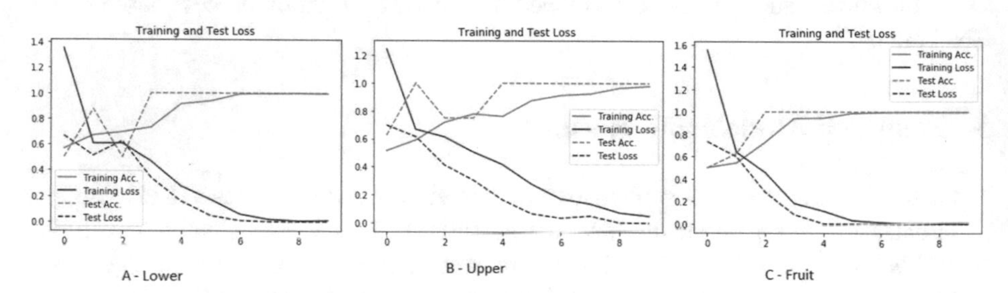

Fig. 4. Single Input CNN Model Accuracy (binary classification)

Second Experiment. The dataset described in Table 1 is the input for the first CNN model, the model architecture consists of 11 layers. The input layer are three images (lower, upper, and fruit) each one has dimension (200, 200).

In this experiment the three datasets (LPDS, UPDS, and FPDS) applied and the accuracy is near to 99% as shown in Fig. 5, also the loss is near to zero. This result is based on the three images added to the inputs parallel, the result is binary and classify two families based on supervising training. The accuracy is stable and better than the first experiment.

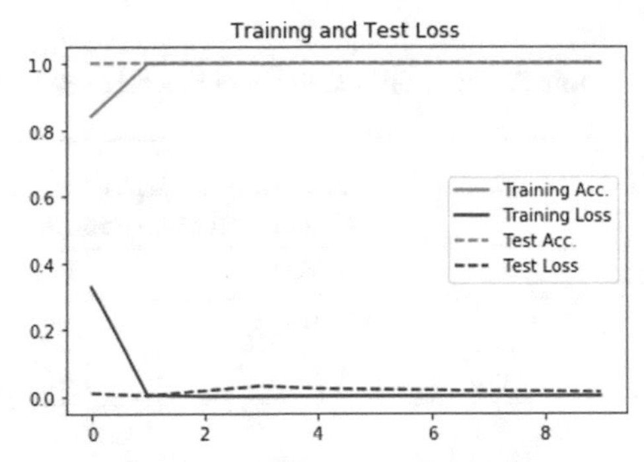

Fig. 5. Three-inputs CNN Model Accuracy (binary classification)

The results of a comparison of different binary classifiers applied on the dataset are shown in Fig. 6, the best accuracy is 99.7% by using the Random Forest method.

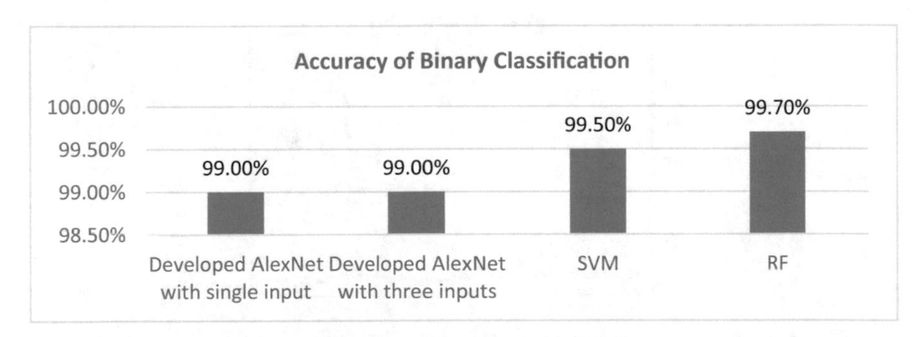

Fig. 6. Comparison of Binary Classification Accuracy

5.2 Species Identification (Categorical Classification)

The categorical classification problem is very important to build the digital library of plants. In this section we implemented the same deep learning models with changing in the output cost functions and number of classes to classify the plants into seventeen plant of the same families.

Third Experiment. In this experiment we applied the same model implemented in the first experiment with changing the number of classes in the output layer to 17 class (Number of plants in the two families), with change the objective function from sigmoid to the activation function calculation, that classify the 17 plant, Softmax function comes to solve categorical classification problem its responsible for the final prediction layer, and with using categorical entropy in loss calculation. We applied this experiment using two dataset size and modifying the developed AlexNet CNN hyperparameters using KERAS python package as shown in Table 2.

Table 2. Developed CNN hyper parameters.

Parameter	Value
Loss	Categorical cross entropy
Learning rate	0.0001
Activation function	Softmax
rho	0.9

The results from this experiment are the classification probabilities for 17 plants using categorical entropy in loss calculation. As shown in Fig. 7 the accuracy and loss for each training and testing of three datasets (LPDS, UPDS, and FPDS) with small dataset samples is very bad, the average of validation accuracy is 6% and the average of validation loss is 282%.

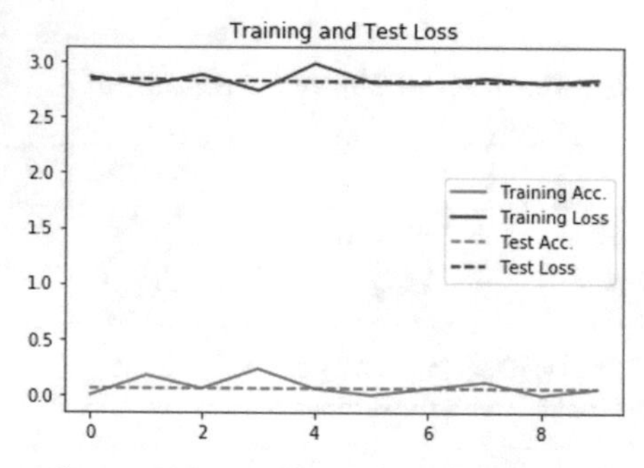

Fig. 7. CNN Plant Categorical Classification of 17 plants without augmentation.

Fourth Experiment (SVM). In this experiment, we were used the SVM method with the parameter's optimization. The best parameters are {'C': 10.0, 'gamma': 1e–08} with a score of 1.00 and using the SKLEARN package from python language. The results from this experiment we were used the SVM method with the parameter's optimization, the testing accuracy of 30% from the dataset is 96.7%.

Fifth Experiment (Random Forest). SKLEARN Python package was used to implement the RF (Random Forest) select the optimal parameters, and to evaluate the accuracy as shown in Table 3.

Random forest method applied to classify 17 plants, 1106 samples the results of important features are shown in Fig. 8, and the testing accuracy of 30% from the dataset is 93%, 96%, and 96% respectively for the fruit, lower, and upper.

Table 3. Random forest parameters

	Max depth	None
Random forest	Min. samples leaf	1
	Min. samples split	2
	Random state	None

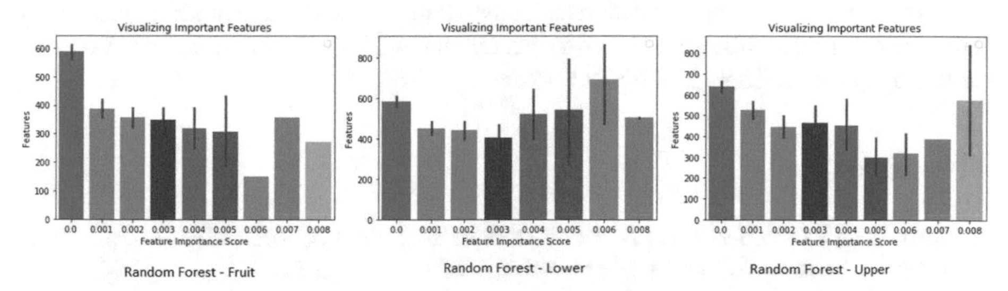

Fig. 8. Random Forest visualizing the important features of 17 plants.

The results of a comparison of different methods implemented on the dataset are shown in Fig. 9 the best accuracy is 98.2% by using the developed CNN model.

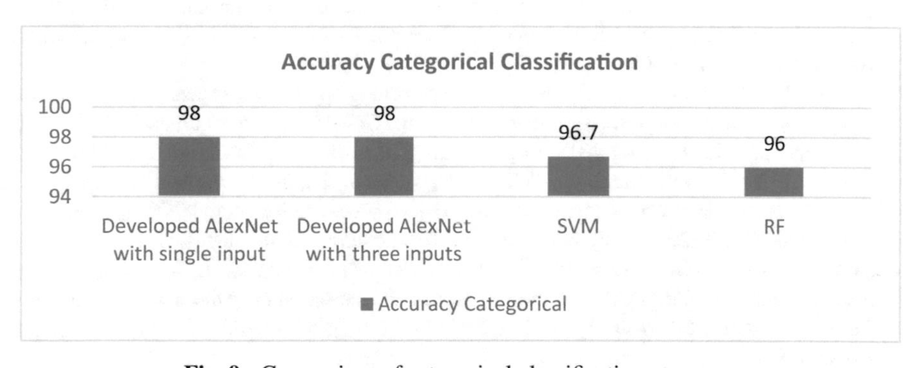

Fig. 9. Comparison of categorical classification accuracy

6 Conclusion and Recommendation for the Future Work

The purpose of the current study was to implement machine learning based tools to serve a plants taxonomy. The wild plants dataset collected from its natural locality in Egypt. The techniques that were compared in the family classifications (binary classification) were the developed convolution neural network (CNN), support vector machine (SVM), and the Random Forest. The highest level of accuracy obtained was 99.7% achieved with the random forest method RF with the two samples classification, while support vector machine (SVM), and CNN obtained 99.5%, and 99% accuracy, respectively. The challenges in the species classification (categorical classification) not in the families, and we obtained the excellent results in this area. The techniques that were compared in the categorical classifications were the developed convolution neural network (CNN), support vector machine (SVM), and the Random Forest. The highest level of accuracy obtained was 98.2% achieved with the developed CNN with the 17 plants samples classification, while support vector machine (SVM), and RF obtained 96.7%, and 96% accuracy, respectively.

In the future, we recommend increasing the samples and implement the digital library using website and mobile application to increase the wild plants samples and to facilitate the biological researchers in the plant taxonomy.

References

1. Jana, B.K., Mukherjee, S.K.: Diversity of cypselar features of seven species of the Genus Crepis L. in. Indian J. Fundam. Appl. Life Sci. **2**(1), 54–58 (2012)
2. Lee, J.W., Chan Yoon, Y.: Fine-Grained Plant Identification using wide and deep learning model 1. In: 2019 International Conference on Platform Technology and Service PlatCon 2019 - Proceedings, no. 2016, pp. 1–5 (2019). https://doi.org/10.1109/PlatCon.2019.8669407
3. Lee, S.H., Chan, C.S., Wilkin, P., Remagnino, P.: Deep-plant: plant identification with convolutional neural networks. In: Proceedings of the International Conference Image Processing ICIP, vol. 2015, pp. 452–456, December 2015. https://doi.org/10.1109/ICIP.2015.7350839
4. Gyires-Tóth, B.P., Osváth, M., Papp, D., Szucs, G.: Deep learning for plant classification and content-based image retrieval. Cybern. Inf. Technol. **19**(1), 88–100 (2019). https://doi.org/10.2478/CAIT-2019-0005
5. Dileep, M.R., Pournami, P.N.: AyurLeaf: a deep learning approach for classification of medicinal plants. In: IEEE Region 10 Annual International Conference Proceedings/TENCON, vol. 2019, pp. 321–325, October 2019. https://doi.org/10.1109/TENCON.2019.8929394
6. Kaya, A., Keceli, A.S., Catal, C., Yalic, H.Y., Temucin, H., Tekinerdogan, B.: Analysis of transfer learning for deep neural network based plant classification models. Comput. Electron. Agric. **158**, 20–29 (2019). https://doi.org/10.1016/j.compag.2019.01.041
7. Picon, A., Alvarez-Gila, A., Seitz, M., Ortiz-Barredo, A., Echazarra, J., Johannes, A.: Deep convolutional neural networks for mobile capture device-based crop disease classification in the wild. Comput. Electron. Agric. **161**, 280–290 (2019). https://doi.org/10.1016/j.compag.2018.04.002
8. Johannes, A., et al.: Automatic plant disease diagnosis using mobile capture devices, applied on a wheat use case. Comput. Electron. Agric. **138**, 200–209 (2017). https://doi.org/10.1016/j.compag.2017.04.013
9. Tan, J.W., Chang, S.W., Abdul-Kareem, S., Yap, H.J., Yong, K.T.: Deep learning for plant species classification using leaf vein morphometric. IEEE/ACM Trans. Comput. Biol. Bioinforma. **17**(1), 82–90 (2020). https://doi.org/10.1109/TCBB.2018.2848653
10. Haupt, J., Kahl, S., Kowerko, D., Eibl, M.: Large-scale plant classification using deep convolutional neural networks. In: CEUR Workshop Proceedings, vol. 2125, pp. 1–7 (2018)
11. Reyes, A.K., Caicedo, J.C., Camargo, J.E., Nari, U.A.: Fine-tuning deep convolutional networks for plant recognition
12. He, K., Zhang, X., Ren, S., Sun, J.: Deep residual learning for image recognition. In: Proceedings of the Computer Society Conference on Computer Vision and Pattern Recognition, vol. 2016, pp. 770–778, December 2016. https://doi.org/10.1109/CVPR.2016.90

13. Choi, S.: Plant identification with deep convolutional neural network: SNUMedinfo at LifeCLEF plant identification task 2015. In: CEUR Workshop Proceedings, vol. 1391, pp. 2–5 (2015)
14. Sun, Y., Zhu, L., Wang, G., Zhao, F.: Multi-input convolutional neural network for flower grading, vol. 2017 (2017)
15. Low, D.G.: Distinctive image features from scale-invariant keypoints. Int. J. Comput. Vis., 91–110 (2004). https://www.cs.ubc.ca/~lowe/papers/ijcv04.pdf
16. Xiao, J., Wang, J., Cao, S., Li, B.: Application of a Novel and Improved VGG-19 Network in the Detection of Workers Wearing Masks Application of a Novel and Improved VGG-19 Network in the Detection of Workers Wearing Masks (2020). https://doi.org/10.1088/1742-6596/1518/1/012041
17. Zhang, S., Huang, W., Huang, Y., Zhang, C.: Neurocomputing Plant species recognition methods using leaf image: Overview, vol. 408, pp. 246–272 (2020). https://doi.org/10.1016/j.neucom.2019.09.113
18. Ullah, M.I., Attique, M., Sharif, M., Ahmad, S., Bukhari, C.: Data in brief a citrus fruits and leaves dataset for detection and classification of citrus diseases through machine learning, vol. 26 (2019). https://doi.org/10.1016/j.dib.2019.104340
19. Mahajan, S., Raina, A., Gao, X.Z., Pandit, A.K.: Plant recognition using morphological feature extraction and transfer learning over SVM and adaboost. Symmetry (Basel) **13**(2), 1–16 (2021). https://doi.org/10.3390/sym13020356
20. Wang, X., Zhang, C., Zhang, S.: Multiscale convolutional neural networks with attention for plant species recognition. Comput. Intell. Neurosci. **2021** (2021). https://doi.org/10.1155/2021/5529905
21. Hearst, B.S.M.A., Dumais, S.T., Osuna, E., Platt, J.: Support vector machines. IEEE Intell. http://www.med.cmu.ac.th/secret/edserv/curriculum/file/2559/ไฟล์ขึ้นเว็บ 2559/BHS 2559/14. Learning and humanistic19 ต.ค. 59 เช้า.pdf?fbclid=IwAR1uKMoC9dIKBu0dvzYzQQvPUKxwxZS7fbQgdA4SBStlPh5996AWWV16hfw.**4**(1), 18–28 (1998)
22. Krizhevsky, A., Sutskever, I., Hinton, G.E.: ImageNet classification with deep convolutional neural networks. In: ACM International Conference Proceedings Series., pp. 145–151 (2020). https://doi.org/10.1145/3383972.3383975
23. Gogul, I., Kumar, V.S.: Flower species recognition system using convolution neural networks and transfer learning. In: 2017 4th International Conference on Signal Processing, Communication and Networking ICSCN 2017, pp. 1–6 (2017). https://doi.org/10.1109/ICSCN.2017.8085675

A Novel Weighted Fractional TDGM Model and Quantum Particle Swarm Optimization Algorithm for Carbon Dioxide Emissions Forecasting

Ani Shabri(✉)

Department of Mathematic, Science Faculty, University Technology of Malaysia, UTM, 81310 Skudai, Johor, Malaysia
ani@utm.my

Abstract. This paper will present a novel weighted fractional TDGM(1,1) (WFTDGM) model based on the combination of the weighted fractional-accumulation generating operator (FAGO) and the TDGM(1,1) model. The suggested WFTDGM model would be able to reduce the traditional TDGM(1,1) model and the fractional TDGM(1,1), or FTDGM model when the parameters are adjusted differently. Hence, the quantum particle swarm optimization algorithm will be used to select the optimal parameters for the proposed model to achieve the best accuracy precision. Whereas the least squares estimate method is used to determine the remaining model parameters. Twenty numerical samples selected from various countries presented in this paper will be used as the case study. When compared to the other conventional grey models such as the GM(1,1), FGM(1,1), TDGM, and FTDGM models, the computational results indicate that the proposed model has the best forecast performance compared to the other models.

Keywords: Grey model · Fractional-accumulation generating operator · Quantum particle swarm optimization algorithm · ANN

1 Introduction

In recent years, climate change has moved to the top of global political agendas, with significant economic repercussions. According to scientific sources, the most major contributor to the global warming phenomena is the release of greenhouse gases (GHGs), especially carbon dioxide (CO2) [1]. Human activity produces CO2 mostly through the burning of fossil fuels and deforestation. According to international statistics, the shipping, international aviation, and transportation sectors have had the most rises in GHG emissions over the last decade, while other sectors have seen declines. Due to these several factors, an accurate CO2 emission forecasting report for the next decade is critical for the concern of current economic and political issues [1]. A handful of techniques have been presented in multiple studies to model and forecast the CO2 emission time series related data.

F. Saeed et al. (Eds.): IRICT 2021, LNDECT 127, pp. 38–49, 2022.
https://doi.org/10.1007/978-3-030-98741-1_4

Several techniques have been implemented in these studies to forecast CO2 emissions data, including statistical models such as Holt-Winters and exponential smoothing [1], the ARIMA model [2, 3], logistic equations [4], and regression models [2, 4, 5]. However, statistical approaches to forecasting accuracy often necessitate a large amount of data that complies with particular statistical assumptions [6]. As the nature of CO2 emissions data fluctuates, some artificial intelligent forecasting methods, such as the artificial neural networks (ANN) [1, 7, 8], fuzzy regression [9], and hybrid models [10], have been applied to forecast CO2 emissions related data. The amount of training data and its representativeness, on the other hand, are limits that affect predicting effectiveness, and both issues have yet to be resolved. In all of the following methodologies, the sample size is a significant issue, restricting their applicability to specific forecasting situations [11].

Grey system theory was proposed by Deng [12] as a solution to problems involving limited, partial, and/or unpredictable data. The grey model, or commonly known in the form of GM (1,1) is commonly used to forecast CO2 emissions, along with its variation such as Pao et al. [15] proposed a nonlinear grey Bernoulli model (NGBM(1,1)), Lin et al. [16] proposed a nonlinear GM(1,1) model, Xu et al. [17] proposed an adaptive grey model, and Wang and Li [18] proposed a grey Verhulst model. Despite the implementation of grey models, these models were developed in response to various challenges, which pushed us to continue developing a more diversely acceptable grey model in the study of CO2 emissions forecasting. Many researchers have worked on different aspects of the GM(1,1) model to improve prediction performance, including attempting to build more accurate background value formulas [19, 20], improving initial guess [21], exploring different accumulation generating operators [22–24], and selecting parameter optimization techniques [25].

In addition, Xie and Liu [26] devised the discrete grey model, abbreviated as DGM(1,1), to solve the GM(1,1) model's inherent flaws caused by converting discrete data into continuous series. Following that, Xie et al. [27] developed the nonhomogeneous discrete grey model (NDGM(1,1)) and to improve the modeling performance of the NDGM(1,1) model, Zhang and Liu [28] suggested the time-varying parameters discrete grey prediction model TDGM(1,1). As a result, it is proved that using time-varying parameters is a practical technique for dealing with the normal volatility and nonlinearity present in most real-world problems.

The accumulated generating operation (AGO) is the central idea of grey system theory, as its purpose is to convert raw data unpredictability into a monotonically rising series. The one-order accumulated generating operation (1-AGO) is commonly served as the identification for the GM(1,1) model. However, the one issue with 1-AGO is that each sample is given the same weightage throughout the whole system [29]. In recent decades, numerous research has suggested that the fractional accumulated generating operation (F-AGO) can improve the performance of the GM(1,1) model. Wu [30, 31] was the first to incorporate the F-AGO with GM(1,1) model, known as the FGM(1,1) model, which results proven to outperform GM (1,1) model. FGM(q,1) model [32], FNGBM(1,1) model [33], fractional non-homogeneous grey model [34], and discrete fractional grey model [35] are some of the additional grey models that have been presented and effectively used in many practical applications based on the concept of F-AGO.

As the AGO is the main focus of this research in this paper, we first try to construct a weighted F-AGO (WF-AGO), which is based on the new information priority concept and the F-AGO. The WF-AGO has two parameters that can change the summing order based on different data sequences and represent information priority variations. The effectiveness and practicality of a new WFTDGM model are compared to the GM(1,1), FGM(1,1), TDGM(1,1), and FTDGM(1,1) models in this study. Furthermore, the quantum particle swarm optimization (QPSO) method is used to find the optimal parameters by generating a nonlinear optimization problem for predicted value [36, 37].

The content of this study is organised as follows: Sect. 2.1 discusses the WF-AGO and its inverse. The WF-AGO linear time-varying parameters discrete grey model is introduced in Sect. 2.2. The proposed QPSO and WTDGM are described in Sect. 2.3. The experimental findings of the CO2 emissions forecast performance of the various grey models evaluated are presented in Sect. 3. Section 4 has a discussion and conclusions.

2 Materials and Methods

2.1 The Weighted Fractional Accumulation Generating Operator and Their Inverse

Assume the time series $x^{(0)} = \left\{x_1^{(0)}, x_2^{(0)}, \ldots, x_k^{(0)}, \ldots, x_n^{(0)}\right\}$ of size n, and the 1st order-fractional accumulation generating operator (1-AGO) of $x^{(0)}$ can be written as $x_k^{(1)} = \sum_{i=1}^{k} x_i^{(0)}$ where $x^{(1)} = \left\{x_1^{(1)}, x_2^{(1)}, \ldots, x_k^{(1)}, \ldots, x_n^{(1)}\right\}$ and $k = 1, 2, \ldots, n$.

The fractional order-accumulation generating operator (F-AGO) is defined as follows:

$$x_k^{(r)} = \sum_{i=1}^{k} \begin{bmatrix} r \\ k-i \end{bmatrix} x_i^{(0)} \tag{1}$$

or in matrix form as $x^{(r)} = A^r x^{(0)}$ where

$$A^r = \begin{pmatrix} \begin{bmatrix} r \\ 0 \end{bmatrix} & 0 & 0 & \cdots & 0 \\ \begin{bmatrix} r \\ 1 \end{bmatrix} & \begin{bmatrix} r \\ 0 \end{bmatrix} & 0 & \cdots & 0 \\ \begin{bmatrix} r \\ 2 \end{bmatrix} & \begin{bmatrix} r \\ 1 \end{bmatrix} & \begin{bmatrix} r \\ 0 \end{bmatrix} & \cdots & 0 \\ \vdots & \vdots & \vdots & \ddots & \vdots \\ \begin{bmatrix} r \\ n-1 \end{bmatrix} & \begin{bmatrix} r \\ n-2 \end{bmatrix} & \begin{bmatrix} r \\ n-3 \end{bmatrix} & \cdots & \begin{bmatrix} r \\ 0 \end{bmatrix} \end{pmatrix} \tag{2}$$

The WF-AGO of $x^{(0)}$ can be written as $x^{(r\lambda)} = \left\{x_1^{(r\lambda)}, x_2^{(r\lambda)}, \ldots, x_k^{(r\lambda)}, \ldots, x_n^{(r\lambda)}\right\}$ where $x_k^{(r\lambda)} = \sum_{i=1}^{k} \begin{bmatrix} r \\ k-i \end{bmatrix} \lambda^{k-i} x_i^{(0)}$. WF-AGO can be represented in matrices formula $x^{(r\lambda)} =$

$A^{r\lambda}x^{(0)}$ where

$$A^{r\lambda}=\begin{pmatrix} \begin{bmatrix} r\\0 \end{bmatrix} & 0 & 0 & \cdots & 0\\ \begin{bmatrix} r\\1 \end{bmatrix}\lambda & \begin{bmatrix} r\\0 \end{bmatrix} & 0 & \cdots & 0\\ \begin{bmatrix} r\\2 \end{bmatrix}\lambda^2 & \begin{bmatrix} r\\1 \end{bmatrix}\lambda & \begin{bmatrix} r\\0 \end{bmatrix} & \cdots & 0\\ \vdots & \vdots & \vdots & \ddots & \vdots\\ \begin{bmatrix} r\\n-1 \end{bmatrix}\lambda^{n-1} & \begin{bmatrix} r\\n-2 \end{bmatrix}\lambda^{n-2} & \begin{bmatrix} r\\n-3 \end{bmatrix}\lambda^{n-3} & \cdots & \begin{bmatrix} r\\0 \end{bmatrix} \end{pmatrix} \tag{3}$$

where $\begin{bmatrix} r\\n \end{bmatrix}=\begin{cases} 1 & n=0\\ \frac{r(r+1)\ldots(r+n+1)}{n!} & n\in N^+ \end{cases}$

When $r=\lambda=1$, the WF-AGO will be reduced in the form of 1-AGO. While when $\lambda=1$, the WF-AGO will be reduced in the form of F-AGO. The inverse of WF-AGO is defined as

$$A^{-r\lambda}=\begin{pmatrix} \begin{bmatrix} -r\\0 \end{bmatrix} & 0 & 0 & \cdots & 0\\ \begin{bmatrix} -r\\1 \end{bmatrix}\lambda & \begin{bmatrix} -r\\0 \end{bmatrix} & 0 & \cdots & 0\\ \begin{bmatrix} -r\\2 \end{bmatrix}\lambda^2 & \begin{bmatrix} -r\\1 \end{bmatrix}\lambda & \begin{bmatrix} -r\\0 \end{bmatrix} & \cdots & 0\\ \vdots & \vdots & \vdots & \ddots & \vdots\\ \begin{bmatrix} -r\\n-1 \end{bmatrix}\lambda^{n-1} & \begin{bmatrix} -r\\n-2 \end{bmatrix}\lambda^{n-2} & \begin{bmatrix} -r\\n-3 \end{bmatrix}\lambda^{n-3} & \cdots & \begin{bmatrix} -r\\0 \end{bmatrix} \end{pmatrix} \tag{4}$$

The relation between $x^{(0)}$ and $x^{(r\lambda)}$ is as shown:

$$x^{(0)}=A^{-r\lambda}x^{(r\lambda)} \tag{5}$$

When $r=\lambda=1,\ x^{(0)}=A^{-1}x^{(1)}$. A^{-1} is the inverse of 1-AGO and can be denoted as

$$A^{-1}=\begin{pmatrix} 1 & 0 & 0 & \cdots & 0\\ -1 & 1 & 0 & \cdots & 0\\ 0 & -1 & 1 & \cdots & 0\\ \vdots & \vdots & \vdots & \ddots & \vdots\\ 0 & 0 & 0 & \cdots & 1 \end{pmatrix} \tag{6}$$

Similarly, when $\lambda = 1$, $x^{(0)} = A^{-r}x^{(r)}$. We refer to A^{-r} as the inverse of F-AGO and can be denoted as

$$A^{-r\lambda} = \begin{pmatrix} \begin{bmatrix} -r \\ 0 \end{bmatrix} & 0 & 0 & \cdots & 0 \\ \begin{bmatrix} -r \\ 1 \end{bmatrix}\lambda & \begin{bmatrix} -r \\ 0 \end{bmatrix} & 0 & \cdots & 0 \\ \begin{bmatrix} -r \\ 2 \end{bmatrix}\lambda^2 & \begin{bmatrix} -r \\ 1 \end{bmatrix}\lambda & \begin{bmatrix} -r \\ 0 \end{bmatrix} & \cdots & 0 \\ \vdots & \vdots & \vdots & \ddots & \vdots \\ \begin{bmatrix} -r \\ n-1 \end{bmatrix}\lambda^{n-1} & \begin{bmatrix} -r \\ n-2 \end{bmatrix}\lambda^{n-2} & \begin{bmatrix} -r \\ n-3 \end{bmatrix}\lambda^{n-3} & \cdots & \begin{bmatrix} -r \\ 0 \end{bmatrix} \end{pmatrix} \tag{7}$$

2.2 The Weighted of Fractional-Order of TDGM Model

The DGM(1,1), given by (Wu et al. 2013) as:

$$x_{k+1}^{(1)} = ax_k^{(1)} + b, \; k = 1, 2, \ldots, n-1 \tag{8}$$

where $x_k^{(1)} = \sum_{i=1}^{k} x_i^{(0)}$ and $x^{(0)} = \left(x_1^{(0)}, x_2^{(0)}, \ldots, x_n^{(0)}\right)$ indicate the original value of size n. The least-square method is used to estimate the parameters of DGM(1,1) model as shown:

$$\begin{bmatrix} a \\ b \end{bmatrix} = \left(X^T X\right)^{-1} X^T Y \tag{9}$$

where

$$Y = \begin{pmatrix} x_2^{(1)} \\ x_3^{(1)} \\ \vdots \\ x_n^{(1)} \end{pmatrix} \text{ and } X = \begin{pmatrix} x_1^{(1)} & 1 \\ x_2^{(1)} & 1 \\ \vdots & \vdots \\ x_{n-1}^{(1)} & 1 \end{pmatrix} \tag{10}$$

The TDGM is denoted by

$$x_{k+1}^{(1)} = (ak + b)x_k^{(1)} + ck + d, \; k = 1, 2, \ldots, n-1 \tag{11}$$

The least-squares estimate method is used to solve the TDGM model's parameters, as defined below:

$$\begin{bmatrix} a \\ b \\ c \\ d \end{bmatrix} = \left(X^T X\right)^{-1} X^T Y \tag{12}$$

where

$$Y = \begin{pmatrix} x_2^{(1)} \\ x_3^{(1)} \\ \vdots \\ x_n^{(1)} \end{pmatrix} \text{ and } X = \begin{pmatrix} x_1^{(1)} & x_1^{(1)} & 1 & 1 \\ 2x_2^{(1)} & x_2^{(1)} & 2 & 1 \\ \vdots & \vdots & \vdots & \vdots \\ (n-2)x_{n-2}^{(1)} & x_{n-2}^{(1)} & n-2 & 1 \\ (n-1)x_{n-1}^{(1)} & x_{n-1}^{(1)} & n-1 & 1 \end{pmatrix} \tag{13}$$

The TDGM model predicted value is as follows:

$$\hat{x}^{(0)} = A^{-1}\hat{x}^{(1)} \tag{14}$$

where $\hat{x}_{k+1}^{(1)} = (ak+b)\hat{x}_k^{(1)} + ck + d, k = 1, 2, \ldots, n-1.$

The WFTDGM is denoted by

$$x_{k+1}^{(r\lambda)} = (ak+b)x_k^{(r\lambda)} + ck + d, \; k = 1, 2, \ldots, n-1 \tag{15}$$

The parameters of the WFTDGM(1,1) model can be estimated using the following formula:

$$\begin{bmatrix} a \\ b \\ c \\ d \end{bmatrix} = \left(X^T X\right)^{-1} X^T Y \tag{16}$$

where

$$Y = \begin{pmatrix} x_2^{(r\lambda)} \\ x_3^{(r\lambda)} \\ \vdots \\ x_n^{(r\lambda)} \end{pmatrix} \text{ and } X = \begin{pmatrix} x_1^{(r\lambda)} & x_1^{(r\lambda)} & 1 & 1 \\ 2x_2^{(r\lambda)} & x_2^{(r\lambda)} & 2 & 1 \\ \vdots & \vdots & \vdots & \vdots \\ (n-2)x_{n-2}^{(r\lambda)} & x_{n-2}^{(r\lambda)} & n-2 & 1 \\ (n-1)x_{n-1}^{(r\lambda)} & x_{n-1}^{(r\lambda)} & n-1 & 1 \end{pmatrix} \tag{17}$$

The predicted value of WFTDGM model is as shown:

$$\hat{x}^{(0)} = A^{-r\lambda}\hat{x}^{(r\lambda)} \text{ or } \hat{x}_k^{(0)} = \sum\nolimits_{i=1}^{k} \begin{bmatrix} -r \\ k-i \end{bmatrix} \lambda^{k-i}\hat{x}_i^{(r\lambda)} \tag{18}$$

$$\text{where } \hat{x}_{k+1}^{(r\lambda)} = (ak+b)\hat{x}_k^{(r\lambda)} + ck + d, \; k = 1, 2, \ldots, n-1 \tag{19}$$

When $r = \lambda = 1$, the WFTDGM model produces the simple form of TDGM(1,1) model, while when $\lambda = 1$ and $0 < r < 1$, it produces the FTDGM model. The WFTDGM model is thus a generalisation of the TDGM(1,1) and FTDGM models.

2.3 Quantum Particle Swarm Optimization Algorithm Weighted of Fractional-Order of WFGM Model

The model's parameter λ and r shall be calculated in advance to construct the WF-AGO sequence. The WFTDGM model's prediction performance is directly influenced by these parameters. To identify the best fitting parameters and forecast accuracy, the mean absolute percentage error (MAPE) is used in this research. To summarize, the minimization problem below can be used to discover the optimal choices for λ and r.

$$\min MAPE = \frac{1}{n}\sum_{k=1}^{n}\frac{\left|\hat{x}_k^{(0)} - x_k^{(0)}\right|}{x_k^{(0)}} \times 100\%$$

$$s.t.\begin{cases} 0 < r \leq 1 \\ 0 < \lambda \leq 1 \\ \begin{bmatrix} a \\ b \end{bmatrix} = \left(X^T X\right)^{-1} X^T Y \\ \hat{x}_{k+1}^{(r\lambda)} = (ak+b)\hat{x}_k^{(r\lambda)} + ck + d \\ \hat{x}_k^{(0)} = \sum_{i=1}^{k}\begin{bmatrix} -r \\ k-i \end{bmatrix}\lambda^{k-i}\hat{x}_i^{(r\lambda)} \\ k = 1, 2, \ldots, n \end{cases} \tag{20}$$

The problem formulation presented above is nonlinear, non-differentiable, and difficult to solve in general. To identify the most optimum solution, we must first identify the parameters *a, b, c,* and *d*. The quantum particle swarm optimization (QPSO) method is used to efficiently obtain a quasi-optimal solution to Eq. (20). The QPSO algorithm incorporates quantum physics into the main Particle Swarm Optimization (PSO) algorithm to ensure global convergence. QPSO outperforms traditional PSO on some benchmark issues [36, 37]. Because Eq. (16) is complicated, it would be difficult to generate analytic findings for the optimum values of r and λ. As demonstrated below, the QPSO is used to discover the optimal values of r and λ.

Since there are just two variables, r and λ, only two-dimensional problem needs to be investigated. Assuming that $E_{i1}(l)$ and $E_{i2}(l)$ are the solutions for the parameters r and λ, respectively. Let $l = 1$, $P_{i1}(1) = E_{i1}(1)$ and $P_{i2}(1) = E_{i2}(1)$ for $i = 1, 2, \ldots, m,$ *in* the first iteration. Next, $(E_{i1}(l), E_{i2}(l))^T$ denotes its coordinate and $E_{i1}(l)$ denotes the position of the ith particle. Furthermore, the ith particle's optimal position at the lth iteration, $P_i(l)$, is referred to as "pbest", while the global optimal position,$P_g(l)$, is referred to as "gbest". Hence, $P_g(l)$ is given by

$$P_g(l) = \begin{pmatrix} P_{g1}(l) \\ P_{g2}(l) \end{pmatrix} \cong \begin{pmatrix} r(l) \\ \lambda(l) \end{pmatrix} = gbest \tag{21}$$

where $g = arg \min_{1 \leq l \leq m} MAPE(P_i(l))$. The position of each particle is updated using the following rule $(E_{i1}(l+1), E_{i2}(l+1))^T$ at the $(l+1)$ th iteration.

$$E_{id}(l+1) = W_{id}(l) \pm \alpha|C_d(l) - E_{id}(l)|.ln\frac{1}{u_{id}(l)} \tag{22}$$

where $W_{id}(l) = \phi_d(l)P_{id}(l) + (1 - \phi_d(l))P_{gd}(l)$, $C_d(l) = \frac{1}{m}\sum_{i=1}^{m} P_{id}(l)$, $\alpha = 0.5 - \frac{0.5(l_{max}-l)}{l}$, $\phi_d(l) = u_{id}(l) \sim U(0, 1), d = 1, 2$ and l_{max} is the maximum iteration number.

We will use the QPSO algorithm to optimize the order number of the WFTDGM model in this section. The procedure for determining the WFTDGM model's optimal solution order is as follows.

Step 1: Determine the initial parameters r and λ, and the data set $x^{(0)}$.
Step 2: Calculate the WF-AGO, $x^{(r\lambda)} = A^{r\lambda}x^{(0)}$.
Step 3: Solve the parameters $\beta = [a, b, c, d]$ using Eq. (16).
Step 4: Calculate the approximated values $\hat{x}_{k+1}^{(r\lambda)}$ and predicated $\hat{x}^{(0)}$ using Eq. (19).
Step 5: Find the optimal parameters r and λ use the QPSO algorithm to minimize the

MAPE as shown below.

i. Set settings such as the particle swarm size, iteration step size, and termination criteria, as well as the position of the population particles.
ii. Calculate the fitness value of each particle using MAPE as the fitness function.
iii. To update the particle position, use Eq. (17).
iv. The fitness number of each particle is calculated, as well as the individual optimal position pbest, $P_{id}(l)$, the global optimal position gbest, $P_{gd}(l)$ and the group ideal center, $C_d(l)$ are changed based on the value of optimal fitness.
v. Repeat step (iv) if the algorithm fails to meet the convergence rule; if it does, continue with step 6.

Step 6: Find the optimal parameters $r*$, $\lambda*$, the associated optimal fitted $\hat{x}_k^{(r\lambda)}$ and the predicted values $\hat{x}^{(0)}$.

Using the procedure outlined above, the modelling flow chart of QPSO-WFTDGM can be drawn as shown in Fig. 1.

3 Experiment Results

Annual total CO2 emissions from the top 20 countries, as published by the International Energy Agency [38] and Hu et al. [39], are used to compare the precision of the proposed WFTDGM model. Data from 2003 to 2013 was used to build the prediction model, and data from 2014 to 2017 was used to test its accuracy.

Annual total CO2 emissions from the top 20 countries, as published by the International Energy Agency [38] and Hu et al. [39], are used to compare the precision of the proposed WFTDGM model. Data from 2003 to 2013 was used to build the prediction model, and data from 2014 to 2017 was used to test its accuracy.

The proposed WFTDGM model's forecasting performance is compared to that of TDGM, FTDGM, and Hu et al. [39] GM(1,1) and FGM(1,1) models result. The population size of QPSO is set to 5 in the proposed WFTDGM model, and the maximum number of iterations is set to 500 times as the stop condition. All of the computations

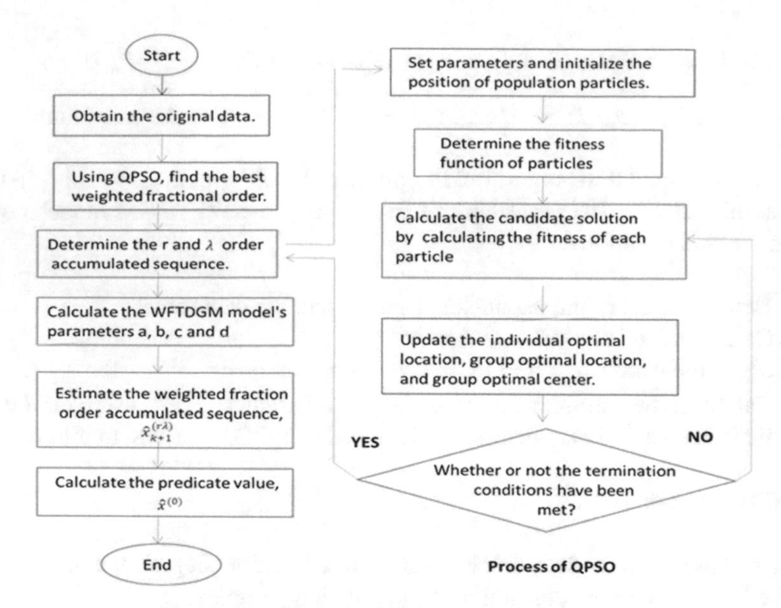

Fig. 1. The QPSO-WFTDGM model's flowchart

were done in Matlab. Table 1 summarizes the MAPE and rank of five different models for the testing data. For 8 of the 20 datasets, the proposed WFTDGM ranked the highest against other models. The average MAPE value of the proposed WFTDGM model is lower than the MAPE values of the other prediction models, as seen in Table 1.

To evaluate the performance of the considered prediction models, the average rank of prediction models denoted by $R_j (j = 1, 2, ..., 5)$ was used to the 20 datasets. When the average rank was lower, the prediction model performed better. As presented in Table 1, $R_1 = 2.95$, $R_2 = 2.55$, $R_3 = 3.0$, $R_4 = 3.1$ and $R_5 = 3.4$ were obtained for TDGM, WFTDGM, FTDGM, FGM(1,1) and GM(1,1), respectively. Table 1 also shows that the proposed WFTDGM model has a lower average rank than the others as the proposed WFTDGM model outperformed the TDGM, FTDGM, GM(1,1), and FGM(1,1) models in terms of efficiency.

Table 1. MAPE and the rank of different prediction models for testing data.

Country	MAPE					The rank of prediction model (R_j)				
	TDGM	WFTD GM	FTD GM	FGM	GM	TDGM	WFTD GM	FTD GM	FGM	GM
China	12.1	11.2	11.3	15.8	23.2	3	1	2	4	5
USA	4.6	6.1	4.6	0.9	2.7	3	5	4	1	2

(continued)

Table 1. *(continued)*

Country	MAPE					The rank of prediction model (R_j)				
	TDGM	WFTD GM	FTD GM	FGM	GM	TDGM	WFTD GM	FTD GM	FGM	GM
Russia	4.2	0.9	4.1	2.7	5.4	4	1	3	2	5
India	3.8	4.5	4.6	3.0	10.2	2	3	4	1	5
Japan	7.2	1.1	7.2	22.6	4.5	4	1	3	5	2
Germany	1.4	1.4	1.4	1.1	1.2	4	3	5	1	2
Canada	2.5	3.0	2.5	3.2	1.7	2	4	3	5	1
Korea	9.8	8.3	8.8	5.4	6.9	5	3	4	1	2
UK	6.3	2.0	6.2	10.6	9.2	3	1	2	5	4
Iran	1.3	2.2	1.4	4.5	4.1	1	3	2	5	4
Mexico	5.8	0.6	5.8	3.5	7.4	4	1	3	2	5
Italy	3.5	3.9	3.5	7.1	3.2	2	4	3	5	1
S. Africa	4.6	2.5	4.5	5.3	5.6	3	1	2	4	5
Saudi	3.5	4.6	5.0	2.9	6.9	2	3	4	1	5
Australia	3.3	3.9	3.4	3.1	3.6	2	5	3	1	4
Indonesia	3.2	3.6	3.6	3.1	3.8	2	3	4	1	5
Brazil	12.3	10.8	12	29.0	12.1	4	1	2	5	3
France	3.8	3.4	3.8	3.8	3.4	4	1	3	5	2
Poland	3.5	3.5	3.5	4.0	4.0	3	2	1	4	5
Spain	11.6	15.2	13.5	14.3	8.3	2	5	3	4	1
Average	5.41	4.63	5.53	7.29	6.4	2.95	2.55	3.00	3.10	3.40

4 Conclusions

The weighted fractional orders with a time-delayed fractional grey model (WFTDGM) were presented in this paper. The optimum values for two different fractional orders were then obtained using the QPSO method. The efficiency of QPSO and WFTDGM was demonstrated using the results of numerical testing with twenty real-world datasets when compared to the original GM(1,1), FGM(1,1), TDGM(1,1), and FTDGM(1,1) models.

According to the findings, the proposed WFTDGM model outperformed the other four conventional grey models. Furthermore, the findings of this paper demonstrated that the proposed WFTDGM model was capable of forecasting CO2 emissions and might be considered a new method to fractional grey modeling in the future, with the ability to build more fractional grey models with reliable results.

Acknowledgments. The authors are grateful to the Ministry of Higher Education Malaysia and Universiti Teknologi Malaysia for fully supporting and funding this research project through the Fundamental Research Grant Scheme under Grant Vot 5F271.

References

1. Tudor, C.: Predicting the evolution of CO2 emissions in bahrain with automated forecasting methods. Sustainability **6**(923), 1–10 (2016)
2. Liu, L., Zong, H., Zhao, E., Chen, C., Wang, J.: Can China realize its carbon emission reduction goal in 2020: from the perspective of thermal power development. Appl. Energy **124**, 199–212 (2014)
3. Pao, H.T., Tsai, C.M.: Modeling and forecasting the CO2 emissions, energy consumption, and economic growth in Brazil. Energy **36**, 2450–2458 (2011)
4. Piecyk, M., McKinnon, A.C.: Forecasting the carbon footprint of road freight transport in 2020. Int. J. Prod. Econ. **128**(1), 31–42 (2010)
5. Hosseini, S.M., Saifoddin, A., Shirmohammadi, R., Aslani, A.: Forecasting of CO2 emissions in Iran based on time series and regression analysis. Energy Rep. **5**, 619–631 (2019)
6. Lee, Y.S., Tong, L.I.: Forecasting energy consumption using a grey model improved by incorporating genetic programming. Energy Convers. Manag. **52**, 147–152 (2011)
7. Mason, K., Duggan, J., Howley, E.: Forecasting energy demand, wind generation and carbon dioxide emissions in Ireland using evolutionary neural networks. Energy **155**, 705–720 (2018)
8. Wen, L., Yuan, X.: Forecasting CO2 emissions in Chinas commercial department, through BP neural network based on random forest and PSO. Sci. Total. Environ. **718**, ID137194 (2020)
9. Pao H.T., Fu H.F., Tseng C.L.: Forecasting of CO2 emissions, energy consumption and economic growth in China using an improved grey model. Energy **40**(1), 400–409 (2012)
10. Sun, W., Wang, C., Zhang, C.: Factor analysis and forecasting of CO2 emissions in Hebei, using extreme learning machine based on particle swarm optimization. J. Clean. Prod. **162**, 1095–1101 (2017)
11. Pi, D., Liu, J., Qin, X.: A grey prediction approach to forecasting energy demand in China. Energy Sources Part A Recover. Util. Environ. Eff. **32**, 1517–1528 (2010)
12. Deng, J.L.: Control problems of grey systems. Syst. Control Lett. **1**, 288–294 (1982)
13. Liu, S., Lin, Y.: Grey Information: Theory and Practical Applications. Springer, London (2010)
14. Liu, S., Yang, Y., Forrest, J.: Grey Data Analysis: Methods, Models and Applications. Springer, Berlin (2017)
15. Pao, H.T., Fu, H.C., Tseng, C.L.: Forecasting of CO2 emissions, energy consumption and economic growth in China using an improved grey model. Energy **40**, 400–409 (2012)
16. Lin, C.S., Liou, F.M., Huang, C.: Grey forecasting model for CO2 emissions: a Taiwan study. Appl. Energy **88**, 3816–3820 (2011)
17. Xu, N., Ding, S., Gong, Y., Bai, J.: Forecasting Chinese greenhouse gas emissions from energy consumption using a novel grey rolling model. Energy **175**, 218–227 (2019)
18. Wang, Z.X., Li, Q.: Modelling the nonlinear relationship between CO2 emissions and economic growth using a PSO algorithm based grey Verhulst model. J. Clean. Prod. **207**, 214–224 (2019)
19. Zeng, B., Li, C.: Improved multi-variable grey forecasting model with a dynamic background-value coefficient and its application. Comput. Ind. Eng. **118**, 278–290 (2018)
20. Ye, J., Dang, Y., Li, N.: Grey-Markov prediction model based on background value optimization and central-point triangular whitenization weight function. Commun. Nonlinear Sci. Numer. Simul. **54**, 320–330 (2018)

21. Wang, Y., Dang, Y., Li, Y., Liu, S.: An approach to increase prediction precision of GM(1,1) model based on optimization of the initial condition. Expert Syst. Appl. **37**(8), 5640–5644 (2010)
22. Song, Z.M., Deng, J.L.: The accumulated generating operation in opposite direction and its use in grey model GOM(1,1). Syst. Eng. **19**(1), 66–69 (2001)
23. Yang, B.H., Zhang, Z.Q.: The grey model has been accumulated generating operation in reciprocal number and its application. Math. Practice Theory **33**(10), 21–25 (2003)
24. Qian, W.Y., Dang, Y.G., Wang, Y.M.: GM(1,1) model based on weighting accumulated generating operation and its application. Math. Practice Theory **39**(15), 48–51 (2009)
25. Li, D.C., Chang, C.J., Chen, C.C., Chen, W.C.: Forecasting short-term electricity consumption using the adaptive grey-based approach-an Asian case. Omega **40**(6), 767–773 (2012)
26. Xie, N.M., Liu, S.F.: Discrete grey forecasting model and its optimization. Appl. Math. Model **33**(2), 1173–1186 (2009)
27. Xie, N.M., Liu, S.F., Yang, Y.J.: On novel grey forecasting model based on nonhomogeneous index sequence. Appl. Math. Model **37**(7), 5059–5068 (2013)
28. Zhang, K., Liu, S.F.: Linear time-varying parameters discrete grey forecasting model. Syst. Eng. Theory Pract. **30**(9), 1650–1657 (2010)
29. Zeng, B., Meng, W.: Research on Fractional Accumulating Generation Operators and Grey Prediction Models. Scientific Press, Beijing (2015)
30. Wu, L.F., Liu, S.F., Yao, L.G.: Grey system model with the fractional accumulation. Commun. Nonlinear Sci. Numer. Simul. **18**(7), 1775–1785 (2013)
31. Wu, L.F., Liu, S.F., Chen, D.: Using gray model with fractional accumulation to predict gas emission. Nat. Hazards **71**(3), 2231–2236 (2014)
32. Mao, S., Gao, M., Xiao, X., Zhu, M.: A novel fractional grey system model and its application. Appl. Math. Model **40**, 5063–5076 (2016)
33. Wu, L., Liu, S., Yao, L., Yan, S.: The effect of sample size on the grey system model. Appl. Math. Model. **37**, 6577–6583 (2013)
34. Wu, W., Ma, X., Zhang, Y., Li, W., Wang, Y.: A novel conformable fractional nonhomogeneous grey model for forecasting carbon dioxide emissions of BRICS countries. Sci. Total. Environ. **707**, ID135447 (2020)
35. Gao, M., Mao, S., Yan, X., Wen, J.: Estimation of Chinese CO2 emission based on a discrete fractional accumulation grey model. J. Grey Syst. **27**, 114–130 (2015)
36. Singh, M.R., Mahapatra, S.S.: A quantum behaved particle swarm optimization for flexible job shop scheduling. Comput. Ind. Eng. **93**, 36–44 (2016)
37. Shen, Q.Q., Shi, Q., Tang, T.P., Yao L.Q.: A novel weighted fractional GM(1,1) model and its applications. 1–20, ID 6570683 (2020)
38. International Energy Agency. Key World Energy Statistics 2019; IEA/OECD: Paris, France (2019)
39. Hu, Y.C., Jiang, P., Tsai, J.F., Yu, C.Y.: An optimized fractional grey prediction model for carbon dioxide emissions forecasting. Int. J. Environ. Res. Public Health **18**(2), 587 (2021)

Text Detergent: The Systematic Combination of Text Pre-processing Techniques for Social Media Sentiment Analysis

Ummu Hani' Hair Zaki(✉), Roliana Ibrahim, Shahliza Abd Halim, and Izyan Izzati Kamsani

School of Computing, Faculty of Engineering, Universiti Teknologi Malaysia, 81300 Skudai, Malaysia
uhani8@graduate.utm.my, {roliana,shahliza,izyanizzati}@utm.my

Abstract. During catastrophes such as natural or man-made disasters, social media services have evolved into a crucial tool utilised by communities to disseminate information. Because a vast number of social media data is being used for many applications, including sentiment analysis, sentiment analysis has become a very useful and demanding problem. Social media data cannot be applied directly because it is raw and unstructured or semi-structured data. Consequently, text pre-processing becomes one of the most important tasks because the process is strongly constrained by its dependable workflow. This reason creates a complex pattern in pre-processing workflows. For this purpose, different text pre-processing techniques have been used on Twitter, Facebook, and YouTube datasets to study the impact of different pre-processing techniques on the accuracy of machine learning algorithms. This paper applied different text pre-processing techniques in a specific sequence based on significance testing. This study examines their influence on sentiment classification accuracy using a machine learning classifier, Support Vector Machines (SVM). Results proved that applying all 14 techniques systematically can achieve up to 82.57% of the accuracy of the SVM classifier with unigram representations. By using *Text Detergent,* the YouTube dataset achieve the highest accuracy compared to Facebook and Twitter datasets. This will potentially improve the quality of the text and leads to better feature extraction, which in turn helps the sentiment analyst produce a better classifier.

Keywords: Social media · Text pre-processing · Support vector machine · Classification · Accuracy

1 Introduction

The data received through social media is either incomplete or noisy, which can lead to serious problems and wastage of precious time in a critical scenario such as disaster events. The information available from social media users is more likely to have grammatical or spelling errors, punctuation signs to emphasize emotions like many exclamation marks, and slang, which makes it challenging for both humans and machines to

F. Saeed et al. (Eds.): IRICT 2021, LNDECT 127, pp. 50–61, 2022.
https://doi.org/10.1007/978-3-030-98741-1_5

decipher the accurate meaning of sentences [1]. In this paper, the term "*noise*" refers to data that provides no useful information for analysis, which in this case is sentiment analysis. Even though sometimes this kind of noise is easily comprehended by humans, a machine cannot detect it, especially in the case of social media data [2]. Some noises can be omitted, substituted, or mixed with others so that they do not have to be included in the machine learning stage. By using suitable text pre-processing techniques in such a way that pre-processing does not degrade classification performance, but rather improves it.

Through our observation and analysis, many pre-processing techniques have been implemented. However, most of them focused only on specific social media services, for example, Twitter. In addition, only a few focus on the sequence of pre-processing techniques. In conclusion, no work has been done on the comparison of different social media service data on the recommended pre-processing techniques. Nonetheless, the great news is, this paper explores exactly how to use "*text detergent*" to clean through the noise of social media data to find the information that matters by applying the most suitable pre-processing steps in a systematic order. The emergence of "*text detergent*" – as a cleansing solution for this noisy data is becoming a key factor through the pre-processing step of social media sentiment analysis.

The key contributions of this paper are (1) utilizing different pre-processing techniques on Facebook, Twitter, and YouTube data and performing analysis on their impact on sentiment classification using disaster based topics; (2) a systematic sequence of pre-processing techniques based on significance testing (*p-value* approach); and (3) comprehensive experiments on disaster based topic datasets are conducted which manifest that the accuracy of the machine learning algorithm is considerably enhanced when combined with a variety of pre-processing techniques in systematic order. The rest of this paper is organized as follows. Section 2 discusses related works; Sect. 3 outlines the research methodology; Sect. 4 presents the experimental results, and Sect. 5 concludes.

2 Related Work

A vast amount of social media data is being used for a variety of purposes, including sentiment analysis [3–7]. Social media data shares many characteristics of big data. The veracity of data causes problems in data pre-processing. Biases, noise, and abnormalities in data are all forms of veracity [8]. The issue of information overload has grown particularly severe, because of the fast development of digital content in the social media community, making it even more difficult to extract meaningful information from noisy data. Allowing those kinds of noises in the text increases the dimensionality, and hence the classification of text becomes more challenging because each word is treated as an individual dimension. To gain the opinion of users from lengthy comments, informal language such as emoticons or abbreviations will complicate the analysis [9]. It is necessary to consider eliminating noise from text to enhance text classification accuracy and speed up the classification process.

Many studies have been conducted on pre-processing techniques for social media data, as seen in Fig. 1 [1, 2, 4, 10–18]. In brief, [2] propose an improved framework for pre-processing of social media feeds for better performance. The framework had an accuracy of 94.07% on a standardized dataset, and 99.78% on a localised dataset when

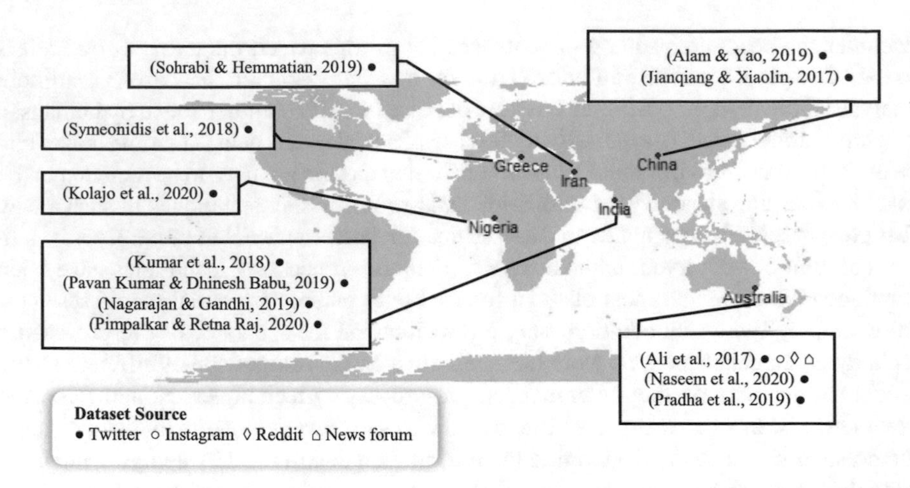

Fig. 1. Research demographic with social media data usage

used to extract sentiments from tweets. In addition, [15] applies the pre-processing techniques that include removal of stop words, expanding abbreviation, spelling correction, and stemming. They combine Particle swarm optimization (PSO), Genetic Algorithm (GA), and Decision Tree (DT) and it has proved to have better performance with an accuracy of over 90% when compared to other existing algorithms.

The result obtained from [16] confirms that Naïve Bayes and SVM were the most common classifiers used and with them performing better among all the classifiers. Even among those two, SVM performed better in most of the cases. According to work by [4], they indicate that after pre-processing of the dataset the F1-score of the classifier is substantially improved. For example, the accuracy and F1-measure of the Twitter sentiment classification classifier are enhanced by [11] when applying pre-processing techniques such as expanding acronyms and replacing negation. However, there were barely any differences when removing URLs, numbers or stop words.

Similarly, [18] presents a quality model to evaluate the quality of social information services. They have constructed three noise removal filters: *Data Overload* (which defines the degree of unwanted data), *Data Relevancy* (which defines the contextual relevancy of the retrieved data), and *Data Corruption* (which defines the level of errors present in the data). They also considered custom stop words to exclude the irrelevant data items for the *Data Relevancy* filter. They also employed a dictionary-based approach for the data correction in the *Data Corruption* filter. The performance of this filter is lower than expected. Only 21.3% of data items were fixed. This demonstrated that applying a *Data Corruption* filter is a time and resource-intensive process that is not always scalable to large datasets.

There are a couple of recommendations by [13] on which techniques are highly advised. If someone wants to pre-process text for a classic machine learning sentiment analysis, they can be considering replacing URLs and user mentions, replacing contractions, removing numbers, replacing repetitions of punctuation and lemmatization.

Meanwhile, [14] looked into how URLs, hashtags, negations, repeated characters, punctuations, stop words and stemming were affected. With the Stanford Twitter Sentiment dataset, the performance of sentiment classification increases when URL removal, username replacing with white space, hashtag removal, negation, character normalization, punctuation removal, stop word elimination and stemming are applied.

A work by [12] exploits several pre-processing techniques such as normalization, removing stop words, and tokenization. In normalization, they combine lowercase, removing accents, removing blank spaces, removing punctuation characters, removing hyphen symbols, and removing watermarks. They prove that the use of the Word2vec method increases the accuracy of the opinion classification in comparison with TF–IDF. Interestingly, [10] utilize pre-processing techniques such as removing emoticons, removing stopwords, stemming, and word vector. These studies show that the accuracy of the Naïve Bayes algorithm was substantially improved after applying the pre-processing steps.

Another proposed method by [1] is that they categorize the techniques into two, which are *category 1* (removing URL, hashtags symbols, punctuations, emoticons, and newlines) and *category 2* (tokenization, expanding slang and acronyms, spelling correction, normalization, removing stop words, stemming and lemmatization). Different from others, not only does [17] investigate the impact of different pre-processing techniques on Twitter, but they also make a recommendation of pre-processing techniques that increase the quality of the text and improve the performance of automated classification. By implementing 12 techniques in a systematic sequence order, the best classifier performance is recommended.

As described above, many studies are based on Twitter text only. There are more social media services with important information that must be analysed, but few pieces of work use multiple social media services [18]. As examined by [19], the most significant and related dataset is produced by Facebook. From an engagement aspect, social media users prefer the YouTube platform. In reading [19]'s article, one may well be convinced that using multiple sources of social media services is a good move in terms of content-wise. Furthermore, pre-processing techniques are interconnected to one another. For example, removing numbers cannot be done before expanding slang and acronyms, because the nature of slang sometimes is a combination of characters and numbers like *gr8* (*great*). Even though [17] applies pre-processing techniques in a systematic order, it only utilizes Twitter, where the applicability is not represented across multiple social media services. Therefore, it is important to have a systematic sequence to implement pre-processing techniques. Given these points, this study does comprehensive experimentation to demonstrate the influence of pre-processing techniques from Twitter, Facebook, and YouTube datasets.

3 Methodology

This section presents the analysis of different pre-processing techniques. The effect of pre-processing is next investigated, followed by a recommended systematic combination of several pre-processing techniques. The algorithms are executed using R language on RStudio utilizing ASUS Nitro 5 notebook (Windows 10 64-bit OS and RAM 16BG)

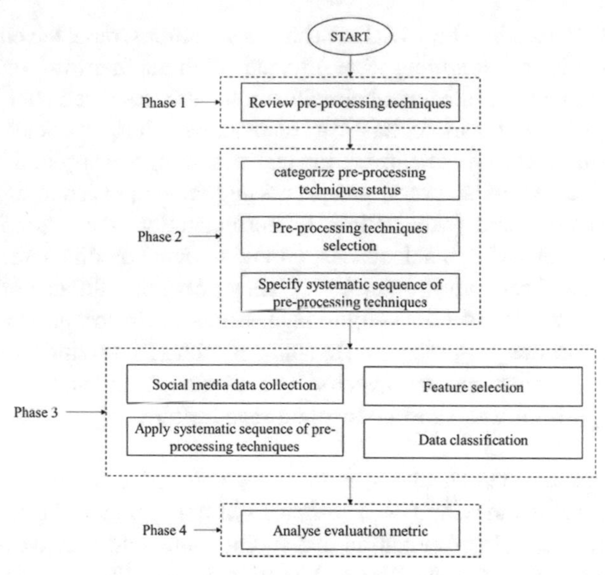

Fig. 2. Methodology flowchart

with R version 4.0.5 and RStudio version 1.4.1717. Figure 2 shows the methodology flowchart.

3.1 Phase 1

In reviewing the pre-processing techniques, we found that there are 21 techniques that researchers usually applied in denoising social media data. The pre-processing techniques are remove stop words [1, 4, 10–18], remove punctuation characters [1, 2, 4, 12–14], [16–18], remove URLs [1, 2, 11, 13, 14, 16–18], remove hashtag [1, 2, 4, 14, 16–18], remove user mention [2, 4, 13, 14, 16–18], stemming [1, 2, 4, 10, 13–16], expand slang and acronyms [1, 2, 11–13, 15, 17], lemmatization [2, 4, 13, 16, 17], spelling correction [1, 2, 13, 15–17], data elongation [2, 11, 13, 14, 17, 18], remove numbers [4, 11, 13, 17], replace contraction [11, 13, 14, 17], lowercase [4, 12, 13, 16, 17], replace emoticon [1, 2, 10, 17], language filter [1, 10, 18], remove encoded text [2, 13, 16, 17], replacing repetitions of punctuation [2, 13], search term inclusion (dictionary based approach) [18], word segmentation [17], remove watermark [12], word negation [13], part-of-speech [2, 13].

3.2 Phase 2

In phase 2, three tasks will be done to develop a systematic step of employing pre-processing techniques for social media data.

Categorize Pre-processing Status. In this task, we are categorizing the pre-processing techniques into three categories such as (1) *Prime* indicates the technique is selected in the study and has high accuracy, (2) *Measured* indicates the technique is selected in the study but does not have distinct accuracy, and (3) *Not Measured* indicates the technique is not selected in that study at all.

Pre-processing Techniques Selection. The systematic sequence will utilize the techniques with *Prime* status. To pick which *Prime* techniques will be included in the systematic sequence, hypothesis testing is conducted. Based on frequency distribution in Fig. 3, the mean usage of *Prime* techniques is 4 times.

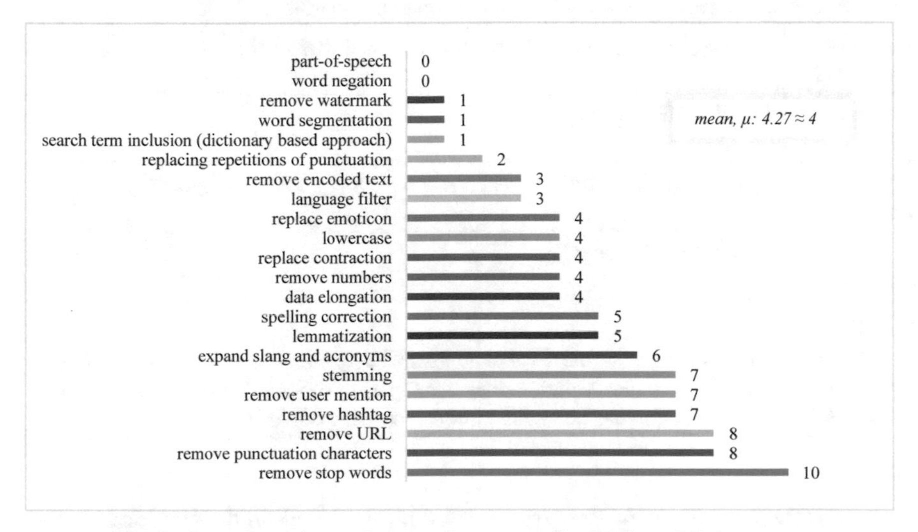

Fig. 3. Pre-processing techniques frequency distribution of *Prime* status

At the 0.05 level of significance, we want to test if the *Prime* technique is used less than 4 times, on average is significant. We are executing null hypothesis significance testing (*p-value* approach) [20] in Microsoft Excel as calculated in Table 1.

Table 1. Hypothesis test (significance test)

Sample statistic and test statistic calculation			
Formulate hypothesis	H_0:$\mu \geq 4$ times	H_a:$\mu < 4$ times	
Sample standard deviation, s	2.797648982	Sigma, σ	NA
Test Statistic To Use:	*t*	Sample size, n	22
The sample mean, $\bar{x}$	4.272727273	Degree of freedom	21

(*continued*)

Table 1. (*continued*)

Sample statistic and test statistic calculation			
Type of test	1 tail left	Significance level, α	0.05
Test Statistic, *t*	0.457242601	Standard error, SE	0.596460767

Probability value (*p-value*) and critical value (*c-value*) calculation	
Rejection Rule p-value	*p-value* $\leq \alpha$, *Reject* H_0 *& accept* H_a | *Fail to Reject* H_0
p-value 1 tail left	0.673904139 *(accept* H_0*)*
Rejection Rule c-value	*Test Statistic* $\geq$ *c-value, Reject* H_0 *& accept* $H_{a,}$ | *Fail to Reject* H_0
c-value 1 tail left	-1.720742903 *(accept* H_0*)*
Conclusion	
There is sufficient evidence from the *c-value* approach and *p-value* approach test to support H_0 (reject H_a). therefore, to pick which *Prime* techniques to be included in the systematic sequence, the selected techniques must have frequency usage of 4 or more	

Specify Systematic Steps of Pre-processing Phase. Based on the significance test in Table 1, there are 14 techniques to be included in the systematic sequence. After identifying how the pre-processing techniques are working, we are sorting the sequence of the techniques. The sequence of techniques is specified based on the degree of noise. The degree of noise is categorized into four such as (1) *Punctuation*, (2) *Spelling*, (3) *Number*, and (4) *Context* as illustrated in Fig. 4. The lesser the degree number, the urgent for it to be denoise. Corpus that contains *Punctuation* must first be removed. And then followed by the enhancement of the *Spelling* component into a standard term. After that, remove the number because it does not give a significant impact on sentiment analysis. Finally, to provide basic dataset comprehension to the analyst, the *Context* component shall be executed.

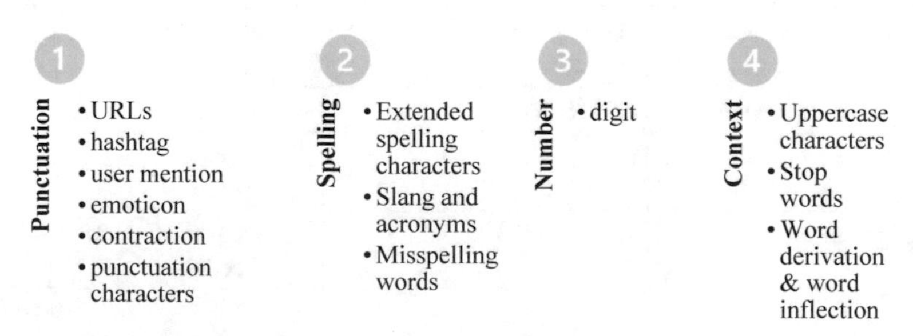

Fig. 4. The degree of noise in social media data text

3.3 Phase 3

The experiment was conducted using the dataset from Facebook, Twitter, and YouTube social media services.

Social Media Data Collection. Three social media datasets are employed for experimentation. The dataset is downloaded from Kaggle[1]. All datasets are consisted of Twitter[2] (331,091 rows), Facebook[3] (89,866 rows), and YouTube[4] (718,458). For Twitter dataset, it is collected using the *#CovidVaccine* hashtag. While the Facebook dataset is Facebook posts made by *Anti-Vaccine and Chilf Care* groups. As for the YouTube dataset, the data has been collected from the comments of listed trending YouTube videos in the UK. However, for this experimental work, we only used 1,500 rows of data for each dataset were 500 rows for each sentiment score (positive, negative, and neutral).

Apply Systematic Sequence of Pre-processing Techniques. Table 2 shows the example of the working mechanism for each technique. Not all techniques perform well when combined with others; even where they perform well when used standalone, some combinations of pre-processing techniques do not interact well. It is not only about the selection of pre-processing techniques that are important, but also their sequence must be logical too as referred to in Fig. 4.

Table 2. The noise mapped with respective pre-processing techniques

Noise	Pre-processing technique
URLs	Remove URLs
Hashtag symbol	Remove hashtag
User mention	Remove user mention
Emoticon	Replace emoticon
Word contraction	Replace contraction
Punctuation characters	Remove punctuation characters
Extended spelling character	Data elongation
Slang and acronyms	Expand slang and acronyms
Misspelling word	Spelling correction
Number	Remove number
Uppercase text	Lowercase

(continued)

[1] https://www.kaggle.com.
[2] https://www.kaggle.com/kaushiksuresh147/covidvaccine-tweets.
[3] https://www.kaggle.com/alechelyar/facebook-antivaccination-dataset.
[4] https://www.kaggle.com/datasnaek/youtube?select=GBcomments.csv.

Table 2. (*continued*)

Noise	Pre-processing technique
Stop words	Remove stop words
Word derivation & word inflection	Lemmatization
Word derivation & word inflection	Stemming

Feature Selection. The pre-processed dataset represents using the n-gram representation model. In this paper, the n-gram that is applied is unigram. Feature selection is carried out using TF-IDF (Term Frequency weighting with Inverse Document frequency) to find the number of terms that appeared in each dataset [21].

Data Classification. In identifying which machine learning algorithm is suitable for this experiment, this paper is using *algorithm explorer*[5]. To classify sentiment polarity, this paper is applying a classification technique to perform supervised learning tasks by using the Support Vector Machine (SVM). Experimentation was carried out utilising a combination of training and testing ratios such as 50:50, 60:40, and 70:30. The AFINN lexicon is used in this work [22]. In this experiment, we are converting all positive integers to 1, all negative integers to –1 and all zeros remain 0.

4 Results

In this section, we discover the outcomes achieved when a variety of types of pre-processing techniques are applied on Twitter, Facebook, and YouTube datasets.

4.1 Phase 4

We are applying a systematic sequence of pre-processing techniques based on Table 2 list order. The feature representation includes a unigram for each process.

Analyze Evaluation Metrics. To discover and investigate the relationship between techniques, a systematic combination study was carried out to investigate the effect between the Prime techniques by combining each of them based on the sequence. The influence of pre-processing techniques on classification accuracy is seen in Fig. 5. Accuracy refers to the correctness of classification obtained overall. The ratio is measured between the correctly classified instances with a total number of instances [15]. The SVM classifier gives better accuracy in unigram when the training and testing ratio is increased. Figure 5 indicates that when utilising a 70:30 split ratio, the SVM classifier on unigram gives higher accuracy. In addition, It plotted that the Twitter dataset is having lower accuracy compared to the Facebook dataset while the YouTube dataset gave the highest accuracy across three split ratios.

[5] https://samrose3.github.io/algorithm-explorer/.

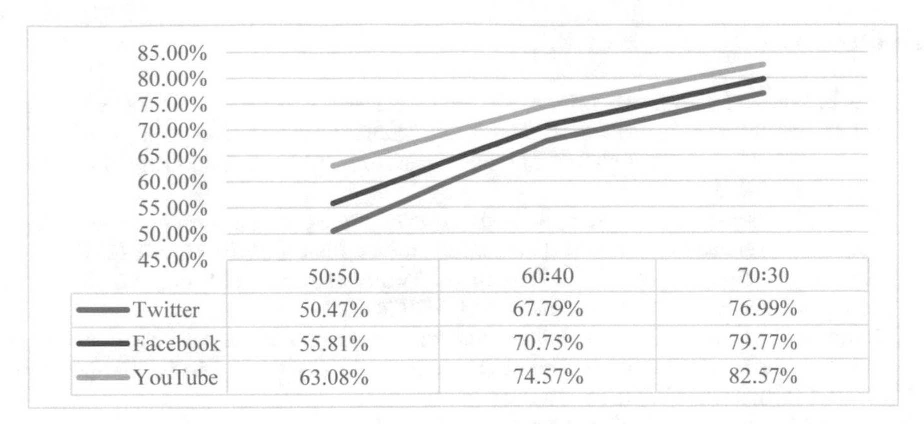

	50:50	60:40	70:30
Twitter	50.47%	67.79%	76.99%
Facebook	55.81%	70.75%	79.77%
YouTube	63.08%	74.57%	82.57%

Fig. 5. Classification accuracy by training and testing ratio

5 Discussion

Figure 5 shows the reported percentage of accuracy of the SVM classifier in the Twitter, Facebook, and YouTube datasets across 50:50, 60:40, and 70:30 proportions of training and testing data. Overall, the accuracy of the thrice dataset has considerably grown. The reported accuracy of Twitter begins at 50.47% with a 50:50 ratio. It rose steadily to reach about 67.79% with a 60:40 ratio. In the 70:30 ratio, it continues to increase to 76.99%. Figure 5 also shows that there is a correlation between training and testing data proportion. Figure 5 demonstrates that YouTube is by far has the highest accuracy when applying the systematic sequence of pre-processing techniques throughout the proportion of training and testing data. This show that the systematic sequence is most suitable when using the YouTube dataset. YouTube achieves 82.57% of accuracy with a 70:30 proportion of training and testing data. The lowest accuracy is from the Twitter dataset, 50.47% with 50:50 with 70:30 proportion of training and testing data. Facebook datasets stay in the middle in terms of accuracy. By implementing the systematic sequence of pre-processing techniques, on average, Twitter is having 65.08% accuracy while Facebook has 68.77% and YouTube 73.41%. Above all, using multiple sources of social media services provide immense perspective for sentiment analysis particularly in denoising the high dimensional data text.

6 Conclusion

Multiple sources of social media services in sentiment analysis suggests a good move in terms of significance, relatedness, and engagement content-wise. Sentiment classification can be improved by applying systematic and suitable text pre-processing techniques in such a manner that pre-processing does not degrade classification performance, but rather improves it. After a thorough experiment and observation of the interactions of various pre-processing techniques, a sequence of optimum pre-processing techniques is proposed that results in the best classifier performance.

References

1. Pavan Kumar, C.S., Dhinesh, L.D.: Novel text preprocessing framework for sentiment analysis. In: Satapathy, S.C., Bhateja, V., Das, S. (eds.) Smart Intelligent Computing and Applications. SIST, vol. 105, pp. 309–317. Springer, Singapore (2019). https://doi.org/10.1007/978-981-13-1927-3_33
2. Kolajo, T., Daramola, A.A., Seth, A.: A framework for pre-processing of social media feeds based on integrated local knowledge base. Inf. Process. Manag. **57**(6), 102348 (2020)
3. Karami, A., Shah, V., Vaezi, R., Bansal, A.: Twitter speaks: a case of national disaster situational awareness. J. Inf. Sci. **46**(3), 313–324 (2020)
4. Pimpalkar, A.P., Retna Raj, R.J.: Influence of pre-processing strategies on the performance of ML classifiers exploiting TF-IDF and BOW features. ADCAIJ Adv. Distrib. Comput. Artif. Intell. J. **9**(2), 49–68 (2020)
5. Sharma, S., Jain, A.: Role of sentiment analysis in social media security and analytics. Wiley Interdiscip. Rev. Data Min. Knowl. Discov. **10**(5) (2020)
6. Ali, K.: Sentiment Analysis as a Service. RMIT University (2019)
7. Khader, M., Awajan, A., Al-Naymat, G.: The impact of natural language preprocessing on big data sentiment analysis. Int. Arab J. Inf. Technol. **16**(3), 506–513 (2019). ASpecial Issue
8. Sivarajah, U., Kamal, M.M., Irani, Z., Weerakkody, V.: Critical analysis of Big Data challenges and analytical methods. J. Bus. Res. **70**, 263–286 (2017)
9. Naresh, A., Venkata Krishna, P.: An efficient approach for sentiment analysis using machine learning algorithm. Evol. Intel. **14**(2), 725–731 (2020). https://doi.org/10.1007/s12065-020-00429-1
10. Alam, S., Yao, N.: The impact of preprocessing steps on the accuracy of machine learning algorithms in sentiment analysis. Comput. Math. Organ. Theory **25**(3), 319–335 (2018). https://doi.org/10.1007/s10588-018-9266-8
11. Jianqiang, Z., Xiaolin, G.: Comparison research on text pre-processing methods on Twitter sentiment analysis. IEEE Access **5**, 2870–2879 (2017)
12. Sohrabi, M.K., Hemmatian, F.: An efficient preprocessing method for supervised sentiment analysis by converting sentences to numerical vectors: a twitter case study. Multimed. Tools Appl. **78**(17), 24863–24882 (2019). https://doi.org/10.1007/s11042-019-7586-4
13. Symeonidis, S., Effrosynidis, D., Arampatzis, A.: A comparative evaluation of pre-processing techniques and their interactions for Twitter sentiment analysis. Expert Syst. Appl. **110**, 298–310 (2018)
14. K. Kumar, H.M., Harish, B.S.: Classification of short text using various preprocessing techniques: an empirical evaluation. In: Kumar Sa, P., Bakshi, S., Hatzilygeroudis, I.K., Sahoo, M.N. (eds.) Recent Findings in Intelligent Computing Techniques, vol. 3, pp. 19–30. Springer, Singapore (2018). Doi: https://doi.org/10.1007/978-981-10-8633-5_3
15. Nagarajan, S.M., Gandhi, U.D.: Classifying streaming of Twitter data based on sentiment analysis using hybridization. Neural Comput. Appl. **31**(5), 1425–1433 (2018). https://doi.org/10.1007/s00521-018-3476-3
16. Pradha, S., Halgamuge, M.N., Tran Quoc Vinh, N.: Effective text data preprocessing technique for sentiment analysis in social media data. In: Proceedings of the 2019 11th International Conference Knowledge System Engineering, KSE 2019 (2019)
17. Naseem, U., Razzak, I., Eklund, P.W.: A survey of pre-processing techniques to improve short-text quality: a case study on hate speech detection on twitter. Multimed. Tools Appl. **80**, 35239–35266 (2020)
18. Ali, K., Dong, H., Bouguettaya, A., Erradi, A., Hadjidj, R.: Sentiment analysis as a service: a social media based sentiment analysis framework. In: 2017 IEEE International Conference on Web Services (ICWS), pp. 660–667 (2017)

19. Hair Zaki, U.H., Ibrahim, R., Abd Halim, S.: A social media services analysis. Int. J. Adv. Trends Comput. Sci. Eng. **8**(1.6), 69–75 (2019)
20. Infanger, D., Schmidt-Trucksäss, A.: P value functions: an underused method to present research results and to promote quantitative reasoning. Stat. Med. **38**(21), 4189–4197 (2019)
21. Na, J., Sui, H., Khoo, C., Chan, S., Zhou, Y.: Effectiveness of simple linguistic processing in automatic. In: Knowledge Organization and the Global Information Society: Proceedings of the Eighth International ISKO Conference, pp. 49–54 (2004)
22. Nielsen, F.Å.: A new ANEW: evaluation of a word list for sentiment analysis in microblogs. CEUR Workshop Proc. **718**, 93–98 (2011)

Improve Short-term Electricity Consumption Forecasting Using a GA-Based Weighted Fractional Grey Model

Ani Shabri[1](✉), Ruhaidah Samsudin[2], and Waseem Alromema[3]

[1] Faculty of Science, Universiti Teknologi Malaysia, 81300 Johor Bahru, Johor, Malaysia
ani@utm.my

[2] Faculty of Engineering, Universiti Teknologi Malaysia, 81300 Johor Bahru, Johor, Malaysia
ruhaidah@utm.my

[3] Computer Science and Information Systems, Applied College, Taibah University, Medina, Saudi Arabia
wromema@taibahu.edu.sa

Abstract. This study proposed a weighted fractional grey model (WFGM) based on a genetic algorithm for forecasting annual electricity consumption. WFGM has two parameters that can be used to adjust the order of the summation based on different data sequences and reflect the new information priority. The key issue with the WFGM model is determining two optimum fractional-order values to improve the accuracy of electricity consumption forecasts. The Genetic Algorithm (GA) is used to select the best values for the weighted fractional-order accumulation, which is one of the most important aspects determining the grey model's prediction accuracy. The additional linear parameters of grey models are estimated using the least squares estimation method. Finally, two real data sets of electricity consumption from Malaysia and Thailand are presented to validate the proposed model. Numerical results show that the new proposed prediction model is very efficient and has the best prediction accuracy compared to the models of GM(1,1) and FGM(1,1).

Keywords: First grey model · Weighted fractional · Genetic algorithm · Forecasting

1 Introduction

As the goal to enhance the energy system's reliability and efficiency of operation become more important, research focus on the area of forecasting electricity consumption has been deemed to be vital to avoid costly errors which might have a critical impact on the environment.

In the last several decades, numerous methods including the least squares support vector machines (LS-SVMs) [1, 2, 3], linear regression models [1, 4], ARIMA models [5], neural networks [1, 6, 7], genetic algorithms [8] and support vector machines (SVMs) [9] have been applied in the study of electricity consumption forecast. However,

F. Saeed et al. (Eds.): IRICT 2021, LNDECT 127, pp. 62–72, 2022.
https://doi.org/10.1007/978-3-030-98741-1_6

these methods mentioned above required a large chunk of data sets with complicated calculations to conducting an adequate prediction experiment.

The grey system theory has been publicized to be an effective strategy in handling the uncertainty problems with limited and incomplete data in recent years. The grey system theory has been widely applied in diverse fields, which includes the study of agricultural output, electricity production, and consumption, transportation, industrialisation, military, as well as medicine [10–13]. Though the accuracy of the GM(1,1) model prediction accuracy is often inconsistent and unsatisfied.

Researchers have found ways to improve the GM(1,1) model's performance, with a majority of work focusing on modifying residual model errors, optimizing the starting values, improving the model background value conformation, as well as merging several prediction models [14–18]. The factional order accumulation-based grey model or FGM has had a wide-ranging impact on the overall grey model efficiency [19–22]. As the FGM offers a better forecasting performance than the GM(1,1) model, they have been applied as a predictive tool extensively by researchers from multiple disciplines [23–25]. As most of the current FGM models only employ a single fractional order, numerous academicians have noted that it reduces the impacts of fractional order accumulation, making FGM less versatile if multivariable data is to be used [26].

A study conducted by Shen et al. [26] introduced the WFGM, which is to construct on the quantum particle swarm optimization technique, by utilizing four numerical examples from various practical applications to obtain the best fitting accuracy. By comparing the GM(1,1) and FGM(1,1) models, the result from the WFGM possessed a better result due to the efficiency of the model. As the WFGM has been proven to be a clear choice, this paper will incorporate the Genetic Algorithm, GA into the WFGM to form a novel GA-WFGM forecasting model to approach the electricity consumption data. To solve the nonlinear optimization problem, we will use the GA natural algorithm intelligent method in determining the ideal parameters for WFGM.

This paper shall be constructed as follows: the weighted fractional accumulated generating matrices and the inverse matrices are to be introduced in Sect. 2. Followed by the weighted fractional grey model in Sect. 3. Section 4 will further explain the application of GA to determine the best fractional order value for the WFGM model. The findings for both Malaysia and Thailand case studies are presented in Sect. 5. Lastly, Sect. 6 will conclude the overall the finding for GA-WFGM model.

2 The Weighted Fractional Accumulated Generating Matrices and Their Inverse Matrices

The original sample size is denoted as $x^{(0)} = \left\{x_1^{(0)}, x_2^{(0)}, \ldots, x_k^{(0)}, \ldots, x_n^{(0)}\right\}$ of size n, and the weighted fractional accumulation generating operator (WF-AGO) of $x^{(0)}$ is defined as

$$x^{(r\lambda)} = \left\{x_1^{(r\lambda)}, x_2^{(r\lambda)}, \ldots, x_k^{(r\lambda)}, \ldots, x_n^{(r\lambda)}\right\}$$

where

$$x_k^{(r\lambda)} = \sum_{i=1}^{k} \begin{bmatrix} r \\ k-i \end{bmatrix} \lambda^{k-i} x_i^{(0)}, \ k = 1, 2, \ldots, n. \tag{1}$$

$x^{(r\lambda)} = A^{r\lambda} x^{(0)}$ is a simple equation to express the WF-AGO, where

$$A^{r\lambda} = \begin{pmatrix} \begin{bmatrix} r \\ 0 \end{bmatrix} & 0 & 0 & \cdots & 0 \\ \begin{bmatrix} r \\ 1 \end{bmatrix}\lambda & \begin{bmatrix} r \\ 0 \end{bmatrix} & 0 & \cdots & 0 \\ \begin{bmatrix} r \\ 2 \end{bmatrix}\lambda^2 & \begin{bmatrix} r \\ 1 \end{bmatrix}\lambda & \begin{bmatrix} r \\ 0 \end{bmatrix} & \cdots & 0 \\ \vdots & \vdots & \vdots & \ddots & \vdots \\ \begin{bmatrix} r \\ n-1 \end{bmatrix}\lambda^{n-1} & \begin{bmatrix} r \\ n-2 \end{bmatrix}\lambda^{n-2} & \begin{bmatrix} r \\ n-3 \end{bmatrix}\lambda^{n-3} & \cdots & \begin{bmatrix} r \\ 0 \end{bmatrix} \end{pmatrix} \tag{2}$$

When $r = \lambda = 1$,then $x_k^{(1)} = \sum_{i=1}^{k} x_i^{(0)}$ can also be written as $x^{(1)} = Ax^{(0)}$. $x^{(1)}$ is the first order-accumulation generating operator (1-AGO), where A is defined as

$$A = \begin{pmatrix} 1 & 0 & \cdots & 0 \\ 1 & 1 & \cdots & 0 \\ \vdots & \vdots & \ddots & \vdots \\ 1 & 1 & \cdots & 1 \end{pmatrix} \tag{3}$$

When $\lambda = 1$ then $x_k^{(r)} = \sum_{i=1}^{k} \begin{bmatrix} r \\ k-i \end{bmatrix} x_i^{(0)}$ can also be written as $x^{(r)} = A^r x^{(0)}$. $x^{(r)}$ is the fractional order-accumulation generating operator (F-AGO), where A^r is defined as

$$A^r = \begin{pmatrix} \begin{bmatrix} r \\ 0 \end{bmatrix} & 0 & 0 & \cdots & 0 \\ \begin{bmatrix} r \\ 1 \end{bmatrix} & \begin{bmatrix} r \\ 0 \end{bmatrix} & 0 & \cdots & 0 \\ \begin{bmatrix} r \\ 2 \end{bmatrix} & \begin{bmatrix} r \\ 1 \end{bmatrix} & \begin{bmatrix} r \\ 0 \end{bmatrix} & \cdots & 0 \\ \vdots & \vdots & \vdots & \ddots & \vdots \\ \begin{bmatrix} r \\ n-1 \end{bmatrix} & \begin{bmatrix} r \\ n-2 \end{bmatrix} & \begin{bmatrix} r \\ n-3 \end{bmatrix} & \cdots & \begin{bmatrix} r \\ 0 \end{bmatrix} \end{pmatrix} \tag{4}$$

where $\begin{bmatrix} r \\ n \end{bmatrix} = \begin{cases} 1 \ n = 0 \\ \frac{r(r+1)\ldots(r+n+1)}{n!} \ n \in N^+ \end{cases}$

The inverse WF-AGO is denoted as

$$A^{-r\lambda} = \begin{pmatrix} \begin{bmatrix} -r \\ 0 \end{bmatrix} & 0 & 0 & \cdots & 0 \\ \begin{bmatrix} -r \\ 1 \end{bmatrix}\lambda & \begin{bmatrix} -r \\ 0 \end{bmatrix} & 0 & \cdots & 0 \\ \begin{bmatrix} -r \\ 2 \end{bmatrix}\lambda^2 & \begin{bmatrix} -r \\ 1 \end{bmatrix}\lambda & \begin{bmatrix} -r \\ 0 \end{bmatrix} & \cdots & 0 \\ \vdots & \vdots & \vdots & \ddots & \vdots \\ \begin{bmatrix} -r \\ n-1 \end{bmatrix}\lambda^{n-1} & \begin{bmatrix} -r \\ n-2 \end{bmatrix}\lambda^{n-2} & \begin{bmatrix} -r \\ n-3 \end{bmatrix}\lambda^{n-3} & \cdots & \begin{bmatrix} -r \\ 0 \end{bmatrix} \end{pmatrix} \tag{5}$$

The relationship between $x^{(0)}$ and $x^{(r\lambda)}$ can be deduced as follows,

$$x^{(0)} = A^{-r\lambda}x^{(r\lambda)}$$

When $r = \lambda = 1$, $x^{(0)} = A^{-1}x^{(1)}$ where A^{-1} is the inverse form of 1-AGO, defined as

$$A^{-1} = \begin{pmatrix} 1 & 0 & 0 & \cdots & 0 \\ -1 & 1 & 0 & \cdots & 0 \\ 0 & -1 & 1 & \cdots & 0 \\ \vdots & \vdots & \vdots & \ddots & \vdots \\ 0 & 0 & 0 & \cdots & 1 \end{pmatrix} \tag{6}$$

Likewise, when $\lambda = 1$, $x^{(0)} = A^{-r}x^{(r)}$. We refer to A^{-r} as the inverse form of F-AGO, defined as

$$A^{-r\lambda} = \begin{pmatrix} \begin{bmatrix} -r \\ 0 \end{bmatrix} & 0 & 0 & \cdots & 0 \\ \begin{bmatrix} -r \\ 1 \end{bmatrix}\lambda & \begin{bmatrix} -r \\ 0 \end{bmatrix} & 0 & \cdots & 0 \\ \begin{bmatrix} -r \\ 2 \end{bmatrix}\lambda^2 & \begin{bmatrix} -r \\ 1 \end{bmatrix}\lambda & \begin{bmatrix} -r \\ 0 \end{bmatrix} & \cdots & 0 \\ \vdots & \vdots & \vdots & \ddots & \vdots \\ \begin{bmatrix} -r \\ n-1 \end{bmatrix}\lambda^{n-1} & \begin{bmatrix} -r \\ n-2 \end{bmatrix}\lambda^{n-2} & \begin{bmatrix} -r \\ n-3 \end{bmatrix}\lambda^{n-3} & \cdots & \begin{bmatrix} -r \\ 0 \end{bmatrix} \end{pmatrix} \tag{7}$$

3 The Weighted of Fractional-Order Grey Model

The $r\lambda$ -order differential equation of grey model is defined as [25]

$$\frac{dx^{(r\lambda)}}{dt} + ax^{(r\lambda)} = b \tag{8}$$

When both sides of Eq. (8) are integrated inside the interval $[k - 1, k]$, the result will be prompted as

$$\int_{k-1}^{k} \frac{dx^{(r\lambda)}}{dt} dt + a \int_{k-1}^{k} x^{(r\lambda)} dt = \int_{k-1}^{k} b dt \tag{9}$$

Hence, the Eq. (9) become

$$x_k^{(r\lambda)} - x_{k-1}^{(r\lambda)} + a z_k^{(r\lambda)} = b \tag{10}$$

where the background value $z_k^{(r\lambda)} = \int_{k-1}^{k} x^{(r\lambda)} dt$ is defined by

$$z_k^{(r\lambda)} = 0.5 x_k^{(r)} + 0.5 x_{k-1}^{(r)}, \quad \forall k = 2, 3, \ldots, n \tag{11}$$

The Eq. (11) can be expressed as

$$x_k^{(r\lambda)} - x_{k-1}^{(r\lambda)} = b - a z_k^{(r\lambda)} \tag{12}$$

To estimate the parameters of the model in Eq. (12), the least-square method shall be applied. The model's parameters are calculated using the equation and follows

$$\begin{bmatrix} a \\ b \end{bmatrix} = \left(X^T X\right)^{-1} X^T Y$$

where

$$Y = \begin{pmatrix} x_2^{r\lambda} - x_1^{r\lambda} \\ x_3^{r\lambda} - x_2^{r\lambda} \\ \vdots \\ x_n^{r\lambda} - x_{n-1}^{r\lambda} \end{pmatrix} \text{ and } X = \begin{pmatrix} -z_2^{(1)} & 1 \\ -z_3^{(1)} & 1 \\ \vdots & \vdots \\ -z_n^{(1)} & 1 \end{pmatrix} \tag{13}$$

The solution for Eq. (8) is defined by

$$\hat{x}_{k+1}^{(r\lambda)} = \left(x_1^{(0)} - \frac{b}{a}\right) e^{-ak} + \frac{b}{a} \tag{14}$$

Lastly, the predicted values of WFGM can be calculated using the inverse r-order fractional accumulated operation as follows:

$$\hat{x}^{(0)} = A^{-r\lambda} \hat{x}^{(r\lambda)}, \text{ k } = 1, 2, \ldots, \text{ n} \tag{15}$$

When $r = \lambda = 1$, the WFGM model will be reduced to GM(1,1) model, whereas when $\lambda = 1$ it shall be reduced to the FGM model. As such, the WFGM model is a generalization form for both the GM(1,1) and FGM models.

4 Genetic Algorithm for Determining the Optimal Value of Fractional Order of WFGM Model

The value for the fractional order, λ of the WFGM model, has been predetermined as 1 for most research. Though in most cases, the value of $\lambda = 1$ might not be suitable for all data sets. Furthermore, the fractional order r has a direct impact on the outcome of WFGM. Therefore, we shall implement the GA to search for the best values for λ and r to solve the issue of nonlinear optimization. The mean absolute percentage error (MAPE) will be used as the GA's fitness function. Figure 1 below depicts the GA-WFGM model, where the optimization procedure for WFGM utilizing GA is presented (for more details, please refer [27]). In summary, the constrained optimization algorithm to obtain the optimal parameters r and λ can be described as follows:

$$\min MAPE = \frac{1}{n}\sum_{k=1}^{n} \frac{\left|\hat{x}_k^{(0)} - x_k^{(0)}\right|}{x_k^{(0)}} \times 100\%$$

$$s.t.\begin{cases} 0 < r \le 1 \\ 0 < \lambda \le 1 \\ \begin{bmatrix} a \\ b \end{bmatrix} = \left(X^T X\right)^{-1} X^T Y \\ \hat{x}_k^{(r)} = \left(x_1^{(0)} - \frac{b}{a}\right) e^{-a(k-1)} + \frac{b}{a} \\ \hat{x}^{(0)} = A^{-r\lambda} \hat{x}^{(r\lambda)},\ k = 1, 2, \ldots, n \end{cases}$$

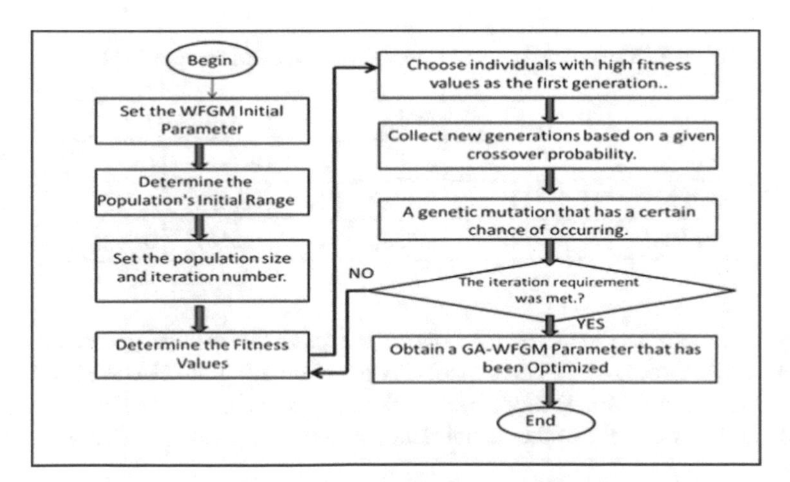

Fig. 1. The flow chart of the GA-WFGM model optimized using a genetic algorithm.

5 Experiment Results

The effectiveness of the proposed GA-WFGM model is evaluated using the electricity consumption data (per capita electricity (kWh)) for Malaysia and Thailand. The data was extracted from the World Bank Data portal, presented in Table 1. The electricity consumption data for the range between 2000 to 2014 (referred to as the in-sample data) is utilized for modeling, while the data from 2015 to 2019 (referred to as the out-of-sample data) is utilized to test the models' forecast performance.

5.1 Performance Measures

To quantify the accuracy of prediction models, various performance measures have been proposed in the literature. The accuracy of GA-WFGM was evaluated using the MAPE. The MAPE can be defined as follows:

$$\text{MAPE} = \frac{1}{n}\sum\nolimits_{k=1}^{n} \frac{\left|\hat{x}_k^{(0)} - x_k^{(0)}\right|}{x_k^{(0)}} \times 100\%$$

where $\hat{x}_k^{(0)}$ is predicted value and $x_k^{(0)}$ actual value. The lower the MAPE value, the better the prediction.

5.2 Obtained Results and Comparison

The purpose of implementing the GA algorithm in this study is to find the best parameters for FGM and WFGM models. The linear parameters for all grey models are estimated using the least-square technique. Table 1 below shows the optimal parameter values for all GM(1,1), FGM and, GA-WFGM models.

Table 1. The optimal parameters of GM(1,1), FGM and GA-WFGM.

	GM(1,1)		FGM		GA-WFGM	
Data	r	λ	r	λ	r	λ
Malaysia	1	1	0.6980	1	0.9878	0.9228
Thailand	1	1	0.7386	1	0.2445	0.8606

Figures 2 compare the actual values to the predicted values generated from all GM(1,1), FGM and, GA-WFGM models. When comparing the GA-WFGM model to both the FGM and GM(1,1) models, it is clear that the simulated values for the GA-WFGM model fit closely to the actual data for both Malaysia and Thailand real-case studies.

Tables 2 and 3 summarize the MAPE results for all GM(1,1), FGM, and GA-WFGM models for Malaysia and Thailand respectively. Tables 2 and 3 are also seen to present the smallest MAPE value for the GA-WFGM model, both in-sample and out-of-sample data, suggesting that the proposed model can accomplish its goal to minimize the forecast error. In the sense of predictive performance, the results indicate that GA-WFGM with optimally weighted fractional order is able to perform better than the GM(1,1) and FGM models.

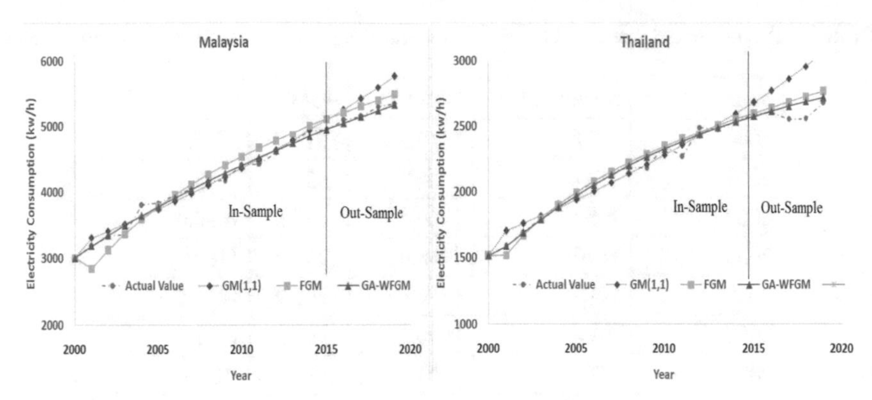

Fig. 2. Comparison of the real values to the predicted values generated by the three grey models.

Table 2. The predicted value and MAPE results for the grey models from Malaysia country

Year	Actual Value	GM(1,1)	FGM	GA-WFGM
2000	3014	3013.9	3013.9	3013.9
2001	3196	3316.3	2855.6	3195.8
2002	3341	3420.2	3128.7	3355.8
2003	3373	3527.3	3377.7	3506.5
2004	3813	3637.7	3596.8	3650.7
2005	3844	3751.7	3792.1	3789.5
2006	3969	3869.1	3968.9	3923.6
2007	4062	3990.3	4131.0	4053.4
2008	4179	4115.3	4281.0	4179.1
2009	4187	4244.2	4421.0	4301.0
2010	4433	4377.1	4552.7	4419.3
2011	4435	4514.2	4677.3	4534.0
2012	4613	4655.5	4795.6	4645.4
2013	4784	4801.3	4908.5	4753.5
2014	4937	4951.7	5016.6	4858.4
In-Sample	MAPE	1.969	3.350	1.312
2015	4959	2683.7	2600.8	4960.3
2016	5106	2772.2	2644.7	5059.3
2017	5164	2863.6	2687.0	5155.4
2018	5307	2958.0	2727.7	5248.7
2019	5353	3055.5	2767.1	5339.4
Out-Sample	MAPE	4.958	2.636	0.490

Table 3. The predicted value and MAPE results for the grey models from Thailand country

Year	Actual Value	GM(1,1)	FGM	GA-WFGM
2000	1517	1517.3	1517.3	1517.3
2001	1589	1704.2	1521.6	1589.4
2002	1693	1760.4	1670.5	1690.0
2003	1796	1818.4	1796.0	1789.4
2004	1910	1878.4	1902.9	1883.5
2005	1994	1940.3	1996.2	1971.4
2006	2078	2004.3	2079.4	2053.4
2007	2154	2070.3	2154.8	2129.7
2008	2186	2138.6	2223.9	2200.7
2009	2182	2209.1	2287.9	2266.8
2010	2345	2281.9	2347.6	2328.3
2011	2271	2357.2	2403.7	2385.5
2012	2491	2434.9	2456.7	2438.8
2013	2475	2515.1	2507.0	2488.3
2014	2539	2598.1	2554.9	2534.4
In-Sample	MAPE	2.690	1.468	1.232
2015	2588	2683.7	2600.8	2577.2
2016	2607	2772.2	2644.7	2617.1
2017	2554	2863.6	2687.0	2654.2
2018	2559	2958.0	2727.7	2688.8
2019	2679	3055.5	2767.1	2720.9
Out-Sample	MAPE	10.368	3.414	2.280

6 Conclusion

To overcome the issue in forecasting the electricity consumption data, an improved weighted fractional-gray model is proposed. The optimal value of the weighted fractional-order values was considered to improve the WFGM modeling and forecasting performance. The GA approach is selected to determine the optimal values of the WFGM model's weighted fractional order accumulation. To demonstrate the effectiveness of the proposed GA-WFGM model, two real-world data sets comprised of Malaysia and Thailand were compared against the traditional GM(1,1) and, FGM models. Hence according to the findings, the proposed GA-WFGM model has greatly increased the forecast accuracy when compared to the other two models in electricity consumption data, therefore, confirming the superiority of the proposed model.

Acknowledgments. The authors are grateful to the Ministry of Higher Education Malaysia and Universiti Teknologi Malaysia for fully supporting and funding this research project through the Fundamental Research Grant Scheme under Grant Vot 5F271.

References

1. Fazil, K., Taplamacioglu, M.C., Cam, E., Hardalac, F.: Forecasting electricity consumption: a comparison of regression analysis, neural networks and least squares support vector machines. Int. J. Electr. Power Energy Syst. **67**, 431–438 (2015). https://doi.org/10.1016/j.ijepes.2014.12.036
2. Sulaiman, M.H., Mustafa, M.W., Shareef, H., Khalid, S.N.A.: An application of artificial bee colony algorithm with least squares support vector machine for real and reactive power tracing in deregulated power system. Int. J. Electr. Power Energy Syst. **37**(1), 67–77 (2012). https://doi.org/10.1016/j.ijepes.2011.12.007
3. Wang, S., Yu, L., Tang, L., Wang, S.: A novel seasonal decomposition based least squares support vector regression ensemble learning approach for hydropower consumption forecasting in China. Energy **36**(11), 6542–6554 (2011). https://doi.org/10.1016/j.energy.2011.09.010
4. Abdel-Aal, R.E., Garni, A.Z.: Forecasting monthly electric electricity consumption in Eastern Saudi Arabia using univariate time series analysis. Energy **22**, 1059–1069 (1997). https://doi.org/10.1016/S0360-5442(97)00032-7
5. Bianco, V., Manca, O., Nardini, S.: Electricity consumption forecasting in Italy using linear regression models. Energy **34**, 1413–1421 (2009). https://doi.org/10.1016/j.energy.2009.06.034
6. Ekonomou, I.: Greek long-term electricity consumption prediction using artificial neural network. Energy **35**, 512–517 (2010). https://doi.org/10.1016/j.energy.2009.10.018
7. Geem, Z.W., Roper, W.E.: Energy demand estimation of South Korea using artificial neural network. Energy Policy **37**, 4049–4054 (2009)
8. Ceylan, H., Ozturk, H.K.: Estimating energy demand of Turkey based on economic indicators using genetic algorithm approach. Energy Convers Manage. **45**, 2525–2537 (2004). https://doi.org/10.1016/j.enconman.2003.11.010
9. Kavaklioglu, L.: Modeling and prediction of Turkey's electricity consumption using support vector regression. Appl. Energy, **88**, 368–375 (2011). https://doi.org/10.1016/j.enconman.2009.06.016
10. Zeng, B., Li, C.: Forecasting the natural gas demand in China using a self-adapting intelligent greymodel. Energy **112**, 810–825 (2016). https://doi.org/10.1016/j.energy.2016.06.090
11. Lihua, Z., Suliang, D., Butterworth, J., Ma, X., Dong, B., Liu, A.: Grey forecasting model for active vibration control systems. J. Sound Vib. **322**(4–5), 690–706 (2009). https://doi.org/10.1016/j.jsv.2008.11.036
12. Xiao, X.P., Mao, S.H.: Grey fForecasting and Decision Methods. Science Press, Beijing, China (2013)
13. Wang, Z.X.: An optimized Nash nonlinear grey Bernoulli model for forecasting the main economic indices of high technology enterprises in China. Comput. Ind. Eng. **64**(3), 780–787 (2013). https://doi.org/10.1016/j.cie.2012.12.010
14. Wu, L., Liu, S., Yang, Y.: A gray model with a time varying weighted generating operator. IEEE Trans. Syst. Man Cybern. Syst. **46**(3), 427–433 (2016). https://doi.org/10.1109/TSMC.2015.2426133
15. Wei, Y., Zhang, Y.: An essential characteristic of the discrete function transformation to increase the smooth degree of data. J. Grey Syst. **19**(3), 293–300 (2007)

16. Zeng, B., Duan, H., Bai, Y., Meng, W.: Forecasting the output of shale gas in China using an unbiased grey model and weakening buffer operator. Energy **151**, 238–249 (2018). https://doi.org/10.1016/j.energy.2018.03.045
17. Xie, N., Liu, S.: Interval grey number sequence prediction by using non-homogenous exponential discrete grey forecasting model. J. Syst. Eng. Electron. **26**(1), 96–102 (2015). https://doi.org/10.1109/JSEE.2015.00013
18. Ma, X., Liu, Z.: The kernel-based nonlinear multivariate grey model. Appl. Math. Model. **56**, 217–238 (2018). https://doi.org/10.1016/j.apm.2017.12.010
19. Mao, S., Gao, G., Xiao, X., Zhu, M.: A novel fractional grey system model and its application. Appl. Math. Model. **40**(7–8), 5063–5076 (2016). https://doi.org/10.1016/j.apm.2015.12.014
20. Wu, L., Liu, S., Yao, L., Yan, S., Liu, D.: Grey system model with the fractional order accumulation. Commun. Nonlinear Sci. Numer. Simul. **18**(7), 1775–1785 (2013). https://doi.org/10.1016/j.cnsns.2012.11.017
21. Wu, L.F., Liu, S.F., Yang, Y.J.: Grey double exponential smoothing model and its application on pig price forecasting in China. Appl. Soft Comput. J. **39**, 117–123 (2016). https://doi.org/10.1016/j.asoc.2015.09.054
22. Wu, L.F., Liu, S.F., Yang, Y.J., Ma, L., Liu, H.: Multi-variable weakening buffer operator and its application. Inf. Sci. **339**, 98–107 (2016). https://doi.org/10.1016/j.ins.2016.01.002
23. Gao, M., Mao, S., Yan, X., Wen, J.: Estimation of Chinese CO2 emission based on a discrete fractional accumulation grey model. J. Grey Syst. **27**(4), 114–130 (2015). https://doi.org/10.3724/SP.J.1248.2014.017
24. Mao, S., Gao, M., Xiao, X., Zhu, M.: A novel fractional grey system model and its application. Appl Math Modell. **40**, 5063–3076 (2016). https://doi.org/10.1016/j.apm.2015.12.014
25. Wu, L., Liu, S., Yao, L., Yan, S., Liu, D.: Grey system model with the fractional order accumulation. Commun. Nonlinear Sci. Numerical Simul. **18**, 1775–1785 (2013). https://doi.org/10.1016/j.cnsns.2012.11.017
26. Shen, Q.Q., Shi, Q., Tang, T.P., Yao, L.Q.: A novel weighted fractional GM(1,1) model and its applications mathematics. Math. Comput. Sci. **6570683**, 1–20 (2020). https://doi.org/10.1155/2020/6570683
27. Wang, C.H., Hsu, L.C.: Using genetic algorithms grey theory to forecast high technology industrial output. Appl. Math. Comput. **195**(1), 256–263 (2008). https://doi.org/10.1016/j.amc.2007.04.080

Efficient Human Activity Recognition System Using Long Short-Term Memory

Athraa Almusawi(✉) and Ali H. Ali

Department of Electronic and Communications Engineering, University of Kufa, Najaf, Iraq
{athraat.almusawi,alih.alathari}@uokufa.edu.iq

Abstract. Human activity recognition (HAR) is a popular and challenging area of research, driven by a diverse set of applications. This paper aims to build a system with the fewest sensors in locations thoughtful enough to distinguish six activities using a Long Short-Term Memory (LSTM) approach to give high performance. We used two wearable Inertial Measurement Units (IMU) sensors with a gyroscope, accelerometer, and magnetometer fixed in the waist and the right ankle of the subject body. For this purpose, ten random subjects were asked to do six activities (walking, sitting, walking upstairs, standing, walking downstairs, and laying) indoors for data acquisition. Then we analyzed these data and used LSTM to classify the labelled dataset with a different number of hidden units, and the best result was with the number of 150 hidden units. After that, we trained the dataset and registered the test accuracy of 98.44%. Thus, the performance of the proposed method achieved the highest accuracy with low computing costs.

Keywords: Wearable sensors · Human activity recognition · Long short-term memory network · Data acquisition · Deep learning

1 Introduction

Human activity recognition (HAR) is a significant area of research worldwide, driven by various applications in a wide variety of contexts, including industrial automation, sports, medical, security…, etc. [1]. HAR methods are categories based on the data type generated: sensor-based HAR and vision-based HAR [2]. Vision-based HAR analyses videos or images captured by the camera that contain human motions [3]. Sensor-based HAR utilizes wearable or ambient sensors [4]. In addition, there is also a hybrid type of HAR that combines the vision-based GRB camera and sensor-based sensors from wearable devices in the smart home with ambient sensors and gives an accuracy of 92.33% [5].

Wearable sensors are one of the most commonly used HAR modalities [3]. Sensors are typically integrated onto a single platform carried by individuals; sensor devices are frequently configured at Smartphones, smartwatches, inertial units, bright clothes, and purpose-built platforms [6]. The position of sensors on the body is essential for HAR [7]. HAR classification could be done offline or online [8]. When the user does not require

F. Saeed et al. (Eds.): IRICT 2021, LNDECT 127, pp. 73–83, 2022.
https://doi.org/10.1007/978-3-030-98741-1_7

immediate feedback, offline classification (non-real-time) is sufficient [9]. However, the deep learning algorithm is supported in the majority of the proposed studies [10].

Deep learning is a machine learning branch that automatically extracts features from raw sensor data, unlike traditional classical learning requiring a human-engineered feature to perform optimally [11]. While CNN is the most widely used method for HAR [12], long short-term memory LSTM is more suitable for complex sequences of sensor inputs [13]. Some researchers believed that combining CNN and recurrent neural networks RNN(LSTM) would produce better results, based on the recent success of RNN in time series domains [29]. A neural network learning capabilities can become more sophisticated as the number of nodes and layers increases [9]. As well, Espinilla et al. confirm that redundant features do exist, and they generally introduce noise into the classification process, resulting in reduced performance efficiency [14]. To solve this problem, some researchers add steps to dimensionality reduction before applying a learning algorithm such as Linear Discriminant Analysis (LDA) or Principal Component Analysis (PCA),.. etc. [10]. The challenge in HAR is to achieve high recognition accuracy at a low computational cost [12].

This paper develops an automated system that can efficiently classify human activities by reducing computations and the number of sensors. We designed a cost-effective device consisting of two IMU sensors. Furthermore, we proposed to use only the two-layer LSTM algorithm in the dataset we collected from the IMU sensors. The same hardware obtained in all the results includes a 2.6GHz Intel Core i7 CPU and 16GB RAM.

The paper is organized as follows. Explanation of HAR dataset acquisition is in Sect. 3. Section 4 contains the description of the raw data pre-processing. Section 5 introduces LSTM Architecture. Section 6 describes and explains the results of the datasets that were used in LSTM algorithms. Finally, Sect. 7 concludes the outcomes of the experiments and future work.

2 Related Work

Human activity recognition is becoming an increasingly appealing study subject in recent years, owing to the rapid development of wearable or body sensor technologies [15]. In one of the earliest HAR studies, Albaba et al. proposed convolutional neural networks (CNN) deep learning algorithm on the WISDM dataset [16] was reached an accuracy of 81% [17].

Lawal and Bano experimented with datasets acquisition from various locations on the body to determine the optimal position, concluding that the shin and waist were the optimal locations for the sensors [7].

San Buenaventura et al. performed seven ambulatory activities for 3–4 min (sitting, walking, jogging, standing, biking, walking downstairs, and walking upstairs). The smartphones are located on-body of ten subjects: the left pants pocket, the belt, the right pants pocket, wrist, and the upper arm [18].

Oluwalade et al. used the popular WISDM dataset for activity recognition. The dataset fed into the LSTM model with 128 LSTM units, followed by a dropout layer (0.3 units), dense layer (64 units), dense layer (32 units), and finally a dense layer with

15 units (for the number of classes). They employed Softmax as the activation function, ReLU in the preceding levels, and the Adam optimizer in the final layer. Categorical cross-entropy to determine the loss. With a batch size of 32, the model trained for 226 epochs achieved 74.3% [19].

Fu et al. proposed the IPL-JPDA method to classify seven activity acquisitions by 1-axis air pressure sensors, 3-axis acceleration, 3-axis gyroscope, and 3-axis Euler angle sensors fixed in the Left thigh of seven subjects. In pre-processed data used Sliding window technology, PCA, Pseudo-Labels, and Joint Probability Domain Adaptation. In result registered an accuracy of 93.2% [1].

Leonardis et al. proposed traditional learning techniques Naïve Bayes (NB), K-Nearest Neighbor (KNN), Decision Tree (DT), Feedforward Neural Network (FNN), and Support Vector Machines (SVM) to classify data acquired from magnetic and inertial measurement units (MIMU) sensors attached to the right thigh of 15 subjects. They extracted manual 342 features and two-step feature selection (genetic algorithm and correlation-based), reduced them to 69 features and achieved more than 90% accuracy. However, the deep learning algorithm is supported in the majority of the proposed studies [10].

In this work, we introduce an automated system capable of efficiently classifying human activities through fewer computations and sensors. We developed a low-cost device using two IMU sensors. Additionally, we proposed to employ only the two-layer LSTM algorithm in the IMU sensor dataset.

3 Data Acquisition

We designed a wearable device content two IMU sensors to dataset acquisition. The first sensor was 3-axis Accelerometer/Compass LSM303, and the other sensor was 9 Degrees of Freedom LSM9DSO, which has all three types of IMU sensors: a gyroscope, accelerometer, and magnetometer. These sensors were based on a flora chip manufactured by Adafruit.

A wearable sensor on-body placement is critical for recognition accuracy [7]. Therefore, these two body-worn sensors are placed on the subject body in two ways. The first experiment fixed LSM9DSO at the right wrist and LSM303 at the waist, as shown in Fig. 1(a). we refer to data collected from this experiment as "Dataset1". In the second experiment, the LSM303 sensor was placed at the waist, and the LSM9DSO sensor at the right ankle, as Fig. 1(b) and Fig. 1(c); in this experiment, we refer to data collected as "Dataset2". These two sensors used protocol 12C to collect data on the flora chip, then we sent Dataset via Bluetooth to the computer. Finally, the information is recorded on the computer by an internal program.

Ten subjects (aged 10 to 58, five males and five females) were asked to do six activities (walking, sitting, walking upstairs, standing, walking downstairs, and laying)) indoors with a fixed order, each activity lasting 11 s. Finally, the entire wireless communication system can acquire datasets of the subject activity using the sensors and the personal computer. Due to the three-axis data provided by each sensor, the raw signals had a total of 12 dimensions (i.e., x, y, and z). Therefore, we gathered 3000 samples at a sampling rate of 10 Hz (10 samples per second), together with the timestamp-associated activity labels (hand-labelled by the observer).

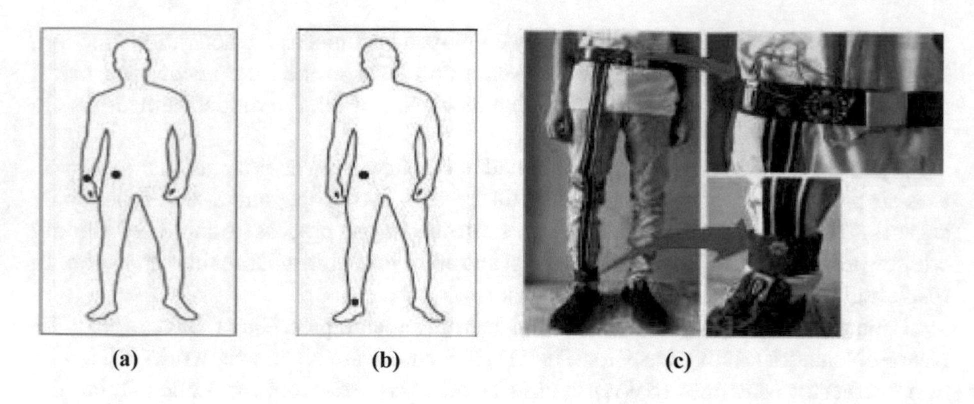

Fig. 1. Sensor position on the subject: **(a)** Initial placement of sensors in the first experiment. **(b)** Initial placement of sensors in the second experiment. **(c)** Actual image of initial placement of sensors in the second experiment.

4 Pre-processing

After data collection, the second step is pre-processing. Noise in the data can be caused by humans or a network system error that fails to provide reliable sensor readings [20], so the first step is to delete the missing or noise data. Then we adjust the standardization to standardized the data and remove the randomized data from input x using Standard Score (z-score) as equation below

$$Z=(x-m)/\delta \tag{1}$$

where δ and m denote the standard deviation and mean of the dataset, respectively [21]. Finally, we divided the HAR dataset into three random sections: training 70%, testing 15%, and Validation 15%; For testing purposes, the epoch with the best validation-set performance is used [22].

5 Architecture

The LSTM architecture is an RNN developed for modelling temporal sequences and solving long-term dependency problems [23]. The LSTM solves the long-term memory problem by utilizing two hidden states denoted by 'h' and 'c'. Internally, the LSTM controls information via four gates: the forget gate f, the input gate i, the cell gate C, and output gate O, as shown in the equations below [24]

$$f_t = \sigma(W_f.[h_{t-1}, x_t] + b_f) \tag{2}$$

$$i_t = \sigma(W_i.[h_{t-1}, x_t] + b_i) \tag{3}$$

$$\tilde{C}_t = tanh(W_C.[h_{t-1}, x_t] + b_C) \tag{4}$$

$$C_t = f_t * C_{t-1} + i_t * \tilde{C}_t \quad (5)$$

$$O_t = \sigma(W_O.[h_{t-1}, x_t] + b_O) \quad (6)$$

$$h_t = O_t * tanh(\tilde{C}_t) \quad (7)$$

In the last step, product the output with tanh to normalized data. After that, the Fully Connection layer integrates all the features from the LSTM layer with each activation unit of the next layer as follows [21]

$$Fc_{\mathcal{K}}^{(\ell+1)} = \sum_j c_j^{\ell} W_{j\mathcal{K}}^{\ell} + \alpha_{\mathcal{K}}^{\ell} \quad (8)$$

where $W_{j\mathcal{K}}^{l}$ is a matrix containing the weight values between the $j^{th}$and $\mathcal{K}^{th}$ nodes of the ℓth and $(\ell+1)^{th}$ layers. c_j^l is the j^{th}node data in the ℓth layer. Some of the output values may be greater than one or negative. Their sum may not reach one, but after applying the Softmax layer, all components will be between [0,1], and their sum is one as equation follows [25]

$$softMax(\vec{z})_i = \frac{e^{zi}}{\sum_{j=1}^{N} e^{zj}} \quad (9)$$

The Classification layer must come after the Softmax layer, take the values from the SoftMax, and mutually assign each input to one of the N classes using the following entropy formula [26]

$$L(n, y) = -\sum_{i=1}^{N} n_i \, log(p_i) \quad (10)$$

where n_i equal one of the target class and p_i the predicted output value from the last layer. We have used MATLAB R2020b for train data, Table 1 display some important LSTM parameters.

Table 1. Parameter range for LSTM implementation.

LSTM parameter	Value
Number of layers	2
Number of features	12
Number of class	6
Execution Environment	GPU
Mini Batch Size	20
Max Epochs	20
Estimation	Adaptive Moment (adam)

The Confusion Matrix (CM) is a matrix N × N, the columns displayed for model prediction, and the rows represent the actual classification. CM Consists of True Positive (TP), False Negative (FN), False Positive (FP), and True Negative (TN). CM gives us a comprehensive view of the types of errors our system makes and the quality of its performance. Measurement performance of all activities are computed for multiclass data by average Recall, Precision, and average Accuracy, as equations below [11]

$$Recall = {}^{1}/_{N} \times \sum_{j=1}^{N} \frac{TP_j}{TP_j + FN_j} \times 100\% \quad (11)$$

$$precision = {}^{1}/_{N} \times \sum_{j=1}^{N} \frac{TP_j}{TP_j + FP_j} \times 100\% \quad (12)$$

$$Accurcy = \frac{\sum_{j=1}^{n} TP_j + TN_j}{Total} \times 100\% \quad (13)$$

$$F_1 - score = 2 \times \frac{Recall \times Precision}{Recall + Precision} \times 100\% \quad (14)$$

However, accuracy is an important performance metric that indicates how well a model performs across all classes.

6 Results

In this section, we present and discuss the result of the LSTM model for classifying our HAR dataset. Both datasets were included in five layers with 150 hidden units for training, classification, and finding accuracy. Table 2 shows the summary of the chosen number of hidden units on "Dataset2".

Table 2. Validation and Testing Accuracy in frass number of hidden units and Precision, Recall, and F1-score for "Dataset2". The bold numbers in the raw represent the best accuracy.

Number of hidden units	Validation accuracy	Testing accuracy	Precision	Recall	F1-score
50	97.11%	96.22%	96.32%	96.40%	96.36%
80	97.11%	97.33%	97.36%	97.58%	97.47%
100	96.67%	97.56%	97.71%	97.61%	97.66%
120	96.67%	96.00%	96.24%	96.17%	96.21%
150	**97.11%**	**98.44%**	**98.41%**	**98.63%**	**98.52%**
180	96.00%	96.67%	96.85%	96.84%	96.85%
200	98.00%	97.78%	97.83%	97.97%	97.90%
220	97.11%	96.89%	96.93%	97.09%	96.36%

Table 3 shows the confusion matrix of the LSTM model for our HAR "Dataset1". Previous works indicated that the most critical activities to be analyzed are the "downstairs" and "upstairs" activities; Due to the similarity of these two activities, all algorithms have difficulty distinguishing them [13]. According to our dataset confusion matrix, these two activities are slightly confused with one another, while the "Downstairs" activity is confused with "walking."

Table 4 show the confusion matrix of the LSTM model for our HAR "Dataset2". From the confusion matrix, we can see that the two "downstairs" and "upstairs" activities are not confused and that the "downstairs" activity is slightly confused with the "walking" activity.

Table 3. Confusion matrix of LSTM model on our HAR "Dataset1". The bold numbers in the diagonal represent correctly classified occurrences; the bold number in the bottom right represents total accuracy. Note that: DownStairs = 1, Laying = 2, Sitting = 3, Standing = 4, UpStairs = 5, and Walking = 6.

		Predicted class						
		1	2	3	4	5	6	Recall (%)
True Class	1	**55**	0	0	0	1	10	83.3%
	2	0	**62**	0	0	0	0	100%
	3	0	0	**78**	0	0	0	100%
	4	0	0	0	**75**	0	0	100%
	5	0	0	0	0	**77**	2	97.5%
	6	8	0	0	2	1	**79**	87%
	Precision (%)	87.3%	100%	98.7%	97.4%	97.5%	86.8%	**94.67%**

Table 4. Confusion matrix of LSTM model on our HAR "Dataset2". The bold numbers in the diagonal represent correctly classified occurrences; the bold number in the bottom right represents total accuracy. Note that: DownStairs = 1, Laying = 2, Sitting = 3, Standing = 4, UpStairs = 5, and Walking = 6.

		Predicted class						
		1	2	3	4	5	6	Recall (%)
True Class	1	**62**	0	0	0	0	4	93.9%
	2	0	**62**	0	0	0	0	100%
	3	0	0	**78**	0	0	0	100%
	4	0	0	0	**75**	0	0	100%
	5	0	0	0	0	**78**	1	98.7%
	6	1	0	0	0	1	**88**	97.8%
	Precision (%)	98.4%	100%	100%	100%	98.7%	94.6%	**98.44%**

As can be seen from the results, the LSTM algorithm performs slightly worse on "Dataset1" than on "Dataset2" for the classes "Sitting" and "Standing" and slightly worse for the activities "Upstairs" and "downstairs." On the other hand, the "Walking" activity has significantly inferior performance. As a result, we may conclude that forecasting the "Walking" activity is considerably more complex than predicting other activities.

For "Dataset1", the test accuracy was 94.67%, training accuracy was 100%, Precision was 94.76%, Recall was 94.83%, validation accuracy was 93.11%, and F1-score was 94.8% when hidden unit 50, max epochs 120, and mini-batch size 10. Figure 2 and Fig. 3 show the accuracy and loss of LSTM on Dataset1 during iteration in the R2020b MATLAB window.

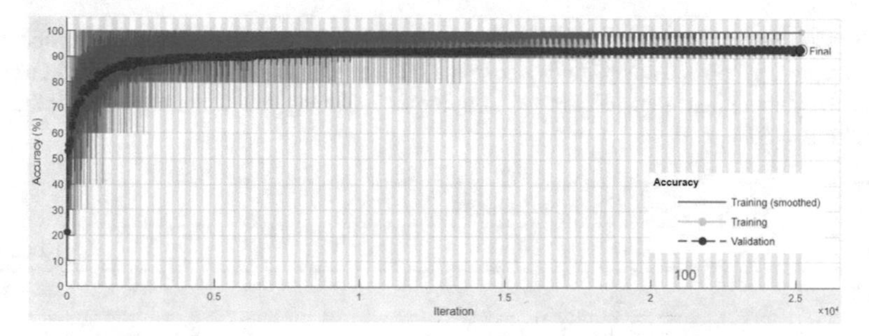

Fig. 2. Validation and Training vs. iteration of Dataset1 using the LSTM model.

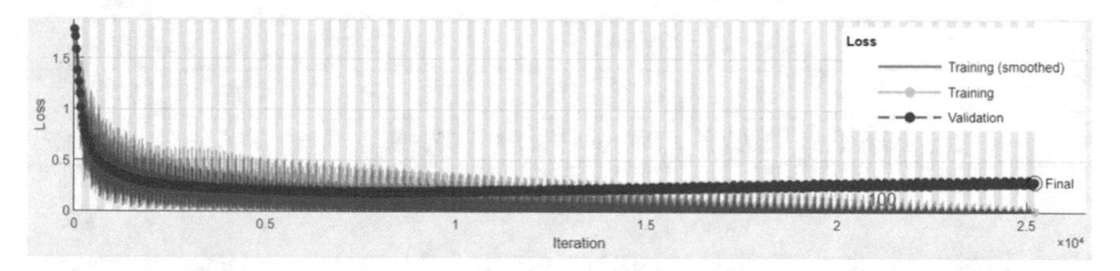

Fig. 3. Validation and training Lost vs. iteration of "Dataset1" using the LSTM model.

For "Dataset2", the testing accuracy of 98.44%, training accuracy 100%, validation accuracy 97.11%, Precision 98.48%, Recall 98.63%, and F1-score 98.52% when hidden unit 150, max epochs 20, and mini-batch size 20. Figure 4 and Fig. 5 show the accuracy and loss of LSTM on Dataset2 during iteration in the R2020b MATLAB window.

However, adopting two IMU sensors placed at the waist and the right ankle improves performance for identifying the six activities when using the LSTM model. As shown in Table 4, the total classification accuracy was 98.48%; and the recognition performance of walking and walking Downstart is better than using two IMU sensors placed at the waist and the right wrist in Table 3.

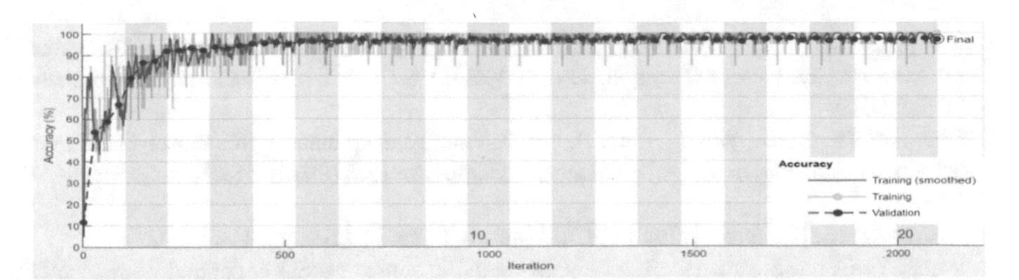

Fig. 4. Validation and Training vs. iteration of "Dataset2" using the LSTM model.

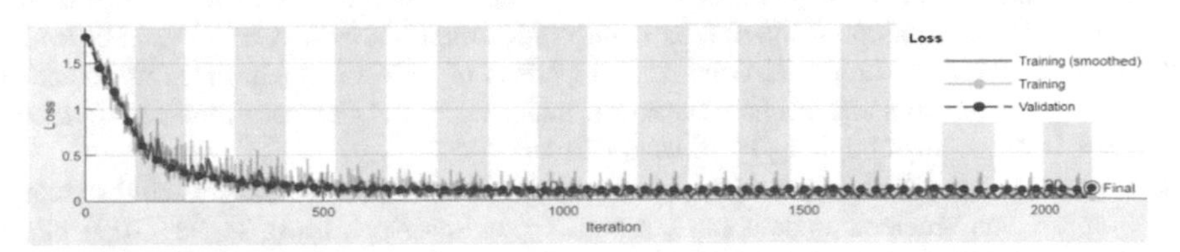

Fig. 5. Validation and training Lost and vs. iteration of "Dataset2" using the LSTM model.

7 Conclusions

This paper proposed a deep learning recurrent neural network architecture for human activity recognition from wearable sensors. It consists of three stages: data acquisition, data analysis, and classification. In addition, two datasets Collected of IMU sensors with gyroscope, accelerometer, and magnetometer placed different positions on subjects, indoor. For this purpose, ten subjects do six activities (walking, sitting, walking upstairs, standing, walking downstairs, and lay-ing). The first dataset was collected from sensors placed in the right wrist and the waist to get "Dataset1", and the second dataset was collected from sensors placed in the right ankle and the waist to get "Dataset2". Each dataset standardizes and divided into three sections: training 70%, testing 15%, and validation 15%. To classify the "Dataset1" used LSTM and requested test accuracy of 94.67% with 50 hidden units. The "Dataset2" classification used LSTM with a different number of hidden units; the number of 150 hidden units registered the highest accuracy was 98.44%. However, adopting two IMU sensors placed at the waist and the right ankle better performance for recognizing the six activities than using two IMU sensors placed at the waist and the right wrist.

References

1. Fu, Z., He, X., Wang, E., Huo, J., Huang, J., Wu, D.: Personalized human activity recognition based on integrated wearable sensor and transfer learning. Sensors (Switzerland) **21**(3), 1–23 (2021). https://doi.org/10.3390/s21030885
2. Minh Dang, L., Min, K., Wang, H., Jalil Piran, M., Hee Lee, C., Moon, H.: Sensor-based and vision-based human activity recognition: a comprehensive survey. Pattern Recognit. 108, 107561 (2020) https://doi.org/10.1016/j.patcog.2020.107561

3. Wang, J., Chen, Y., Hao, S., Peng, X., Hu, L.: Deep learning for sensor-based activity recognition: a survey. Pattern Recognit. Lett. **119**, 3–11 (2019). https://doi.org/10.1016/j.patrec.2018.02.010
4. Chen, K., Zhang, D., Yao, L., Guo, B., Yu, Z., Liu, Y.: deep learning for sensor-based human activity recognition: overview, challenges and opportunities (2020) http://arxiv.org/abs/2001.07416
5. Aparecida, R., Romero, F.: Inertial Units and Ambient Sensors, pp. 1–32 (2021)
6. Wang, Y., Cang, S., Yu, H.: A survey on wearable sensor modality centred human activity recognition in health care. Expert Syst. Appl. **137**, 167–190 (2019). https://doi.org/10.1016/j.eswa.2019.04.057
7. Lawal, I.A., Bano, S.: Deep human activity recognition with localisation of wearable sensors. IEEE Access **8**, 155060–155070 (2020). https://doi.org/10.1109/ACCESS.2020.3017681
8. Suto, J., Oniga, S., Lung, C., Orha, I.: Comparison of offline and real-time human activity recognition results using machine learning techniques. Neural Comput. Appl. **32**(20), 15673–15686 (2018). https://doi.org/10.1007/s00521-018-3437-x
9. Slim, S.O., Atia, A., Elfattah, M.M.A., Mostafa, M.S.M.: Survey on human activity recognition based on acceleration data. Int. J. Adv. Comput. Sci. Appl. **10**(3), 84–98 (2019). https://doi.org/10.14569/IJACSA.2019.0100311
10. . De Leonardis, G., et al.: Human activity recognition by wearable sensors: Comparison of different classifiers for real-time applications. In: MeMeA 2018 - 2018 IEEE Int. Symp. Med. Meas. Appl. Proc., vol. 3528725544, pp. 1–6 (2018). doi: https://doi.org/10.1109/MeMeA.2018.8438750
11. Nweke, H.F., Teh, Y.W., Al-garadi, M.A., Alo, U.R.: Deep learning algorithms for human activity recognition using mobile and wearable sensor networks: State of the art and research challenges. Expert Syst. Appl. **105**, 233–261 (2018). doi: https://doi.org/10.1016/j.eswa.2018.03.056
12. Zebin, T., Scully, P.J., Ozanyan, K.B.: Human activity recognition with inertial sensors using a deep learning approach. Proc. IEEE Sensors, no. 1 (2017). https://doi.org/10.1109/ICSENS.2016.7808590
13. Milenkoski, M., Trivodaliev, K., Kalajdziski, S., Jovanov, M., Stojkoska, B.R.: Real time human activity recognition on smartphones using LSTM networks. In: 2018 41st International Convention on Information and Communication Technology, Electronics and Microelectronics, MIPRO 2018 - Proceedings, pp. 1126–1131 (2018). https://doi.org/10.23919/MIPRO.2018.8400205
14. Espinilla, M., et al.: Human activity recognition from the acceleration data of a wearable device. which features are more relevant by activities? Proceedings **2**(19), 1242 (2018). https://doi.org/10.3390/proceedings2191242
15. Hassan, M.M., Huda, S., Uddin, M.Z., Almogren, A., Alrubaian, M.: Human activity recognition from body sensor data using deep learning. J. Med. Syst. **42**(6), 1–8 (2018). https://doi.org/10.1007/s10916-018-0948-z
16. Weiss, G.M.: WISDM Smartphone and Smartwatch Activity and Biometrics Dataset. UCI Mach. Learn. Repos. WISDM Smartphone Smartwatch Act. Biometrics Dataset Data Set, vol. 7, pp. 133190–133202 (2019)
17. Albaba, M., Qassab, A., Yilmaz, A.: Human activity recognition and classification using of convolutional neural networks and recurrent neural networks. Int. J. Appl. Math. Electron. Comput. **8**(4), 185–189 (2020). https://doi.org/10.18100/ijamec.803105
18. San Buenaventura, C.V., Tiglao, N.M.C., Atienza, R.O.: Deep learning for smartphone-based human activity recognition using multi-sensor fusion. In: Chen, J.-L., Pang, A.-C., Deng, D.-J., Lin, C.-C. (eds.) WICON 2018. LNICSSITE, vol. 264, pp. 65–75. Springer, Cham (2019). Doi: https://doi.org/10.1007/978-3-030-06158-6_7

19. Oluwalade, B., Neela, S., Wawira, J., Adejumo, T., Purkayastha, S.: Human activity recognition using deep learning models on smartphones and smartwatches sensor data. In: Heal. 2021 - 14th Int. Conf. Heal. Informatics; Part 14th International Joint Conference on Biomedical Engineering Systems and Technologies BIOSTEC 2021, pp. 645–650 (2021). https://doi.org/10.5220/0010325906450650
20. Munoz-Organero, M.: Outlier detection in wearable sensor data for human activity recognition (HAR) based on DRNNs. IEEE Access **7**, 74422–74436 (2019). doi: https://doi.org/10.1109/ACCESS.2019.2921096
21. Uddin, M.Z., Hassan, M.M.: Activity recognition for cognitive assistance using body sensors data and deep convolutional neural network. IEEE Sens. J. **19**(19), 8413–8419 (2019). https://doi.org/10.1109/JSEN.2018.2871203
22. Lyu, L., He, X., Law, Y.W., Palaniswami, M.: Privacy-preserving collaborative deep learning with application to human activity recognition. In: International Conference on Information and Knowledge Management Proceedings, vol. Part F1318, pp. 1219–1228 (2017). https://doi.org/10.1145/3132847.3132990
23. Holzinger, A., Kieseberg, P., Tjoa, A.M., Weippl, E. (eds.): CD-MAKE 2017. LNCS, vol. 10410. Springer, Cham (2017). https://doi.org/10.1007/978-3-319-66808-6
24. Zhao, Y., Yang, R., Chevalier, G., Xu, X., Zhang, Z.: Deep residual bidir-LSTM for human activity recognition using wearable sensors. Math. Probl. Eng. **2018** (2018). https://doi.org/10.1155/2018/7316954
25. Sharma, S., Sharma, S., Anidhya, A.: Understanding activation functions in neural networks. Int. J. Eng. Appl. Sci. Technol. **4**(12), 310–316 (2020)
26. Aljarrah, A.A., Ali, A.H.: Human activity recognition by deep convolution neural networks and principal component analysis. In: Balas, V.E., Solanki, V.K., Kumar, R. (eds.) Further Advances in Internet of Things in Biomedical and Cyber Physical Systems. ISRL, vol. 193, pp. 111–133. Springer, Cham (2021). https://doi.org/10.1007/978-3-030-57835-0_10

Job Training Recommendation System: Integrated Fuzzy AHP and TOPSIS Approach

Okfalisa[1](✉), Rizal Siburian[1], Yelfi Vitriani[1], Hidayati Rusnedy[2], Saktioto[3], and Melfa Yola[4]

[1] Department of Informatics Engineering, Universitas Islam Negeri Sultan Syarif Kasim Riau, Pekanbaru, Indonesia
okfalisa@gmail.com
[2] Faculty of Computer Science, Universitas Putra Indonesia YPTK Padang, Padang, Indonesia
[3] Faculty of Science, Universitas Riau, Pekanbaru, Indonesia
[4] Department of Industrial Engineering, Universitas Islam Negeri Sultan Syarif Kasim Riau, Pekanbaru, Indonesia

Abstract. A penitentiary serves as a job training mechanism to intensify and delve into jailbirds' talent and interest for workforce preparedness. Unfortunately, the job training commonly fails to reach the jailbird's potential benefits in getting the proper workforce position. Therefore, this study tries to develop an integrated multi-attribute decision making Fuzzy Analytical Hierarchy Process (Fuzzy-AHP) together with The Technique for Order of Preference by Similarity to Ideal Solution (TOPSIS) to assist the jailbird in finding the appropriate training place on age, latest education, work experience, talents and interests as domain criteria. Fuzzy-AHP employs the weighting criteria, whereas TOPSIS takes a role as an alternative ranking tool. Six alternatives are suggested based on their preferences, including cooking, sewing, building, furniture, farming, and raising livestock. This recommended system has been successfully proposed fifty jailbirds for their optimal training job. Hence, there is optimism that this profession will enhance their future level of life.

Keywords: Fuzzy-AHP · Job training · TOPSIS · Decision support system · Recommended system

1 Introduction

The ex-jailbirds face various challenges when returning to their society, including the broken family relationships, social abuse that assume the ex-jailbirds would never move to be the right people, and mental health issues. Nevertheless, the greatest insists upon finding the right job in a friendly and accepting environment. The workforce grows into the influencing key factor for ex-jailbirds after incarceration [1]. It is due to the unemployed person is substantial returns to crime (recidivism) if he lacks sufficient skills and competencies. Moreover, the negative societal stigma makes it challenging for ex-offenders to get respectable work [2–4]. Therefore, job training or vocational education

F. Saeed et al. (Eds.): IRICT 2021, LNDECT 127, pp. 84–94, 2022.
https://doi.org/10.1007/978-3-030-98741-1_8

for jailbirds is crucial in leading to the qualification provision and eligible workforce enhancement as rehabilitative contributions of Correctional Institution services [5].

Bierens and Carvalho (2011) identified that the effectiveness persuades the recidivism reduction of employment supported programs, the jailbirds' age management [6, 7], the successful finding of the post-release workforce, or particular work in progress. However, Duwe (2017) notes that the increased recidivism rates significantly impact both social and economic circumstances and community [8–10]. On the contrary, it was discovered that the proposed job training fails to provide substantial percussion on jailbirds or even ex-jailbirds. It is due to the limitation of supporting tools and approaches and the lack of training tailored to the convicts' abilities, talents, and interests.

Chang [10] first introduced Fuzzy-AHP to complement the Analytical Hierarchy Process (AHP) approach. As one of the Multi-Criteria Decision Making (MCDM) schema, AHP assessed the relative significance of criteria in decision-making problems [11]. One of the most convincing drawbacks of AHP is the limitation of decision-makers in expressing their precise figures of opinion or evaluation. Meanwhile, Fuzzy logic plays an essential role in capturing decision makers' uncertainty judgment [12, 13]. Hasan et al. (2018) supported the advantages of fuzzy AHP to compute the inconsistency rate of criteria through the pairwise comparisons matrix for job satisfaction assessment [14]. They successfully rated the hierarchy job satisfaction criteria scoring in less than 0.1 for variables and sub-variables. With AHP, fuzzy extends the uncertainty of incomplete information interpretation in AHP to serve more logical judgment in solving decision-making issues [15]. The application of AHP and Fuzzy-AHP in many fields of decision-making problems, such as business, industrial, energy, farming, health, and education, has been identified. Okfalisa et al. (2021) has successfully compared AHP and Fuzzy-AHP for smartphone selection [16]. AHP has been studied to measure the different factors of Small Medium Enterprises (SMEs) digitalization preparedness from multiple perspectives and judgments [17]. Wang et al. (2019) integrated the Fuzzy-AHP and SWOT analysis approach to choosing renewable energy resources [18]. Yucesan et al. (2019) hybrid the Fuzzy-AHP and Fuzzy-TOPSIS for hospital service quality assessment [19]. Pilevar et al. (2020) conducted the land suitability assessment using Fuzzy-AHP and GIS techniques [20]. The fuzzy-AHP method prioritizes the criteria by determining the pairwise comparisons on a nine-point scale. Pairwise comparison ratios are expressed in absolute numbers, namely a scale of 1–9, which has the advantage of simplicity and ease of use [21]. A nine-point scale was used to compare pairs of each selected criterion. Meanwhile, this pairwise comparison indicates the priority of the criteria being compared [22].

The Technique for Order Preference by Similarity to Ideal Solution (TOPSIS) method was developed by Hwang and Yoon in 1981 [23]. This technique is initiated as the most commonly used MCDM technique for finding the ideal point category [24]. Herein, the ranking of alternatives is determined by calculating the distance between the ideal solution and the negative ideal solution. Hence, the selection of optimal alternatives is simultaneously administered by the shortest distance from the ideal solution and the longest distance from the negative ideal solution. [25]. In a nutshell, TOPSIS hands over the full use of original data and accurate results to reflect the gaps between various evaluation schemes instead of the other approaches [26]. TOPSIS works well optimum in priority alternatives, while Fuzzy-AHP flourishing pursues the criteria assessment in multi-tier hierarchies [27]. Dogan et al. (2019) utilized the integration of the above methods for vehicle corridor selection [28], Li et al. (2020) applied for assessing successful B2C e-commerce websites [29], Kahraman et al. (2018) devoted to outsources manufacturers evaluation [30]. Chou et al. (2020) applied to identify critical organizational capabilities [31]. Thus, integrating these approaches is potentially adopted to clear up the job training recommendation system for jailbirds. Whereas Fuzzy-AHP employs the weighting job training criteria, and TOPSIS deploys to rank the potential job training as alternatives based on the jailbirds' criteria and conditions.

2 Research Method

This study accommodates two potential Decision Support System methods, whereby the Fuzzy-AHP handling the weighting criteria as well as the TOPSIS equips for alternative rankings. The Fuzzy-AHP follows the algorithm stage by [16].

Stage 1: Structuring the problem hierarchy and pairwise matrix comparisons between criteria with the Triangular Fuzzy Number (TFN) scale to find consistent values ($CR \leq 0.1$) on the comparison matrix. Furthermore, the value of the AHP comparison matrix will be changed into the Fuzzy-AHP value. TFN Scale is explained in Table 1.

Table 1. The TFN comparison scale [21]

Level significance	Linguistic set	TFN	Invers
1	Equal relative importance	(1, 1, 1)	(1, 1, 1)
2	Equally to moderately more important	(1/2, 1, 3/2)	(2/3, 1, 2)
3	Moderately more important	(1, 3/2, 2)	(1/2, 2/3, 1)
4	Moderately to strongly important	(3/2, 2, 5/2)	(2/5, ½, 2/3)
5	Strongly important	(2, 5/2,3)	(1/3, 2/5, 1/2)
6	Strongly to very strongly more important	(5/2, 3, 7/2)	(2/7, 1/3, 2/5)
7	Very strongly more important	(3, 7/2, 4)	(1/4, 2/7, 1/3)
8	Very strongly to extremely more important	(7/2, 4, 9/2)	(2/9, ¼, 2/7)
9	Extremely important (high priority)	(4, 9/2, 9/2)	(2/9, 2/9, ¼)

Stage 2: Calculating the value of Fuzzy Synthesis (Si) (See Eq. 1) and the consideration parameters including TFN number (M), number of criteria (m), row (i), column (j), and parameter (g) in low (l), middle (m), and upper (u) categorization.

$$(Si) : \sum_{j=1}^{m} M_{gi}^{j} \times \left[\sum_{i=1}^{n} \sum_{j=1}^{m} M_{gi}^{j}\right]^{-1} \quad (1)$$

Stage 3: Computing the vector value (V), M2 = (l2, m2, u2) ≥ M1 = (l1, m1, u1) are defined as a vector value.

$$V(M_2 \geq M_1) = sup\left[min(\pi M_1(x)),\ min(\pi M_2(y))\right]$$

$$\mathrm{VM_2 \geq M_1} = \left\{\begin{array}{c} 1 \ \ \text{if}\ \mathrm{m_2 \geq m_1} \\ 0 \ \ \text{if}\ \mathrm{l_1 \geq u_2} \\ \frac{\mathrm{l_{1-u_2}}}{\mathrm{(m_2-u_2)-(m_2-l_2)}} \end{array}\right\} \tag{2}$$

Stage 4: De-fuzzification Ordinary Value (d′) For k = 1, 2, n; k ≠ I, it obtains the vector weight value:

$$\mathrm{W' = \left(d'(A1),\ d'(A2), \ldots d'(An)\right)T} \tag{3}$$

Stage 5: Normalizing value of fuzzy vector weights (W), where W is defined as a non-fuzzy number.

$$\mathrm{W = (d(A1),\ d(A2), \ldots, d(An))T} \tag{4}$$

The following stage of TOPSIS approaches [31]:

Stage 1: Determining the normalized decision matrix (rij).

$$\mathrm{r_{ij}} = \frac{\mathrm{x_{ij}}}{\sqrt{\sum_{\mathrm{i=1}}^{\mathrm{m}} \mathrm{x_{ij^2}}}} \tag{5}$$

Stage 2: Calculating the weighted normalized decision matrix. The positive ideal solution + and the negative ideal solution can be determined based on the normalized weight rating (*yij*).

$$\mathrm{y_{ij} = w_i r_{ij}} \tag{6}$$

Stage 3: Calculate the positive ideal solution matrix and the negative ideal solution matrix.

$$\mathrm{A^+ = \left(y1^+, y2^+, \ldots, yn^+\right)} \tag{7}$$

$$\mathrm{A^- = \left(y1^-, y2^-, \ldots, yn^-\right)} \tag{8}$$

Assumption:

$$\mathrm{y_j^+} = \left\{\begin{array}{l} \max\ \mathrm{y_{ij}}\ \ \text{if j is a benifit attribute} \\ \min\ \mathrm{y_{ij}}\ \ \text{if j is the attribute cost} \end{array}\right.$$

$$\mathrm{y_j^-} = \left\{\begin{array}{l} \max\ \mathrm{y_{ij}}\ \ \text{if j is a benifit attribute} \\ \min\ \mathrm{y_{ij}}\ \ \text{if j is the attribute cost} \end{array}\right. \tag{9}$$

Stage 4: Calculating the distance (d) between the values of each alternative with the positive ideal solution matrix (d*) and the negative ideal solution matrix (d−).

$$d_j^* = \sqrt{\sum_{j=1}^{n} \left(v_{ij} - v_j^*\right)^2},\ i = 1, \ldots, m \tag{10}$$

$$d_j^- = \sqrt{\sum_{j=1}^{n} \left(v_{ij} - v_j^-\right)^2},\ i = 1, \ldots, m \tag{11}$$

Stage 5: Calculating preference values for each alternative (CC).

$$CC_i = \frac{d_i^-}{d_i^* + d_i^-},\ i = 1, \ldots, m \tag{12}$$

3 Results and Discussion

3.1 Criteria and Sub-criteria Analysis

By referencing literature reviews and interviews with penitentiary staff responsible for jailbird's job training, the criteria and sub-criteria for this DSS mechanism are defined in Table 2.

Table 2. The criteria formulation.

No	Criteria	Sub-criteria	Range	Weight	Attribute	References
1	Age (C01)	Old age adult	>55	1	Cost	[6, 7]
		Young-age adult	17–25	2		
		Middle-age adult	26–55	3		
2	Latest education (C02)	Low	Not educate	1	Benefit	[2, 3]
		Moderately low	Elementary school	2		
		Moderate	Junior high school	3		
		Moderately High	senior high school	4		
		High	Diploma/Bachelor	5		
3	Work experience (C03)	Low	<1 year	1	Benefit	[1, 5]
		Moderate	2–3 year	2		
		High	≥3 year	3		

(continued)

Table 2. (*continued*)

No	Criteria	Sub-criteria	Range	Weight	Attribute	References
4	Talents (C04)	Abstract	Pattern and design skill	1	Benefit	[8–10]
		Speed accuracy	Laboratory and office skill	2		
		Mechanic	Mechanical skill	3		
5	Interest (C05)	Professional	Science and art interest	1	Benefit	[8–10]
		Commercial	Enterprise interest	2		
		Physical	Physical and mechanical interest	3		

Meanwhile, six alternatives are listed as optimum recommended training for the jailbirds, including cooking (A01), sewing (A02), building (A03), furnishing (A04), farming (A05), and raising (A06).

3.2 Criteria and Sub-criteria Analysis

The hierarchy problems for the job training recommendation system can be depicted in Fig. 1.

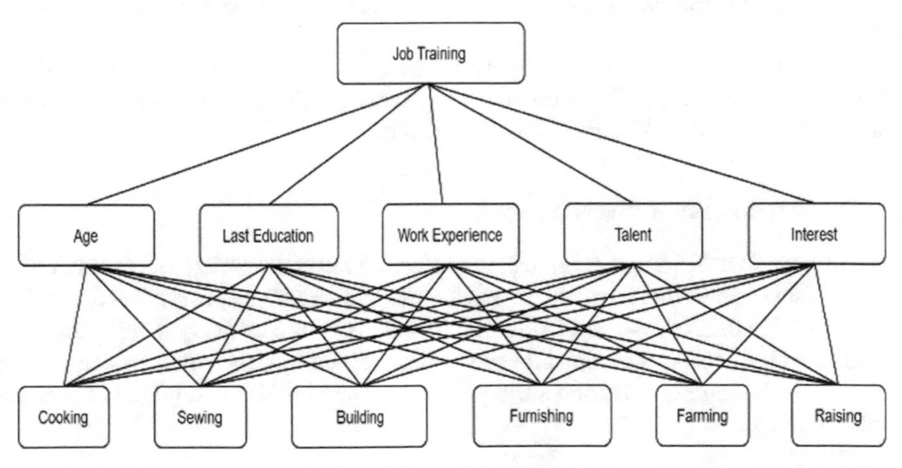

Fig. 1. Hierarchy problems.

Referring to Eq. (1), Table 3 explained that the values of CR $\leq$ 0,1. These values indicated the consistency of the proposed criteria. Thus the synthesis of fuzzy calculations for the Low (l), Middle (m), and Upper (u) scales can proceed. Next, following

Table 3. Fuzzy synthesis values.

Fuzzy synthesis value (Si)						
CI	CR	RI	Criteria	L	M	U
0.11	0.098	1.12	C01	0.122	0.250	0.455
			C02	0.090	0.167	0.375
			C03	0.095	0.186	0.348
			C04	0.108	0.218	0.401
			C05	0.090	0.179	0.401

Table 4. Normalization of criteria weighting values.

Criteria	W′ (vector weight)	W (fuzzy vector weight)
C01	1	0.236
C02	0.753	0.178
C03	0.780	0.184
C04	0.898	0.212
C05	0.799	0.189
Total	7.433	1

Eqs. (2) to (5), the criteria weighting and normalized fuzzy vector weights are described in Table 4.

The criterion weight value is normalized on a scale of 0–1. Table 3 informed that C01 (age) is the most significant criteria in influencing job training selection. It is then followed by C04, C05, C03, and C02, respectively.

3.3 Criteria and Sub-criteria Analysis

Following the TOPSIS stage at Eq. (6), the value of matrix normalization is obtained as bellows. Table 4 points out that matrix value for alternative A01 against C01 at 0.258, C02 at 0.521, C03 at 0.224, C04, and C05 at 0.243 and 0.333, respectively. These values are generated as the basic calculations for the next stage TOPSIS algorithm by considering each criterion's weight values and attribute (Table 2) and jailbird's weighted assessment (Tables 4 and 5).

Table 5. Normalization matrix value.

Alternatives	Criteria standard value					Criteria respondent #1 value				
	C01	C02	C03	C04	C05	C01	C02	C03	C04	C05
A01	0.258	0.521	0.224	0.243	0.333	0.061	0.278	0.041	0.154	0.126
A02	0.516	0.521	0.447	0.243	0.167	0.122	0.278	0.082	0.154	0.063
A03	0.516	0.391	0.447	0.485	0.500	0.122	0.209	0.082	0.309	0.189
A04	0.516	0.521	0.671	0.728	0.333	0.122	0.278	0.124	0.463	0.126
A05	0.258	0.130	0.224	0.243	0.500	0.061	0.070	0.041	0.154	0.189

Hence, following the calculation of positive and negative ideal solutions and the distance between both ideal solutions as determined at Eq. (7–13), the preferences values of each alternative for fifty respondents are presented in Table 6.

Table 6. Preference values for an alternative.

Respondents	Alternative	Positive	Negative	Pref	Rank
Respondent#1	A01	0.326	0.226	0.409868	3
	A02	0.342	0.213	0.383671	4
	A03	0.185	0.246	0.571663	2
	A04	**0.088**	**0.387**	**0.815185**	**1**
	A05	0.382	0.140	0.268312	5
	A06	0.382	0.140	0.268312	6
Respondent#2	A01	0.241	0.170	0.414214	5
	A02	0.308	0.084	0.213495	6
	A03	0.170	0.226	0.570101	2
	A04	**0.155**	**0.251**	**0.618348**	**1**
	A05	0.232	0.226	0.492856	3
	A06	0.232	0.226	0.492856	4
…	…	…	…	…	…
Respondent#50	A01	0.205	0.195	0.487492	3
	A02	0.221	0.161	0.421441	6
	A03	0.164	0.187	0.532393	2
	A04	**0.138**	**0.247**	**0.641807**	**1**
	A05	0.239	0.176	0.42445	4
	A06	0.239	0.176	0.42445	5

Table 6 resolved that alternative A04 (furnishing) is suggested as the first rank optimal job training for the jailbird at a value of 0.815. It is then followed by A03 (building), A01 (cooking), A02 (sewing), A05 (farming), and A06 (raising), respectively.

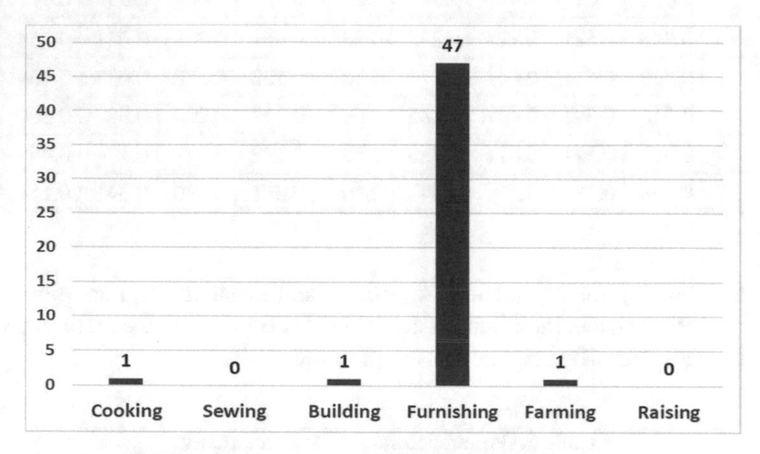

Fig. 2. The recapitulation of system recommendation.

Moreover, the respondents for this job training recommendation system are fifty jailbirds at Bangkinang penitentiary class two. As shown in Fig. 2, it reveals forty-seven jailbirds are the first rank suggested to join the furnishing job training mechanism. Meanwhile, only one jailbird is the first ranked advised to cooking, building, and farming. None jailbirds are the first list proposed for sewing and building. Regarding the efficacy of Fuzzy-AHP and TOPSIS integration, similar results are also found by Hasan et al. (2018) and Ali et al. (2018) in analyzing the ranking of legality factors based on job satisfaction [32] and career decision making in the maritime industry [33], respectively.

4 Conclusion

An integration of Fuzzy-AHP and TOPSIS has been successfully applied for solving the job training recommendation system for Bangkinang's jailbirds. The system proposed the optimal rank of alternatives from cooking, building, farming, furnishing, sewing, and raising hinge on the significant fuzzy weight of criteria on their assessment as well as age, latest education, work experience, talents, and interests. This job training endorsement can be utilized as an advisement tool to lead the jailbirds in singling out their personalities, talents, and interests to the future directly into the right and prospect jobs. Hence, the ex-jailbirds that escort a criminal can be reduced, and their forthcoming life will be raised.

References

1. Mcroberts, O.M.: Prisoner Reentry and the Institutions of Civil Society: Bridges and Barriers to Successful Reintegration Religion, Reform, Community: Examining the Idea of Church-Based Prisoner Reentry, March 2002

2. Hirschfield, P.J., Piquero, A.R.: Normalization and legitimation: modeling stigmatizing attitudes toward ex-offenders. Criminology **48**(1), 27–55 (2010)
3. Uggen, C., Vuolo, M., Lageson, S., Ruhland, E., Whitham, H.K.: The edge of stigma: an experimental audit of the effects of low-level criminal records on employment. Criminology **52**(4), 627–654 (2014)
4. Decker, S.H., Ortiz, N., Spohn, C., Hedberg, E.: Criminal stigma, race, and ethnicity: the consequences of imprisonment for employment. J. Crim. Justice **43**(2), 108–121 (2015). Elsevier Ltd.
5. Cale, J., et al.: Australian prison vocational education and training and returns to custody among male and female ex-prisoners: a cross-jurisdictional study. Aust. N. Z. J. Criminol. **52**(1), 129–147 (2019)
6. Maden, A., Skapinakis, P., Lewis, G., Scott, F., Burnett, R., Jamieson, E.: Gender differences in reoffending after discharge from medium-secure units: national cohort study in England and Wales. Br. J. Psychiatry **189**(AUG), 168–172 (2006)
7. Payne, J.: Recidivism in Australia: findings and future research. AIC Res. Publ. Policy Ser. (80), 140 (2007)
8. Duwe, G.: The use and impact of correctional programming for inmates on pre- and post-release outcomes. Natl. Inst. Justice **10097**(2010), 1–41 (2017)
9. Andrews, D.A., Bonta, J.: Rehabilitating criminal justice policy and practice. Psychol. Publ. Policy Law **16**(1), 39–55 (2010)
10. Okfalisa, Anugarah, S., Anggraini, W., Absor, M., Fauzi, S.S.M., Saktioto: Integrated analytical hierarchy process and objective matrix in balanced scorecard dashboard model for performance measurement. Telkomnika (Telecommun. Comput. Electron. Control) **16**, 2703–2711 (2018)
11. Mdallal, A., Hammad, A.: Application of fuzzy analytical hierarchy process (FAHP) to reduce concrete waste on construction sites. In: Proceedings, Annual Conference - Canadian Society for Civil Engineering, June 2019
12. Kaya, T., Kahraman, C.: Multicriteria renewable energy planning using an integrated fuzzy VIKOR & AHP methodology: the case of Istanbul. Energy Elsevier **35**(6), 2517–2527 (2010)
13. Dogan, O.: Process mining technology selection with spherical fuzzy AHP and sensitivity analysis. Expert Syst. Appl. **178**(May), 114999 (2021). Elsevier Ltd.
14. Liu, Y., Eckert, C.M., Earl, C.: A review of fuzzy AHP methods for decision-making with subjective judgements. Expert Syst. Appl. **161**, 113738 (2020). Elsevier Ltd.
15. Okfalisa, Rusnedy, H., Iswavigra, D.U., Pranggono, B., Haerani, E., Saktioto: Decision support system for smartphone recommendation: the comparison of fuzzy AHP and fuzzy ANP in multi-attribute decision making. Sinergi **25**(1), 101 (2020)
16. Okfalisa, Anggraini, W., Nawanir, G., Saktioto, Wong, K.Y.: Measuring the effects of different factors influencing on the readiness of SMEs towards digitalization: a multiple perspectives design of decision support system. Decis. Sci. Lett. **10**(3), 425–442 (2021)
17. Wang, Y., Xu, L., Solangi, Y.A.: Strategic renewable energy resources selection for Pakistan: based on SWOT-Fuzzy AHP approach. Sustain. Cities Soc. **52** (2020)
18. Yucesan, M., Gul, M.: Hospital service quality evaluation: an integrated model based on Pythagorean fuzzy AHP and fuzzy TOPSIS. Soft Comput. **24**(5), 3237–3255 (2020). Springer, Heidelberg
19. Pilevar, A.R., Matinfar, H.R., Sohrabi, A., Sarmadian, F.: Integrated fuzzy, AHP and GIS techniques for land suitability assessment in semi-arid regions for wheat and maize farming. Ecol. Indic. **110**(August 2019), 105887 (2020). Elsevier
20. Zoghi, M., Rostami, G., Khoshand, A., Motalleb, F.: Material selection in design for deconstruction using Kano model, fuzzy-AHP and TOPSIS methodology. Waste Manag. Res. (2021)

21. Avikal, S., Singh, A.K., Kumar, K.C.N., Badhotiya, G.K.: A fuzzy-AHP and TOPSIS based approach for selection of metal matrix composite used in design and structural applications. Mater. Today Proc. **46**, 11050–11053 (2021). Elsevier Ltd.
22. Zeng, J., Lin, G., Huang, G.: Evaluation of the cost-effectiveness of Green Infrastructure in climate change scenarios using TOPSIS. Urban Forestry Urban Green. **64**(December 2020), 127287 (2021). Elsevier GmbH
23. Amini, A., Alinezhad, A., Yazdipoor, F.: A TOPSIS, VIKOR and DEA integrated evaluation method with belief structure under uncertainty to rank alternatives. Int. J. Adv. Oper. Manag. **11**(3), 171 (2019)
24. Palczewski, K., Sałabun, W.: The fuzzy TOPSIS applications in the last decade. In: 23rd International Conference on Knowledge-Based and Intelligent Information and Engineering System, Procedia Computer Science, vol. 59, pp. 2294–2303 (2019)
25. Leng, L., et al.: Performance assessment of coupled green-grey-blue systems for Sponge City construction. Sci. Total Environ. **728** (2020)
26. Ekmekcioğlu, Ö., Koc, K., Özger, M.: Stakeholder perceptions in flood risk assessment: a hybrid fuzzy AHP-TOPSIS approach for Istanbul, Turkey. Int. J. Disaster Risk Reduction **60**(May) (2021)
27. Dogan, O., Deveci, M., Canıtez, F., Kahraman, C.: A corridor selection for locating autonomous vehicles using an interval-valued intuitionistic fuzzy AHP and TOPSIS method. Soft. Comput. **24**(12), 8937–8953 (2019). https://doi.org/10.1007/s00500-019-04421-5
28. Li, R., Sun, T.: Assessing factors for designing a successful B2C E-Commerce website using fuzzy AHP and TOPSIS-Grey methodology. Symmetry **12**(3) (2020)
29. Kahraman, C., Öztayşi, B., Onar, S.C.: An integrated intuitionistic fuzzy AHP and TOPSIS approach to evaluation of outsource manufacturers. J. Intell. Syst. **29**(1), 283–297 (2020)
30. Chou, T.Y., Chen, Y.T.: Applying fuzzy AHP and TOPSIS method to identify key organizational capabilities. Mathematics **8**(5) (2020)
31. Swindiarto, V.T.P., Sarno, R., Novitasari, D.C.R.: Integration of fuzzy C-means clustering and TOPSIS (FCM-TOPSIS) with Silhouette analysis for multi criteria parameter data. In: 2018 International Seminar on Application for Technology of Information and Communication: Creative Technology for Human Life, iSemantic 2018, pp. 463–468. IEEE (2018)
32. Denavi, H.D. Mirabi, M., Rezaei, A.: Ranking of leagility factors based on job satisfaction through a combinatory model of fuzzy TOPSIS and AHP (case study: M.R.I Hospital, Shiraz, Iran). Open J. Bus. Manag. **06**(01), 21–38 (2018)
33. Kaya, A.Y., Asyali, E., Ozdagoglu, A.: Career decision making in the maritime industry: research of merchant marine officers using Fuzzy AHP and Fuzzy TOPSIS methods. Zeszyty Naukowe Akademii Morskiej w Szczecini **55**(127), 95–103 (2018)

Improvement of Population Diversity of Meta-heuristics Algorithm Using Chaotic Map

Samuel-Soma M. Ajibade[1,2(✉)], Mary O. Ogunbolu[3], Ruth Chweya[4], and Samuel Fadipe[5]

[1] Department of Computer Engineering, Istanbul Ticaret Universitesi, Istanbul, Turkey
asamuel@ticaret.edu.tr
[2] Department of Computer Science, Universiti Teknologi Malaysia, Johor Bahru, Malaysia
[3] Department of Computer Science, Lead City University, Ibadan, Oyo State, Nigeria
bunmi810@yahoo.com
[4] School of Information Science and Technology, Kisii University, Kisii, Kenya
rchweya@kisiiuniversity.ac.ke
[5] Lagos State University, Ojo, Lagos, Nigeria
samuel.fadipe@lasu.edu.ng

Abstract. Particle swarm optimization (PSO) is a global optimization and nature-inspired algorithm known for its good quality and easily applied in various real-world optimization challenges. Nevertheless, PSO has some weaknesses such as slow convergence, converging prematurely and simply gets stuck at local optima. This study aims to solve the problem of deprived population diversity in the search process of PSO which causes premature convergence. Therefore, in this research, a method is brought to PSO to keep away from early stagnation which explains premature convergence. The aim of this research is to propose a chaotic dynamic weight particle swarm optimization (CHPSO) wherein a chaotic logistic map is utilized to enhance the populace diversity within the search technique of PSO with the aid of editing the inertia weight of PSO in an effort to avoid premature convergence. This study additionally investigates the overall performance and feasibility of the proposed CHPSO as a function selection set of rules for fixing problems of optimization. 8 benchmark functions had been used to assess the overall performance and seek accuracy of the proposed (CHPSO) algorithms and as compared with a few other meta-heuristics optimization set of rules. The outcomes of the experiments show that the CHPSO achieves correct consequences in fixing an optimization and has established to be a dependable and green metaheuristics algorithm for selection of features.

Keywords: Particle swarm optimization · Premature convergence · Inertia weight · Population diversity · Poor diversity

1 Introduction

Nowadays, in every facets of life, we deal with voluminous or massive data which cut across every field of study. Datamining is a procedure of extracting and discovering

F. Saeed et al. (Eds.): IRICT 2021, LNDECT 127, pp. 95–104, 2022.
https://doi.org/10.1007/978-3-030-98741-1_9

styles in large datasets concerning methods on the intersection of machine learning, facts, database structures. Data Mining strategies are utilized to locate hidden designs and relations on an intensive measure of facts that is probably beneficial in making of choices [1]. Because of the way that the greater part of the datasets created have an enormous number of redundant and insignificant elements, there could be broad lessening in the exactness of preparing the classifiers and furthermore a decrease in the training speed of the classifiers. This issue is prominently called "curse of dimensionality" in information mining methods and this makes the computational intricacy of fostering the classifiers to upsurge [2, 3]. To beat the issues of exorbitant dimensionality, feature selection is used to reduce the assortment of capacities and improve the fine of the feature set by discarding unseemly and excess capacities. The complete space of exploring consists of all the feasible subsets of capabilities and this shows that the request space degree is $2n$ wherein n is the quantity of the actual capabilities [4].

To eliminate the weaknesses of filter and wrapper techniques, Metaheuristics algorithm was introduced. Recently, metaheuristics-based techniques have involved several considerations because of their good performance in resolving the issues of feature selection and have been widely applied because of their potential global search ability [2]. PSO has been utilized as an efficient method in feature selection [5]. However, it has a few drawbacks, for example, premature convergence [6], high computational complexity [6], slow convergence [7]. Furthermore, the search direction of PSO is to approach the global optimum, which makes the information exchange in the group in a single direction, such that the particles quickly gather in a small search area, resulting in the poor swarm diversity [8], which makes it easy to fall into local optima and get poor convergence accuracy. The swarm diversity information can reflect the distribution of the entire particle swarm. The lack of swarm diversity will cause the swarm to converge prematurely to some local optimums whilst tackling complex optimization difficulties [9]. Additionally, it has the inadequacies of premature convergence with weakness in fine-tuning close local optimum positions [10]. Another confinement is choosing similar features in the final feature subset which winds up not giving optimal solution for feature selection because PSO does not efficiently deal with the relationship between exploitation (local search) and exploration (global search), therefore it generally converges to a local minimum so quick and reduces the convergence speed [6].

2 Review of Literature

2.1 Particle Swarm Optimization (PSO)

PSO is an optimization algorithm which was invented by Kennedy and Eberhart in 1995 [6] that imitates the social practices of persons in swarms of fish and fowls. PSO has been shown to be less exorbitant computationally and can quickly merge with the other metaheuristics techniques like Genetic Algorithm (GA), Ant Colony Optimization (ACO), Differential Evolution (DE) [2] etc. Additionally, PSO is easy to execute and it has minimum parameters that are being fine-tuned and it is much lesser computationally costly in memory and speed requirements. It is therefore vastly used as an efficient method for feature selection and various domains. Despite the fact that the PSO is extremely proficient in dealing with looks for ideal subsets of component, it tragically has different difficulties, for example, premature convergence that exist in complex issues of optimization [5], they likewise ignore the quantity of elements in their course of looking while it exclusively lay accentuation on limiting the error rate of classification. Another shortcoming that it has is that it chooses features that are indistinguishable in the finishing up include subset [7]. Furthermore, the PSO does not make use of correlation information which belongs to the features that heads process of searching, and this causes similar features to be chosen in the concluding feature subset, thereby decreasing the classifier performance [8]. It is easy and requires only few control parameters [13]. The PSO technique distinguishes the global ideal arrangement by refreshing the flying velocity and the area of every person in the swarm as per Eqs. (1) and (2).

$$\begin{aligned} v_{id}(t+1) = {} & v_{id}(t) + r_1(t) \times c_1 \times \left(pbest_{id}(t) - x_{id}(t)\right) \\ & + r_2(t) \times c_2 \times (gbest(t) - x_{id}(t)) \end{aligned} \tag{1}$$

$$x_{id}(t+1) = x_{id}(t) + v_{id}(t+1) \tag{2}$$

where c_1 and c_2 are the acceleration parameters, which are set to 2.0 commonly; r_1 and r_2 are two uniform distributed values in the range [0, 1]. Therefore, making use of the inertia weight w, the Eq. (1) is improved to Eq. (3) as shown below:

$$\begin{aligned} V_{id}(t+1) = {} & \omega \times v_{id}(t) + r_1(t) \times c_1 \times \left(pbest_{id}(t) - x_{id}(t)\right) + r_2(t) \times c_2 \\ & \times (gbest(t) - x_{id}(t)) \end{aligned} \tag{3}$$

The best current location of particle i is recorded as pbest and the global best location is recorded as gbest. Also, the location of the particle of the coming generation relies essentially upon the present location, which is known as, xid(t), and the flying speed, known as, vid(t + 1). The initial term in the right-hand side of Eq. (3) utilizes ω, which stands for the inertia weight and the two terms are excitations towards promising areas in the pursuit space as announced by the global and personal best locations.

2.2 Inertia Weight

The chaotic map is brought to regulate the inertia weight ω of PSO. The tuning of inertia weight ω using chaotic maps is able to enhance the potential of PSO escape from neighborhood optima when solving multimodal functions. According to [9] and [10], the logistic map is chosen to music inertia weight ω of PSO. Due to the ergodicity, irregularity and non-repetition homes of logistic map, it has the potential to improve population variety within the seek system and additionally will increase the capacity to converge at global most useful, hereby keeping off untimely convergence. The range of the logistic map is always [0, 1] and any wide variety within that variety can be selected because the preliminary cost. Nevertheless, it has to be famous that the preliminary value is capable of have important results on the sample of fluctuation of a few chaotic maps together with logistic map. This type of chaotic maps is selected with various attitudes, while the initial cost is set to 0.7 for all of them [11]. The inertia weight ω is represented in Eq. (4).

$$\omega = \varphi * cos\left(\frac{Mj}{M\,max}\right) * \pi + \tau \tag{4}$$

2.3 Chaotic Logistic Map

The chaos is a deterministic, arbitrary like technique that is seen in non-linear, dynamic, which is non-period, non-merging and limited. Numerically, chaos occurs as a simple and random deterministic dynamical framework and the system which entail chaos can be seen as a source of randomness. Several chaotic maps have been introduced in literature and these chaotic maps differs by their mathematical equations. In recent times, the chaotic maps have been broadly used in optimization because of their dynamic conduct distinctive confused guides having diverse numerical conditions are utilized. Since a decade ago, clamorous guides have been broadly refreshing in the field of enhancement because of their dynamic conduct that aids the optimization techniques in investigating the search space globally. In the chaotic maps, numbers within the range of [0, 1] can be used as the initial value. Nonetheless, the initial value used can impact the instability pattern of some chaotic maps. The chaotic maps positively influence the convergent rate of the algorithms because the maps initiate chaos in the feasible ahead and is likely just for an initial short time and stochastic for longer time frame. Some of the well-known chaotic maps are:

Cubic Map: The cubic map generates values in the interval [−1.5, 1.5]. It is almost similar to Sine map. It is defined as:

$$\mathrm{X_{k+1}} = 3\mathrm{x_k}\left(1 - \mathrm{X_k^2}\right) \tag{5}$$

where $\mathrm{X_k}$ is the kth chaotic number, with k denoting the iteration number.

Sine Map: The sine map is a unimodal map and it is represented by:

$$\mathrm{X_{k+1}} = \frac{a}{4}\sin(\pi \mathrm{x_k}) \tag{6}$$

where $\mathrm{X_k}$ is the kth chaotic number, with k denoting the iteration number.

Logistic Map: The equation of logistic map is a non-linear dynamic of population which is biological evidencing chaotic behaviour. The map is represented by:

$$\mathrm{X_{k+1}} = \mathrm{ax_k}(1 - \mathrm{X_k}) \tag{7}$$

where $\mathrm{X_k}$ is the kth chaotic number, with k denoting the iteration number.

In the method of using the logistic chaotic map:

i. A chaotic random sequence Z is generated between [0, 1] by utilizing the logistic map formula, thereafter pass the carrier map in Eq. (8), by incorporating the chaos into *gbest*, a nearby area, in order to accomplish the local chaotic search:

$$Z \to Y : X = gbest + R \times \cos(Z) \tag{8}$$

where R is the search radius which is used to control the range of local chaotic search. $R \in [0.1, 0.4]$.

3 Methodology

The framework of the research contains all the procedures involved in order to accomplish the research objectives. The framework of this research comprises of 2 stages. The phase 1 of the framework described the process of data pre-processing techniques that were used. Phase 2 focused on the initialization of PSO where chaotic logistic map was introduced into PSO in order to avoid premature convergence.

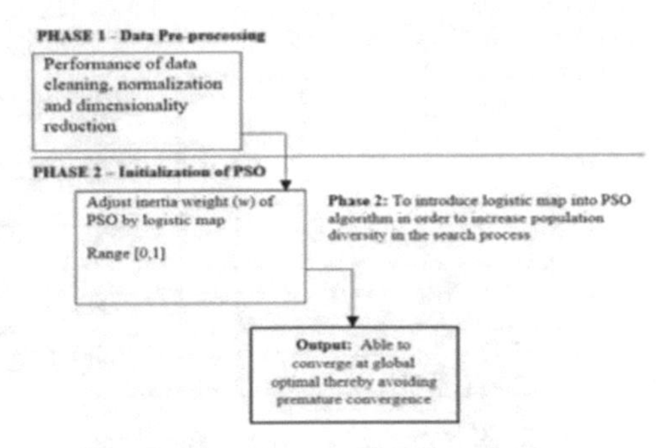

Fig. 1. Research operational framework.

In the Fig. 1, Phase 1 which is data pre-processing addresses the issue of the interference of different data attribute scaling. The attributes in the datasets for this study are directly meaningful to the original domain, or are designed for the use of their current operational system. Usually, these raw attributes reduce the performance of machine learning classification power, because those with higher values exercise dominance over the attributes with lower values. Therefore, normalization (a linear) transform was employed on all the original attributes to generate new attributes with better properties with uniform distribution. This will help the predictive power of the classifiers. It improves the accuracy of the classifier as well as reduces the computational time. Phase 2 which is Initialization of PSO contains the research activities which involves introducing chaotic maps to adjust the inertia weight in order to increase the diversity of population in the search process of PSO to avoid premature convergence and improve the convergence performance of PSO. In spite of its convergence rate, the population maintenance of PSO is little, thereby causing it to converge prematurely. Hence, in order to lessen this impact and also improve the convergence performance, CHPSO is developed by introducing chaos into PSO algorithm. The performance of this technique was measured using eight benchmark functions as shown in Fig. 2.

4 Result and Discussion

The occasions which a cost function is reviewed to be calculated can be considered as a basis to gauge the convergence performance of the algorithms that is most commonly used in literature [12], this is known as the Number of Function Evaluation (NFE). The average number of function evaluation (Avg NFE) is the average number of function calls to reach at the termination criteria in 30 number of runs. The Pop size (NP) is set to 50, while the dimension setting values are 30 and 50 as used by [13]. A smaller NFE specifies higher convergence speed.

No	Function	Formula	Value	Dim	Range	Properties
1	Sphere	$f(x)=\sum_{i=1}^{n}x_i^2$	0	30	[-100, 100]	Unimodal, Separable
2	Rosenbrock	$f(x)=\sum_{i=1}^{n-1}[100(x_{i+1}-x_i^2)^2+(x_i-1)^2]$	0	30	[-30, 30]	Unimodal, Inseparable
3	Quartic	$f(x)=\sum_{i=1}^{n}ix_i^4+random[0,1)$	0	30	[-1.28, 1.28]	Unimodal, Inseparable
4	Griewank	$f(x)=\frac{1}{4000}\sum_{i=1}^{n}x_i^2-\prod_{i=1}^{n}\cos\frac{x_i}{\sqrt{i}}+1$	0	30	[-600, 600]	Multimodal, Inseparable
5	Sumsquare	$f(x)=\sum_{i=1}^{n}ix_i^2$	0	30	[-5.12, 5.12]	Unimodal, Separable
6	Schwefel	$f(x)=\sum_{i=1}^{n}-x_i\sin\left(\sqrt{\lvert x_i\rvert}\right)$	0	30	[-500, 500]	Multimodal, Separable
7	Rastrigin	$f(x)=\sum_{i=1}^{n}x_i^2-10\cos(2\pi x_i)+10$	0	30	[-5.12, 5.12]	Multimodal, Separable
8	Michalewicz	$f(x)=-\sum_{i=1}^{n}\sin(x_i)(\sin(ix_i^2/\pi))^{2m}$	-4.688	5	[0, π]	Multimodal, Separable

Fig. 2. Numerical benchmark functions.

4.1 Comparison of NFE, Mean Fitness Value and Standard Deviation for Proposed CHPSO and Other Algorithms

To assess the proposed algorithm's performance, eight benchmark test capabilities are utilized in this study and the benchmark functions are defined. All the chosen functions are well-known within the global optimization literature. The test function comprises of unimodal and multimodal functions. Table 1 offers the average NFE of GA, PSO and CHPSO algorithm for eight benchmarks feature for dimension 30.

Table 1. Avg NFE of GA, PSO and the proposed CHPSO for D = 30

Function	GA	PSO	CHPSO
$f1$	20014	16984	**7124**
$f2$	20019	17169	**3879**
$f3$	20013	20001	**9898**
$f4$	14574	17146	**8145**
$f5$	12491	18633	**6635**
$f6$	20000	20001	**16252**
$f7$	20055	8226	**10163**
$f8$	13682	20001	**6689**

A smaller NFE indicates higher convergence rate, hence Table 1 displays that the proposed CHPSO algorithm has a higher convergent rate when compared with the original PSO and GA because the population diversity of PSO was improved to give the proposed CHPSO a better performance. CHPSO obtains a better result in all the functions for dimension 30. This depicts that PSO converges at local optima for all the functions. It is shown in Fig. 3.

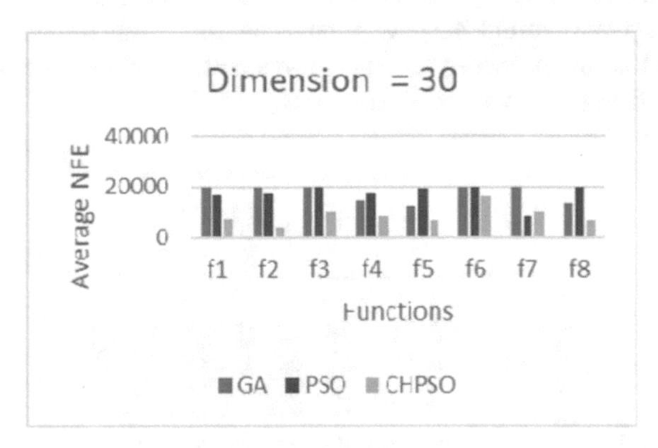

Fig. 3. Average NFE of GA, PSO and the proposed CHPSO for D = 30.

Table 2 compares the average NFE of PSO, GA and CHPSO algorithm for eight benchmarks functions for dimension 50.

Table 2. Avg NFE of GA, PSO and the proposed CHPSO for D = 50

Function	GA	PSO	CHPSO
*f*1	20025	11702	**10905**
*f*2	20016	12525	**8191**
*f*3	20013	20000	**19948**
*f*4	18308	18627	**18462**
*f*5	19536	20000	**8239**
*f*6	18999	20000	**20001**
*f*7	20018	**1335**	13711
*f*8	16941	20000	**19976**

A smaller NFE indicates higher convergence rate, hence Table 2 shows that the proposed CHPSO algorithm has a higher convergent rate when compared with the original PSO and GA because the population diversity of PSO was improved to give the proposed CHPSO a better performance. CHPSO obtains a better result in all the functions except *f7* where PSO obtains a better performance for dimension 50 because the *f7* (Rastrigin function) is quite difficult to resolve as it presents various local optima locations where an optimization algorithm possesses higher chances of being trapped in the local optima. It is shown in Fig. 4.

Tables 3 and 4 show average mean fitness values and standard deviation by GA, PSO and the proposed CHPSO for dimensions 30 and 50 respectively in 30 independent runs.

As proven in Table 3, 8 classical benchmark functions are used. It is found that for the 8 standard features taken within the have a look at the proposed CHPSO algorithm executed a higher result via giving best mean fitness and standard deviation for all functions except (f2) wherein PSO gave great mean fitness function value. The result in the table means that the proposed CHPSO gave a better performance than the original PSO in that it converges at worldwide solutions.

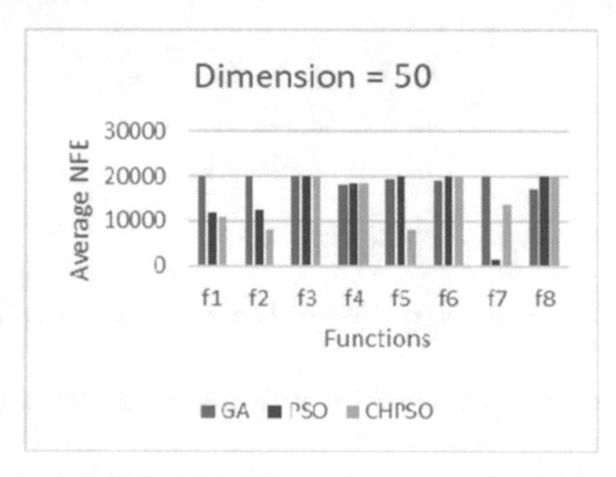

Fig. 4. Average NFE of GA, PSO and the proposed CHPSO for D = 50.

Table 3. Avg NFE of GA, PSO and the proposed CHPSO for D = 30

D = 30						
Function	GA		PSO		CHPSO	
	Mean	SD	Mean	SD	Mean	SD
*f*1	4.09E−16	1.94E−15	1.2E−201	1.98E−22	**5.49E−23**	**0.640088**
*f*2	1.866335	3.29E−14	**7.63E−15**	**1.487041**	6.9E−22	3.74E−21
*f*3	1.53E−23	7.9E−23	0.216669	122.8667	**238.7992**	**0.408601**
*f*4	3.49063	5.192793	0.398026	4.165899	**2.255447**	**2.006048**
*f*5	0.530645	0.568466	0.051125	1.801896	**5.603973**	**0.280023**
*f*6	0.068839	0.042799	0.04746	2.621595	**0.054535**	**0.039852**
*f*7	4.48E−11	2.45E−10	2E−16	3.87E−06	**4.97E−06**	**9.25E−16**
*f*8	6.62E−06	2.97E−06	0.329245	1.891857	**5.39E−15**	**8.99E−15**

As shown in Table 4, 8 classical benchmark features are used. It is located that for the 8 general capabilities taken in the observe the proposed CHPSO set of rules done a better end result through giving the best mean fitness and standard deviation for all features except (f3) in which GA gave best mean fitness function value. The result in the table implies that the proposed CHPSO gave a better performance than the authentic PSO in that it converges at global resolutions.

Generally, from the result illustrated in the tables above, the proposed CHPSO algorithm proves to be more efficient and reliable in escaping premature convergence than the GA and original PSO because the weakness of converging at a local optimum for the original PSO comes to play when solving complex both unimodal and multimodal problems since it still has poor swarm diversity as seen in the result.

Table 4. Avg NFE of GA, PSO and the proposed CHPSO for D = 50

D = 50						
Function	GA		PSO		CHPSO	
	Mean	SD	Mean	SD	Mean	SD
$f1$	7.7795E−06	2.21E−06	3.53E−06	5.1975	**3.75E−18**	**1.73E−17**
$f2$	4.07E−18	3.45E−06	70.28041	23.27691	**1.62E−06**	**2.44E−06**
$f3$	**2.894472**	**3.469198**	2931.641	1015.749	372.8988	812.7194
$f4$	22.39456	25.14135	226.1307	66.2979	**8.3794177**	**2.211705**
$f5$	4.775809	3.084979	47.41923	11.92975	**2.327313**	**5.310664**
$f6$	0.44720163	0.078309	48.44681	15.95185	**0.141085**	**0.079965**
$f7$	4.8E−08	2.61E−07	4.8407E−06	0.001491	**0.001162**	**4.04E−20**
$f8$	0.60455	0.675166	0.00187485	1.346292	**4.48E−08**	**4.58E−08**

5 Conclusion

This study discusses the implementation of the phases of this research. After the preprocessing stage, the PSO was improved by introducing chaotic map to adjust the inertia weight so as to increase the population diversity of PSO, thereby avoiding premature convergence. This new improved algorithm is known as CHPSO. In CHPSO, the logistic map is merged with PSO to adjust the inertia weight ω hence improves the convergence speed and avoid premature convergence. The result of the comparison on NFE indicates that CHPSO had higher overall performance than GA and PSO but DE slightly outperformed the CHPSO algorithm.

References

1. Ajibade, S.S.M., Ahmad, N.B.B., Shamsuddin, S.M.: A novel hybrid approach of AdaboostM2 algorithm and differential evolution for prediction of student performance. Int. J. Sci. Technol. Res. **8**(07), 65–70 (2019)

2. Makinde, O., Chakraborty, B.: On some classifiers based on multivariate ranks. Commun. Stat. Theory Methods **47**(16), 3955–3969 (2018)
3. Azmi, M.S., Arbain, N.A., Muda, A.K., Abas, Z.A., Muslim, Z.: Data normalization for triangle features by adapting triangle nature for better classification. In: 2015 IEEE Jordan Conference on Applied Electrical Engineering and Computing Technologies (AEECT), pp. 1–6. IEEE, November 2015
4. Ajibade, S.S.M., Ahmad, N.B., Shamsuddin, S.M.: An heuristic feature selection algorithm to evaluate academic performance of students. In: 2019 IEEE 10th Control and System Graduate Research Colloquium (ICSGRC), pp. 110–114. IEEE, August 2019
5. Mirjalili, S., Song Dong, J., Lewis, A., Sadiq, A.S.: Particle swarm optimization: theory, literature review, and application in airfoil design. In: Mirjalili, S., Song Dong, J., Lewis, A. (eds.) Nature-Inspired Optimizers. SCI, vol. 811, pp. 167–184. Springer, Cham (2020). https://doi.org/10.1007/978-3-030-12127-3_10
6. Chen, K., Zhou, F., Liu, A.: Chaotic dynamic weight particle swarm optimization for numerical function optimization. Knowl.-Based Syst. **139**, 23–40 (2018)
7. Lin, G.-H., Zhang, J., Liu, Z.-H.: Hybrid particle swarm optimization with differential evolution for numerical and engineering optimization. Int. J. Autom. Comput. **15**(1), 103–114 (2016). https://doi.org/10.1007/s11633-016-0990-6
8. Wang, D., Tan, D., Liu, L.: Particle swarm optimization algorithm: an overview. Soft. Comput. **22**(2), 387–408 (2017). https://doi.org/10.1007/s00500-016-2474-6
9. Felippe, W.N., Carneiro, L.F.: A discrete particle swarm algorithm for sizing optimization of steel truss structures. Paper presented at the World Congress of Structural and Multidisciplinary Optimisation (2017)
10. Rehman, T., Khan, F., Khan, S., Ali, A.: Optimizing satellite handover rate using particle swarm optimization (PSO) algorithm. J. Appl. Emerg. Sci. **7**(1), 53–63 (2017)
11. Ajibade, S.S.M., Ahmad, N.B.B., Zainal, A.: A hybrid chaotic particle swarm optimization with differential evolution for feature selection. In: 2020 IEEE Symposium on Industrial Electronics and Applications (ISIEA), pp. 1–6. IEEE, July 2020
12. Kennedy, J., Eberhart, R.: Particle swarm optimization. In: Proceedings of ICNN 1995-International Conference on Neural Networks, vol. 4, pp. 1942–1948. IEEE, November 1995
13. AlNuaimi, N., Masud, M.M., Serhani, M.A., Zaki, N.: Streaming feature selection algorithms for big data: a survey. Appl. Comput. Inform. (2020)

Adaptive and Global Approaches Based Feature Selection for Large-Scale Hierarchical Text Classification

Abubakar Ado[1(✉)], Mustafa Mat Deris[1], Noor Azah Samsudin[1], and Abdurra'uf Garba Sharifai[2]

[1] Faculty of Computer Science and Information Technology, Universiti Tun Hussein Onn Malaysia, Batu Pahat, Malaysia
adamrogo@yahoo.com

[2] Department of Computer Science, Yusuf Maitama Sule University, Kano, Nigeria

Abstract. High-feature dimensions is one of the obvious challenges facing large-scale hierarchical classification problem. One promising way to overcome such problem is reducing the features size by removing irrelevant, noise and redundant features. Filter-based feature selection methods are commonly used to construct smaller subset of most relevant features in either adaptive or global approach at each non leaf node within the hierarchy. Both the Feature selection approaches do not only reduce time and space complexity but also improve classification accuracy of the learning models. In this study, the effectiveness of the main approaches for constructing relevant features subset, that is adaptive and global approaches are analyzed using the two filter-based methods suitable for text classification. Experiment evaluation conducted on 20NG, IPC, and DMOZ-small datasets shows that implementing feature selection adaptively has more capability of selecting most relevant features, thus, achieving the best classification accuracy. Moreover, further evaluation shown integrating feature selection with LSHC records improve performance when compared to without feature selection.

Keywords: Feature selection · Filter-based method · Adaptive · Global · Large-scale

1 Introduction

The advancement of digital technology has resulted in tremendous growth of digital data from numerous sources including web directories, social networks and so on, most of which are in text format [1]. Apart from large volume problem, current text data generated known as large-scale data also faces with problems of high features size and large number of classes. Yahoo! Directory, Directory Mozilla, and International Patent Record are some few examples of such large-scale text datasets that are associated with hundred millions of features and millions of instances distributed between thousands of classes [2]. Classification of such kind of data into a large number of label classes has achieved significance predominantly in the perspective of Big Data [3]. Statistical and

F. Saeed et al. (Eds.): IRICT 2021, LNDECT 127, pp. 105–116, 2022.
https://doi.org/10.1007/978-3-030-98741-1_10

machine learning have emerged in few decades as a key approach for analyzing such kind of large-scale data. Thus, the continued exponential growth of text data and its complexities have made text classification problems more cumbersome [4, 5], while at the same time resulting in new problems for the text classification task. These problems make it very difficult to handle using the conventional learning frameworks.

Several recent applications need a classification with extremely large number of instances, features and classes to effectively analyze and extract valuable information [6]. In order to achieve this, there is a need to define a structure taxonomy upon the data first [6]. Usually, hierarchical structures provide a suitable means to organize data. Hierarchical classification (HC) is one specific problem of interest that effectively handles this large-scale taxonomy. A considerable number of Large Scale Hierarchical Classification (LSHC) approaches have been proposed to deal with the problems and challenges that have arisen, such as minimizing training time, faster class prediction, performance improvement, and reducing memory footprint utilization [1].

To reduce the processing time and memory requirements, one of the common approach is to integrate suitable dimensional reduction technique in combination with model training [1, 7]. Dimensional reduction is the known popular approach recently use to overcome the problems associated with large-scale problem (by reducing the storage and processing time requirement). The main idea behind this approach is to scale up or improve the performance of machine learning models by squeezing the feature dimensionality of a given large-scale dataset from high-dimensions into lower dimensions [8, 9]. This effective method scales up the learning model by allowing it to be trained only on the resultant lower features subset rather than the original features set [10], while maintaining or improving the classification accuracy of the model. This is possible for LSHC problems by utilizing only the features subset that are useful in discriminating among the classes at every internal node within the hierarchy. Even though, HC-models that consider parent-child relationship show improvement in classification accuracy but are computational expensive [1, 11].

In this paper, we analyze the two main filter methods based on the adaptive and global FS approaches for solving the LSHC problem. We independently integrate the considered filter methods at the preprocessing phase in the classification framework before training the models. The study wishes to answer the following research questions: What is the effect of feature selection on classification performance? Which of the feature subset construction approaches (adaptive or global) in congestion with filter methods (IG or Chi2) shows the greatest impact on classification performance?

The remaining body of this paper is systematically partitioned as follows: In Sect. 2, literature review is systematically presented. Hierarchical classification method, considered filter-based methods, and feature construction based approaches are briefly discussed in Sect. 3. Properties of the datasets used and experimental set up are devoted to Sect. 4. Experimental results and analysis are systematically placed in Sect. 5. Finally, the study ends with a conclusion and highlights of possible future work which are given in Sect. 6.

2 Literature Review

2.1 Hierarchical Classification (HC)

Following the popularity of hierarchies across various application domains, especially in text categorization, a group of researchers from the Institute of Informatics, Greece and Laboratoire d'Informatique de Grenoble, France, tried to boost the motivation of HC by jointly organizing a competition known as the Large Scale Hierarchical Text Classification (LSHTC) challenge [12]. Their efforts resulted in a sequence of competitions (2009, 2011, 2012, and 2014) that enabled them to set benchmarks for the problem [13–15]. This is achieved by evaluating the effectiveness of the methods by processing large-scale datasets with large instances and classes number. These days, datasets with defined hierarchies are widely utilized in various application domains, such as ImageNet (system for indexing hundreds of millions of images), audio hierarchy (system for organizing and classifying signals of music), international patent classification (system for surfing patent documents), DMOZ hierarchy (system for classifying and organizing internet pages), and gene hierarchy (system for classifying and organizing gene sequences) [6]. HC also known as structured classification, is a sort of classification task in which the instances' classes have a pre-defined hierarchical information, which is usually expressed as a tree (single label) or a directed acyclic graph (Multi-label) [16]. Therefore, HC takes advantage of taxonomy structure to break large scale classification problems into a subset of smaller tasks, one for every node in the tree taxonomy.

There are generally two main approaches adopted for designing HC models. The first approach, which is the simpler one called *flat classification*, does not consider inter-dependency relationships between the classes in the process of model training. The second approach, which is more complex and is called *Hierarchical Classification* considers inter-dependency relationships between the classes in the process of model training. The later approach can be further categorized into two: the Local Classifier approach and Global Classifier approach. The first approach (LC) considers local parent-child relationships in the processing of model [1]. This approach is further subdivided into three approaches based on how hierarchies are explored from the parent to the child [17], namely: Local Classifier per Node (LCN), Local Classifier per Parent Node (LCPN), and Local Classifier per Level (LCL) [12]. The second approach, known as the Global Classification (GC) approach, takes the classification problem as a whole and trains a single global classification model at the same time, taking the hierarchy information into consideration [12]. This approach is more complex and computational expensive than the Local approach. Both the approaches followed a similar approach in predicting new examples.

2.2 Dimensional Reduction (DR)

Dimensionality reduction [9, 18] is a process of converting or transforming high-dimensional space into low-dimensional space. With the recent increase in high-dimensional data, proposing and employing different reduction techniques has become necessary in various application domains [19], especially in text classification. Dimensional reduction constructs a lower discrepant features set by taking input features set (high-dimensional) and transforms it into a lower features representation (low-dimension) while preserving the important information as much as possible [20]. The resultant low feature representation of the input data aids to tackle dimensionality curse issue and can be easily visualized, analyzed and processed. Dimensional reduction can be broadly categorized in to three groups namely, Feature Selection, Feature Extraction, and Feature Hashing.

Feature Selection (FS) reduces the size of features set by selecting small subset of most informative features and eliminating those features that are known to be noise, irrelevant, and redundant from a given input set of features [21, 22]. The methods that utilizes FS technique basically adopts either the strategy of subsets performance evaluation or feature ranking strategy [23]. *Features Extraction (FE)* [24–26] and *Feature Hashing (FH)* [27–29] transform or project the original input features into lower feature space [30], while preserving Euclidean distance. The techniques reduce the dimensionality by taking the whole set of original features and projecting them into a smaller index space, whereby the discriminating features lie within the low-dimensional space. This study revolves around FS. Therefore, the following section will detail more on the approaches of FS.

2.3 Feature Selection Approaches

Generally, FS methods are broadly grouped into filter methods, wrapper methods, and embedded methods [21, 31, 32]. Filter methods are independent that they do not interact with classifier when constructing an informative feature subset. They rely on metrics for evaluating and ranking the importance of a feature prior to the classification. The methods can attain quick feature sorting to effectively filter out a high number of non-relevant or noise features [32]. They select features subset by considering the usefulness of a feature according to evaluation metrics [21, 32]. Wrapper methods are dependent on classifiers that they frequently interact with the classification algorithm in order to construct a subset of informative features [21, 32]. They evaluate a particular feature subset by training and testing a given classifier, and they are tailored to a particular classifier [33]. The methods in this group have poor computational efficiency but result in high classification accuracy. These methods are not usually favored in text classification task [34]. Embedded Methods integrate classifiers with feature selection technique during the training phase and optimally search feature subset by designing an optimization function [21, 35]. Like wrapper methods, embedded methods frequently interact with the classifier but have better computational efficiency than wrapper methods and are also tailored to a specific classifier [34].

Upon all the FS approaches explained so far, filter approaches are shown to be computational inexpensive, good storage compression, and preserves sparsity [27, 36]. These make them scalable and more advantageous in large scale problems. Therefore, this study integrates filter-based based FS methods into the Large-scale HC problem framework. However, few studies in the past consider reducing features dimensionality prior to training HC, which shown to achieve significant improvement.

3 Material and Methods

3.1 Hierarchical Classification Method

The HC method uses the hierarchical structure of a given dataset to split the classification problem into simpler task problems, one per internal node of the tree hierarchy. Any classification model can be extended and used as a baseline model to perform HC by placing a distinct classifier at each non-leaf node of the tree structure. To predict category label y_i for unknown input instance x_i, the classification process which referred as to Top-Down approach greedily moves down the tree structure until it reaches the target leaf node y_i. As presented in Algorithm 1. The process starts at the root node $\mathcal{Q}$ and chooses the best child nodes $c(n)$ recursively until it reaches a category label $y_i \in \ell$ (terminal node). Where ℓ is a set of leaf nodes. In this study, we used LR (Logistic Regression) and SVM (Support Vector Machine) as the baseline models for training.

Algorithm 1: Top-Down Hierarchical Classification

Input: Input: instance x_i , parameters $w_c^{\mathcal{Q}}$
Output: ℓ_s
Set $\mathcal{Q} = 0$ \\ Start from the root node
Repeat
$\mathcal{Q} = argmax_{\{c:(\mathcal{Q},c)\in E\}(w_c^{\mathcal{Q}})^T \hat{}x_i}$ \\ Transverse through the most weighted child
Until $|c(n)| = 1$ \\ Until a node with single category label is reach.
Return ℓ_s \\ Return the predicted label

3.2 Information Gain Method

The Information Gain (IG) is an information theory-based method commonly used in statistics to model word association [36, 38]. IG measures the amount of information presence or absence of a feature and its contribution in making the appropriate classification prediction on labelled classes. The method computes and assigns a score to each feature by considering the variation between the entropy obtained based on the presence or absence of feature/term in a class [4, 39]. High IG score indicates the discriminating capability of a feature and ranked top. The general formula for calculating IG of a given feature t is given in Eq. (1).

$$I(t, c) = \sum_{c\in\{c_i,\bar{c}_i\}} \sum_{t\in\{t_k,\bar{t}_k\}} P(t, c) * \log\left(\frac{P(t, c)}{P(t) * P(c)}\right) \quad (1)$$

Where $P(t,c)$ is the probability of class c and occurrence of the feature t, $P(t)$ is the probability of class containing feature t, $P(c)$ is the probability of class c. $\overline{t_k}$ *and* $\overline{c_k}$ donate feature not present, and class not present, respectively.

3.3 Chi-square Method

Chi-Square (Chi2) is a statistical-based and important non-parametric test method used to Compare more than two attributes for a randomly chosen data [34]. It is commonly known as independence test, and the method is applied to test if the concurrence of a particular term and a particular category are not dependent [36]. Chi2 generates a value that reveals the relationship between a term and category during feature filtering. The Chi2 score of a give term t_k for a category c_i is calculated as:

$$Chi - square(t_k c_i) = \frac{NP(t_k)^2 (P(c_i|t_k) - P(c_i))^2}{P(t_k)(1 - P(t_k))P(c_i)(1 + P(c_i))} \quad (2)$$

Where $P(t_k)$ is the probability of a document that contains term t_k, $P(c_i)$ is the probability of documents that belongs to class c_i; $P(c_i|t_k)$ is the conditional probabilities of a document that belongs to c_i; given that it contained t_k.

3.4 Adaptive and Global Approaches

There are two different approaches for constructing discrepant features subset at each internal node in the hierarchy which are adaptive and global approach. For adaptive approach, variable number and different features are selected at each non leaf node within the hierarchy to construct the subset of discrepant features. The size and the features elected at the parent node should not necessary be the same as that of children nodes (likewise among the sibling nodes). For the global approach, the same number of features is selected at every node in the entire hierarchy, and also the same set of discrepant features is selected for every tree branch in the hierarchy. The approach construct discrepant features subset by selecting equal features for each tree branch rooted to the leaf node. The two approaches are nearly equivalent in terms of computational complexity because model tuning and optimization need almost equal runtime, which makes up the main computational fraction [1].

4 Dataset and Experiment Settings

We have conducted experimental evaluation using three benchmark text datasets, including 20Newsgroup (20NG) [40], International Patient Classification (IPC) [41], and Directly Mozilla (DMOZ-small) [15]. Table 1 presents the key summary properties of the datasets. We believe all the datasets are sparse and highly dimensional.

For all the experiments, we utilized the standard train-test partitions available in order to preserve comparability with previously evaluations presented, see Table 1. We further split the training set into 90% as the main training set (to train Top-Down models) and 10% as the small validation set (to fine tune the regularization parameter). The model is trained with a set of a parameter values ranges from 0.01 to 1000 in steps of "x10", and utilized the validation dataset to select the best value. The models are trained again using the whole training dataset (including the validation dataset) using the best choosing parameter value, we measure the models' performance using the unseen test dataset. Conventionally, we build bag of words (BOW) and vectored the features with

l_2-*norm* using TF-IDF transformation. As for the FS, we select the best initial threshold by varying the size of features ranging from 10% to 80% of the entire features set in steps of 10. From the preliminary results, we chose the threshold at which the model attained the best performance. We use Top-down approach with Logistic Regression (LR) as the baseline classifier. Therefore, training multi-class LR in respect of ith child (C_i) of a corresponding internal node n, the respective objective function is formulated as given in Eq. (3)

$$LR\_f_n^c = \min_{w_n^c}\left[\lambda \sum_{i=1}^{T_n} \log\left(1 + \exp\left(-(y_i)_n^c \left(w_n^c\right)^T x_i\right)\right) + \left\|w_n^c\right\|_2^2\right] \tag{3}$$

Where $\lambda > 0$ denotes penalty parameter value for mis-classification, $\|\cdot\|_2^2$ denotes regularization term, and T_n is the total number of instances. To get the optimal weight vector w_n^c, one of the above equations is solve (based on the model used) for every child C_i belonging to the corresponding node n within the taxonomy $\mathcal{H}$. The entire set of parameters for $\mathcal{C}$(n) that is $W_n = \left[w_n^c\right]_{c\in C(n)}$ constructs the multi-class learned model at that particular node while total parameters for all non-leaf nodes that is $W = [W_n]_{n\in N}$ constructs the TD-learned model.

Table 1. Properties of the datasets used.

Dataset	#Training doc	#Testing doc	#Features	#Classes	#Nodes	Height
20NG	11269	7505	61188	20	28	4
IPC	46324	28926	1123497	451	553	4
DMOZ-small	6323	1858	51033	1139	2388	6

The performance of the HC methods is reported using suitable metrics commonly used for HC in literature, namely, Micro-f1 (gives equal importance to every document), Macro-f1 (gives equal importance to every category), Hierarchical-f1 and Hierarchical-error [6], which are computed as follows:

$$Micro - F1 = \frac{2PR}{P + R} \tag{4}$$

$$Macro - F1 = \frac{1}{|\ell|} \sum\nolimits_{n=1}^{|\ell|} \frac{2P_nR_n}{P_n + R_n} \tag{5}$$

$$hF1 = \frac{2 \times hP \times hR}{hP + hR} \tag{6}$$

$$HE = \frac{1}{N} \sum\nolimits_{i=1}^{m} E\left(\hat{y}_i, y_i\right) \tag{7}$$

Where P and R denote precision and recall, respectively, P_n and R_n are the precision and recall for leaf node n, $|\ell|$ denotes total number of labels or classes, *hP, hR, hF1,* and *HE* represent hierarchical precision, hierarchical recall, hierarchical-f1, and hierarchical-error, respectively, $A(y_i)$ denotes all the ancestors of the categories plus the true label, $A(\widehat{y_i})$ denotes all the ancestors of the categories plus the predicted label, and $E(\widehat{y_i}, y_i)$ denotes the length of undirected path from y_i to the label category.

5 Results Analysis

Table 1 shows the micro-f1 and macro-f1 comparison of IG and Chi2 methods by considering both adaptive and global approaches against All Features (AF). The face bolded indicates the best results on comparing between adaptive and global FS while figures with subscript plus sign (+) indicates the best results when considering AF. The results from the table shows that Chi2 outperformed IG in all comparisons except on micro-F1 of IPC. This is because IG usually assigns higher weight to lengthier documents when computing features importance and in addition, it favors those terms that are distributed in several categories, while those terms have less discriminating capability in text classification problem. Chi2 selects more rare terms than IG, even though IG also select rare terms as much as possible but its chosen criteria does not essentially choose the terms that improve classification accuracy. We can see from the both tables that adaptive approach based FS achieves better performance for all datasets when compare with global approach. This shows that selecting the same set and number of features for all internal nodes will not significantly improve classification accuracy. For instance, a particular feature in the parent node could be more informative in discriminating the children nodes but it could be less informative when it comes to discriminating the grandchildren. On comparing against AF we can see that adaptive based FS still achieves best performance across all the datasets (with around 2% accuracy improvement). In general, adaptive FS is significantly better due to its ability to selects small subset of variable number features that are more important for discriminating data-sparse nodes that exist in LSHC datasets.

Figure 1 shows the hierarchical error comparison based on TD-LR for 20NG, IPC and DMOZ-Small datasets with feature selection (Chi2) and all features (AF). We consider only Chi2 due to its outstanding performance in the previous experiment and also due to space limit. We can see that less error is committed when the classifiers are used with feature selection compared to AF (without feature selection). This is because feature selection methods able to filter out irrelevant features that may interrupt the modelling of linear classifier in process of discriminating children nodes at each level within the hierarchy. Moreover, adaptive based FS gives the lowest error, this reveals its capability to select the most discrepant number of features at each non leaf nodes in the hierarchy. Another observation is that global based FS achieves almost similar error when compared with all features (AF) on DMOZ-small dataset while achieves significant improvement on 20NG and IPC datasets (Table 2).

Table 3 and 4 show the level-wise performance and hierarchical-f1 analysis for AFS, GFS, and AF using IPC and DMOZ-Small datasets. From the tables we can observe the poor performance of the models in terms of hierarchical-f1 (hF1) relative to the baseline level three and level five of IPC and DMOZ-small, respectively. As stated by other studies, we also attribute the obtained result to the backside of top-down hierarchical approach; errors occur at upper level of the hierarchy are not recoverable at the subsequent

Table 2. Performance comparison of adaptive and global approaches upon IG and Chi2 based filter method in terms of micro-f1 and macro-f1 using TD-LR

Dataset	Metric	IG		Chi		AF
		Adaptive	Global	Adaptive	Global	
20NG	micro-F1	77.09	77.01	**78.12**$^{+}$	**77.90**	76.10
	macro-F1	77.03	76.93	**77.94**$^{+}$	**77.83**	75.84
IPC	micro-F1	**48.94**$^{+}$	46.45	48.55	**46.90**	46.83
	macro-F1	42.23	39.62	**42.46**$^{+}$	**40.07**	40.75
DMOZ-small	micro-F1	42.02	40.94	**42.22**$^{+}$	**41.04**	39.91
	macro-F1	27.81	26.68	**28.02**$^{+}$	**26.77**	25.80

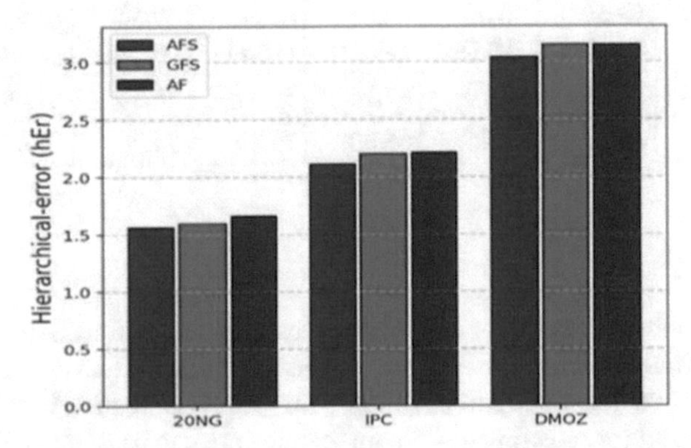

Fig. 1. Performance comparison of feature selection based on adaptive, global and all features in terms of hierarchical-error using TD-LR.

lower levels and, therefore propagate down to the leaf level, affecting the performance of TD-models. We can also observe that higher score is obtained at uppermost level compared to the lower level. This is because at upper levels each of the children nodes that has to be categories is a multiple combination of leaf classes which could not be accurately modelled using the linear classifiers. Furthermore, AFS achieves the best results on level wise comparison (maximum accuracy improvement of about 6.61% and 5.55% using IPC and DMOZ-small dataset. When compared to GFS, this demonstrates its ability to select the most relevant and informative features. In general, from the tables we can see that the performance with feature selection is better than without feature selection.

Table 3. Level-wise analysis for adaptive and global based feature selection and all features in terms of hierarchical-fi based on TD-LR using IPC dataset.

	L1	L2	L3	hF1
AFS	92.82 **(+4.92)**	89.94 **(+6.61)**	79.20 **(+2.8)**	68.41 **(+2.48)**
GFS	90.57	85.73	77.85	66.84
AF	87.90	83.33	76.40	65.93

Table 4. Level-wise analysis for adaptive and global based feature selection and all features in terms of hierarchical-fi based on TD-LR using DMOZ-small dataset.

	L1	L2	L3	L4	L5	hF1
AFS	92.54 **(+3.51)**	90.00 **(+5.55)**	88.01 **(+3.11)**	84.40 **(+5.11)**	77.34 **(+2.44)**	68.85 **(+0.86)**
GFS	91.13	88.70	87.14	80.47	76.84	67.09
AF	89.03	84.45	85.30	79.29	74.90	67.99

6 Conclusion

The main approaches for constructing relevant features subset for LSHC problem that is adaptive and global approach are analyzed in this study. For extensive comparative, two filter based feature selection methods suitable for text classification in respect to IG and Chi2 are considered for selecting discrepant features prior to training of TD-LR baseline classifier. Series of experiments conducted on 20NG, IPC, and DMOZ-small benchmark datasets, results show that using Chi2 method in an adaptive approach achieves maximum improvement of around 2% accuracy when compared with the other approaches across all the datasets. Further analysis showed that integrating feature selection method with LSHC achieved significant improvement against all features (without feature selection).

References

1. Ado, A., Samsudin, N.A., Mat Deris, M.: A new feature hashing approach based on term weight for dimensional reduction. In: IEEE International Congress of Advance Technology and Engineering (ICOTEN), pp. 1–7 (2021)
2. Naik, A., Rangwala, H.: Embedding feature selection for large-scale hierarchical classification. In: IEEE International Conference on Big Data (Big Data), pp. 1212–1221 (2016)
3. Babbar, R., Partalas, L., Gaussier, E., Amini, M., Amblard, C.: Learning taxonomy adaptation in large-scale classification. J. Mach. Learn. Res. **17**, 1–37 (2016)
4. Ado, A., Deris, M.M., Noor Azah, S., Aliyu, A.: A new feature filtering approach by integrating IG and T-test evaluation metrics for text classification. Int. J. Adv. Comput. Sci. Appl. **12**(6), 500–510 (2021)

5. Pilnenskiy, N., Smetannikov, I.: Feature selection algorithms as one of the Python data analytical tools †. Futur. Internet Artic. **54**(12), 1–14 (2020)
6. Naik, A., Rangwala, H.: Large Scale Hierarchical Classification: State of the Art. Springer Briefs in Computer Science, pp. 1–104. Springer, Cham (2018). https://doi.org/10.1007/978-3-030-01620-3
7. Zhou, D., Xiao, L., Wu, M.: Hierarchical classification via orthogonal transfer. In: International Conference on Machine Learning (ICML), pp. 801–808 (2011)
8. Ikeuchi, K.: Computer Vision: A Reference Guide, 2014th edn, vol. 2. Springer, Boston (2014). https://doi.org/10.1007/978-0-387-31439-6
9. Krishnan, R., Samaranayake, V.A., Jagannathan, S.: A hierarchical dimension reduction approach for big data with application to fault diagnostics. J. Big Data Res. **18**, 100121 (2019)
10. Cunningham, J.P., Ghahramani, Z.: Linear dimensionality reduction: survey, insights, and generalizations. J. Mach. Learn. Res. **16**(1), 2859–2900 (2015)
11. Gopal, S., Yang, Y.: Recursive regularization for large-scale classification with hierarchical and graphical dependencies. In: ACM SIGKDD, pp. 257–265 (2013)
12. Alan, R., Jaques, P.A., Francisco, J.: An analysis of hierarchical text classification using word embeddings. Inf. Sci. (Ny) **471**, 216–232 (2019)
13. Naik, A., Rangwala, H.: Filter based taxonomy modification for improving hierarchical classification. arXiv:1603.00772v3 [cs.AI], vol. 3, pp. 1–14 (2016)
14. Charuvaka, A., Rangwala, H.: HierCost: improving large scale hierarchical classification with cost sensitive learning. In: Appice, A., Rodrigues, P.P., Santos Costa, V., Soares, C., Gama, J., Jorge, A. (eds.) ECML PKDD 2015. LNCS (LNAI), vol. 9284, pp. 675–690. Springer, Cham (2015). https://doi.org/10.1007/978-3-319-23528-8_42
15. Partalas, I., et al.: LSHTC: a benchmark for large-scale text classification. CoRR, vol. abs/1503, pp. 1–9 (2015)
16. Ramírez-corona, M., Sucar, L.E., Morales, E.F.: Hierarchical multilabel classification based on path evaluation. Int. J. Approx. Reason. **68**, 179–193 (2016)
17. Silla, C.N., Freitas, A.A.: A survey of hierarchical classification across different application domains. Data Min. Knowl. Discov. **22**(1–2), 31–72 (2011)
18. Zhang, S., Chen, X., Li, P.: Principal component analysis algorithm based on mutual information credibility. In: 2019 International Conference on Computation and Information Sciences, ICCIS, pp. 536–545 (2019)
19. Ayesha, S., Hanif, M.K., Talib, R.: Overview and comparative study of dimensionality reduction techniques for high dimensional data. Inf. Fusion **59**(01), 44–58 (2020)
20. Juvonen, A., Sipola, T., Hämäläinen, T.: Online anomaly detection using dimensionality reduction techniques for HTTP log analysis. Comput. Netw. **91**, 46–56 (2015)
21. Rong, M., Gong, D., Gao, X.: Feature selection and its use in Big Data: challenges, methods, and trends. IEEE Access **7**, 19709–19725 (2019)
22. Sharif, W., Samsudin, N.A., Deris, M.M., Khalid, S.K.A.: A technical study on feature ranking techniques and classification algorithms. J. Eng. Appl. Sci. **13**(9), 7074–7080 (2018)
23. El-Hasnony, I.M., Barakat, S.I., Elhoseny, M., Mostafa, R.R.: Improved feature selection model for Big Data analytics. IEEE Access **8**, 66989–67004 (2020)
24. Lhazmir, S., El Moudden, I., Kobbane, A.: Feature extraction based on principal component analysis for text categorization. In: 6th IFIP International Conference on Performance Evaluation and Modelling in Wired and Wireless Networks, PEMWN 2017, pp. 1–6 (2018)
25. Hira, Z.M., Gillies, D.F.: A review of feature selection and feature extraction methods applied on micraarray data. Adv. Bioinform. 1–13 (2015)
26. Subasi, A.: Practical Guide for Biomedical Signals Analysis Using Machine Learning Techniques, 1st edn. Elsevier Inc., Amsterdam (2019)

27. Freksen, C.B., Kamma, L., Larsen, K.G.: Fully understanding the hashing trick. In: International Conference on Neural Information Processing System, NIPS 2018, pp. 5394–5404 (2018)
28. Shi, Q., et al.: Hash kernels. In: Proceedings of Machine Learning Research, MLR, pp. 496–503 (2009)
29. Weinberger, K., Dasgupta, A., Langford, J., Smola, A., Attenberg, J.: Feature hashing for large scale multitask learning. In: 26th Annual International Conference on Machine Learning, ICML 2009, pp. 1113–1120 (2009)
30. Khalid, S., Khalil, T., Nasreen, S.: A survey of feature selection and feature extraction techniques in machine learning. In: 2014 Science and Information Conference, SAI 2014, pp. 372–378 (2014)
31. Gu, N., Fan, M., Du, L., Ren, D.: Efficient sequential feature selection based on adaptive eigenspace model. Neurocomputing **161**, 199–209 (2015)
32. Li, M., Wang, H., Yang, L., Liang, Y., Shang, Z.: Fast hybrid dimensionality reduction method for classification based on feature selection and grouped feature extraction. Expert Syst. Appl. **150**(July), 1–10 (2020)
33. EL Aboudi, N., Benhlima, L.: A review on wrapper feature selection approaches. In: International Conference of Engineering and MIS (ICEMIS), pp. 1–5 (2016)
34. Şahin, D.Ö., Kılıç, E.: Two new feature selection metrics for text classification. J. Control Meas. Electron. Comput. Commun. **60**(2), 162–171 (2019)
35. Das, A.K., Sengupta, S., Bhattacharyya, S.: A group incremental feature selection for classification using rough set theory based genetic algorithm. Appl. Soft Comput. J. **64**(April), 400–411 (2018)
36. Jagadeesan, M., Understanding sparse JL for feature hashing. In: Proceeding of Advances in Neural Information Processing Systems, NeurlPS 2019, pp. 1–31 (2019)
37. Haris, B. S., Revanasidappa, M.B.: A comprehensive survey on various feature selection methods to categorize text documents. Int. J. Comput. Appl. **164**(8), 1–7 (2017)
38. Ado, A., Samsudin, N.A., Deris, M.M., Ahmed, A.: Comparative analysis of integrating multiple filter-based feature selection methods using vector magnitude score on text classification. In: 11th Annual International Conference on Industrial Engineering and Operations Management (IEOM), pp. 4664–4676 (2021)
39. Zhou, H., Han, S., Liu, Y.: A novel feature selection approach based on document frequency of segmented term frequency. IEEE Access **6**, 53811–53821 (2018)
40. Dhillon, I.S., Mallela, S., Kumar, R.: A divisive information-theoretic feature clustering algorithm for text classification. J. Mach. Learn. Res. **3**, 1265–1287 (2003)
41. WIPO: Guide to the International Patent Classification (2016)

Ensemble Method for Online Sentiment Classification Using Drift Detection-Based Adaptive Window Method

Idris Rabiu[1,4](✉), Naomie Salim[1], Maged Nasser[1], Faisal Saeed[2], Waseem Alromema[3], Aisha Awal[4], Elijah Joseph[4], and Amit Mishra[5]

[1] School of Computing, Univerti Teknologi Malaysia, 81310 Bahru, Johor, Malaysia
irabiu@ibbu.edu.ng
[2] College of Computer Science and Engineering, Taibah University, Medina, Saudi Arabia
[3] Computer Science and Information Systems, Applied College, Taibah University, Medina, Saudi Arabia
[4] Ibrahim Badamsi Babangida University, Lapai, Niger State, Nigeria
[5] Baze University, Abuja, Nigeria

Abstract. Textual data streams have been widely applied in real-world applications where online users' expressed their opinions for online products. Mining this stream of data is a challenging task for researchers as a result of changes in data distribution, a phenomenon widely known as concept drift. Most of the existing classification methods incorporated drift detection methods that depend on the classification errors. However, these methods are prone to higher false-positive or missed detections rates. Thus, there is a need for more sensitive detection methods that can detect the maximum number of drifts in the data stream to improve classification accuracy. In this paper, we present a drift detection-based adaptive windowing for ensemble classifier, an adaptive unsupervised learning algorithm for sentiment classification, and opinion mining. The proposed algorithm employs four different dissimilarity measures to quantify the magnitude of concept drift in data streams, to improve the classification performance. Series of the experiments were conducted on the real-world datasets and the results demonstrated the efficiency of our proposed model.

Keywords: Data streams · Sentiment analysis · Concept drift · Ensemble classification

1 Introduction

Data streams are a well-ordered sequence of samples that were generated continuously in real-time [1]. Examples of data streams include recommender systems, computer network traffic streams, financial time series, and various sensor data among others. Besides, the sentiment classification in stream data mining applications, each of which is made up of an instance and a class label is most widely explored using the stream classification models [2]. Unlike the traditional stationary settings, stream data are very

F. Saeed et al. (Eds.): IRICT 2021, LNDECT 127, pp. 117–128, 2022.
https://doi.org/10.1007/978-3-030-98741-1_11

different due to the problems such as the increase in data volume, read-only once, different types of concept drift, and imbalanced situations [3].

In the text stream analysis, especially review-based sentiment classification, these issues become more challenging as review contents are unpredictable and mostly a user's perception changes often times [4, 5]. Sometimes, users express their opinions for a given item based on their characteristics which may change over time. For example, in a phone product, a user may have a positive sentiment about the phone, and at a specific time if some features change (i.e., some add or remove), then suddenly some terms associated with the new features may be appeared or disappeared in the user's review for the phone, revealing a different sentiment. In such a dynamic environment, the classifier performance degrades as a result of these shifts in the underlying distribution of data [6, 7]. Concept drifts are generally categorized as abrupt and gradual concept drifts dependent on the speed [8]. A number of approaches have been presented to address concept drifts, which are basically comprised of three groups, such as window-based, weight-based, and ensemble-based methods [5]. Among these methods, the ensemble-based method is particularly popular and effective, but it calls for a more powerful design to accommodate the high speed and dynamic data streams environments. Moreover, the ensemble method combines various base methods leveraging the advantages of their joint performances, to increase the predictive power that any of the individual methods can achieve [9, 10]. In recent times, several efforts have proposed the ensemble approach and much success has been recorded [10–12]. However, most of these methods only integrate base classifiers to improve the predictive performance of data streams, they do not explicitly consider concept drift detection [13–15].

In this paper, a novel drift detection-based adaptive windowing (DDAW) is proposed for ensemble classifier in online user sentiment classification that incorporates drift detectors intending to simultaneously identify different types of concept drifts, rather than using a static ensemble of the classifier. To this end, the contribution of this paper is summarized in three folds:

i. Concept drift detection technique is deployed to provide fast reaction to sudden changes. Moreover, a two-window method is used to handle drift detection tasks.
ii. To quantify the drift magnitude, different dissimilarity measures are explored based on their performances to measure the changes between two windows, that is, the reference window and the current window, respectively. Besides, the framework for a novel adaptive ensemble classification method is presented, which considers concept drift to improve the predictive performance of the ensemble classifier.
iii. A series of experiments were performed on two real-world datasets and the results show the superiority of our model over the state-of-the-art models in terms of accuracy.

The rest of this paper is as follows: Sect. 2 provides short review of the related works. The proposed method is presented in Sect. 3, while the experimental settings and results are presented in Sect. 4 to assess the performance of the proposed model. Finally, the paper is concluded in Sect. 5.

2 Related Works

In this section, we present a review of the related works for change detection. Accordingly, this paper investigates how to exploit the textual data features to detect and handle concept drift of user opinions which have widely appeared in real-world online applications, and posed a significant challenge for classification accuracy [16]. In most cases, concept drift detection methods work together with a base classifier such as NB and LibSVM (SVM) models to improve classification accuracy [17–19]. Generally, the stream classification models are aimed to train the prediction models using both the historical data and current examples in the stream to predict the true class of incoming examples [20, 21]. However, the data instances arrive at a higher rate, which classifiers need to process with stringent constraints of time and memory. To address these issues, ensemble paradigms are designed for streaming environments for enhancing classification accuracy [11]. The existing ensemble methods mainly address the issue of improving the accuracy of prediction by training individual classifiers on different portions of data instances and combining them via voted weighting schemes to predict the incoming instances [11]. Unfortunately, such methods could not deal with concept drift properly.

Essentially, there are two types of works concerning the concept drift detection, which are categorized into evolving-based and trigger-based learners [4]. With evolving learning approach, the learners are updated periodically independent of whether the change has occurred or not. This means that evolving learners do not detect changes explicitly and therefore they do not influence the decision on how the new model should be reconstructed [5]. Under this category, two approaches are distinguished, namely instance selection and instance weighting. Instance selection involves selecting the instances that are more appropriate to the current concept. The most common variant of the instance selection method is the time window approach that moves in varying sizes or a fixed size over the newly arrived instances [22]. Instance weighting approach on the other hand processes weighting of the instances by employing the decay functions according to their age and relevance to the current concept [22].

The second category of adaptation method which is more prevalent is the trigger-based learners. The trigger-based approach works in conjunction with detection models which produced signals, indicating the need to update the current model. Trigger-based models are of two types. The first group produced the signals based on information about classifier's performance while the second group is by monitoring changes in data distributions using dissimilarity measures. Based on the first group, some references [23–25] used the difference between the accuracy of the recent instances and that of the overall data to detect the concept drift. Also, [5] for example proposed a model to detect concept drift using the classifier's error rate based stream data as the change indicator. The monitoring approach is that when the error rate exceeds the threshold, a concept drift is signaled, and a model update is required. However, the problem with this method is that if the sliding window is mall it produces too many false alarms. But, if the sliding window is too large, it does not perform well on graduate drifts. Another type of drift detection approach is by using the batch mode for monitoring two distributions. Distributions over these two windows are compared based on dissimilarities measures and performing statistical tests with the null hypothesis H_0, indicating that the distributions are equal, and alternative hypothesis H_1, indicating that change has occurred [26]. This is rarely used in the previous works. A common advantage of this approach is that it doesn't depend on the classification error rate to signal drift detection, unlike the above-mentioned methods. As a result, our method takes advantage of these approaches and the ensemble of the classifier, which is aimed to detect different types of drifts simultaneously.

3 Proposed Ensemble Method for Sentiment Classification Using DDAW

This section presents the proposed DDAW approach for sentiment classification, which uses an unsupervised concept drift detection method that triggers the drift points as they occur more timely and efficiently. A trigger-based approach observes all the possible drift points in the data streams and then adapts the model accordingly. DDAW is specifically designed to deal with the concept drift of online users' sentiments and opinions based on their review data. It aims at enhancing the ability of the ensemble model to deal with the drift of user opinions and maximizing the accuracy of the model. To this end, the proposed model comprises two components: the drift detection component and the classification component. Each of these components is detailed as follows:

3.1 Drift Detection Component

As noted in the literature, most of the concept drift detection methods work with the classifiers or learning models. Also, most of these change detections techniques focus on detecting changes in the error rate of the classifiers, without considering changes in the distribution of data [27, 28]. To build our DDAW, we adopt the two-window scheme as shown in Fig. 1, which is also the most extensively used method by comparing the data distribution between two consecutive windows [11].

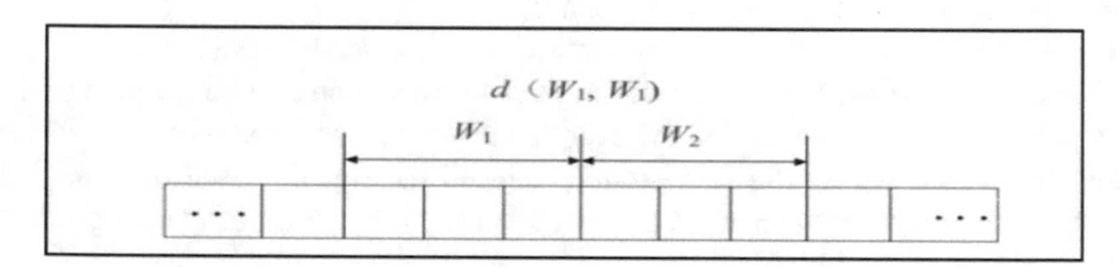

Fig. 1. Two-window scheme for change detection model

From Fig. 1, W_1 and W_2 represent the reference and current windows, respectively. And the size of each window is n. In stream mining, the problem of drift detection is to test the null hypothesis H_0 against alternative hypothesis H_1 as shown below:

$$\begin{cases} H_0 \ d(W_1, W_2) \leq \varepsilon \\ H_1 \ d(W_1, W_2) > \varepsilon \end{cases}$$

Where ε is a distance-based threshold that determines if the change has occur, and $d(W_1, W_2)$ is a distance function that measures the similarity of two windows. When the dissimilarity between two windows is greater than a given threshold, then, a change has occurred. In this study, four distance measures are considered to be used to compare the current window and the reference window based on their efficiency for drift detection, such as Hellinger distance (HD), Kullback–Leibler divergence (KD), Total variation distance (TVD), and the Kolmogorov–Smirnov statistic (KS distance) [26]. The steps for the drift detection method is presented in Algorithm 1.

Algorithm 1: Drift Detection-based Adaptive Windowing

```
Input:
   D: A set of review textual data
    Window size n
Output: Drift detection
Begin
1. Initialize t = 0;
2. Set reference window W_1 = {d_{t+1}, ..., d_{t+n}};
3. Set detection window W_2 = {d_{t+n+1}, ..., d_{t+2n}};
4.     for each instance in D do
5.          Calculate d(W_1, W_2) according to any of equation (4.6) to (4.11);
6.          Calculate ε according to Theorem 1;
7.             if d(W_1, W_2) > ε then
8.                    t ++;
9.                    Report drift at time t;
10.                   Clear all windows and go to step 2;
11.             else
12.                    Slide W_2 by 1 point;
13.             end if
14.       end for
15. end
```

3.2 Ensemble Method for Sentiment Classification Using DDAW

In recent times, ensemble approach is mostly used for stream data classification to enhance the accuracy [11, 20, 29]. As illustrated in Fig. 2, the proposed ensemble method maintains a pool of classifiers, where each classifier represents the existing concept to be used to predict the class of incoming instances based on the weighted voting weighted scheme. In addition, a change detector was employed to track the distribution between two consecutive windows, one representing the older instance and the other the more recent instances. Once a drift occurs, a new classifier is trained on the new data and added to the pool to represent a new concept identified.

To generate the final prediction, it assumed that, as new models were added, the previously added classifiers lose their weights and thus contribute little to the final result, and need to be pruned from the ensemble classifier. Moreover, it is worth noting that, as new classifiers are being added, the total number of classifiers in the ensemble is checked if it has exceeded the predefined maximum limit K (number of classifiers

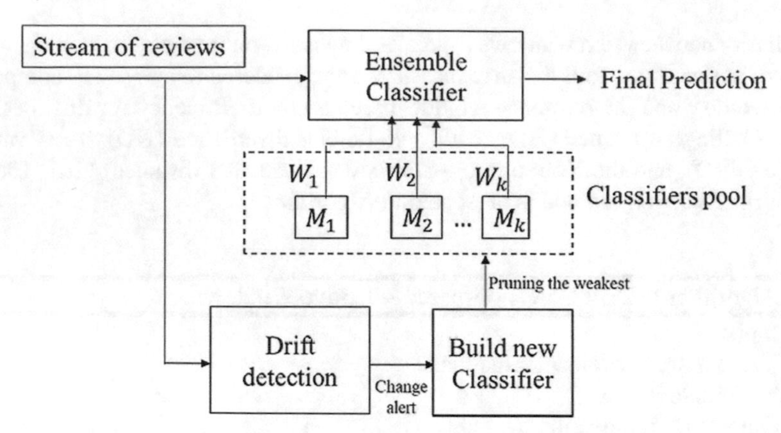

Fig. 2. The structure of the proposed ensemble learning models

maintained for prediction), then the classifier with the least weight is removed from the ensemble before adding a new classifier.

Weighting Mechanism. As noted in the previous sections, the idea is to train an ensemble of classifiers from a different portion of the data stream. Then, based on their performance on current data, the weights of each classifier are updated. When a new model is built as a result of drift detection, the weaker models are pruned and only the top k-classifiers are kept. This implies that two key strategies play a vital role in this approach. These comprise of weighting the member classifiers and pruning the weakest classifier - removing the worst-performing classifier. For each incoming instance d, each ensemble member $M_i \in E$ is weighted according to Eq. 1 when concept drift is detected.

$$W_i = \frac{1}{MSE_r + MSE_i + \alpha} \tag{1}$$

Where W_i is the weight of classifier M_i, and α is added to avoid division by zero. MSE_r and MSE_i are the root mean square error of the model M_i performance on the data in the reference window and data in the current window, respectively. The steps for the ensemble method for sentiment classification with drift detection can be given in Algorithm 2 as follows:

Algorithm 2: Ensemble method using DDAW algorithm

```
Input:
      D : A set of review textual data;
      k: the size of ensemble classifier
Output:
      E: the ensemble of classifier
1 Begin
2    E ← Ø;
3    for all instances dt in D do
4    W ← W ∪ {dt};
5       if change detected = = true (according to equation (4.6) and (4.11)) then
6          create a new classifier M';
7          update the weight of all classifiers in an ensemble based on eq. (4.12)
8          if |E| < k then
9                E ← E ∪ M';
10              else prune the worst classifier;
11         else
12              reuse the classifier in E;
13         end if
14       end if
15    end for
16 end
```

---

4 Experimental Results and Discussions

In this section, we first present the results and discussed the performance of the different settings of our proposed DDAW model using four different distance measures and then identifies the best performing setting for further comparison with other baseline methods on two real-world datasets, Amazon shopping [30] and 20-Newsgroup [31]. To evaluate our proposed model, we employ the false-positive rate, miss detection rate, and accuracy [32]. Each of these measures is detailed as follows:

False-Positive Rate - describes the percentage of non-draft detected as drift, which is defined as the number of non-drift samples detected as drifts divided by the total number of non-drift samples, shown in Eq. 2.

$$False\ Alarm\ Rate = \frac{FP}{FP + TN} \tag{2}$$

Miss Detection Rate - describes the percentage of drift samples detected as non-drift, which is defined as the number of drift samples classified as non-drifts divided by the total number of drifts samples, as shown in Eq. 3.

$$Miss\ Rate = \frac{FN}{FN + TP} \tag{3}$$

Accuracy - describes the overall accuracy of the detection method to detect between the concept drift and non-concept drift preferences as shown in Eq. 4.

$$Accuracy = \frac{TP + TN}{TP + TN + FP + FN} \tag{4}$$

The baseline methods include reactive drift detection method RDDM [33], Page-Hinkley [34], and AEE [35] which are widely used in concept drift detection, and several studies in this field use them as baseline algorithms.

4.1 Performance of the Different DDAW Versions

Table 1 and Fig. 3 demonstrate different performances of our proposed DDAW model for drift detection with different versions across all the datasets in terms of False Positive, Miss Rate, and Accuracy across all the datasets. The False Positive Rate indicates the rate of identified drifts when none occurred, while the Miss Detection Rate indicates the rate of missed drifts when they actually occurred. The lower values indicate that the methods actually identify drifts correctly.

Table 1. Results of the DDAW Variants in terms of False rate, Miss rate and Accuracy.

Model	Amazon			20-Newsgroup		
	F	M	A	F	M	A
DDAW-KL	0.034	0.017	0.091	0.044	0.062	0.487
DDAW-TVD	0.033	0.014	0.115	0.046	0.068	0.592
DDAW-KSD	0.024	0.013	0.198	0.035	0.056	0.794
DDAW-HD	**0.013**	**0.005**	**0.293**	**0.025**	**0.032**	**0.937**

From Table 1, it can be observed that the DDAW-HD version outperforms all the other versions of the model, namely, DDAW-KL, DDAW-TVD, and DDAW-KSD in all cases. Specifically, it can be seen that compared to the DDAW-KL version which utilized Kullback–Leibler divergence, the DDAW-HD outperformed it with significant improvements of 2.5%, 4.1%, and 3.1%, 3.5% in terms of the False Positive and Miss Detection rates respectively. Compared to the DDAW-TVD, which uses Total variation distance, the DDAW-HD recorded gains of 2.9%, 4.4%, and 2.6%, 2.7% in terms of the False Positive and Miss Detection rates respectively. Meanwhile compared to the DDAW- KSD which performs better than the other two measures, the DDAW-HD recorded gains of 1.9%, 2.1%, and 2.5%, 2.7% in terms of the False Positive and Miss Detection rates respectively. This directly indicates the robustness of Hellinger distance as a distance measure of quantifying the concept drift between two distributions, which in turns reaffirms many of the previous findings signifying the benefit of the Hellinger distance over the other measures [26, 36].

4.2 Performance Comparison with Existing Methods

In comparison with the existing methods, the best performing version of the proposed DDAW model according to Table 1 and Fig. 3 was selected to make further comparison with the existing methods in Table 2 and Fig. 4. Essentially, for the fact that DDAW-HD performs better among the other versions of the DDAW method, we only report the result

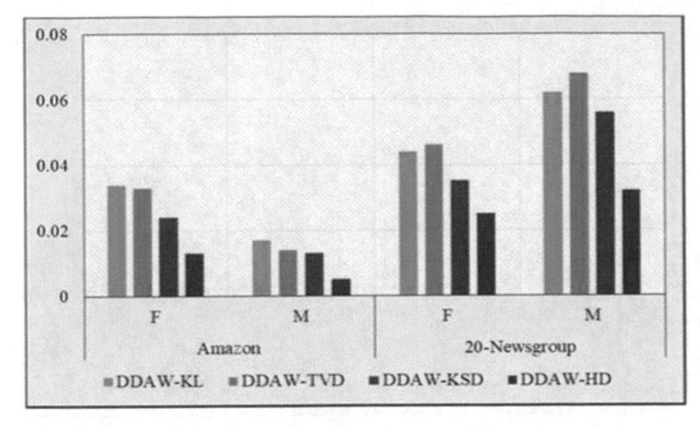

Fig. 3. Graphical representation of the results of different versions of our model

on the DDAW-HD to make a comparison with RDDM, PH, and AEE methods. From Table 2 and Fig. 4, it can be seen that our proposed DDAW-HD model outperformed all the existing methods across all the datasets.

Table 2. Performance of DDAW compared with the baselines

Model	Amazon			20-Newsgroup		
	F	M	A	F	M	A
AEE	0.053	0.041	0.297	0.130	0.132	0.460
RDDM	0.048	0.034	0.293	0.092	0.124	0.467
PH	0.044	0.037	0.304	0.070	0.110	0.753
DDAW-HD	**0.013**	**0.005**	**0.409**	**0.025**	**0.032**	**0.937**

Compare to the RDDM model, our DDAW-HD approach performs better with a reduced error rate of 18.23%, 24.5%, and 13.40%, 6.8% on the Amazon and 20-Newsgroups datasets in terms of False Positive and Miss Detection rates, respectively. More importantly, our DDAW-HD approach performs better compared to the PH model which is the best performing model among the baselines on drift detections. Specifically, our DDAW-HD approach outperformed the PH model with a reduced error rate of 13.76%, 4.5%, and 7.3%, 4.18% on the 20-Newsgroups and Amazon datasets in terms of False Positive and Miss Detection rates, respectively. This can be attributed to the fact that the baselines are based on error rates of classifications, which results in missing several concept drifts as the learners cannot respond to the error rates timely and accurately in most cases.

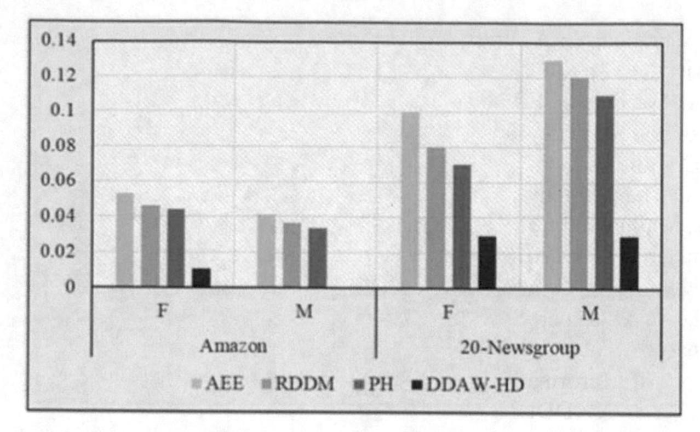

Fig. 4. Graphical representation of the DDAW results compared with baselines

5 Conclusion

The availability of concept drift detection techniques offers many different potentials for extracting the possible changes between concepts depending on whether the change is mine through model performance or by comparing data distribution over two windows, using different similarity measures. In this study, we exploit the second approach and used different similarity measures to compare text data streams for concept drift detection. In this paper, we proposed the DDAW algorithm for concept drift detection based on the distance measures to quantify concept drift. It was found that our DDAW model with Hellinger distance measure (DDAW-HD performs better than other versions and the baseline methods. We believe this is due to the different ways it produces the desired distance. In addition, Hellinger distance is known to be an excellent and easy-to-use numerical estimation tool for high-dimensional data. Finally, from these results, we may conclude that distance measures play a significant role in quantifying concept drift. Moreover, it is believed that more robust approaches can be explored by incorporating our detection measures into the techniques such as deep learning models to increase the performance of sentiment classification models.

References

1. Aggarwal, C.C.: Recommender Systems The Textbook. Springer, Cham (2016). https://doi.org/10.1007/978-3-319-29659-3
2. Gaber, M.M., Zaslavsky, A., Krishnaswamy, S.: A survey of classification methods in data streams. In: Data Streams (2007)
3. Widmer, G.: Learning in the presence of concept drift and hidden contexts. Mach. Learn. (1996). https://doi.org/10.1007/bf00116900
4. Žliobaitė, I., Pechenizkiy, M., Gama, J.: An overview of concept drift applications. In: Japkowicz, N., Stefanowski, J. (eds.) Big Data Analysis: New Algorithms for a New Society. SBD, vol. 16, pp. 91–114. Springer, Cham (2016). https://doi.org/10.1007/978-3-319-26989-4_4
5. Gama, J., Zliobaite, I., Bifet, A., et al.: A survey on concept drift adaptation. ACM Comput. Surv. **46** (2014)

6. Sujatha, P., Saradha, S.: A study of data mining concepts and techniques. Int. J. Appl. Eng. Res. (2014)
7. Pinage, F.A., dos Santos, E.M., da Gama, J.M.P.: Classification systems in dynamic environments: an overview. Wiley Interdiscip. Rev. Data Min. Knowl. Discov. (2016). https://doi.org/10.1002/widm.1184
8. Tsymbal, A.: The problem of concept drift: definitions and related work (2004)
9. Rokach, L., Maimon, O.: The Data Mining and Knowledge Discovery Handbook, pp. 1203–1224. Springer, Boston (2010). https://doi.org/10.1007/978-0-387-09823-4
10. Min, J.K., Hong, J.H., Cho, S.B.: Combining localized fusion and dynamic selection for high-performance SVM. Expert Syst. Appl. (2015). https://doi.org/10.1016/j.eswa.2014.07.028
11. Sun, Y., Shao, H., Wang, S.: Efficient ensemble classification for multi-label data streams with concept drift. Information (2019). https://doi.org/10.3390/info10050158
12. Minku, L.L., Yao, X.: DDD: a new ensemble approach for dealing with concept drift. IEEE Trans. Knowl. Data Eng. **24**, 619–633 (2012). https://doi.org/10.1109/TKDE.2011.58
13. Katakis, I., Tsoumakas, G., Vlahavas, I.: Tracking recurring contexts using ensemble classifiers: an application to email filtering. Knowl. Inf. Syst. (2010). https://doi.org/10.1007/s10115-009-0206-2
14. Krawczyk, B., Cano, A.: Adaptive ensemble active learning for drifting data stream mining. In: IJCAI International Joint Conference on Artificial Intelligence (2019)
15. Jędrzejowicz, J., Jędrzejowicz, P.: GEP-based ensemble classifier with drift-detection. In: Bramer, M., Petridis, M. (eds.) SGAI 2018. LNCS (LNAI), vol. 11311, pp. 121–131. Springer, Cham (2018). https://doi.org/10.1007/978-3-030-04191-5_9
16. Al-Ghossein, M., Murena, P.A., Abdessalem, T., et al.: Adaptive collaborative topic modeling for online recommendation. In: RecSys 2018 - 12th ACM Conference on Recommender Systems, pp 338–346. Association for Computing Machinery, Inc., (2018)
17. Bifet, A., Frank, E., Holmes, G., Pfahringer, B.: Accurate ensembles for data streams: combining restricted hoeffding trees using stacking. J. Mach. Learn. Res. (2010)
18. Tomás, C.C., Oliveira, E., Sousa, D., et al.: Proceedings of the 3rd IPLeiria's international health congress. BMC Health Serv. Res. (2016). https://doi.org/10.1186/s12913-016-1423-5
19. Zhang, H., Wu, J., Norris, J., et al.: Predictors of preference for caesarean delivery among pregnant women in Beijing. J. Int. Med. Res. (2017). https://doi.org/10.1177/0300060517696217
20. Gomes, H.M., et al.: Adaptive random forests for evolving data stream classification. Mach. Learn. **106**(9–10), 1469–1495 (2017). https://doi.org/10.1007/s10994-017-5642-8
21. Arya, M., Choudhary, C.: Improving the efficiency of ensemble classifier adaptive random forest with meta level learning for real-time data streams. In: Bhateja, V., Satapathy, S.C., Zhang, Y.-D., Aradhya, V.N.M. (eds.) ICICC 2019. AISC, vol. 1034, pp. 11–21. Springer, Singapore (2020). https://doi.org/10.1007/978-981-15-1084-7_2
22. Gemaque, R.N., Costa, A.F.J., Giusti, R., dos Santos, E.M.: An overview of unsupervised drift detection methods. Wiley Interdiscip. Rev. Data Min. Knowl. Discov (2020)
23. Nishida, K., Yamauchi, K.: Detecting concept drift using statistical testing. In: Corruble, V., Takeda, M., Suzuki, E. (eds.) DS 2007. LNCS (LNAI), vol. 4755, pp. 264–269. Springer, Heidelberg (2007). https://doi.org/10.1007/978-3-540-75488-6_27
24. Misra, S., Biswas, D., Saha, S.K., Mazumdar, C.: Applying Fourier inspired windows for concept drift detection in data stream. In: 2020 IEEE Calcutta Conference, CALCON 2020 - Proceedings (2020)
25. Yu, S., Abraham, Z.: Concept drift detection with hierarchical hypothesis testing. In: Proceedings of the 17th SIAM International Conference on Data Mining, SDM 2017 (2017)
26. Goldenberg, I., Webb, G.I.: Survey of distance measures for quantifying concept drift and shift in numeric data. Knowl. Inf. Syst. **60**(2), 591–615 (2018). https://doi.org/10.1007/s10115-018-1257-z

27. Costa, F.G.d., Duarte, F.S.L.G., Vallim, R.M.M., Mello, R.F.d.: Multidimensional surrogate stability to detect data stream concept drift. Expert Syst. Appl. **87**, 1339–1351 (2017). https://doi.org/10.1016/j.eswa.2017.06.005
28. Gama, J., Sebastião, R., Rodrigues, P.P.: On evaluating stream learning algorithms. Mach. Learn. **90**(3), 317–346 (2012). https://doi.org/10.1007/s10994-012-5320-9
29. Polikar, R.: Ensemble based systems in decision making. IEEE Circuits Syst. Mag. (2006)
30. McAuley, J., Leskovec, J.: Hidden factors and hidden topics: understanding rating dimensions with review text. In: RecSys 2013 - Proceedings of the 7th ACM Conference on Recommender Systems (2013)
31. Zhang, Y., Chu, G., Li, P., et al.: Three-layer concept drifting detection in text data streams. Neurocomputing (2017). https://doi.org/10.1016/j.neucom.2017.04.047
32. Du, L., Song, Q., Jia, X.: Detecting concept drift: an information entropy based method using an adaptive sliding window. Intell. Data Anal. **18**, 337–364 (2014). https://doi.org/10.3233/IDA-140645
33. Barros, R.S.M., Cabral, D.R.L., Gonçalves, P.M., Santos, S.G.T.C.: RDDM: reactive drift detection method. Expert Syst. Appl. (2017). https://doi.org/10.1016/j.eswa.2017.08.023
34. Sebastião, R., Fernandes, J.M.: Supporting the page-hinkley test with empirical mode decomposition for change detection. In: Kryszkiewicz, M., Appice, A., Ślęzak, D., Rybinski, H., Skowron, A., Raś, Z.W. (eds.) ISMIS 2017. LNCS (LNAI), vol. 10352, pp. 492–498. Springer, Cham (2017). https://doi.org/10.1007/978-3-319-60438-1_48
35. Kolter, J.Z., Maloof, M.A.: Using additive expert ensembles to cope with concept drift. In: ICML 2005 - Proceedings of the 22nd International Conference on Machine Learning (2005)
36. Ditzler, G., Polikar, R.: Hellinger distance based drift detection for nonstationary environments. In: IEEE SSCI 2011: Symposium Series on Computational Intelligence - CIDUE 2011: 2011 IEEE Symposium on Computational Intelligence in Dynamic and Uncertain Environments (2011)

Rainfall Forecasting Using the Group Method of Data Handling Model: A Case Study of Sarawak, Malaysia

Azlina Narawi[1,2](✉), Dayang Norhayati Abang Jawawi[2], and Ruhaidah Samsudin[2]

[1] Universiti Teknologi MARA Cawangan Sarawak, Kampus Samarahan 2, 94300 Kota Samarahan, Sarawak, Malaysia
azlina_14@uitm.edu.my

[2] School of Computing, Faculty of Engineering, Universiti Teknologi Malaysia, 81310 Skudai, Johor, Malaysia
{dayang,ruhaidah}@utm.my

Abstract. Time series forecasting has led to the emergence of various forecasting models applied to arrays of time series problems, such as rainfall forecasting, dengue forecasting, tourism forecasting, and others. The Artificial Neural Network (ANN) is a popular Artificial Intelligence (AI) model extensively employed in much research for time series forecasting due to its nonlinear modeling ability. The group method of data handling (GMDH) is an AI model with the characteristics of heuristic self-organizing capability. This model has shown successful results in many areas. Nowadays, rainfall forecasting remains a vital interest and is still actively researched, where researchers use different soft computing techniques. The ANN has been popularly studied for rainfall forecasting because of its ability to efficiently train a large amount of data and completely detect complex connections between nonlinear dependent and independent variables. However, research on rainfall forecasting using the GMDH model is limited. Hence, this paper designates the GMDH model and its application to rainfall forecasting. The conventional GMDH model uses the polynomial transfer function. The sigmoid transfer function is proven to solve the multicollinearity issue caused by the quadratic polynomial of the GMDH model. Hence, this research tackled the multicollinearity issue of using different transfer functions in GMDH modeling and forecasting. The study compares the results of using polynomial and sigmoid transfer functions for the GMDH model development. This research uses the Malaysia rainfall dataset of the Sarawak regions from 2010 until 2019 as a case study to evaluate the effectiveness of the GMDH models in this research. The results exhibit that the polynomial transfer function is dominant in achieving the smallest RMSE and MSE values in all regions.

Keywords: Group method of data handling · GMDH · Time series · Rainfall · Forecasting

F. Saeed et al. (Eds.): IRICT 2021, LNDECT 127, pp. 129–140, 2022.
https://doi.org/10.1007/978-3-030-98741-1_12

1 Introduction

Forecasting of time series involves historical data to make a prediction. Forecasting time series data is a challenging problem, and it has attracted many researchers over the years, making it an active research area. Time series forecasting has led to the emergence of various forecasting models applied to arrays of time series problems, such as in rainfall forecasting [3, 15], dengue forecasting [14], tourism forecasting [6], and others. In forecasting of time series, the challenge is due to the pattern in the data. It is rare to find time series data that are purely linear or nonlinear. They are usually a mixture of both patterns [35]. The complex underlying nonlinear relationship in the data is not straightforward to understand. Numerous models have been employed by past researchers in conducting time series forecasts.

However, research on Artificial Intelligence (AI) model development has received much attention recently. The Artificial Neural Network (ANN) is a popular AI model extensively employed in much research for time series forecasting due to its capability in nonlinear modeling [25, 37]. On the other hand, the group method of data handling (GMDH) has gained research attention recently, which offers several advantages over the ANN. The GMDH is a self-organizing heuristic AI model introduced by a Russian mathematician, Ivakhnenko, in 1968. It can automatically structure its networks without human interventions. At first, Prof. Alexey G. Ivakhnenko introduced the GMDH model in the 1960s to identify the nonlinear relations between the input and output variables, modeling complex systems, pattern recognition, data clustering, and prediction [16]. Farlow (1981) reported that Ivakhnenko's inspiration to develop GMDH came from his frustration with the causal model, which requires practitioners to know the system beforehand [12]. The GMDH model works for small datasets, where according to Tamura and Kondo (1978) is a valuable practical technique to identify nonlinear input-output relationships in complex systems, even if small datasets are involved [31]. Contrarily the ANN requires a massive amount of historical data. The setting of parameters is seen to be one of the main issues when implementing the ANN model, including the number of neurons and layers. On the other hand, the GMDH model can self-organize its structure in the training procedure; the initial guessing of the neurons number in a layer and the number of layers is unrelated [32]. Before forecasting, essential parameters in the GMDH model must be set the highest layers number, highest neurons number, and the selection pressure [13]. The ANN tends to overfit while the GMDH can resist overfitting [32]. The GMDH can avoid biases and misjudgments due to its ability to automatically self-organize without any human involvement, allowing it to discover the optimal solution for a given problem [2]. The GMDH model can generate explicit expressions, whereas the ANN generates implicit models (black box in nature). This unique feature of the GMDH model helps find the most influential variables and has been previously applied as an input selector [33].

The GMDH model has gradually received researchers' attention and has been explored in much research. It is an AI model that has comparatively related structures to the ANN. In previous literature, comparisons between ANN and GMDH have frequently been made where their performances vary. For instance, in the research work of [34] in comparing the GMDH and ANN performance, it was claimed that the ANN performed better than the GMDH. Instead, according to [13] the GMDH was far more successful than the ANN in prediction. Nevertheless, Varahrami (2012) stated that the GMDH is more reliable than the ANN when the system at hand is very complex, and the underline input-output relationship is not entirely comprehensible or if the system exhibits a chaotic pattern [35].

The GMDH model's advantages encourage us to implement the model for rainfall forecasting. Nowadays, rainfall forecasting remains a vital interest and is still actively researched, where researchers use different soft computing techniques like the ANN, Genetic Algorithm, Support Vector Regression, Particle Swarm Optimization, and Fuzzy logic [5, 9, 17, 21, 28, 36]. The ANN has been popularly researched for rainfall forecasting because it can train a large amount of data efficiently and can detect complex connections between nonlinear dependent and independent variables altogether [11]. On the other hand, Onwubolu et al. (2007) applied the GMDH model for rainfall forecasting [27]. They spread the self-organizing enhanced GMDH (e-GMDH) model for daily pressure, daily temperature, and monthly rainfall. The weather data used were the daily temperature and pressure from 2000 until 2007 and a chaotic rainfall dataset for the city of Suva from 1990 to 2002. The e-GMDH enhanced the polynomial GMDH with several better features like thresholding schemes coefficient rounding and pruning through a half-randomized selection method. The research results reported that the e-GMDH outperformed the polynomial neural network and the enhanced polynomial neural network for daily temperature. However, for the monthly rainfall and daily temperature, the e-GMDH did not perform well compared to the other methods.

Table 1 summarizes various methods used in rainfall forecasting.

Table 1. Summary of methods used in rainfall forecasting.

Authors	Data	Rainfall predicting variables	Methods	Accuracy measure
[30]	The South Tangerang, Indonesia 6 years data	Rainfall and temperature	ANFIS technique	RMSE MSE
[10]	Iran rainfall data Mean annual rainfall data (25 years, 1990–2014)	Stations, latitude, elevation, min, max, mean, coefficient of variation	A hybrid rainfall forecasting model using support vector regression and firefly (SVR-FFA) The hybrid SVR-FFA was reported to outperform the SVR and GP-based multigene genetic programming MGGP significantly	RMSE NSE

(*continued*)

Table 1. (*continued*)

Authors	Data	Rainfall predicting variables	Methods	Accuracy measure
[23]	Predictand data from Kuching airport rainfall station	Monthly averages of GCM climatological variables (predictors), and observed local monthly average precipitation data (predictand)	Cuckoo Search Optimization Neural Network model to forecast. Benchmarked the Levenberg-Marquardt (LM) optimisation method and Scale Conjugate Gradient (SCG). The CS algorithm with the Feedforward Neural Network besides Recurrent Neural Network, CSOFNN and CSORNN respectively. The CS algorithm outperformed the SCG and LM optimization methods	RMSE MAE MB (mean bias) R (correlation coefficient)
[7]	42 cities data in Europe and the USA	Rainfall amount	Decomposition Genetic Programming (DGP) performed on a different regression equation based on the rainfall level. The DGP was reported to significantly outperform all other algorithms	RMSE MSE
[24]	The Iranian meteorological dataset from 1981 to 2012	The monthly rainfall	The proposed combined monthly rainfall prediction models using Artificial Neural Network–Autoregressive Conditional Heteroscedasticity as well as Gene Expression Programming–Autoregressive Conditional Heteroscedasticity abbreviated as ANN-ARCH and GEP-ARCH respectively. The hybrid models had outperformed the ANN and GEP models. The ANN-ARCH model was reported to surpass the GEP-ARCH model	RMSE R2 (coefficient of determination)

The conventional GMDH model by Ivakhnenko uses the polynomial transfer function. Nevertheless, Jirina (1994) proposed a logistic sigmoid transfer function to replace the polynomial function to solve the multicollinearity caused by the quadratic polynomial of the GMDH model. Further, through their experimental results, Kondo and Pandya (2003) reported that the GMDH model that uses the sigmoid transfer function performed better than the GMDH model that uses the radial basis function and ANN. They testified that using sigmoid as the transfer function helps identify the nonlinear system as the neural network architecture handled to fit the complex nonlinear system [22]. On the other hand, the implementation of different transfer functions was done by Tauser and Buryan (2011), who implemented eight different functions, namely polynomial, harmonic (cosine), square root, inverse polynomial, logarithmic, arc tangent and exponential in their GMDH network [32]. Hence, this research would investigate the effectiveness of the polynomial and sigmoid transfer functions for the GMDH model in solving the multicollinearity issues, particularly for rainfall forecasting.

2 The Group Method of Data Handling Model

Prof. Ivakhnenko invented a model that focuses solely on input and output relationships and requires no human interventions. Thus, the GMDH model is considered a data-driven model. Ivakhnenko proposed the basic GMDH model, which is especially useful in identifying complex as well as the unknown nonlinear system as testified by [12, 21], and [35]. Like the ANN, the GMDH model entails the three layers: input, hidden, and output. Simple neurons are created via a two-variable combination in every hidden layer that implements its transfer function of a quadratic polynomial. The neurons in the following layer will receive the outputs from this layer. However, the reduction of inefficient neurons will happen via some threshold value. The best-performing neurons will be retained, while the lowest-achieving ones will be removed. In the final layer, only one neuron exists; thus, this last layer's output will represent the entire network's output. The GMDH basic process is like the principle of a traditional neural network created using the forward propagation of signals via neurons. The strong point of GMDH lies in its capability to naturally organize its structures in a heuristic manner [2]. GMDH has the criteria for automatically generating the neuron number in a layer and the layer number with no human intervention. It also has a self-organizing feature, which allows it to discover the ideal solution for a given problem while avoiding bias and misjudgments [2]. Thus, this feature of the GMDH also contributed to it having a small number of parameters tuned: the highest neurons number, the highest layers number, and pressure of selection, making it a reliable and straightforward AI model [13].

In the conventional GMDH, the connection between inputs and outputs variable can be modelled by the Kolmogorov-Gabor polynomial [16] as presented in the equation below;

$$y = a_0 + \sum_{i=1}^{n} a_i x_i + \sum_{i=1}^{n}\sum_{j=1}^{n} a_{ij} x_i x_j + \sum_{i=1}^{n}\sum_{j=1}^{n}\sum_{k=1}^{n} a_{ijk} x_i x_j x_k + \ldots \quad (1)$$

According to Tamura and Kondo (1978), the complete description in Eq. 1 is most widely used because nearly all real-life systems can be described using the equation above [31]. The Kolmogorov-Gabor polynomial plays a big role in GMDH modelling as it acts as a universal approximator to estimate unknown functions in a system [20]. Essentially, the complete description above is formed by joining the following second order polynomials of paired variables in each layer.

$$y_k = a_0 + a_1 x_i + a_2 x_j + a_3 x_i^2 + a_4 x_j^2 + a_5 x_i x_j \tag{2}$$

The above equation is identified as the Partial Description (PD), and yk is the intermediate variable. In Step 1: The data is divided into training and testing sets. The coefficient approximation is made via the training data while the testing data is required to select intermediate variables. Next, Step 2: Based on the combination of two input variables x_i and x_j the parameters a_0, a_1, a_2, a_3, a_4 and a_5 in Eq. 2 are estimated using least square method via training data. Step 3: The regularity criterion for the checking data is calculated by using the PD estimated in Step 2. In traditional GMDH, MSE is used as the regularity criterion. The intermediate variables which give the smallest MSE will be selected as useful variables. Lastly, Step 4: Variables x_i and x_j are replaced by y_i and y_j respectively. Steps 2 to 5 are repeated until the performance of the variables cannot be further improved. Figure 1 shows the GMDH block diagram, where x_1, x_2, … x_m are training data and m is the frequency of observations.

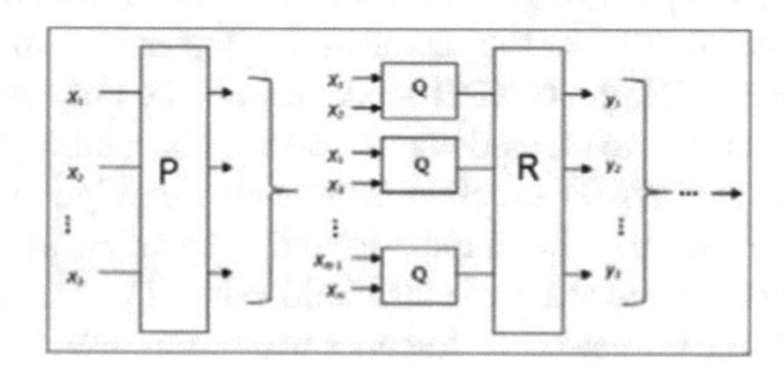

Fig. 1. The basic GMDH block diagram.

The diagram in Fig. 1 can be briefly described:

P: All the training data are merged into pairs to form a partial quadratic polynomial.
Q: The partial quadratic polynomial coefficients are computed using least square method.
R: The performance of the outputs obtained from the neuron is measured using MSE. A threshold will be used to filter the outputs based on their performances.

On the other hand, this study also employs the logistic sigmoid transfer function as an alternative to the polynomial transfer function. Besides the polynomial transfer function, which was used in the GMDH models [4, 8, 21, 32], the sigmoid transfer function is also popularly employed in the GMDH models [4, 18, 21, 22].

The GMDH model employs the logistic sigmoid function using the following equation:

$$y_{sig} = \frac{1}{1 + e^{-z_k}} \tag{3}$$

The calculation for the transfer function of the logistic sigmoid is using the following formula:

$$z_k = log\left(\frac{\emptyset'}{1 - \emptyset'}\right) \tag{4}$$

where, ϕ' is the normalized output variable (0–1) and ϕ is the output variable. Then the model calculates the coefficient z_k using regression.

3 Methods

3.1 Dataset

This study uses the monthly rainfall average for January 2010 until December 2019 for Sarawak regions, including Kuching, Sri Aman, Sibu, Miri, and Bintulu. The dataset was obtained from the Department of Meteorology Malaysia. Figure 2 shows the monthly average rainfall for Kuching, Miri, Bintulu, Sibu, and Sri Aman from 2010 until 2019. Generally, the rainfall distribution is higher in Kuching than other regions, with the highest value of 20.19 and an overall average of 12.38. Meanwhile, the lowest distribution occurs in Miri, with the highest value of 12.09 and an overall average of 7.88.

A dataset needs to undergo the pre-processing data stage before entering a forecasting model. In this research, with the aims to perform time series forecasting, the steps

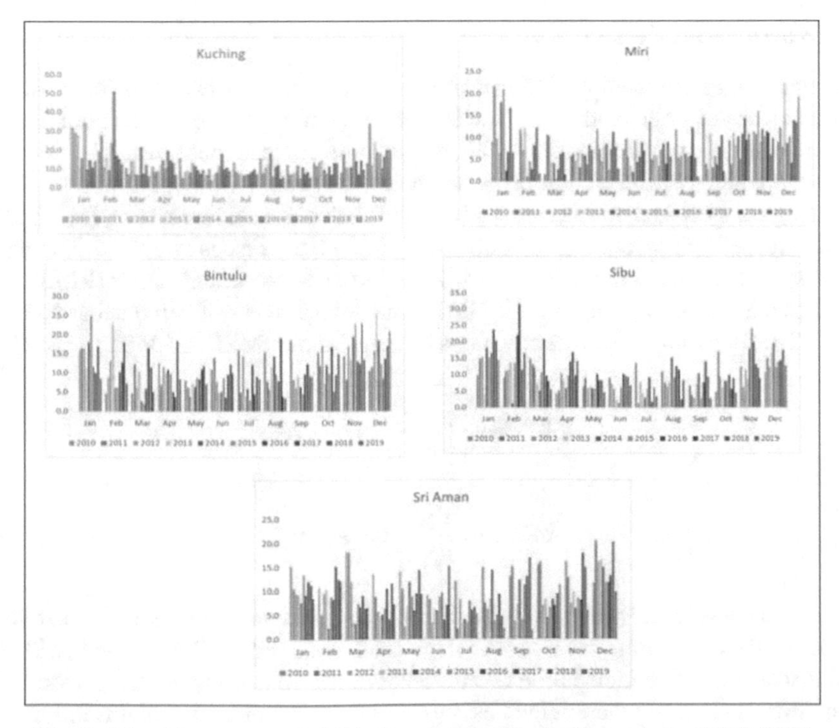

Fig. 2. Monthly average rainfall in Sarawak Region for the period of 2010–2019

concerned include data transformation, division of the data into the training and testing sets, lagging the data, and choosing suitable inputs.

For data transformation, the data is rescaled into a specific smaller range such as between 0 to 1, −1 to 1, and others. Smaller numbers are essential to avoid calculating huge numbers. In this research, the data is normalized into the range of 0 to 1, using the following formula [26]:

$$Y^1 = \frac{Y - b}{a - b} \tag{5}$$

where Y^1 is the normalized data, Y is the actual data, a is the maximum values of the actual data and b is the minimum values of actual data.

Enormous computation problems may exist when forecasting uses the daily rainfall data for ten years to predict daily rainfall. As an alternative, we selected monthly rainfall averages. The data is further divided into training and testing sets. Further, division the data into the training and testing sets where the training sets are used to develop the model, while the testing sets are used to test the model accuracy. After a model has been developed using the training sets, the model is tested by making predictions against the testing sets. If all the data are used for both model development and forecast, the model might experience overfitting. In this study, the chosen meteorological parameters will be trained and tested to forecast rainfall. The training data size is 90%, whereas 10% for testing.

3.2 Experimental Results

Performance measurement is vital to evaluate the dispersion between the observed data and the forecasted data. Additionally, it is used to accurately examine the reliability and strength of the model in forecasting. Moreover, performance measurements enable the comparisons between different forecasting models possible to be made. RMSE and MSE are among the well-known measures often used in time series forecasting [1, 19, 29].

Each model's performance for both the training and test data is evaluated and selected according to the Mean Squared Error (MSE) and Root-Mean-Square Error (RMSE). The results of rainfall forecasting via the GMDH model are also evaluated using MSE and RMSE. The following shows the equations for calculating RMSE and MSE, respectively.

$$RMSE = \sqrt{\frac{1}{n}\sum_{t=1}^{n}(y_t - \hat{y}_t)^2} \tag{6}$$

$$RMSE = \frac{1}{n}\sum_{t=1}^{n}(y_t - \hat{y}_t)^2 \tag{7}$$

Where y_t is the original value, $\hat{y}_t$ is the is the forecasted value and n is the size of the sample. In the evaluation process, smaller values obtained for RMSE and MSE of a given distribution are better. These two measures are used to compare the performances of the GMDH models, wherein the best model reflects the one that obtains the smallest RMSE and MSE. Tables 1 and 2 present the MSE and RMSE results obtained in this study. The GMDH models which use the polynomial and sigmoid transfer functions are denoted as GMDH-Poly and GMDH-Sig, respectively. The best results in Tables 2 and 3 are in bold.

Table 2. MSE Performance results for the training and testing sets.

Region	Train MSE		Test MSE	
	GMDH-Poly	GMDH-Sig	GMDH-Poly	GMDH-Sig
Kuching	**0.0094721**	0.0172605	0.0172605	**0.0086596**
Miri	**0.0214740**	0.0241085	**0.0241085**	0.0764576
Bintulu	**0.0301350**	0.0393166	**0.0393166**	0.0528348
Sibu	**0.0142780**	0.0238548	0.0238548	**0.0193620**
Sri Aman	**0.0286880**	0.0320923	**0.0320923**	0.0611177

Table 3. RMSE performance results for the training and testing sets.

Region	Train RMSE		Test RMSE	
	GMDH-Poly	GMDH-Sig	GMDH-Poly	GMDH-Sig
Kuching	**0.0973250**	0.1313793	0.0962950	**0.0930569**
Miri	**0.1465400**	0.1552690	**0.2131400**	0.2765097
Bintulu	**0.1735900**	0.1982842	**0.1833100**	0.2298583
Sibu	**0.1194900**	0.1544501	0.1642800	**0.1391474**
Sri Aman	**0.1693800**	0.1791433	0.7049500	**0.2472199**

From Tables 2 and 3, it is observed that, the GMDH-polynomial obtained the smallest MSE and RMSE values for every region for the training sets. However, for the testing set the GMDH-sigmoid obtained the smallest MSE for Kuching and Sibu. The GMDH-polynomial obtained the smallest testing MSE for Miri, Bintulu and Sri Aman. Further, the results for RMSE for testing sets show that the GMDH-sigmoid obtained the smallest values for Kuching, Sibu and Sri Aman whereas the GMDH-polynomial obtained the smallest testing RMSE for Miri and Bintulu. Table 3 summarizes the performances of the GMDH-polynomial and GMDH-sigmoid. The '*' symbol denotes the best result obtained in the study.

Table 4 generally shows that the GMDH-polynomial dominates the MSE and RMSE for training and testing sets.

Table 4. Performance comparison for the training and testing sets

Region	GMDH-Poly				GMDH-Sigmoid			
	Train MSE	Test MSE	Train RMSE	Test RMSE	Train MSE	Test MSE	Train RMSE	Test RMSE
Kuching	*		*			*		*
Miri	*	*	*	*				
Bintulu	*	*	*	*				
Sibu	*	*	*			*		*
Sri Aman	*	*	*					*

4 Conclusion

Rainfall forecasting is one of the time series problems which is still studied frequently. The ANN is a popular model in this study area. On the other hand, the GMDH model has increasingly attracted research attention due to its ability to self-organize and have advantages over the ANN model. The conventional GMDH model uses the polynomial as a transfer function was reported in previous work not being able to solve multicollinearity issues. This research experimented with the different transfer functions using the polynomial and the sigmoid functions for rainfall data of the Sarawak region in Malaysia. The results demonstrate that the polynomial transfer function has dominated the performance result compared to the sigmoid transfer function. Different transfer functions will be considered in future studies. In addition, a GMDH model that is integrated with another optimization strategy will be studied.

Acknowledgement. Special thanks to the Meteorology Department of Malaysia for its data contribution.

References

1. Ahmad, A.S., et al.: A review on applications of ANN and SVM for building electrical energy consumption forecasting. Renew. Sustain. Energy Rev. **33**(1), 102–109 (2014)
2. AlBinHassan, N.M., Wang, Y.: Porosity prediction using the group method of data handling. Geophysics **76**(5), O15–O22 (2011)
3. Altunkaynak, A., Nigussie, T.A.: Prediction of daily rainfall by a hybrid wavelet-season-neuro technique. Elsevier J. Hydrol. **529**(2015), 287–301 (2015)
4. Basheer, H., Khamis, A.B.: A hybrid group method of data handling (GMDH) with the wavelet decomposition for time series forecasting: a review. ARPN J. Eng. Appl. Sci. **11**(18), 10792–10800 (2016)
5. Caraka, R.E., Chen, R.C., Toharudin, T., Tahmid, M., Pardamean, B., Putra, R.M.: Evaluation performance of SVR genetic algorithm and hybrid PSO in rainfall forecasting. ICIC Express Lett. Part B: Appl. ICIC Int. **11**(7 July 2020), 631–639 (2020). ISSN 2185-2766
6. Claveria, O., Torra, S.: Forecasting tourism demand to Catalonia: neural networks vs. time series models. Econ. Model. **36**, 220–228 (2014)

7. Cramer, S., Kampouridis, M., Freitas, A.A.: Decomposition genetic programming: an extensive evaluation on rainfall prediction in the context of weather derivatives. Elsevier Appl. Soft Comput. **70**(2018), 208–224 (2018)
8. Dag, O., Yozgatligil, C.: GMDH: an R package for short term forecasting via GMDH-type neural network algorithms. R J. **8**(1), 379–386 (2016)
9. Danandeh Mehr, A.: Seasonal rainfall hindcasting using ensemble multi-stage genetic programming. Theoret. Appl. Climatol. **143**(1–2), 461–472 (2020). https://doi.org/10.1007/s00704-020-03438-3
10. Danandeh Mehr, A., Nourani, V., Karimi Khosrowshahi, V., Ghorbani, M.A.: A hybrid support vector regression-firefly model for monthly rainfall forecasting. Int. J. Environ. Sci. Technol. (IJEST) **16**(1), 335–346 (2019)
11. Darji, M.P., Dabhi, V.K., Prajapati, H.B.: Rainfall forecasting using neural network: a survey. In: 2015 International Conference on Advances in Computer Engineering and Applications (ICACEA), India (2015)
12. Farlow, S.J.: The GMDH algorithm of Ivakhnenko. Am. Stat. **35**(4), 210–215 (1981)
13. Ghazanfari, N., Gholami, S., Emad, A., Shekarchi, M.: Evaluation of GMDH and MLP networks for prediction of compressive strength and workability of concrete. Bulletin de la Société Royale des Sciences de Liège **86**(special edition), 855–868 (2017)
14. Guo, P., et al.: Developing a dengue forecast model using machine learning: a case study in China. Research Article, PLOS Neglected Trop. Dis. (2017)
15. Hernández, E., Sanchez-Anguix, V., Julian, V., Palanca, J., Duque, N.: Rainfall prediction: a deep learning approach. In: Martínez-Álvarez, F., Troncoso, A., Quintián, H., Corchado, E. (eds.) HAIS 2016. LNCS (LNAI), vol. 9648, pp. 151–162. Springer, Cham (2016). https://doi.org/10.1007/978-3-319-32034-2_13
16. Ivakhnenko, A.G.: Polynomial theory of complex systems. IEEE Trans. Syst. Man Cybern. **4**, 364–378 (1971)
17. Janarthanan, R., Balamurali, R., Annapoorani, A., Vimala, V.: Prediction of rainfall using fuzzy logic. Elsevier Mater. Today Proc. **37**, 959–963 (2021)
18. Jirina, M.: The modified GMDH: sigmoidal and polynomial neural net. IFAC Proc. Vol. **27**(8), 611–613 (1994)
19. Khosravia, K., et al.: A comparative assessment of flood susceptibility modeling using multi-criteria decision-making analysis and machine learning methods. Elsevier J. Hydrol. **573**(2019), 311–323 (2019)
20. Kock, A.B., Terasvirta, T.: Forecasting with nonlinear time series models. In: CREATES Research Paper, 2010-1, pp. 1–31 (2010)
21. Kondo, T.: GMDH neural network algorithm using the heuristic self-organization method and its application to the pattern identification problem. In: Proceedings of the 37th SICE Annual Conference 1998, International Session Papers, pp. 1143–1148. IEEE (1998)
22. Kondo, T., Pandya, A.S.: Structural identification of the multi-layered neural networks by using revised GMDH-type neural network algorithm with a feedback loop. In: SICE 2003 Annual Conference (IEEE Cat. No. 03TH8734), vol. 3, pp. 2768–2773. IEEE (2003)
23. Kueh, S.M., Kuok, K.K.: Forecasting long term precipitation using cuckoo search optimization neural network models. Environ. Eng. Manag. J. **17**(6), 1283–1291 (2018)
24. Mehdizadeh, S., Behmanesh, J., Khalili, K.: New approaches for estimation of monthly rainfall based on GEP-ARCH and ANN-ARCH hybrid models. Water Resour. Manag. **32**(2), 527–545 (2017). https://doi.org/10.1007/s11269-017-1825-0
25. Neto, P.S.G.D.M., Firmino, P.R.A., Siqueira, H., Tadano, Y.D.S., Alves, T.A., JOÃO Oli, F.L.D.: Neural-based ensembles for particulate matter forecasting. IEEE Access **9** (2021). Electronic ISSN 2169-3536
26. Nourani, V., Komasi, M.: A geomorphology-based ANFIS model for multi-station modeling of rainfall-runoff process. J. Hydrol. **490**, 41–55 (2013)

27. Onwubolu, G.C., Buryan, P., Garimella, S., Ramachandran, V., Buadromo, V., Abraham, A.: Self-organizing data mining for weather forecasting. In: IADIS European Conference Data Mining (2007)
28. Refonaa, J., Lakshmi, M., SrinivasaRao, R.S.S., Prasad, E.: Rainfall prediction using genetic algorithm. Int. J. Recent Technol. Eng. (IJRTE) **8**(2S3) (2019). ISSN 2277-3878
29. Shabri, A., Samsudin, R.: A hybrid GMDH and Box-Jenkins models in time series forecasting. Appl. Math. Sci. **8**(62), 3051–3062 (2014)
30. Suparta, W., Samah, A.A.: Rainfall prediction by using ANFIS times series technique in South Tangerang, Indonesia. Elsevier Geodesy Geodyn. **11**, 411–417 (2020)
31. Tamura, H., Kondo, T.: Revised GMDH algorithm using prediction sum of squares (PSS) as a criterion for model selection. Trans. Soc. Instrum. Control Eng. **14**(5), 519–524 (1978)
32. Tauser, J., Buryan, P.: Exchange rate predictions in international financial management by enhanced GMDH algorithm. Prague Econ. Papers **20**(3), 232–249 (2011)
33. Teng, G., Xiao, J., He, Y., Zheng, T., He, C.: Use of group method of data handling for transport energy demand modeling. Energy Sci. Eng. **5**(5), 302–317 (2017)
34. Ugrasen, G., Ravindra, H.V., Prakash, G.N., Keshavamurthy, R.: Estimation of machining performances using MRA, GMDH and artificial neural network in wire EDM of EN-31. Procedia Mater. Sci. **6**, 1788–1797 (2014)
35. Varahrami, V.: Good prediction of gas price between MLFF and GMDH neural network. Int. J. Finance Acc. **1**(3), 23–27 (2012)
36. Wu, J., Zhou, J.: Support vector regression based on particle swarm optimization and projection pursuit technology for rainfall forecasting. In: 2009 International Conference on Computational Intelligence and Security (2009)
37. Zhang, G.P.: Time series forecasting using a hybrid ARIMA and neural network model. Neurocomputing **50**, 159–175 (2003)

Detecting Public Outlook Towards Vaccination Using Machine Learning Approaches: A Systematic Review

Sheikh Md. Hanif Hossain and Suriani Sulaiman(✉)

Department of Computer Science, International Islamic University Malaysia (IIUM), Kuala Lumpur, Malaysia
ssuriani@iium.edu.my

Abstract. Vaccination is an effective measure to prevent the spread of harmful diseases. The prevalence towards vaccine hesitancy, however, has been growing throughout the years and expressed openly in various social media platforms. Research works on automating the detection of public's opinion towards vaccination in social media has recently gained significant popularity with the rise of the COVID-19 pandemic. This paper presents a systematic review on the machine learning approaches used by researchers to detect the inclination of the public towards vaccination. We analyzed the research work conducted within the past five years and summarized their findings. Our systematic review reveals that Support Vector Machine is the most widely used machine learning technique in identifying public sentiment towards vaccination producing the best performance with an F1-score of 97.3, while Twitter is found to be the most popular platform for extracting source of data.

Keywords: Machine learning · Vaccine hesitancy · Anti-vaccine · Deep learning · Ensemble learning · Vaccine sentiment detection

1 Introduction

Negative outlook towards vaccination such as vaccine hesitancy or anti-vaccination can lead a country or a society towards greater risks of pandemic. The recent outbreak of the COVID-19 pandemic manifests the importance of getting vaccinated to lower the risks of infections. Over the past decades, a variety of vaccines have been developed and proven to be very successful to cure diseases. However, there is a growing group of individuals who perceive vaccination as unsafe and unnecessary, either due to political gains, cultural, psychosocial, spiritual and cognitive factors [1, 2] or personal preference and doubts [3].

Vaccine misinformation and hesitancy are spreading over social media at a tremendously fast pace which leads to more individuals openly demonstrating negative sentiments towards vaccination [4]. It is thus crucial to stop the influence of vaccine related misinformation and hesitancy on majority of the public through social media, that may further develop as healthcare threats in countering diseases that can be safely prevented

F. Saeed et al. (Eds.): IRICT 2021, LNDECT 127, pp. 141–150, 2022.
https://doi.org/10.1007/978-3-030-98741-1_13

through vaccine intakes. Research communities are actively working on this issue to find efficient ways to prevent such spreading [5, 6].

Many machine learning approaches have been proposed to detect anti-vaccines [7] and vaccine misinformation in social media [8, 9]. Some of them are very promising and can be implemented in real life to prevent the spread of misinformation regarding vaccines. However, a systematic review for the detection of vaccine misinformation and hesitancy using machine learning approaches can help researchers to identify the current research gaps and possible areas of improvement in this field. For these reasons, we conducted a systematic review to investigate the types of machine learning algorithms used in the detection of public outlook towards vaccination, their efficiency in detecting vaccine hesitancy, the platforms in which the data are collected and ways to improve current approaches. The main contributions of this systematic review are as follows:

1. A source of reference for more accurate and recent information on previously implemented machine learning approaches for the detection of public outlook towards vaccination.
2. A guide for researchers to make better research decisions in terms of choosing suitable machine learning models and data sources for vaccine hesitancy detection.

The rest of this article is organized as follows; Sect. 2 outlines the theoretical background of the study, Sect. 3 describes the systematic review process, Sect. 4 provides the summary of results while Sect. 5 concludes the review and proposes future works.

2 Theoretical Background

Vaccination is crucial for us as it protects us from serious diseases like Diphtheria, Hepatitis and COVID-19. However, there have been many negative sentiments towards vaccination since the time the vaccine was invented. Some of them relate to vaccine hesitancy, vaccine misinformation and anti-vaccination. WHO defines vaccine hesitancy as a "delay in acceptance or refusal of vaccines despite availability of vaccination services" [10]. Vaccine misinformation refers to the propagation of misinformation about a vaccine without having fundamental understanding about it. Anti-vaccine means someone, or some groups, who decides to simply refuse vaccination for some reasons which may include political gains. All these negative sentiments regarding vaccination are circulating rapidly through social media.

Machine learning (ML) refers to an algorithm which learns based on examples. Deep learning (DL) is a branch of machine learning which utilizes more advanced algorithms to learn from the examples. Both ML and DL are being used in computer related classification problems such as image classification, text classification and hate speech detection [11]. Deep learning has recently been gaining popularity among research communities. Many researchers are trying to detect vaccine misinformation by using this method.

3 Systematic Review

When developing machine learning algorithms, researchers often look for current implementation and data sources in the field. The right selection of algorithms and data is crucial for successful research. This systematic review has the following goals:

1. To identify state-of-the-art machine learning algorithms for detecting vaccine hesitancy and misinformation.
2. To identify the data sources that have been used for the detection of public outlook towards vaccination.
3. To suggest future improvement for research work in vaccine hesitancy detection based on machine learning methods.

This systematic review has one restriction. We decided to include peer-reviewed scientific research work which has explicit and comprehensive implementation of machine learning algorithms. Hence, general studies or descriptive analyses without ML implementations are excluded. This review testifies the following research questions:

1. RQ1: What are the most used machine learning algorithms for detecting vaccine hesitancy and misinformation?
2. RQ2: What is the source of data used to train the machine learning model?

To examine RQ1, we have gathered all the related papers and the algorithms that are being used to detect public outlook towards vaccination using machine learning approaches. Based on the frequency of the algorithm used, we determine the most popular algorithm. As for RQ2, we compare the type of data being used versus the accuracy of the algorithm. After we have selected the related papers based on specific search queries and exclusion criteria discussed below, a summarization of the papers is done by reviewing the paper carefully from beginning to end. To keep our systematic review solid, we come up with the following exclusion criteria:

1. EC1: Publications must have been published in indexed journals or indexed conference proceedings and they must be peer reviewed.
2. EC2: Publications must contain research work on machine learning algorithms.
3. EC3: Publications must be in English and unique (i.e., published only once). For repeated copies of a publication, only one copy is preserved.
4. EC4: Publications must be published within the past 5 years from the year of systematic review.

Vaccine hesitancy and resistance have been described in various terms. Some authors like to use the term "anti-vaccination", "anti-vaccine", "vaccine hesitancy" or "vaccine misinformation". The term machine learning is found to appear together with closely related methods such as "deep learning", "ensemble learning" and "transfer learning". Thus, our systematic review has the following search criteria:

- TITLE-ABS-KEY ((vaccine OR vaccination OR anti-vaccination OR vaccine hesitancy OR vaccine resistance) AND (machine learning OR deep learning OR ensemble learning OR transfer learning))

This search query returns vaccine related papers which contain the term 'machine learning' and 'vaccine' in the title, abstract or keywords. After we applied the search terms in google scholar, Scopus, MDPI, Elsevier and IEEE databases, we downloaded the papers by reading the titles and the abstracts. The total number of downloaded papers is 31 and after applying the exclusion criteria (EC) mentioned above, only 13 papers were retained for the final systematic review. The summary of all the final papers is presented in the following section. We organize the summary of the papers into three categories; machine learning based model, deep learning based model and ensemble learning based model.

3.1 Machine Learning Models

Using machine learning to compare pro-vaccine and anti-vaccine discourse among the public on social media was proposed by [12]. [12] categorized vaccine related tweets into three; pro-vaccine, anti-vaccine and neutral. A logistic regression model was used and achieved an F1-score of 95.7. Similar study was conducted by [13]. Tweets related to measles, mumps, and rubella (MMR) vaccines were collected and classified into three categories: pro-vaccine, anti-vaccine and neutral. Several supervised machine learning models were trained. Among them, the support vector machine (SVM) performed the best with an F1-score of 73.13 on the test dataset.

An automated classification of web pages about early childhood vaccination using supervised machine learning was discussed in [14]. Webpages were manually classified as reliable or not reliable and a naïve bayes classifier was trained. The model achieved an overall F1-score of 88.0.

A project called MAVIS [15] aimed to study the social media sentiments published in Spanish language on disease and vaccination. Data was collected from Twitter and Instagram and trained with a random forest model. By applying the SMOTE method to balance the dataset, the best accuracy was an ROC of 85.1. Almost identical research was conducted by [16] in which the researchers conducted sentiment analysis on Human Papillomavirus (HPV) vaccine related tweets using machine learning. 6,000 HPV vaccines related tweets were manually annotated and trained with support vector machine (SVM) algorithms. An F1-score of 74.42 was achieved with an optimized feature set. Another similar approach was proposed to identify vaccine hesitancy in social media by [17]. The dataset spanning approximately 8 years from 1 June 2011 to 30 April 2019 consists of 1,499,227 vaccine-related tweets published on Twitter. A support vector machine (SVM) was trained using the dataset and the model achieved 85% accuracy on the test set. Further analysis from the dataset showed that the number of negative and positive tweets was increasing over time while the number of neutral tweets was decreasing.

3.2 Deep Learning Models

Public outlook towards vaccination was analyzed using twitter data by [18]. At first, the authors classified tweets into two groups; relevant and not relevant. The relevant tweets were then further categorized into pro-vaccination, anti-vaccination and neutral outlook. The neural network model's performance was the best in terms of classifying vaccine outlook with an F1 score of 58.0. Sentiment analysis was performed on related tweets for HPV vaccine using transfer learning [19]. Among the previously compared models, the fine-tuned Bidirectional Encoder Representations from Transformers (BERT) model performed the best in analyzing vaccine sentiments with an average F1 score of 76.9.

Identification of anti-vaccination tweets using machine learning was proposed by [20] and [21] during COVID-19 pandemic. Several machine learning and deep learning models were trained and evaluated using twitter dataset. The performance of the BERT model with an F1-score of 95.5 was achieved by [20] which was the best compared to the other models used whereas [21] reported the performance of the BERT model with an F1-score of 79.2.

The detection of stigmatized behavior towards vaccination using predictive modelling was discussed in [22]. Facebook comments were extracted and categorized into anti-vaccination and pro-vaccination. Several machine learning models were trained and tested using the dataset. Among them, the fastText model performed the best with an average accuracy of 75% to classify anti-vaccine and pro-vaccine related comments.

3.3 Ensemble Learning Models

The use of multimodal deep learning for the detection of medical misinformation on vaccination was proposed by [23]. In this research, [23] collected the dataset from Instagram, which consists of images, hashtags as well as text descriptions. The models have three branches; hashtag branch with word-level feature extractor, text branch with sentence level feature extractor and an image branch with visual feature extractor. A semantic and task level attention mechanism layer were used to produce better output of the model. Each branch was trained with a different deep learning model. An ensemble model was then produced by adding another branch called the three-branch model which includes features from all prior three branches. Output of these four-prediction models were combined as four-dimensional features. Finally, an SVM algorithm with radial basis function (RDF) kernel was trained with these four features. The ensemble model achieved an F1-score of 97.3.

Vaccination behavior detection involves prediction of a person who received or was about to receive a vaccine. To detect vaccination behavior, an ensemble-based machine learning method, rule-based method and a deep learning method were proposed by [24]. The ensemble machine learning method consists of three algorithms; logistic regression, support vector machine and random forest. Tweets from twitter were used as the source of data. A tweet identified to be positive must be classified as positive by at least two classifiers. The F1-score for this method was reported to be 80.75. In the rule-based approach, if a tweet contains certain positive keywords (e.g., give, take, gave, receive), the tweet was classified as positive. Otherwise, it was classified as negative.

F1-score of 40.84 was achieved for this method. Five deep learning models such as sentence vector, dense neural network, Bidirectional Long Short-term Memory (BiLSTM), Convolutional Neural Network (CNN) and Long Short-term Memory Language Model (LSTM-LM) were trained separately to identify vaccination behaviors. Among these deep learning models, LSTM-LM performed the best with an F1- score of 80.87.

4 Systematic Review Results

Table 1 summarizes the findings of our systematic literature review. For research papers with comprehensive analysis, we include only one machine learning model per research if there were more than one machine learning models being evaluated. The following criteria are taken into considerations while selecting the model for each research:

- The model which produced the best performance among other models.
- The model that was implemented to detect public outlook or sentiment.

Table 1. Summary of findings on the use of machine learning approaches in the detection of public outlook towards vaccination in the order of the most recent year of publications.

Ref.	Year	Model	Best performance	Data source	Related vaccine
[12]	2021	Logistic Regression	F1-score: 95.7	Twitter	Multiple/general
[14]	2021	Naïve Bayes	F1-score: 88	Webpage	Multiple/general
[17]	2021	SVM	Accuracy: 85	Twitter	Multiple/general
[23]	2021	SVM	F1-score: 97.3	Instagram	Multiple/general
[20]	2021	BERT	F1-score: 95.5	Twitter	COVID-19
[21]	2021	BERT	F1-score: 79.2	Twitter	COVID-19
[15]	2020	Random Forest	ROC: 85.1	Twitter	Multiple/general
[19]	2020	BERT	F1-score: 76.9	Twitter	HPV
[18]	2019	Neural Network	F1-score: 58	Twitter	Multiple/general
[24]	2019	LSTM-LM	F1-score: 80.87	Twitter	COVID-19
[22]	2019	fastText	Accuracy: 75	Facebook	Multiple/general
[13]	2018	SVM	F1-score: 73.13	Twitter	Multiple/general
[16]	2017	SVM	F1-score: 74.42	Twitter	HPV

This systematic review focuses on discussing the machine learning models used to detect public outlook towards vaccination, the performance of the models and the sources of collected data. After reviewing each paper in detail, we have come up with several insights which are reported in the figures that follow.

Figure 1 demonstrates the frequency of machine learning models used to detect the public outlook towards vaccination as described in the reviewed papers. SVM was found to be the most frequently used machine learning model followed by BERT.

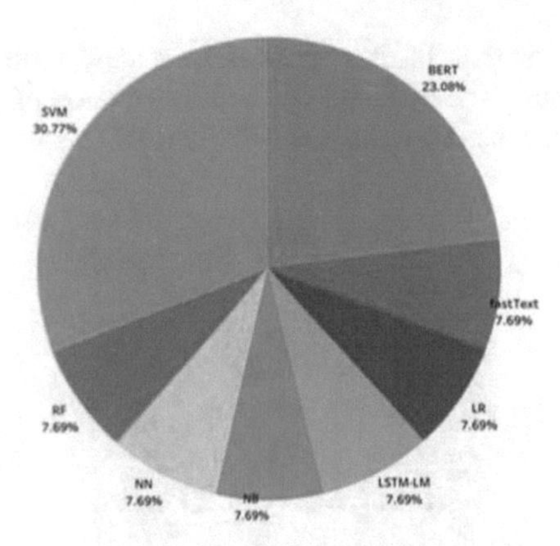

Fig. 1. Frequency of machine learning models used in the detection of public outlook towards vaccination.

In terms of the performance, SVM was also found to be the model that achieved the highest score in terms of accuracy and F-measure. Text classification problems usually have high dimensional feature spaces and are linearly separable [25]. SVM has overfitting protection and can find linear separators very easily, thus the SVM model performs the best in detecting public outlook from textual data. Figure 2 illustrates the performance of the models used in the reviewed literatures in the detection of public outlook towards vaccination. Both Figs. 1 and 2 answered our RQ1.

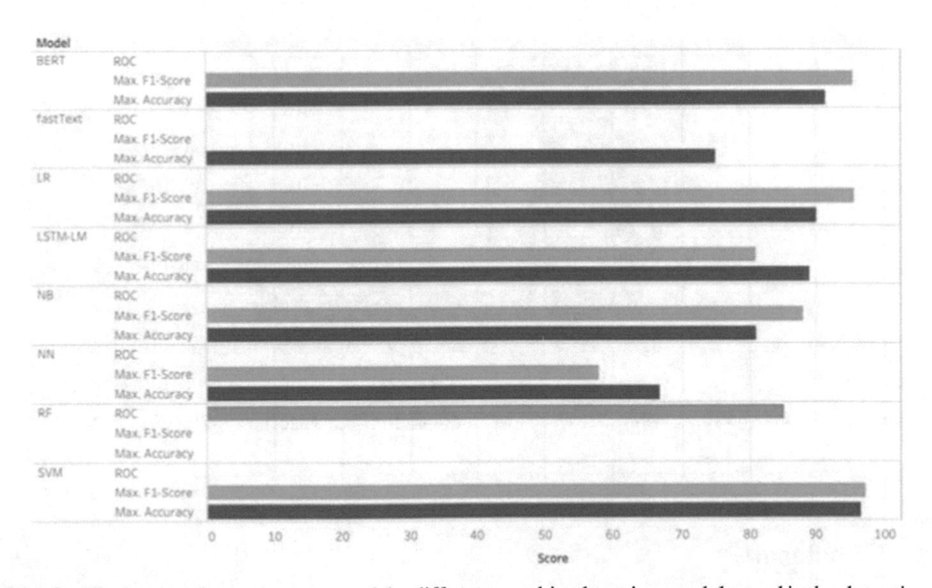

Fig. 2. The best performance scores of the different machine learning models used in the detection of public outlook towards vaccination

Figure 3 demonstrates that Twitter is the most widely used social media platform by researchers in extracting the data source for the detection of public outlook through machine learning approaches. Figure 3 answered our RQ2.

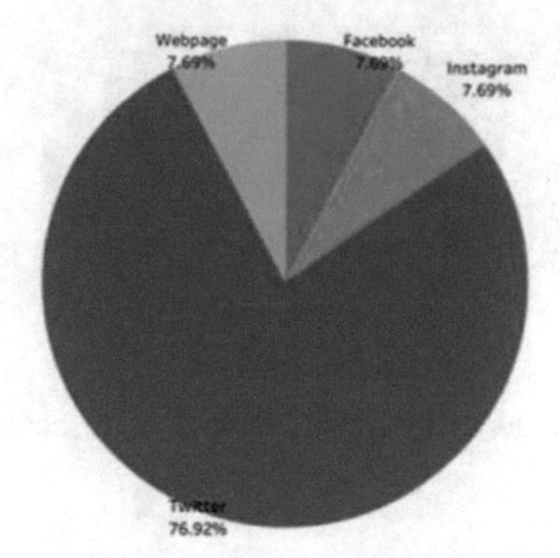

Fig. 3. Data sources from social media platforms for analyzing public outlook towards vaccination

Figure 4 illustrates the mostly studied types of vaccine for detecting public views towards vaccination using machine learning approaches. Three studies, [20, 21, 24] specifically focused on COVID-19 vaccine while two more studies, [16, 19] focused on the HPV vaccine. The rest of the studies discussed other types of vaccines such as MMR or various other vaccines in general.

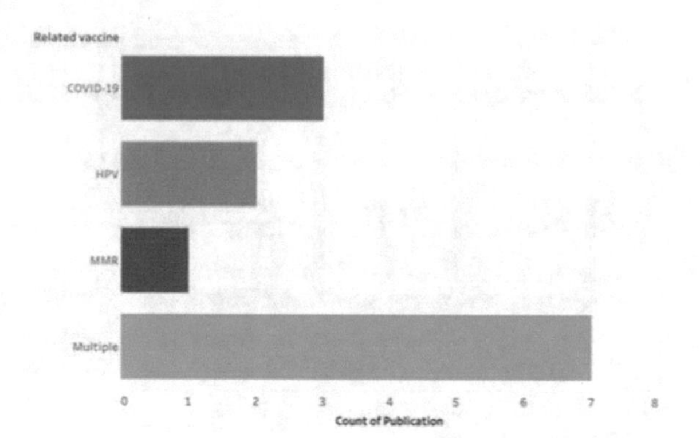

Fig. 4. Number of research conducted per vaccine type

5 Conclusion

An effective machine learning model is required to accurately detect the public outlook towards vaccination on social media which can be a great contribution to the entire healthcare system in battling vaccine hesitancy. From this systematic review, we can sense that deep learning and ensemble-based models perform better than classical machine learning models. Incorporating image and hashtag information into the training data can be useful to achieve better accuracy. However, more research work is required in deep learning and ensemble methods along with image and hashtag information to detect public outlook. Further improvements to the current machine learning implementations in this field can also be done by including data from multiple sources to train the model. Machine learning models with multiple data sources from various social media platforms of diverse input types, are expected to perform and generalize better with reduced bias, beside presenting more meaningful insights. Integrating emotional features expressed in texts extracted from the inherently dynamic nature of social media may also add more significant features in improving classification performance and model accuracy.

References

1. Kennedy, J.: Populist politics and vaccine hesitancy in Western Europe: an analysis of national-level data. Eur. J. Publ. Health **29**(3), 512–516 (2019). https://doi.org/10.1093/eurpub/ckz004. PMID: 30801109
2. Dube, E., Laberge, C., Guay, M., Bramadat, P., Roy, R., Bettinger, J.: Vaccine hesitancy: an overview. J. Hum. Vaccines Immunotherapeutics **9**(8), 1763–1773 (2013)
3. Pullan, S., Dey, M.: Vaccine hesitancy and anti-vaccination in the time of COVID-19: a Google trends analysis. Vaccine **39**(14), 1877–1881 (2021). https://doi.org/10.1016/j.vaccine.2021.03.019
4. Muric, G., Wu, J., Ferrara, E.: COVID-19 vaccine hesitancy on social media: building a public Twitter dataset of anti-vaccine content, vaccine misinformation and conspiracies, May 2021. http://arxiv.org/abs/2105.05134
5. Ruiz, J.B., Featherstone, J.D., Barnett, G.A.: Identifying vaccine-hesitant communities on Twitter and their geolocations: a network approach. In: Proceedings of the 54th Hawaii International Conference on System Sciences, pp. 3964–3969. HICSS, Hawaii (2021)
6. Yousefinaghani, S., Dara, R., Mubareka, S., Papadopoulos, A., Sharif, S.: An analysis of COVID-19 vaccine sentiments and opinions on Twitter. Int. J. Infect. Dis. **108**, 256–262 (2021). https://doi.org/10.1016/j.ijid.2021.05.059
7. Garay, J., Yap, R., Sabellano, M.J.: An analysis on the insights of the anti-vaccine movement from social media posts using k-means clustering algorithm and VADER sentiment analyzer. In: IOP Conference Series: Materials Science and Engineering, vol. 482, no. 1 (2019). https://doi.org/10.1088/1757-899X/482/1/012043
8. Kwok, S.W.H., Vadde, S.K., Wang, G.: Tweet topics and sentiments relating to COVID-19 vaccination among Australian Twitter users: machine learning analysis. J. Med. Internet Res. **23**(5), e26953 (2021). https://doi.org/10.2196/26953
9. Du, J., et al.: Use of deep learning to analyze social media discussions about the Human Papillomavirus Vaccine. JAMA Netw. Open **3**(11), e2022025 (2020). https://doi.org/10.1001/jamanetworkopen.2020.22025
10. MacDonald, N.E.: Vaccine hesitancy: definition, scope and determinants. Vaccine **33**(34), 4161–4164 (2015)
11. Salur, M.U., Aydin, I.: A novel hybrid deep learning model for sentiment classification. IEEE Access **8**, 58080–58093 (2020). https://doi.org/10.1109/ACCESS.2020.2982538
12. Argyris, Y.A., Monu, K., Tan, P.-N., Aarts, C., Jiang, F., Wiseley, K.A.: Using machine learning to compare provaccine and antivaccine discourse among the public on social media: algorithm development study. JMIR Publ. Health Surveill. **7**(6), e23105 (2021). https://doi.org/10.2196/23105

13. Yuan, X., Crooks, A.T.: Examining online vaccination discussion and communities in Twitter. In: ACM International Conference Proceeding Series, pp. 197–206 (2018). https://doi.org/10.1145/3217804.3217912
14. Meppelink, C.S., Hendriks, H., Trilling, D., Van Weert, J.C.M., Shao, A., Smit, E.S.: Reliable or not? An automated classification of webpages about early childhood vaccination using supervised machine learning. Patient Educ. Couns. **104**(6), 1460–1466 (2021). https://doi.org/10.1016/j.pec.2020.11.013
15. González, A.R., et al.: Creating a metamodel based on machine learning to identify the sentiment of vaccine and disease-related messages in Twitter: the MAVIS study. In: IEEE 33rd International Symposium on Computer-Based Medical Systems (CBMS), vol. 1, pp. 245–250 (2020). https://doi.org/10.1109/CBMS49503.2020.00053
16. Du, J., Xu, J., Song, H., Liu, X., Tao, C.: Optimization on machine learning based approaches for sentiment analysis on HPV vaccines related tweets. J. Biomed. Semant. **8**(1), (2017). https://doi.org/10.1186/s13326-017-0120-6
17. Piedrahita-Valdés, H., et al.: Vaccine hesitancy on social media: sentiment analysis from June 2011 to April 2019. Vaccines **9**(1), 1–12 (2021). https://doi.org/10.3390/vaccines9010028
18. Baru, C.: Analyzing public outlook towards vaccination using Twitter. Inst. Electr. Electron. Eng. IEEE Comput. Soc. (2019)
19. Zhang, L., Fan, H., Peng, C., Rao, G., Cong, Q.: Sentiment analysis methods for HPV vaccines related tweets based on transfer learning. Healthcare **8**(3), 307 (2020). https://doi.org/10.3390/healthcare8030307
20. To, Q.G., et al.: Applying machine learning to identify anti-vaccination tweets during the covid-19 pandemic. Int. J. Environ. Res. Publ. Health **18**(8), 4069 (2021). https://doi.org/10.3390/ijerph18084069
21. Liu, S., Li, J., Liu, J.: Leveraging transfer learning to analyze opinions, attitudes, and behavioral intentions toward COVID-19 vaccines: social media content and temporal analysis. J. Med. Internet Res. **23**(8), e30251 (2021)
22. Straton, N., Ng, R., Hyeju, J., Vatrapu, R.K., Mukkamala, R.R.,: Predictive modelling of stigmatized behaviour in vaccination discussions on Facebook. In: IEEE International Conference on Bioinformatics and Biomedicine (BIBM) (2019)
23. Wang, Z., Yin, Z., Argyris, Y.A.: Detecting Medical misinformation on social media using multimodal deep learning. IEEE J. Biomed. Health Inform. **25**(6), 2193–2203 (2021). https://doi.org/10.1109/JBHI.2020.3037027
24. Joshi, A., Dai, X., Karimi, S., Sparks, R., Paris, C., MacIntyre, C.R.: Shot or not: Comparison of NLP approaches for vaccination behaviour detection. In: Proceedings of the 2018 EMNLP Workshop SMM4H: The 3rd Social Media Mining for Health Applications Workshop and Shared Task, pp. 43–47. Association for Computational Linguistics, Brussels (2019). https://doi.org/10.18653/v1/w18-5911
25. Joachims, T.: Text categorization with support vector machines: Learning with many relevant features. In: Nédellec, C., Rouveirol, C. (eds.) ECML 1998. LNCS (LNAI), vol. 1398, pp. 137–142. Springer, Heidelberg (1998). https://doi.org/10.1007/BFb0026683

Forecasting Carbon Dioxide Emission for Malaysia Using Fractional Order Multivariable Grey Model

Assif Shamim Mustaffa Sulaiman[1(✉)], Ani Shabri[1], and Rashiq Rafiq Marie[2]

[1] Department of Mathematical Science, Faculty of Science, Universiti Teknologi Malaysia, Skudai, Malaysia
assifshamim@graduate.utm.my, ani@utm.my

[2] Information System Department, College of Computer Science and Engineering, Tahibah University, Medina, Kingdom of Saudi Arabia

Abstract. Forecasting the amount of carbon dioxide (CO_2) emissions has been crucially important to the civilisation of society to ensure that we can inhabit this planet in years to come. Hence, the study that focuses on the prediction on the amount of CO_2 releases into the environment has always been the focal point in any international level climate change conferences to ensure the target set would be considerably reached in the future. As the conventional multivariable grey model or GM (1,*N*) model has widely been used in the study to forecast short-term sample size data, this model possessed issues when dealing with prioritization of information as the weightage was evenly spread across all data points, causes an ineffective forecasting result. This study will use the fractional order multivariable grey model, or FAGM (1,*N*) model to predict the amount of CO_2 emissions for Malaysia within the 10 years timeframe data set. As the FAGM (1,*N*) model focuses on the prioritization of newer information, the proposed model will be able to forecast the CO_2 emissions better compared to the GM (1,*N*) model even with a small sample size data.

Keywords: Carbon dioxide emissions · Short-term forecast · Fractional order multivariable grey model

1 Introduction

The term "grey" in the grey system theory often deals with incomplete and uncertain data, which frequently has a small sample size [1]. With the monotonic addition property that permits data to be built up the system, as well as the ease of use mechanism, it is evident that researchers would employ this method when dealing with any type of short-term data for forecasting purposes [2]. The grey forecasting model has been widely used in a range of sectors to undertake short-term forecasts, ranging from demographic type data [3], to forecasting environmentally impacted data [4–7]. As a result, the grey forecasting model has been proven to be a useful tool for forecasting.

F. Saeed et al. (Eds.): IRICT 2021, LNDECT 127, pp. 151–159, 2022.
https://doi.org/10.1007/978-3-030-98741-1_14

The capacity to weigh and distribute the value of information evenly from the accumulation generating coefficient (AGO) process is one of the notable benefit when applying the grey forecasting model. However, it's also vital to remember that the system's newer sets of data should be given more weight than the older data that the standard GM (1,1) model is not capable of. The rolling mechanism introduced by Chang et al. able to restructure the forecast ability when the newest information replaces the oldest information in the system [8, 9]. Though the contribution of the research brings a significant impact on the grey forecasting model, however, the process is strenuous. As a result, fractional order accumulation, an enhanced variation of grey forecasting model, may reflect the importance of newer information in the system, and will be studied further in this paper.

The fractional order form of grey forecasting model, better known as the FAGM (1,1) model, was introduced by Wu et al. [10]. It replaces the typical one-order AGO (1-AGO) process in the GM (1,1) model with a fractional order accumulation (r^{th}-order accumulated generating sequence). The FAGM (1,1) model's two main ideas are information disparities and the prioritization of newer information. Firstly, newer information should be considered differently than older information, and each piece of information in the system will be evaluated differently if the rth-order accumulation generating sequence is used. Second, newer information will be prioritized over older information by giving newer information more weight, which will minimize primitive sequence randomness and increase the model's forecast accuracy significantly.

Many academics have used the FAGM (1,1) model in their research, and the findings have been positive when compared to the classic GM (1,1) model. Wang et al. employed the FAGM (1,1) model to investigate gear fault trend prediction [11]. The results strongly suggest that the FAGM (1,1) model outperformed other commonly used forecasting models model in terms of model error. Another study by Sahin & Sahin looked at the number of confirmed COVID-19 cases in three major nations by implementing the FANGBM (1,1) model, which is a nonlinear grey Bernoulli variant of FAGM (1,1) [12]. This study's in-sample employs a 35-day daily case range and forecasts the following 30 days. The FANGBM (1,1) model gave the lowest MAPE, RMSE, and model errors values when compared to the GM (1,1) and NGBM (1,1) models.

We will now look into specific studies that use the FAGM (1,1) model to forecast CO_2 emissions related data. Based on the proposed novel FAGM (1,1) model by Wu et al., the authors use the FAGM (1,1) model to investigate Taiwan's CO_2 emissions data [10]. The result reveals that when the r value for the FAGM (1,1) model is 0.1 (for r^{th}-order accumulation generating sequence), the FAGM (1,1) model produced the lowest MAPE value for in-sample data, suggesting that with suitable r value, the better the fitting error of the GM (1,1). They further analysed the model with different r values and discovered that it yielded low MAPE values for both the in-sample and out-sample. This shows that the overall amount of CO_2 emissions for each subsequent year has a close link, as evidenced by the strong correlation in the grey system.

There are a few studies on the CO_2 emissions forecast that attempted to enhance the current FAGM (1,1) model. A study to analysed China's CO_2 emissions from 1999 to 2012, Gao et al. presented the discrete FAGM (1,1) model called FAGM (1,1,D) [13]. The fractional accumulation value in the FAGM (1,1) model is optimised using a technique known as the particle swarm optimization, PSO method. The MAPE value was used as the optimization objective in the model, while the value of r was used as the search parameter. According to the findings, both the FAGM (1,1) and FAGM (1,1,D) models produce low MAPE values, with forecasted values for the next three years that are practically indistinguishable between the two models when compared to other conventional grey models.

Next, an optimised FAGM (1,1) model is used to forecast the top 20 nations with the biggest CO_2 emissions contributors. The authors employ the genetic algorithm method, GA method, to identify the appropriate model parameters rather than the traditional least squares (OLS) method [14]. The proposed GA-FAGM (1,1) model has various distinguishing characteristics, including the use of a single variable model as a development basis and fractional order accumulation during control variable determination. In comparison to existing grey forecasting methods, the suggested GA-FAGM (1,1) model provided the smallest MAPE value in 11 of the 20 nations studied, demonstrating the superiority of the FAGM (1,1) model in forecasting emissions related data.

Hence, this research will implement the FAGM (1,N) model to forecast Malaysia's CO_2 emissions data in order to demonstrate its superiority over the traditional GM (1,N) model. This paper will be structured as accordingly: The technique of the FAGM (1,N) model and the usage of assessment metrics will be presented in Sect. 2, and the results of the models' performance will be shown in Sect. 3 along with discussions. Finally, Sect. 4 will bring this paper to a close.

2 Methodology

2.1 Fractional Order Multivariable Grey, FAGM (1,N) Model

The grey forecasting model, which was first developed by Deng, has been widely employed in a variety of fields, with a large range of grey forecasting models [15]. The multivariable grey model, also known as the GM (M,N), belongs to the grey forecasting model family, with M indicating the order's number and N indicating the variable's number. This study focuses on the fractional order accumulation form of the grey forecasting model, often known as the FAGM (1,N) model. As this paper is using the emissions in Malaysia data, the initial series of the emissions is denoted as

$$X^{(0)} = \left(X^{(0)}(1), X^{(0)}(2), X^{(0)}(3), \ldots, x^{(0)}(n)\right) \tag{1}$$

where i = 1, 2, ..., N denoting the total variable's numbers and n denoting data entries for modelling sets of data. The rth-AGO in Eq. (1) is implemented to give prioritization of new information by distributing difference weightage among the information of the system based on the relevancy of information. The new sequence series of $X^{(r)}$ is given in Eq. (2).

$$X^{(r)} = \left(X^{(r)}(1), X^{(r)}(2), X^{(r)}(3), \ldots, X^{(r)}(n)\right) \tag{2}$$

where

$$x^{(r)} = \sum_{i=1}^{k} x^{(r-1)}(i);\ k = 1, 2, \ldots, n \tag{3}$$

The rth-AGO of the initial series, $X^{(0)}$ is denoted as

$$\alpha^{(r)}X^{(0)} = \left(\alpha^{(r)}x^{(0)}(1), \alpha^{(r)}x^{(0)}(2), \ldots, \alpha^{(r)}x^{(0)}(n)\right) \tag{4}$$

where

$$\alpha^{(r)}x^{(0)}(k) = \alpha^{(r-1)}x^{(0)}(k) - \alpha^{(r-1)}x^{(0)}(k-1) \tag{5}$$

and k = 2, …, n.

By assuming the initial series $X^{(0)}$ is a series of non-negative sequence, for r = 1,2,…,n,

$$X^{(r)}(k) = \left(x^{(r)}(1), x^{(r)}(2), \ldots, x^{(r)}(n)\right) \tag{6}$$

Equation (6) is denote as the rth-AGO sequence of $X^{(0)}$, hence we will obtain

$$x^{(r)}(k) = \sum_{i=1}^{k} \binom{k-i+r-1}{k-i} x^{(0)}(i),\ k = 1, 2, \ldots, n \tag{7}$$

where

$$\binom{k-i+r-1}{k-i} = \frac{(k-i+r-1)(k-i+r-2)\ldots r}{(k-1)!} \tag{8}$$

As the order of r (0 < r ≤ 1) of $X^{(0)}$ AGO, we have

$$\begin{aligned} \alpha^{(r)}X^{(0)} &= \alpha^{(1)}X^{(1-r)}(k) \\ &= \left(\alpha^{(1)}X^{(1-r)}(1), \ldots, \alpha^{(1)}X^{(1-r)}(n)\right) \end{aligned} \tag{9}$$

Hence,

$$x^{(r-1)}(k) + az^{(r)}(k) = \sum_{i=2}^{N} bx^{(r)}(k) \tag{10}$$

is the general form of FAGM (1,N) model. The parameter a is denote to as developing coefficient of the grey system, whereas b is the control variable of the system. When the $r = 1$, the FAGM (1,N) model will be simplified to the GM (1,N) model in its traditional form.

The sequence of $z^{(r)}(k)$

$$z^{(1)} = \left\{z^{(1)}(2), z^{(1)}(3), z^{(1)}(4), \ldots, z^{(1)}(k)\right\} \tag{11}$$

is referred as the mean equation from Eq. (2), as shown in Eq. (12)

$$z^{(1)}(k) = \omega x^{(1)}(k) + (1-\omega)x^{(1)}(k-1) \tag{12}$$

where conventionally the value of $\omega = 0.5$.

The FAGM (1,*N*) model uses the ordinary least square (OLS) method to calculate both parameters *a* and *b* using Eq. (13).

$$[a,b]^{T} = \left(B^{T}B\right)^{-1}B^{T}Y_{N} \tag{13}$$

where.

$$B = \begin{bmatrix} -z^{(r)}(2) \; x_2^{(r)}(2) \ldots x_N^{(r)}(2) \\ -z^{(r)}(3) \; x_2^{(r)}(3) \ldots x_N^{(r)}(3) \\ \vdots \quad \vdots \quad \ddots \quad \vdots \\ -z^{(r)}(n) \; x_2^{(r)}(n) \ldots x_N^{(r)}(n) \end{bmatrix}, \text{ and } \; Y = \begin{bmatrix} x^{(r-1)}(2) \\ x^{(r-1)}(3) \\ \vdots \\ x^{(r-1)}(n) \end{bmatrix} \tag{14}$$

Let

$$\hat{a} = [a, b_1, b_2, \ldots, b_N]^T = (B^T B)^{-1} B^T Y$$

the whitenization solution of FAGM (1,*N*) model for equation $\frac{dx_1^{(1)}}{dt} + ax_1^{(1)} = \sum_{i=2}^{N} bx^{(1)}$ is

$$\begin{aligned} x^{(1)}(t) &= e^{-at}\left[\sum_{i=2}^{N} \int bx^{(1)}(t)e^{at} + x^{(1)}(0) - \sum_{i=2}^{N} \int b\,x^{(1)}(0)dt\right] \\ &= e^{-at}\left[x_1^{(1)}(0) - t\sum_{i=2}^{N} b\,x^{(1)}(0) + \sum_{i=2}^{N} b\,x^{(1)}(t)e^{at}dt\right] \end{aligned} \tag{15}$$

The forecasted values of the series point $X_i^{(1)}$ from r^{th}-AGO is expressed as

$$\hat{x}_1^{(0)}(k+1) = \left(x_1^{(0)} - \frac{1}{a}\sum_{i=2}^{N} b\,x^{(1)}(k+1)\right)e^{-at} + \frac{1}{a}\sum_{i=2}^{N} b\,x^{(1)}(k+1) \tag{16}$$

where value of $X_1^{(1)}(0)$ takes on the value of $X_1^{(0)}(1)$.

Lastly, the restored values of inverse accumulation of FAGM (1,*N*) model is

$$\hat{x}_1^{(0)}(k+1) = \hat{x}_1^{(1)}(k+1) - \hat{x}_1^{(1)}(k) \tag{17}$$

2.2 Forecast Accuracy Measurement

The mean absolute percentage error (MAPE), which measures the proximity between the actual and forecasted values, is the accuracy precision measurement used to evaluate the performance of the proposed FAGM (1,*N*) model, using Eq. (18).

$$\text{MAPE} = \frac{1}{m}\left(\left|\frac{\sum(\hat{x}^{(1)} - x^{(0)})}{x^{(0)}}\right|\right) \times 100\% \tag{18}$$

The number of observations of the system is denoted by *m*. In conclusion, we may conclude that the smaller the value of MAPE, the higher the level of accuracy of the proposed model.

2.3 Conceptual Framework

A conceptual framework depicts the cause-and-effect relationship for the task in question, which was carried out to meet the research objectives depicted in Fig. 1. This paper is initiated by the data collection process of CO_2 emissions, population, Gross Domestic Product (GDP), and energy consumption. Next, we will begin the process of model building by performing the calculation of FOA method, or r^{th}-order AGO using a pre-determined ω value of 0.5 into the GM (1,*N*) model. The step taken to search for the optimal *r* value, the value of MAPE of modelling will serve as the objective of this study. When we have found the best MAPE value, we will use the *r* value into the FAGM (1,*N*) model to forecast, and the error forecast will be recorded. A new set of forecasted value using the proposed FAGM (1,*N*) model is obtained and compared against the traditional multivariable grey model, GM (1,*N*) model.

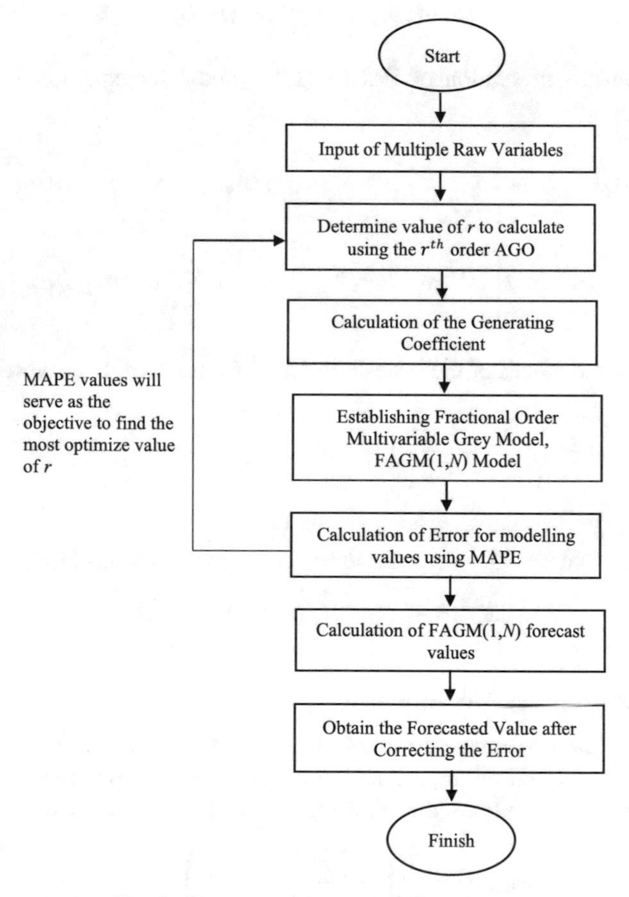

Fig. 1. Conceptual framework flowchart

3 Result and Discussion

This paper uses the data for CO_2 emissions in Malaysia, with subsequent factors such as population, GDP, and energy consumption from the year 2010 to 2019. The data for CO_2 emissions and energy consumption are extracted from the International Energy Agency (IEA), whereas population and GDP are extracted from World Bank Data. To validate the proposed models, data from 2010 to 2016 will serve as the testing set of data while the remaining subsequent 3 years will be for the forecasting purpose.

Table 1. Original Malaysia's CO_2 Emissions data from year 2010 to 2019

Year	Carbon dioxide emissions (Mt)	Population (million people)	GDP (million USD)	Energy consumption (Mtoe)
2010	189.9	28.2	225,017	24.0
2011	191.5	28.7	297,952	23.6
2012	192.8	29.1	314,443	24.1
2013	208.7	29.5	323,277	28.1
2014	220.2	29.9	338,062	29.3
2015	220.2	30.3	301,355	27.5
2016	216.3	30.7	301,255	28.3
2017	210.8	31.1	319,112	28.9
2018	228.0	31.5	358,715	28.3
2019	236.6	31.9	364,681	29.5

Table 1 above depicts the original Malaysia's CO_2 emissions along with its subsequent variables. This paper will demonstrate the effectiveness of implementing the FAGM (1,4) model against the conventional GM (1,4) model for comparison. Using Eq. (1), we will denote the Malaysia's CO_2 emissions as $x_1^{(r)}$ and its subsequent variables will be denoted as $x_2^{(r)} \ldots x_4^{(r)}$. The values for r are non-negative within the range of 0.1 to 2, which reflects the rth-order accumulated generating sequence using the FAGM (1,4) model. Both GM (1,4) and FAGM (1,4) models use the OLS method to calculate the parameters for both equations, using Eq. (13). The values of parameters for both models are shown in Table 2 below.

Table 2. Parameter's values for GM (1,4) and FAGM (1,4) models

Parameters	GM (1,4)	FAGM (1,4)
a	1.8197	1.9370
b_2	3.7931	7.3467
b_3	−0.0001	0.0002
b_4	5.0546	5.3378

The value of r selected for this paper is 0.9. The selection of the r value is determined by setting the MAPE as the optimization objective and r as the search parameter. Essentially, the value of r shall be used when the MAPE value prompted is the smallest. Hence, Table 3 displays the forecasted values for both the GM (1,4) and FAGM (1,4) models. The MAPE values for FAGM (1,4) model outperform the GM (1,4) model by showcasing a smaller value, 2.72% against GM (1,4) model which is 5.33%. This can be achieved as the rth- order accumulated generating sequence in the FAGM (1,4) is able to transform the values in the data to prioritize the newer information compared to the older information by applying more weightage on newer information. As a result, the authors conclude that the FAGM (1,4) model is superior to the GM (1,4) model. Figure 1 below illustrates the graph of actual versus the forecasted values of CO_2 emissions in Malaysia.

Table 3. Forecasted values for GM (1,4) and FAGM (1,4) models

Year	Original values	GM (1,4)		FAGM (1,4)	
		Forecasted values	APE (%)	Forecasted values	APE (%)
2010	189.9	189.9		189.9	
2011	191.5	168.0		174.2	
2012	192.8	214.6		219.1	
2013	208.7	220.8		222.4	
2014	220.2	220.8		224.2	
2015	220.2	216.5		216.5	
2016	216.3	221.6		219.8	
2017	210.8	223.8	**6.14%**	224.3	6.41%
2018	228.0	217.4	4.66%	227.6	**0.20%**
2019	236.6	224.3	5.20%	232.9	**1.55%**
MAPE (%)			5.33%		**2.72%**

4 Conclusion

The primary goal of this work is to demonstrate that using the FAGM (1,N) model to undertake a short-term forecast based on CO_2 emissions data is superior. The criteria that set apart between the GM (1,N) model with FAGM (1,N) model is its ability to prioritize new information that is better reflected with the rth-order accumulated generating sequence when the in-sample size of the data is small. To minimize the MAPE values for the FAGM (1,N) model, the MAPE will serve as the optimization objective with the r act as the search parameter. Upon determining the most suitable r value, it can be used to forecast and compare against the conventional GM (1,N) model. The indication of MAPE value proved that FAGM (1,4) model is the better model used to forecast Malaysia's CO_2 emissions data. With these hints, it may be served as guidelines for us on what are the effects of global warming, and the increase of the number of CO_2 emissions into the environment may harm the future generations to have a safe and conducive living place to inhabit. As we approach a tipping point of no return that will catastrophe our chances of surviving on this planet, more actions and initiatives should be implemented from all sectors to ensure a promising land for the next decades incoming.

References

1. Xiao, L., Wang, H., Duan, M.: The optimization of grey model GM (1,1) based on posterior error. In: 2020 5th International Conference on Control Robot cybernetics CRC 2020, pp. 87–91
2. Hu, Y.-C.: Energy demand forecasting using a novel remnant GM(1,1) model. Soft. Comput. **24**(18), 13903–13912 (2020). https://doi.org/10.1007/s00500-020-04765-3
3. Ma, L., Li, J., Zhao, Y.: Population forecast of China's rural community based on CFANGBM and improved aquila optimizer algorithm, 1–30 (2021)
4. Qian, W., Sui, A.: A novel structural adaptive discrete grey prediction model and its application in forecasting renewable energy generation. Expert Syst. Appl. **186**, 115761 (2021)
5. Duan, H., Liu, Y.: Research on a grey prediction model based on energy prices and its applications. Comput. Ind. Eng. **162**, 107729 (2021)
6. Xiong, P., Li, K., Shu, H., Wang, J.: Forecast of natural gas consumption in the Asia-Pacific region using a fractional-order incomplete gamma grey model. Energy **237**, 121533 (2021)
7. Zhao, Y.-F., Wang, Z.-X., He, L.-Y.: Forecasting the seasonal natural gas consumption in the US using a gray model with dummy variables. Appl. Soft Comput. **113**, 108002 (2021)
8. Chang, S.C., Lai, H.C., Yu, H.C.: A variable P value rolling grey forecasting model for Taiwan semiconductor industry production. Technol. Forecast Soc. Change **72**, 623–640 (2005)
9. Mustaffa, A.S., Shabri, A.: An improved rolling NGBM(1,1) model with GRG nonlinear method of optimization for fossil carbon dioxide emissions in Malaysia and Singapore. In: 2020 11th IEEE Control and System Graduate Research Colloquium (ICSGRC 2020), pp 32–37 (2020)
10. Wu, L., Liu, S., Yao, L., Yan, S., Liu, D.: Grey system model with the fractional order accumulation. Commun. Nonlinear Sci. Numer. Simul. **18**, 1775–1785 (2013)
11. Wang, J., Sun, C., Sun, Q., Yan, H.: Gear fault trend prediction based on FGM(1, 1) model. In: Proceeding of 2017 32nd Youth Academic Annual Conference of Chinese Association of Automation, YAC 2017, pp. 827–831 (2017)
12. Şahin, U., Şahin, T.: Forecasting the cumulative number of confirmed cases of COVID-19 in Italy, UK and USA using fractional nonlinear grey Bernoulli model. Chaos Solitons Fractals (2020). https://doi.org/10.1016/j.chaos.2020.109948
13. Gao, M., Mao, S., Yan, X., Wen, J.: Estimation of Chinese CO2 emission based on a discrete fractional accumulation grey model. J. Grey Syst. **27**, 114–130 (2015)
14. Hu, Y.C., Jiang, P., Tsai, J.F., Yu, C.Y.: An optimized fractional grey prediction model for carbon dioxide emissions forecasting. Int. J. Environ. Res. Publ. Health **18**, 1–13 (2021)
15. Ju-Long, D.: Control problems of grey systems. Syst. Control Lett. **1**, 288–294 (1982)

A Hybrid Algorithm for Pattern Matching: An Integration of Berry-Ravindran and Raita Algorithms

Abdulwahab Ali Almazroi[1], Fathey Mohammed[2](✉), Muhammad Ahsan Qureshi[1], Asad Ali Shah[1], Ibrahim Abaker Targio Hashim[3], Nabil Hasan Al-Kumaim[4], and Abubakar Zakari[5]

[1] College of Computing and Information Technology at Khulais, Department of Information Technology, University of Jeddah, Jeddah, Saudi Arabia
aalmazroi@uj.edu.sa

[2] School of Computing, Universiti Utara Malaysia (UUM), 06010 Sintok, Kedah, Malaysia

[3] Department of Computer Science, College of Computing and Informatics, University of Sharjah, Sharjah 27272, UAE

[4] Faculty of Technology Management and Technopreneurship, Center of Technopreneurship Development (CTeD), Universiti Teknikal Malaysia Melaka (UTeM), 75460 Melaka, Malacca, Malaysia

[5] Department of Computer Science, Kano University of Science and Technology, Wudil P.M.B 3244, Kano, Nigeria

Abstract. Due to the quick actions of technology, a complicated and huge volume of data deriving from biological sciences are generated which makes string matching patterns a challenging task. This direction has the aim to make the utilization of an individual algorithm for string searching nearly ineffectual as the number of tries and the number of observations continues to increase. So, the solution is in the grouping of more than one algorithm to create a hybrid algorithm for quicker performance. The proposed hybrid algorithm uses the best features of Raita algorithm and Berry-Ravindran algorithm. The reason for choosing these two algorithms is because they achieve better performance in "number of attempts" and "number of character comparisons" tests. New Hybrid Algorithm (BRR) is able to produce better results by decreasing the effort and character comparisons. The data types used to evaluate performance are English text, DNA, and protein. In number of attempts evaluation, for DNA, English, and protein text datasets, the improvement of the hybrid algorithm was 18%, 50%, and 50% in comparison to Berry-Ravindran algorithm and it was 71%, 74%, and 70% in comparison to Raita algorithm. The results show that regardless of the size of the data used, the mix of algorithms yields better results and improved performance than the original algorithm.

Keywords: Hybrid algorithm · Pattern · String searching · String matching

F. Saeed et al. (Eds.): IRICT 2021, LNDECT 127, pp. 160–172, 2022.
https://doi.org/10.1007/978-3-030-98741-1_15

1 Introduction

Since the beginning of computer science, the problem of string-matching has gained a lot of interest from researchers, and it plays a basic role in assuring pattern matching and string search from multiple biological resources, such as protein and DNA data [1–4]. The importance of string matching involves a wide range of interests, such as applications, biometrics, internet search engines, spell checkers, text processing, and more [5–9].

In simple terms, the string-matching algorithm is a technique for finding occurrences of a pattern in a text-based based document [10]. The main problem with the algorithms is knowing the way to slide the window during the search phase so as to compare the pattern in a big text pool [11].

The algorithms typically work through scanning a set of texts in a window [12]. If a match or mismatch happens, the window includes the length of the pattern. Formerly, characters in the text and the pattern were compared; the text in the window is arranged in rows until a match is found. Matches or mismatches typically occur throughout the search phase [13]. When this event occurs, the window moves to the rightmost portion to start aligning the text going right to left at the start of a given search [14].

The biological science data has been increasing due to the rapid advancement in technology in the last few years. Therefore, instead of using one string search algorithm to resolve these complicated search problems, two algorithms are integrated to decrease number of comparisons performed improve the searching time when performing string matching. Therefore, the focus of recent attention has been on the development of hybrid algorithms due to improved performance and better solutions [9, 15–20]. The reason being the fact that scientific data is getting stronger [21].

With regards to this development, a new hybrid algorithm called the hybrid Berry Ravindran-Raita algorithm (BRR) is proposed, which basically involves a process combining the vital features of the Berry-Ravindran (BR) and Raita(R) algorithms to improve search effectiveness. The purpose of selecting these algorithms to create a hybrid algorithm is that the Raita(R) algorithm has the best practical behavior [22] and the performance of the search pattern in English text because it has character dependence.

With respect to Berry-Ravindran (BR) algorithm, it is known to have two good characters with good shift values [8]; by using the bad character table (brBc) during the search stage, the BR is simply shifted to the highest Bit distance.

1.1 Problem Statement

The rapid development of technology has made it necessary to generate complex and large amount of biological data are generated making pattern matching a daunting job. Hence, the developments are intended to make the utilization of an algorithm for string search virtually ineffectual, as the amount of tries and the number of comparisons stays comparatively high. Consequently, a hybrid algorithm may be created by the grouping of more than one algorithm in order to improve performance is the way forward.

2 Related Studies

Early research efforts have confirmed that the good performance of integrating the two algorithms leads to enhanced mixing performance in the search stage, because each algorithm has specific advantages and can improve output when properly combined.

The hybrid algorithm is called KMPBS which uses a combination of two algorithms including the Boyer Moore (BM) and the Knuth-Morris-Pratt (KMP) algorithms [15]. This hybrid algorithm decreases the first or last character that did not attain the condition to decrease the number. Compare and promote the implementation of pattern matching. The improvements are made in the pre-processing and search phases by using KMP's algorithm Next function and the BMHS algorithm's Right p [j] values.

In another study, the combination of the two algorithms forms a hybrid algorithm named ZTFS [18]. This algorithm is a combination of Fast Search (FS) and Zhu-Takaoka (ZT). The hybrid algorithms uses processes from both FS and ZT algorithms, which addresses bad character heuristics and BM good suffix heuristics for demonstrating characters, and ztBc (a) giving maximum shift value. The b) function, as well as the bmGs(j) function, also prefix the pattern in the preprocessing stage.

Another hybrid algorithm that has been put into use includes the Aho-Corasick (AC) and the Backward Hashing (BH) algorithms [17]. These algorithms are suitable for scanning and tracking information about text viruses. One of the methods used by the hybrid algorithm is to use the Prefix Sliding Window (PSW) to index the shift table. Moreover, the Backward Hashing (BH) algorithm checks for lengthier modes in the PSW and is checked since the shift value did not exceed the PSW, as a result, helps save time.

A hybrid ZTBMH was also implemented. This hybrid consists of the Boyer-Moore-Horspool (BMH) and Zhu-Takaoka (ZT) algorithms [23]. The algorithm can be used in searching biological sequence database, specifically for minor letters and lengthy patterns. Performance improvements are obtained by utilizing a function in the preprocessing stage that handles characters' bad character heuristic. Additionally, a function is used that provides the largest shift. value. The search stage uses these functions to calculate the highest shift value in all attempts. In the case of a mismatch, the bad character shift value is used.

The ShiftAnd-BMS algorithm is a hybrid algorithm [16] that searches for regular strings and uncertain strings in English text. The algorithm integrates ShiftAnd and BMS algorithm. The hybrid algorithms performance is enhanced by using several techniques provided by the individual algorithm. Firstly, it uses the shifting technique provided by the BMS algorithm. Secondly, in the case the match is found at the end of pattern then the hybrid algorithm transfers to the ShiftAnd matching instead. This continues till no match is identified at the existing point, then jumps to the next one before the final BMS shift position.

The integration of Skip Search and Berry-Ravindran algorithms was performed to propose a hybrid algorithm to improve search effectiveness. The algorithm performed better in terms of search results as compared to the original algorithms [20].

In another study [19], a grouping of Alpha Skip Search and Berry Ravindran algorithms is experimented on biological data and English textual data. The results of experiment exhibited superiority of this integration over original algorithms on English text and DNA protein datasets.

Researchers also proposed a hybrid algorithm that reduces the number of character comparisons in string matching to improve performance. They named it Fast Online Hybrid Matching Algorithm [24]. This hybrid algorithm uses techniques of three algorithms including 1) quick search, 2) SSABS [25] and ABSBMH [26]. The results showed the proposed hybrid approach performing better than ABSBMH algorithm by taking fewer attempts.

The Atheer algorithm is also a hybrid algorithm that uses a combination of efficient string-matching algorithm [27]. The proposed algorithm uses features of Karp–Rabin, Raita, and Smith algorithms. The proposed hybrid algorithm performed more efficiently in comparison to several algorithms (Horspool, Quick search, Two-way, Fast search, SSABS, TVSBS, AKRAM, and Maximum shift).

An improved hybrid algorithm that performs better than the Atheer algorithm was also proposed [28]. The new hybrid algorithm accomplishes this by using the searching features from the Atheer algorithm, and the shifting techniques of the Berry-Ravindran algorithms. This allowed the hybrid algorithm to perform better in both evaluation metrics including 1) number of attempts and 2) less character comparisons, in contrast to the original algorithms, even when evaluation was performed on multiple datasets.

Researchers proposed a hybrid algorithm capable of reducing character comparisons made [26]. The proposed called ABSBMH algorithm is based on two algorithms. This includes SSABS algorithm and a modified version of the Horspool algorithm. However, the algorithm did little to no improvement in number of attempts evaluation.

Researchers proposed an algorithm that aimed at improving string matching performance in both "number of attempts" and "number of character comparisons" [9]. It was named after the evaluations metrics, and thus called Minimum Attempts and Character Comparisons (MACC) hybrid algorithm. The hybrid algorithm uses a novel technique to improve performance in addition to using index-based shifting and the Berry-Ravindran algorithm. The algorithm performed better than both original algorithms and techniques used in the hybrid algorithm.

3 Materials and Methods

The study first determined the advantages and disadvantages of the string search algorithms before deciding on the R and BR algorithms. Then extract the finest attributes of these algorithms. The shift value from the initial stage (pre-processing) is calculated to choose a larger shift value for window in the search stage.

The hybrid approach ensures that when two or more algorithms are incorporated, the hybrid algorithm provides optimal properties of original algorithms are preserved and performance is improved. BR utilizes two consecutive characters to provide the best shift value. Nevertheless, the drawback of the algorithm is it do not search the initial stage as a first phase. The Raita algorithm is beneficial when searching for patterns specific to English text [22], and in practice it has a good behavior in performance because of the existence of character reliance.

Raita algorithm performs its searching functions by beginning every initial attempt through the comparisons of character between the pattern's last and first characters positioned in the window. When a match occurs, comparisons are done as follows; firstly, comparison among pattern's starting character and the last left character in the window, secondly, the center character is also compared, and lastly, before comparing the rest of the character beginning from the second to the last but one, and then back to the central point character comparisons again when a match is existed.

The BRR may exhibit good performance because tests are performed at every beginning point and at every attempt leading to a higher shift value than the original algorithm, and subsequently the weaknesses are overcome by the hybrid which applied their advantages in the searching stage.

3.1 Hybrid Algorithm Pre-processing Phase

The preprocessing stage has been developed using a hybrid algorithm [29], and at this stage the hybrid algorithm does perform the construction of the bad character table, brBc, that is built through utilizing the Berry-Ravindran formula, as shown in formula. 1:

$$\mathrm{brBc}[\mathrm{m}, \mathrm{n}] = \min \left\{ \begin{array}{ll} 1 & \text{If } \mathrm{x}[\mathrm{m}-1] = \mathrm{m} \\ \mathrm{m}-\mathrm{i}+1 & \text{If } \mathrm{x}[\mathrm{i}] \times [\mathrm{i}+1] = \mathrm{mn} \\ \mathrm{m}+1 & \text{If } \mathrm{x}[0] = \mathrm{n} \\ \mathrm{m}+2 & \text{Otherwise} \end{array} \right\} \tag{1}$$

3.2 Hybrid Algorithm Searching Phase

In this stage, it commences by using the pattern length. The following processes are conducted in this phase:

- The text's m length characters will be scanned to break down the potential starting search points.
- Checking of the last character of the text window. If there is a mismatch with the pattern, then move the Berry-Ravindran shift value by applying the rightmost two next characters immediately once detecting the m-length character.
- If scanned characters in the pattern are found, the character are arranged from the start of the search point and the pattern with the corresponding position in the pattern.
- Matching is started from the end with the character at the far right in the text window, and when it matches, a comparison will be made of the first initial character together with the character in the text window that is at the left-end. Lastly, the match occurs. The second character is compared to the last. Other characters of one character.
- If a given match or mismatch happens, the process involves moving the pattern. This is done by determining the Berry-Ravindran shift value of the two characters following the window, i.e., the right-end character.

4 Analysis

The new hybrid consists of the preprocessing stage of Berry-Ravindran, it represents the $O(m + \sigma^2)$ time complexity [6], so the time complexity of the preprocessing stage is $O(m + \sigma^2)$. The time complexity of the search stage is classified as follows.

4.1 Lemma 1: The Worst-Case Scenario with Respect to Time Complexity is Defined as O(Mn).

Proof: The worst-case interpretation of the hybrid algorithm denotes that the whole character in the text is matched and cannot be larger than m times. The worst-case commonly happens all the way through the process, in case pattern's characters are similar to the characters present in the next text. For instance, with the text T = "aaaaaaaaaaaaa" and the pattern P = "aaaaa", it is noted that O(mn) is the worst-case time complexity.

4.2 Lemma 2: The Best-Case Scenario with Respect to Time Complexity is O(N/(M + 2)).

Proof: In each attempt, when the character being checked in the pattern does not exist, the shift value is going to be $m + 2$, this is calculated by the Berry-Ravindran function in the preprocessing stage. The best-case scenario would arise if the characters used in the pattern do not occur in the text given. For instance, with the text T = "aaaaaaaaaaaaaaa" and the pattern P = "bbbbb", the shift value will equate to $m + 2$, this is performed for each attempt of the search stage, therefore the best-case time complexity is $O(n/(m) + 2))$.

The features used to evaluate the mean time complexity include the alphabet pool size and the likelihood of each character being present in each text. Therefore, the maximum offset to be implemented is expressed as $m + 2$, and the minimum character comparison is normally between $1 - m$, and it is a random sum established on the input data. The average time complexity is often not predictable due to its randomness and no actual estimates.

4.3 Evaluation

In evaluating the performance of the hybrid and original algorithms, three distinct forms of data are utilized as test data for each algorithm, and the graphs obtained from each algorithm are utilized as a comparison between each algorithm. The data selected for the test algorithm is the benchmark for evaluating the performance of the algorithm [18] when given characters and patterns of different sizes. Similarly, the experimental results obtained from the proposed hybrid and 8 executions of the original algorithm.

The data type utilized for the evaluation have various letter sizes, where σ indicates the letter size. This includes DNA data having $\sigma = 4$, protein data having $\sigma = 20$, and English text having $\sigma = 100$. This research acquired English texts and DNA data are from the Gutenberg project [30], while the protein data was acquired from the Swiss-Prot database [31].

The algorithm was executed on a computer having the specifications including 3 GB RAM and an Intel Core 2 Duo processor having 1.93 GHz speed. The evaluation platform was running Microsoft Windows Vista operating system and used the programming editor C++ 2010 Architect. We measured the performance of the new hybrid BRR algorithm using the number of attempts and the number of character comparisons.

Number of Attempts
The starting point for this technique is that the initial character in the pattern is mapped to a particular character within the text and then carry on moving until the text ends to ascertain if a match or mismatch has occurred before the text arrives. The anticipated amount of transfers to the end of the text is called the number of attempts [32].

Number of Character Comparisons
The portion of the text signifies the beginning point in the text moving to the text letter at the end, where the characters of the pattern are taken individually and matched to the text characters to determine if there is a match or no match [14].

5 Results

Results are tested by utilizing data size of 50 MB comprising DNA, English text and protein data types. Moreover, the performances of the algorithms are evaluated by using various pattern lengths. The proposed algorithm was evaluated with pattern lengths 5, 10, 15, 20, 30, 40, 50, 60, 70, 80, 90 and 100 characters. The following Figures reveal the two criteria for the evaluation. The evaluation criteria include 1) number of attempts and 2) number of characters comparisons.

The results acquired from Figs. 1, 2, 3, 4, 5 and 6 illustrate that the BRR hybrid algorithm demonstrates enhanced performance by the attempts number and the character

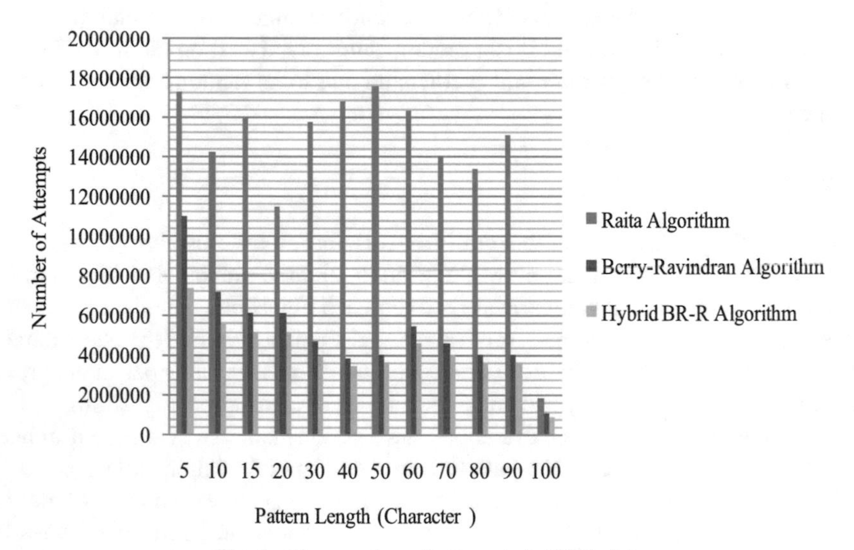

Fig. 1. The number of attempts in DNA data

comparisons number. In view of this, the combination of the algorithms exploits the good properties of each to improve the mixing performance. For instance, the results obtained from the English text, protein, and DNA of the hybrid algorithm confirm the performance is greater to the original algorithm, mainly due to the use of Berry-Ravindran's bad character shift function (brBc) to achieve a larger conversion window. The value thus improves the performance of the hybrid algorithm.

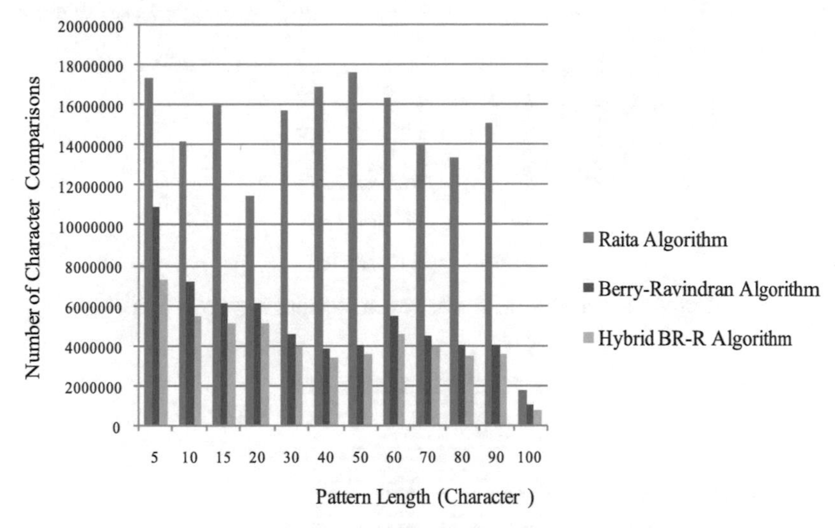

Fig. 2. The number of character comparisons in DNA data

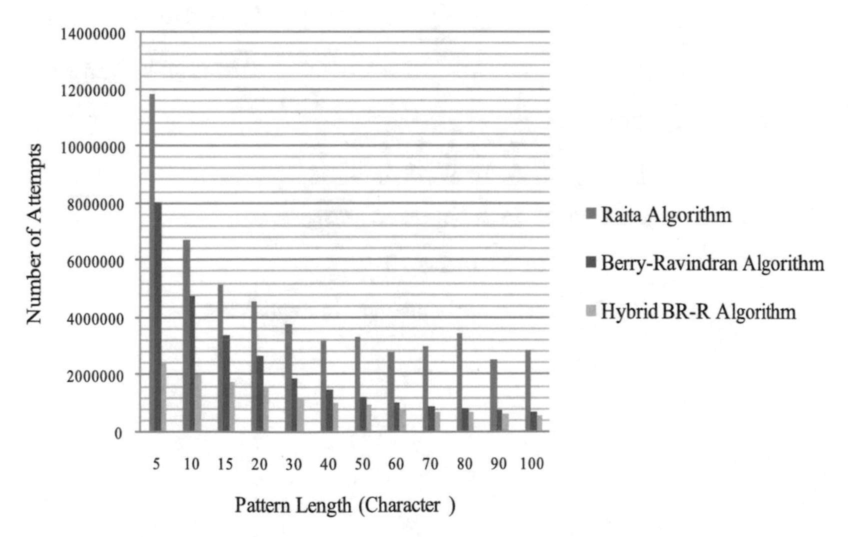

Fig. 3. The number of attempts in protein data

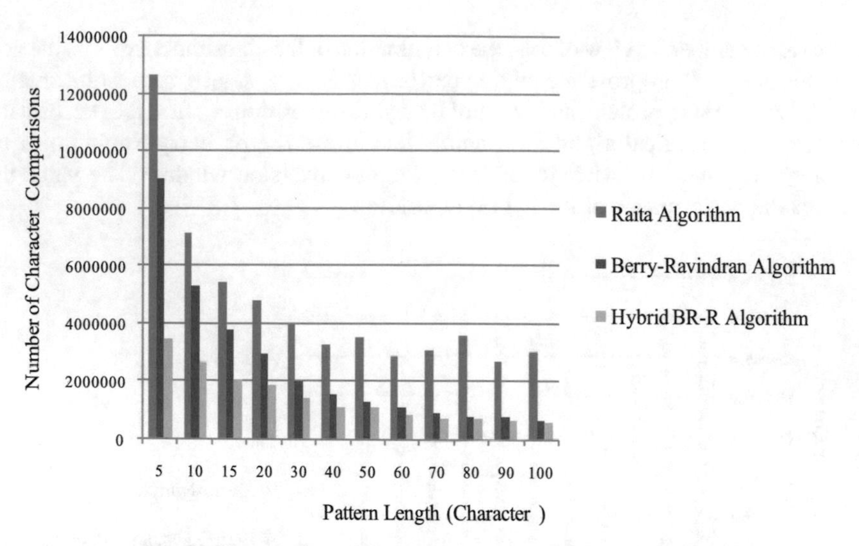

Fig. 4. The number of character comparisons in protein data

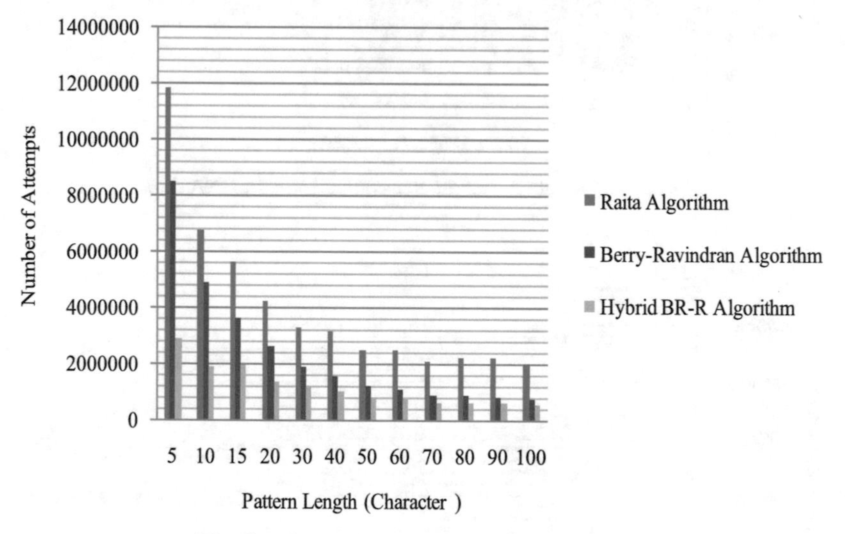

Fig. 5. The number of attempts in English text

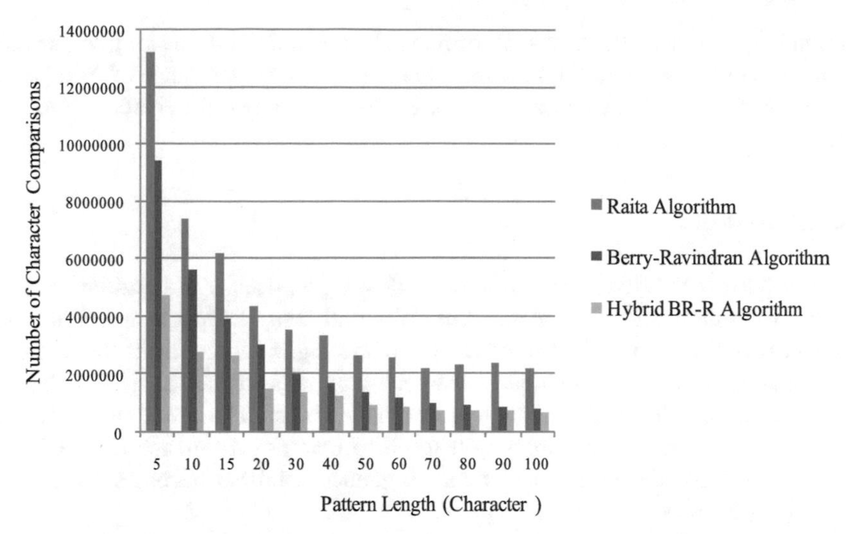

Fig. 6. The number of character comparisons in English text

6 Discussion

As mentioned earlier, the purpose of this study is to incorporate two algorithms to create a hybrid algorithm to improve the performance of string search, as the biological science database becomes larger and larger. To assess the performance of the new BRR hybrid algorithm, the data consisted of three forms: DNA, English text and protein. The results indicate that the BRR has a significant attempts number and a reduction in the number of character comparisons, and further improves the performance of the original algorithm.

The proposed hybrid algorithm produced much better results in comparison to both Berry-Ravindran algorithm and Raita algorithm. The proposed hybrid algorithm results are enhanced by 18%, 50%, and 50% over the Berry-Ravindran algorithm, and are enhanced by 71%, 74%, and 70% over the Raita algorithm, when performing tests on DNA, English text, and protein data types respectively.

The results really describe why the mix of algorithms should be taken seriously because it has a bright future and ensures faster processing, rather than a single algorithm for string searching, which does not meet today's complex data needs. The achievement of the new hybrid algorithm further indicates that in order to achieve the necessary balance in the improved performance, it is very important to choose the appropriate algorithm to form the mixture, because not all algorithms complement each other, so we must carefully study the two algorithms to form Finished before mixing. The results further confirmed the feasibility of integrating two string search algorithms, which brought good benefits by improving search and matching mode performance.

Hence, looking at the results obtained, we strongly recommend the hybrid algorithm to be applied to future string search development, because it is one of the best ways to improve the performance of string search, because the biological science data is increasing, so a powerful search algorithm is needed. Looking at the results obtained, we strongly recommend the hybrid algorithm to be applied to future string search development, because it is one of the best ways to improve the performance of string search, because the biological science data is increasing, so a powerful search algorithm is needed.

7 Conclusion

In this study, a new hybrid algorithm named BRR was proposed. The algorithm integrates the Berry-Ravindran and Raita algorithms. When utilizing distinct forms of data sizes and pattern lengths of 5–100 characters, the hybrid algorithm confirms the number of improved attempts and the amount of character comparisons, so the hybrid algorithm can be used to search for DNA, English text, and protein. The result also proves that the utilization of hybrid algorithms will result to better performance than individual algorithms, because the biological science sequence database becomes complex and huge in today's times.

References

1. Chen, Y.: A new algorithm for subset matching problem. J. Comput. Sci. **3**(12), 924–933 (2007)
2. Mohammad, A., Saleh, O., Abdeen, R.A.: Occurrences algorithm for string searching based on brute-force algorithm. J. Comput. Sci. **2**(1), 82–85 (2006)
3. Kociumaka, T., Pissis, S.P., Radoszewski, J.: Pattern matching and consensus problems on weighted sequences and profiles. Theory Comput. Syst. **63**(3), 506–542 (2019). https://doi.org/10.1007/s00224-018-9881-2
4. Neamatollahi, P., Hadi, M., Naghibzadeh, M.: Simple and efficient pattern matching algorithms for biological sequences. IEEE Access **8**, 23838–23846 (2020)
5. Sleit, A., AlMobaideen, W., Qatawneh, M., Saadeh, H.: Efficient processing for binary submatrix matching. Am. J. Appl. Sci. **6**(1), 78 (2009)
6. Yuen, C.T., Rizon, M., San, W.S., Seong, T.C.: Facial features for template matching based face recognition. Am. J. Appl. Sci. **6**(11), 1897–1901 (2009)
7. Radhakrishna, V., Phaneendra, B., Kumar, V.S.: A two way pattern matching algorithm using sliding patterns. In: 2010 3rd International Conference on Advanced Computer Theory and Engineering (ICACTE), pp. V2-666-V2-670. IEEE (2010). https://doi.org/10.1109/ICACTE.2010.5579739
8. Neamatollahi, P., Hadi, M., Naghibzadeh, M.: Efficient pattern matching algorithms for DNA sequences. In: 2020 25th International Computer Conference, Computer Society of Iran (CSICC), pp. 1–6. IEEE (2020)
9. Mahmud, P., Rana, M.S., Talukder, K.H.: An efficient hybrid exact string matching algorithm to minimize the number of attempts and character comparisons. In: 2018 21st International Conference of Computer and Information Technology (ICCIT), pp. 1–6. IEEE (2018)
10. Deusdado, S., Carvalho, P.: GRASPm: an efficient algorithm for exact pattern-matching in genomic sequences. Int. J. Bioinform. Res. Appl. **5**(4), 385–401 (2009)
11. Hudaib, A., Al-Khalid, R., Suleiman, D., Itriq, M., Al-Anani, A.: A fast pattern matching algorithm with two sliding windows (TSW). J. Comput. Sci. **4**(5), 393 (2008)
12. Raju, V., Vinayababu, A.: Parallel algorithms for string matching problem on single and two-dimensional reconfigurable pipelined bus systems. J. Comput. Sci. **3**(9), 754–759 (2007)

13. Nadarajan, K., Zukarnain, Z.A.: Analysis of string matching compression algorithms. J. Comput. Sci. **4**(3), 205–210 (2008)
14. Kalsi, P., Peltola, H., Tarhio, J.: Comparison of exact string matching algorithms for biological sequences. In: Elloumi, M., Küng, J., Linial, M., Murphy, R.F., Schneider, K., Toma, C. (eds.) BIRD 2008. CCIS, vol. 13, pp. 417–426. Springer, Heidelberg (2008). https://doi.org/10.1007/978-3-540-70600-7_31
15. Xian-feng, H., Yu-bao, Y., Lu, X.: Hybrid pattern-matching algorithm based on BM-KMP algorithm. In: 2010 3rd International Conference on Advanced Computer Theory and Engineering (ICACTE), pp. V5-310-V5-313. IEEE (2010). https://doi.org/10.1109/ICACTE.2010.5579620
16. Smyth, W.F., Wang, S.: An adaptive hybrid pattern-matching algorithm on indeterminate strings. Int. J. Found. Comput. Sci. **20**(06), 985–1004 (2009)
17. Lin, P.-C., Lin, Y.-D., Lai, Y.-C.: A hybrid algorithm of backward hashing and automaton tracking for virus scanning. IEEE Trans. Comput. **60**(4), 594–601 (2010)
18. Cai, G., Nie, X., Huang, Y.: A fast hybrid pattern matching algorithm for biological sequences. In: 2009 2nd International Conference on Biomedical Engineering and Informatics, pp. 1–5. IEEE (2009)
19. Almazroi, A.A.: A fast hybrid algorithm approach for the exact string matching problem via Berry Ravindran and alpha skip search algorithms. J. Comput. Sci. **7**(5), 644–650 (2011)
20. Al-Mazroi, A.A., Rashid, N.A.A.: A fast hybrid algorithm for the exact string matching problem. Am. J. Eng. Appl. Sci. **4**(1), 102–107 (2011)
21. Klaib, A.F., Osborne, H.: BRQS matching algorithm for searching protein sequence databases. In: 2009 International Conference on Future Computer and Communication, pp. 223–226. IEEE (2009)
22. Sheik, S., Aggarwal, S.K., Poddar, A., Sathiyabhama, B., Balakrishnan, N., Sekar, K.: Analysis of string-searching algorithms on biological sequence databases. Curr. Sci. **89**(2), 368–374 (2005)
23. Huang, Y., Pan, X., Gao, Y., Cai, G.: A fast pattern matching algorithm for biological sequences. In: 2008 2nd International Conference on Bioinformatics and Biomedical Engineering, pp. 608–611. IEEE (2008)
24. Islam, T., Talukder, K.H., Faisal, R.H.: A fast on-line hybrid matching algorithm for exact string matching. Barisal Univ. J. Part 1 **4**(2), 399–411 (2017)
25. Sheik, S., Aggarwal, S.K., Poddar, A., Balakrishnan, N., Sekar, K.: A fast pattern matching algorithm. J. Chem. Inf. Comput. Sci. **44**(4), 1251–1256 (2004)
26. Al-Dabbagh, S.S.M., Barnouti, N.H.: A new efficient hybrid string matching algorithm to solve the exact string matching problem. J. Adv. Math. Comput. Sci. **20**(2), 1–14 (2017)
27. AbdulRazzaq, A.A., Nur'Aini Abdul Rashid, M.A., Abu-Hashem, A.A.H.: A new efficient hybrid exact string matching algorithm and its applications. Life Sci. J. **11**(10), 474–488 (2014)
28. Abdul Razzaq, A.A., Rashid, N.A.A., Abbood, A.A., Zainol, Z.: The improved hybrid algorithm for the atheer and Berry-Ravindran Algorithms. Int. J. Electr. Comput. Eng. **8**(6), 4321–4333 (2018). (2088–8708)
29. Klaib, A.F., Osborne, H.: RSMA matching algorithm for searching biological sequences. In: 2009 International Conference on Innovations in Information Technology (IIT), pp. 195–199. IEEE (2009)

30. Kärkkäinen, J., Na, J.C.: Faster filters for approximate string matching. In: 2007 Proceedings of the Ninth Workshop on Algorithm Engineering and Experiments (ALENEX), pp. 84–90. SIAM (2007)
31. Huang, Y., Ping, L., Pan, X., Jiang, L., Jiang, X.: A fast improved pattern matching algorithm for biological sequences. In: 2008 International Symposium on Computational Intelligence and Design, pp. 375–378. IEEE (2008)
32. Jun-bo, W., Fei, K., Yang, L.: A fast single pattern matching algorithm for the longer pattern. In: 2010 2nd International Conference on Future Computer and Communication, pp. V2-128-V2-131. IEEE (2010). https://doi.org/10.1109/ICFCC.2010.5497356

A Survey of the Hybrid Exact String Matching Algorithms

Abdulwahab Ali Almazroi[1](✉), Asad Ali Shah[1,2], Abdulaleem Ali Almazroi[3], Fathey Mohammed[4], and Nabil Hasan Al-Kumaim[5]

[1] College of Computing and Information Technology at Khulais, Department of Information Technology, University of Jeddah, Jeddah, Saudi Arabia
aalmazroi@uj.edu.sa

[2] Department of Computing, School of Electrical Engineering and Computer Science, National University of Sciences and Technology, Islamabad, Pakistan

[3] Department of Information Technology, Faculty of Computing and Information Technology, King Abdulaziz University, Rabigh 21911, Saudi Arabia

[4] School of Computing, Universiti Utara Malaysia (UUM), 06010 Sintok, Kedah, Malaysia

[5] Faculty of Technology Management and Technopreneurship, Center of Technopreneurship Development, Universiti Teknikal Malaysia Melaka, 75460 Melaka, Malacca, Malaysia

Abstract. The matching of search string patterns has become a bigger issue of concern because biological sequence databases are growing rapidly at overwhelming proportions so string matching algorithm is an essential scientific tool to assist in solving composite string search problems. At present, the shift of focus is geared towards hybrid algorithms as they provide better performance in various evaluation metrics. Thus, researchers and experts view a hybrid algorithm as the way forward for resolving string search difficulties. Therefore, the concentration will be on the various kinds of hybrid algorithms that have been implemented, their processes, and their performances. This research has performed a systematic literature review by reviewing over 30 papers and identifying 15 string matching hybrid algorithms. When reviewing these hybrid algorithms, it is found that by combining different original algorithms, the hybrid algorithm can outperform the individual algorithms in different evaluation metrics. The purpose, enhanced concepts, and results of these algorithms have been highlighted in the article. This article has critically reviewed different string matching hybrid algorithms and provided useful information for experts and researchers that can utilize strong-matching hybrid algorithms in their systems.

Keywords: Approximate string match · Exact string match · Hybrid string matching algorithm · Pattern search · String search

1 Introduction

The persistent progress in the area of biological science databases has necessitated the burning desire for enhanced and better-performing string searching algorithms. Over the years, researchers and experts have preferred hybrid string searching algorithms,

F. Saeed et al. (Eds.): IRICT 2021, LNDECT 127, pp. 173–189, 2022.
https://doi.org/10.1007/978-3-030-98741-1_16

which are the combination of two or more algorithms instead of the frequent usage of a single search string algorithm implementations [1–3]. For many years, search string and pattern matching algorithms had been the fundamental basis for computer science applications, biological sciences, text processing, bioinformatics, and artificial intelligence [4]. A String matching algorithm searches for all the possible occurrences of a specific pattern(s) in a very large chunk of a given text of alphabets. In other words, it is the discovery of one or more precise instances of a particular pattern found in a document or text.

String matching-based algorithms comprise two major components including 1) pre-processing phase and 2) searching phase. The pre-processing phase is responsible for reviewing patterns in the given text, while the searching phase involves searching text or the sequence pattern iteratively [5, 6]. Essential information is gathered in the pre-processing phase through iterative procedures of testing and shifting. This information is then passed on to the searching phase for further processing. The searching phase identifies the exact patterns in successive windows. The goal of these algorithms, when processing data, is to lessen the number of attempts and to ensure a greater shift value. This is how a good string matching algorithm is evaluated.

Given the importance of hybrid exact string matching algorithms, researchers and experts need to be aware of the possible algorithms available and the combinations that should be used to produce better results. To the best of our knowledge, there is little research available that has reviewed hybrid exact string matching algorithms extensively. Al-Khamaiseh, Alshagarin [7] survey on string matching algorithms provides an overview and general working on all types of algorithms including exact, approximate, and hybrid algorithms. In comparison, this research focuses on hybrid exact string matching algorithms only. Alhendawi, Baharudin [8] research provides a short survey on string matching algorithms, their pseudocode, and time complexities. However, this research also does not highlight the purpose of the algorithms and their results. This research reviewed existing hybrid exact string matching algorithms and highlighted the combination of algorithms used, where the hybrid system can be used ideally and the results achieved by the system.

At later stages, the attention will be directed towards most of all the hybrid algorithms having been implemented currently and more essentially their usefulness in enhancing the pattern searching. The use of hybrid algorithms is seen as the way forward for solving most of the string searching problems due to voluminous types of scientific data being generated today [9, 10]. There are two main approaches used by string matching algorithms. These include 1) exact string matching algorithms and 2) approximate string matching algorithms. Both are these approaches are discussed in Sect. 2. In Sect. 3, the evaluation approaches applied for testing the hybrid algorithms' performances are highlighted. In Sect. 4, the existing hybrid algorithms are listed, compared, and discussed in terms of enhanced concepts and results. Section 4 covers the discussion while Sect. 5 concludes the paper's findings.

2 String Matching Algorithms

It is the discovery of one or many of all instances of a pattern present in the text provided. In string matching. there are two main approaches. These include 1) exact string matching algorithm and 2) approximate string matching algorithm. Different string search algorithms are grouped under either one of these two approaches, and their distinctions are of great importance as they form the main categorization and performance of all string matching algorithms [7].

2.1 Exact String Matching Algorithm

As the name suggest involves the process of finding out the specific pattern(s) in a given text, for instance, given that, $T = t_1 t_{2...} t_n$, and a pattern made up of $P = p_1 p_2 ... p_m$, the aim for this algorithm is to discover if P appears in and if P can be found in T, where is the location to be found [11, 12]. In recent years, however, research has proven that exact string algorithms are more suitable for string searching as their prediction, estimation, and performance are considered to be exact to searching and matching patterns in a text.

2.2 Approximate String Matching Algorithm

This approach also tries to find the pattern from a given text document, but instead of finding the exact match, it approximates the occurrence instead. In a text document T with pattern P to search for, the notion involves the discovery of the approximate or the nearest occurrences of all P in T. The procedures involve finding all the substrings of a text that are quite close to the given pattern, but may or may not be the same. For example, given a string N_1 and another string N_2, transformations are from N_2 to N_1 normally implemented by three functions namely; deletions, insertions, and substitutions [13].

1. Deletion Operation: Given that N_1 = btcga, and N_2 = btccgga, the deletion of (c) is at the position (4) and the deletion of (g) is at the position (5) from N_2. After the deletion operations, a transformation has taken place where N_2 is transformed to N_1.
2. Insertion Operation: For this function of approximate string matching when given that N_1 = bactgt, and N_2 = bctt, insert (a) in the position (2) and (g) in the position (5) of N_2. After the insertion, N_2 is transformed into N_1.
3. Substitution Operation: When given a text and pattern and N_1 = tactgta, and N_2 = tbctata, the transformation N_2 to N_1 is applied by the substitution operation at positions (2) and (5) respectively of N_2, where at position (2), (b) is substituted by (a), and at position (5), (a) is substituted by (g).

Apart from the above function descriptions for approximate string matching, the other functions are the Hamming distance and Levenshtein or Edit distance. In Hamming distance [14], the function denotes two strings having the same string length. Then it finds the number of locations where both the strings have mismatching characters. The hamming distance function is used in approximate string searching algorithms. In such algorithms d indicates the hamming distance while k indicates the instances where two strings were mismatched. On the other hand, Levenshtein distance calculates the distance, by comparison, two different strings of different sizes. It comprises the smallest number of character insertions, deletions, and substitutions with the central goal of transforming one string into another. It is also known as string searching with k differences or k errors [15].

3 Evaluation Approaches

The evaluation approaches applied for testing the performances for all the hybrid algorithms discussed below all follows similar trends including the varying degree of data set made up of amino acids, DNA, English text, UNIX dictionary (e.g. BR algorithm), nucleotides sequences (e.g. BMBR algorithm) and protein sequences and other data obtained from databases such as Genome (Arabidopsis Thaliana) and Swiss-Prot containing 8740 proteins and used by most of the hybrid algorithms. Moreover, the algorithms reviewed showed that when using the same alphabet size it was set four letters ($\sigma = 4$), while bigger alphabet sizes were set to 20 ($\sigma = 20$) by many algorithms as the test data. The algorithms have been tested in different environments, such as different processing speeds, process generation, different RAM generation and size, different operating systems, and so forth. There are three evaluation metrics for calculating performance in search string algorithms, which are 1) the "number of attempts" conducted by the algorithm, 2) "the number of character comparisons", and 3) the "searching time" taken by the algorithm to find the results. These are the recommended metrics for evaluating search string algorithms and understanding their behavior when changing different parameters such as the alphabet and pattern size.

1. The number of attempts: It is described as the process where the beginning area of the first pattern character is the link to a specific character in the text, and which then carry on shifting till the end of the text document to ascertain if there is a match or mismatch that had occurred at the end of processes. The number of times it is shifted to ascertain that a match is found is known as the number of attempts [16].
2. The number of character comparisons: This evaluation metric calculates by initiating a point inside a given text to the last character of the text, showing how the character of patterns are extracted separately and then equated with the given text to find out the occurrence of a match or mismatch [17].
3. Searching time: Also known in string searching as execution time or elapsed time is the processing times needed by the CPUs to execute functions to complete the search, and matching all the patterns within a given text to determine the time taken to achieve a specific result [18].

4 Review on Hybrid Algorithms

Recent years have seen tremendous emphasis and progression towards the use of hybrid algorithms for string searching. This is because they provide the best performances and results than the application of a single-string algorithm. As data is becoming more complex, hybrid algorithms are seen as the direction to follow because they can march the tedious rigors involved in string searching of voluminous data. The hybrid algorithms summary is provided in Table 1, which shows the hybrid algorithm name, algorithms used, the purpose for which the algorithm should be used, and results obtained during implementations. The algorithms are discussed in greater detail in their respective sections.

Table 1. Summary of string matching hybrid algorithms

The algorithm	Algorithms used	Purpose	Results
Berry-Ravindran Hybrid Algorithm	Quick Search Zhu-Takaoka algorithms	Searching English text	+16.66% performance
SSABS Hybrid Algorithm	Quick Search Raita algorithms	Searching biological sequence	Elapsed time = 40 s
FJS Hybrid Algorithm	Boyer-Moore Knuth-Morris-Pratt	Searching DNA sequence	Faster times when alphabet sizes are $\geq$ 15
TVSBS Hybrid Algorithm	Berry-Ravindran SSABS	Searching biological sequence	TVSBS took 4,984,654 number of attempts
BMBR Hybrid Algorithm	Boyer-Moore Berry Ravindran	Searching biological sequence	Less average time
ZTBMH Hybrid Algorithm	Zhu-Takaoka Boyer-Moore-Horspool	Searching biological sequence nucleotides sequences	Lower average time than BMH, BM, FS, ZT
BRFS Hybrid Algorithm	Fast Search Berry-Ravindran	Useful for small alphabets and long patterns searching biological sequence	More efficient than the original algorithms
BRBMH Hybrid Algorithm	Berry-Ravindran Boyer-Moore Horspool	Searching protein sequence	Achieved the lowest number of character comparisons when compared to other algorithms
BRQS Hybrid Algorithm	Berry-Ravindran Quick Search algorithm	Searching protein sequence	Recorded the better performance at 1240 in comparison to other algorithms
ZTFS Hybrid Algorithm	Zhu-Takaoka Fast-Search algorithms	Nucleotides sequences Long patterns	The average time taken is less than other algorithms

(continued)

Table 1. *(continued)*

The algorithm	Algorithms used	Purpose	Results
RSMA-BR Hybrid Algorithm	Berry-Ravindran Random String Matching	Searching protein sequence	Less average time and number of comparisons performed than QS and BMH
ShiftAndBMS Hybrid Algorithm	ShiftAnd BMS	Searching English text	Execution time better than BMS
BRSS Hybrid Algorithm	Berry-Ravindran Skip Search	Small alphabets Long patterns	Better in all evaluation metrics compared to Berry-Ravindran
BHAC Hybrid Algorithm	Backward Hashing Aho-Corasick	Scanning string information on computer virus	The algorithm performed quicker than the original implementations
KMPBS Hybrid Algorithm	Boyer-Moore Knuth-Morris-Pratt	Searching English text	More efficient in the number of character comparison evaluations than original algorithms

4.1 Berry-Ravindran Hybrid Algorithm

Berry-Ravindran (BR) entails two algorithms involving Quick Search (QS) and Zhu-Takaoka (ZT) algorithms [19, 20], and it is applicable for searching English text specifically tested using UNIX dictionary. The intention for the algorithm was to conduct a random text that can lead to a simulation of a tangible English text, and all the characters used in the UNIX dictionary were in lower cases to increase the possibility of a match.

Enhancement concepts: The improvements are through each of the two algorithms and not one, the shift value for the algorithm is from a two-dimensional table composed of bad character tables of BR and QS. QS algorithm uses another function and not the good suffix function to compute the shifts. It applied a reformed version of the last occurrence function, the function defines the rightmost instance. If it is not present, the pattern is then shifted by $m + 1$ positions. ZT instead applied the good suffix function for the shift, if a mismatch occurs the last occurrence function defines the rightmost occurrence of the text in the pattern, so the computations from both forms good shift values from each algorithm which enables the new algorithm to be more proficient.

Results: The decisions on the BR at the end established through the outcome that the algorithm performances were boosted when the comparison is made because at any pattern length as it shows 16.66% improvement in two evaluation metrics. This includes the character comparison and searching time. It performed better as compared to the other original algorithms such as BM 43.29%, Raita 42.82%, ZT 26.09%, and QS 29.72%.

Additionally, ZT functions better recording a total percentage figure of 26.09% over QS which shows almost 29.72% during the number of comparisons when all the maximum pattern length 22 was calculated.

4.2 SSABS Hybrid Algorithm

SSABS combines two search algorithms namely Quick Search (QS) and Raita algorithms [21, 22] to form a hybrid algorithm and it is useful for searching biological sequence databases. The algorithm was also designed for other database uses, for instance, searching other databases such as Protein databases containing protein sequences and information about protein motifs and features of protein structures from Swiss Prot and Protein Data Bank (PDB), Swiss Institute of Bioinformatics (SIB) and among others.

Enhancement concepts: SSABS algorithm improvements were achieved through these procedures; in the new algorithm there is a fixed point for the direction character comparisons that is done among the window and the search string at every attempt. The pattern is checked against the string from right to left of the window. The shifting of the window is calculated by discovering the location of the bad character in the string when a match or mismatch happens.

Results: Experiment results were on elapse time and in the end, it corroborates that any given length the SSABS algorithm is more valuable on protein sequences with size = 20, and regardless of the size and the string search length involved than the other algorithms the lowest elapsed time of 40 s at the maximum length of character. At the same stage also Raita Algorithm performance is better when reviewed with QS with elapse time of 41 s as against 55 s by QS.

4.3 FJS Hybrid Algorithm

The algorithm is the hybrid of Boyer-Moore (BM) and Knuth-Morris-Pratt algorithms (KMP) [23, 24], and it is used for searching DNA sequence databases. The perfection of this hybrid algorithm FJS was due to the significant accuracy of the BMS and KMP which complement each other very well. Moreover, any BM-derived algorithm is flexible for the active use of indexed alphabets of variable size. The goal of the algorithm is to include the advantages and performance of the BM, which also addresses some of the scenarios where the KMP algorithm performs inadequately.

Enhancement concepts: The improvements are from both algorithms to improve performance in elapsed time. This is done by introducing two arrays namely Sunday's array and KMP array in the pre-processing stage. To avoid numerous string matches, in the case of the worst-case scenario, the KMP-type letter assessments are used over the remaining characters to improve efficiency.

Results: Derived experiment results quoting from the paper on elapse time gives the benefits to the new algorithm owing to the certainty that the FJS displays the best improvements and is executed at faster times when alphabet sizes are ≥ 15 with an average time of 5–10% better than the BM and KMP at about 20 s when pattern size is at maximum 2 MB and almost having a dominant effect when alphabet size is ≥ 8. Meanwhile, BM also executed much quicker than BMH at 28 s as compared to BMH at 42 s, so it was considered the second-best.

4.4 TVSBS Hybrid Algorithm

The algorithm is composed of Berry-Ravindran and SSABS algorithms [17, 25], all of which are hybrid algorithms by their nature of implementation. This algorithm is suitable for searching biological sequence databases specifically nucleotide and amino acid. This algorithm shows great strength and it is easily adapted for exact pattern applications and exhibits the best and worst-case complexities.

Enhancement concepts: The enhancement of the TVSBS algorithm was due to the good functions from BR which are coupled with SSABS. For example, the BR bad character (brBc) function is known to be more efficient at the pre-processing phase. Moreover, character comparisons are done starting from the last character in the pattern, where the window is skipped in the event of finding two characters in succession in the string. This enables the brBc function to achieve the maximum shift values and thereby decreasing the comparisons performed.

Results: Performance indicators during the implementation number of comparison and execution time announced, the TVSBS as the more proficient as the number of comparisons was 4,984,654 compared to SSABS of 8,564,471 when pattern length is 30 and alphabet size was 20, and at any pattern length the new algorithm still performs better. Moreover, the average time of 108 s compared to 110 s when alphabet size is 20.

4.5 BMBR Hybrid Algorithm

The hybrid algorithm consists of Boyer-Moore and Berry Ravindran algorithms [26, 27]. Chicago is normally referred to as BMBR. This hybrid algorithm is very useful in biological sequence databases for search pattern matching. It also absorbs the idea of BR that is noted for attaining maximum shift values and applied the mismatch information at the searching phase Additionally it is an applicable algorithm for small alphabets and long patterns which shows that the longer the pattern the best performance derived from the algorithm.

Enhancement concepts: The concepts of enhancements for this algorithm were made possible by the implementation of two functions from the algorithms. The first is the good suffix heuristics offered by the BM algorithm. The BR algorithm complements the algorithm by providing bad character heuristics. This allows the hybrid algorithm to achieve a better working of the shift function while also attaining the best shift distance, thus, improving performance.

Results: Using the number of comparisons and average time, the results mark BMBR algorithm was the enhanced performance through the figures obtained where the average time taken was lesser than all other the algorithms. The algorithm was compared against BM, BMH, BR, QS, SSABS, and TVSBS algorithms. In the first test, the researchers tested the algorithm by setting the length of the short pattern is to 28. In this scenario the average time is taken by BMBR to other algorithms considered (as per the order mentioned above) is 70%, 61%, 87%, 45%, 48%, and 87% respectively. In the second test, when the length of the long pattern is set to 1024, the average time taken by BMBR to other algorithms is 76%, 44%, 79%, 79%, 35%, and 73% respectively. The original algorithms also exhibited different results with BM better than BR on both short and long patterns recording 70% and 76% while BR was 87% and 79% of average times.

4.6 ZTBMH Hybrid Algorithm

The hybrid algorithm is a hybrid of Zhu-Takaoka (ZT) and that of Boyer-Moore-Horspool (BMH) algorithms [28, 29]. The algorithm is designed to be used in the biological sequence database. However, it also works well nucleotides sequences and long patterns. With this algorithm the longer the length of the pattern, the better it performs.

Enhancement concepts: One of the changes made by the hybrid algorithm to increase the performance was the introduction of a single function in the pre-processing phase. The function utilized both the bad character heuristic and the maximum shift value. In the searching phase, the function computes the maximum shift value after every attempt. Moreover, the window is skipped in the case a match is not found. The algorithm utilizes the bad character shift value in the case of a mismatch.

Results: The elapsed time was applied to gauge the final output and the results confirmed ZTBMH as the best algorithm than the rest of the algorithms including BM, BMH, FS, and ZT. The algorithm better performed better in both average times for short and long patterns. In the first test, when the short pattern length is set to 28, the average time taken by ZTBMH compared to other algorithms (in the order given above) is 50%, 38%, 50%, and 89% respectively. In the second test, where the pattern length is set to 1024, the average time taken by the ZTBMH algorithm compared to other algorithms is 54%, 30%, 54%, and 99% respectively. For individual original algorithms, BMH improved over ZT over 38% for short patterns and 30% for long patterns with ZT recording 89% and 99.

4.7 BRFS Hybrid Algorithm

BRFS hybrid algorithm uses Fast Search (FS) and Berry-Ravindran (BR) algorithms [28, 30]. The hybrid algorithm is ideal when searching databases involving biological sequences, but it can also be used for both short and long patterns. The algorithm follows the style of algorithms, which are noted for having a very good shift value such as Boyer Moore (BM), and applied the good concepts of BR and FS.

Enhancement concepts: The enhancement of BRFS came about through the extraction of two functions. The first is the inclusion of bad character (brBc) suffixes heuristic from the Berry–Ravindran algorithm and good suffix heuristic bmGs(j) from the Boyer Moore (BM) algorithm. These are added at the pre-processing phase. In addition to this, the algorithm also stores the shift value in one-dimensional called the brBc array. In the searching phase, after every attempt, the window skip is commutated through the brBc function and the window for maximum skip when characters do not appear in the pattern.

Results: It was measured on the number of comparisons and elapse time, and the results proved BRFS is more efficient than the original algorithms. The BRFS algorithm was evaluated against other algorithms including BM, BMH, BR, QS, SSABB, and TVSBS algorithms. In the first evaluation test, the pattern length was set to 28 for evaluating performing in short patterns. In this test, the average time taken by the proposed hybrid algorithm attained 70%, 61%, 87%, 45%, 48%, and 87% compared to other algorithms in the order given above respectively. In the second test, the length of the pattern length was set to 1024 to evaluate the hybrid algorithm for long patterns.

In the second test, the average time taken by the hybrid algorithm compared to other algorithms was 76%, 44%, 79%, 33%, 35%, and 73% respectively. Moreover, for each respective algorithm, BR performed better compared to QS by over 8% on the average running number of comparisons with a maximum pattern length of 28.

4.8 BRBMH Hybrid Algorithm

The BMBM hybrid algorithm comprises features from both Berry-Ravindran (BR) and Boyer-Moore Horspool (BMH) algorithms [31, 32]. The hybrid algorithm is a deal when searching protein sequence databases but can also be used in other string search applications. The algorithm improves the performance by using the pre-processing phase of BR and the searching phase of BMH.

Enhancement concepts: As stated before, the BRBMH algorithm uses good features from both BR and BMH algorithms. This includes the bad-character shift function in BMH and BR algorithms. The difference between them is that BMH defines one for text the search window to the text window. This improves the pre-processing phase where the pattern characters are compared by using the shift values instead of counting the text characters. Afterward, the shift values are stored in a one-dimensional array which is easily accessible in the searching phase.

Results: The principle used was elapsed time and the results established, the new hybrid algorithm from the low pattern length of 32 through to the high of 1024, indicated that BRBMH displayed the lowest number of character comparisons when compared to other algorithms, at maximum pattern length of 1024, the character compared by BRBMH was 1239, other algorithms recorded higher values like 1243, 2647 for TVSBS and QS respectively. Moreover, elapse time for BRMMH was about less than 5 s as compared to QS which was executed at a high value of 18 s and BRFS of about less than 10 s.

4.9 BRQS Hybrid Algorithm

The hybrid algorithm uses the good features of the two algorithms. This includes 1) Berry-Ravindran (BR) and 2) Quick Search algorithm (QS) algorithms [33]. This algorithm is suitable for searching protein sequence databases and many other string applications. The purpose of the algorithm was to accomplish maximum effectiveness in the shifting values and the search patterns within the given text. Moreover, the algorithms also decrease the attempts for string search and elapsed time when searching using long patterns.

Enhancement concepts: The BRQS algorithm's performance is improved due to two features. The first feature is the bad-character shift function provided by the Quick-Search algorithm. The second feature used is the BR bad-character shift function that is provided by the Berry-Ravindran algorithm. The difference between both of them is that one is using one character, while the other uses two characters next to the search window. This allows the algorithm to achieve maximum shift values. Moreover, storing the results in a one-dimensional array allows faster accessibility during the searching phase.

Results: From the experiment results publicized on the number of comparisons and elapse time, the BRQS recorded the better performance at 1240 in terms of the number of comparisons when pattern length is at a maximum 1024 better in terms of the number of comparisons and elapse time is below 5 s over the than the original algorithms. Also BRFS, TVSBS results were 1282, 1243 respectively which is better than the QS algorithm having 2647 on the number of character comparisons. On elapse time results BRFS was about 10 s with QS 20 s.

4.10 ZTFS Hybrid Algorithm

ZTFS hybrid algorithm uses the best features of two algorithms. The first one is the Zhu-Takaoka (ZT) algorithm. The second algorithm used by the hybrid algorithm is the Fast-Search (FS) algorithm [30, 34]. The hybrid algorithm is ideal when searching for exact patterns in the biological sequence database. The proposed algorithm is much useful for small alphabets. For example, nucleotides sequences and long patterns.

Enhancement concepts: The performance of the ZTFS hybrid algorithm is improved due to the use of two functions. The first function is the good suffix heuristic provided by the bmGs(j) function of BM. The second is the bad character heuristic ztBc(a, b) function for ZT. The ztBc(a, b) function also supplies the maximum shift values. Moreover, the bmGs(j) function provides the prefix of the pattern during the pre-processing phase. At the searching phase, Zhu-Takaoka bad character shift value is applied. However whenever a mismatch occurs the shift is taken over by the bmGs function.

Results: The algorithm was evaluated against six other algorithms, including FS, TVSBS, and ZT algorithms, for different evaluation metrics. The algorithm achieved better elapsed time results in comparison to other algorithms. When the pattern length is set to 28, for short patterns, the average time taken by ZTFS to other algorithms (as per the order given above) is 51%, 83%, and 90% respectively. The hybrid algorithm was also tested for long patterns by setting the pattern length to 1024. In the test, the average time taken by ZTFS to other algorithms is 53%, 74%, and 97% respectively. Furthermore, FS time taken was 51% for short pattern and 53% for longer pattern during execution so it is better than ZT which shows high figures.

4.11 RSMA-BR Hybrid Algorithm

This hybrid algorithm is the mixture of Berry-Ravindran (BR) and Random String Matching (RSMA) algorithm [1, 35] and can be applied in the protein sequence database. The major objective of this hybrid algorithm is to reduce the number of attempts during the searching phase and to increase the shift values for the patterns. This will allow the hybrid algorithm to perform better in comparison to other algorithms such as Brute Force (BF), KMP, BM, and Boyer Moore Horspool (BMH).

Enhancement concepts: The enrichment RSMA-BR algorithm were made possible by the application of good attributes from both algorithm by the first brBc function which counts shift values on every character in the pattern, then stored them in brBc one-dimensional array at the pre-processing phase, from the searching phase it applies a function known as Random Division (RD) value to do the comparison before counting the Text through a method known as Text Division value (TD).

Results: The results include the number of comparisons and elapse time used as the performance yardstick, and the hybrid algorithm was judged the best, as in any pattern length range from 32 to 1024 than the rest of the algorithm, where at 1024 the of the number of comparisons was 1129 as compared to QS 2647 and BMH 2186. For elapse time, the running times were less than 5 s when compared to QS of about 20 s, BMH of around 18 s, and other algorithms which show high numbers.

4.12 ShiftAndBMS Hybrid Algorithm

The algorithm is the combination of ShiftAnd and BMS algorithms [36, 37]. It is used is for searching English text such as both regular string and indeterminate strings. The idea was the cautious mixture of algorithms by flip-flopping among two or more processes, and from one another according to the local environments sections of text.

Enhancement concepts: the algorithm is improved by using the good features of both BMS and ShiftAnd matching algorithms. In the searching phase, the algorithm uses the BMS shift operation by default. However, it switches to the SwiftAnd function if the match is found at the end of the pattern, allowing it to improve performance. The algorithm switches back to BMS shift operation in the case no match was found in the current comparison.

Results: The printed outcome of the results in the paper on the criteria execution time, illustrate the new algorithm execution time was much better among the other algorithms, having an overall total figure of 11862 ms per million letters when compared to 12341 ms for BMS and 27888 ms for ShiftAnd. During the same time, BMS performed better than ShiftAnd executing at a time of 12341 ms per million letters as compared to ShiftAnd algorithm time at 27888 ms per million letters.

4.13 BRSS Hybrid Algorithm

This hybrid algorithm [12] is the combination of two algorithms. This includes the 1) Berry-Ravindran (BR) and 2) Skip Search (SS) algorithms. The key benefits of using this hybrid algorithm are that the BR algorithm provides the best shift value. This is achieved using the bad character table calculated from the two consecutive characters immediately after the window. Moreover, the SS algorithm is useful for both small and long patterns. Additionally, the hybrid algorithm performs processing on the characters in the pattern before initializing the search phase.

Enhancement concepts: As stated before, the hybrid algorithm has the bad-character shift mechanism from the Berry-Ravindran algorithm to improve performance. The feature checks the window's right side for two successive text characters located. In the pre-processing phase, each character pair is computed. In the searching phase when a match or mismatch occurs, the shift value depends on the two successive text characters located at the window's right side, and is calculated from the Berry-Ravindran bad character table, normally represented bybrBc function. Additional enhancement features also came from SS shift value which computes the bucket list in the pre-processing stage and the derived bucket list results are used in the searching stage to ensure a bigger shift value. But here both BR and SS shift values are compared and the bigger shift value is chosen for shifting the pattern.

Results: The hybrid algorithm performed better in all evaluation metrics in comparison to Berry-Ravindran in DNA, Protein, and English text. The results in these texts are 50%, 43%, and 44% respectively. Moreover, the hybrid algorithm also showed improvements over the Skip Search algorithm. The results show that in DNA, Protein, and English text, the algorithm improved by 20%, 30%, and 18% respectively. Consequently, the SS algorithm is better than the BR algorithm from pattern lengths ranging from 5–100 characters applying all the three different sets of data as well namely DNA, Protein, and English text.

4.14 BHAC Hybrid Algorithm

This hybrid algorithm comprises two algorithms. This includes 1) Backward Hashing (BH) and 2) Aho-Corasick (AC) algorithms [38]. The algorithm is ideal when used for scanning string information in a computer virus search. The BM is appropriate for long patterns while AC searches for a shorter length of the pattern.

Enhancement concepts: The improvements were due to the use of the two algorithm's best features. The first is the superior heuristic which defines the shift distance. This technique indexes the shift table. This is done using the Prefix Sliding Window (PSW) that is required to be performed before initiating the search phase. Moreover, BH is also used in long pattern searches if the characters lie within the PSW. This procedure reduces the elapsed time of the algorithm. Secondly, another improvement is the bad-block heuristic that helps to decrease the false-positive rate while at the same time engineering a bigger shift value and maintaining the Block-size to appreciable levels.

Results: The results from the paper evaluated on execution time implies the hybrid algorithm improved overall throughput. The results showed that was increased from 19.44 Mbps (original algorithm) to 53.81 Mbps (hybrid algorithm). Thus an increase of 277% is achieved showing faster times than the rest of the algorithms when the size of the bloom filter is 512 KB. In the implementation, the results also show that the BH algorithm is also quicker. The time taken by the original implementation is 14.19 s, while the AC algorithm took a time of 15.74 s during execution.

4.15 KMPBS Hybrid Algorithm

KMPBS is a combination of two algorithms. The hybrid algorithm includes 1) Boyer-Moore (BM) and 2) Knuth-Morris-Pratt (KMP) algorithms [39]. The algorithm is good for searching English text. The algorithm is ideal for scenarios where the character is positioned at the end of the window, which allows the algorithm to attain maximum shifts.

Enhancement concepts: The KMPBS improvements were made using the good attributes of the algorithm. This includes the pre-processing phase and the searching phase of the KMP algorithm. Moreover, from the BMHS algorithm, the number of letters from the string are grouped as one character for a single function. The calculation for the Next Function value for KMP string P is used and the BM algorithm applied the next character to determine the value string pattern P to be shifted.

Results: Results obtained from assessing the performance on the number of comparison shows, the KMPBS is more efficient as the number of character comparisons stood at 35 times when pattern length is 267 than KMP algorithm figure of 468 times when the same pattern size was applied. Meanwhile, BM performs better than KMP with 367 times the number of comparisons as compared to KMP which estimated number of comparisons stood at 789 times.

5 Discussion

All the hybrid algorithms reviewed have varying degrees of factors that influence their performances and while some are useful for short alphabets (e.g. BMBR), long patterns (e.g. BH), and large alphabets (FJS). From the review, one essential point that stood out was that the purpose for all the algorithms was the belief of trying to reduce the number of attempts on character comparisons and to decrease searching times hence the mixing of good properties extracted from each algorithm. And these enhancements were accomplished either through the combination of two functions extracted from each algorithm for the pre-processing phases and then later pass on to the searching phases or solely based on only one function extracted from the algorithm for the pre-processing phase (e.g. BR with SSABS, where only brBc function was used for the new algorithm), the main concern for all these processes was to derive the maximum shift values to be used for shifting the window. Some of the hybrid algorithms also do perform better at certain length pattern sizes e.g. FJS when size ≥ 8, and also ZTBMH, ZTFS that demonstrated that the longer the pattern the better the performance of the algorithms.

Moreover, another area for enhanced performance can be attributed to the different types of data and environments such as PC GHz processor, Operating System, type of database (Swiss-Prot Database), string length, pattern occurrence frequency, pattern length, and alphabet size. For example in the BR experiment results the test data set amounted to 1,500,000 separate tests carried out, that of RSMA-BR algorithm data set obtained from the Swiss-Prot database contains about 8740 proteins. The results for the number of comparisons, elapsed time, and the number of attempts, were the major improvements accomplished by each algorithm which was mostly due to the different extraction of the good properties from each of the algorithms. Though most of the algorithms do have limitations, the positive evidence is that whenever algorithms are combined, the overall performance of the algorithm is enhanced significantly than the previous ones. Some are also very suitable for a specific choice of data set but are not a suitable choice for others, for example, FJS which is good for protein molecules containing amino acids but cannot optimize performance for DNA for pattern size starts to get bigger.

6 Conclusion

The research undertaken focuses on almost all various types of hybrid algorithms currently implemented for string searching. The initiative was to review and highlight string matching hybrid algorithms and give a summary of their functions and improvements attributes when the two algorithms are combined and how that can boost the performance of string searching and matching of patterns. The result realized from the research does give a free and fair view of all the hybrid algorithms being in use now. In the future, another research will be conducted on the more recent invention of newer algorithms which is yet to challenge the traditional ones that have been tried and tested.

References

1. Al-Mazroi, A.A., Rashid, N.A.A.: A fast hybrid algorithm for the exact string matching problem. Am. J. Eng. Appl. Sci. **4**(1), 102–107 (2011)
2. Markić, I., Štula, M., Zorić, M., Stipaničev, D.: Entropy-based approach in selection exact string-matching algorithms. Entropy **23**(1), 31 (2021)
3. Prabha, K.S., Mahesh, C., Raja, S.: An enhanced semantic focused web crawler based on hybrid string matching algorithm. Cybern. Inf. Technol. **21**(2), 105–120 (2021)
4. Deusdado, S., Carvalho, P.: GRASPm: an efficient algorithm for exact pattern-matching in genomic sequences. Int. J. Bioinform. Res. Appl. **5**(4), 385–401 (2009). https://doi.org/10.1504/ijbra.2009.02751
5. Qu, J., Zhang, G., Fang, Z., Liu, J.: A parallel algorithm of string matching based on message passing interface for multicore processors. Int. J. Hybrid Inf. Technol. **9**(3), 31–38 (2016). https://doi.org/10.14257/ijhit.2016.9.3.04
6. Moh'd Mhashi, M., Alwakeel, M.: New enhanced exact string searching algorithm. IJCSNS **10**(4), 193–202 (2010)
7. Al-Khamaiseh, K., Alshagarin, S.: A survey of string matching algorithms. Int. J. Eng. Res. Appl. **4**(7), 144–156 (2014). (Version 2)
8. Alhendawi, K., Baharudin, A.S.: String matching algorithms (SMAs): survey & empirical analysis. J. Comput. Sci. Manag. **4**(7), 2637–2644 (2013). (Version 2)
9. Gladkov, L., Leyba, S., Gladkova, N.: The development of hybrid algorithms and program solutions of placement and routing problems. In: Silhavy, R., Silhavy, P., Prokopova, Z., Senkerik, R., Kominkova, Z. (eds.) CSOC 2017. AISC, vol. 575, pp. 406–415. Springer, Cham (2017). https://doi.org/10.1007/978-3-319-57141-6_44
10. Javangula, P., Modarre, K., Shenoy, P., Liu, Y., Nayebi, A.: Efficient hybrid algorithms for computing clusters overlap. Procedia Comput. Sci. **108**, 1050–1059 (2017)
11. Lecroq, T.: Fast exact string matching algorithms. Inf. Process. Lett. **102**(6), 229–235 (2007). https://doi.org/10.1016/j.ipl.2007.01.002
12. Almazroi, A.A.: A fast hybrid algorithm approach for the exact string matching problem via Berry Ravindran and alpha skip search algorithms. J. Comput. Sci. **7**(5), 644 (2011)
13. Yeh, M.-C., Cheng, K.-T.: A string matching approach for visual retrieval and classification. In: Proceedings of the 1st ACM International Conference on Multimedia Information Retrieval, Vancouver, British Columbia, Canada, pp. 52–58. Association for Computing Machinery (2008)
14. Navarro, G.: A guided tour to approximate string matching. ACM Comput. Surv. **33**(1), 31–88 (2001). https://doi.org/10.1145/375360.375365
15. Michailidis, P.D., Margaritis, K.G.: On-line approximate string searching algorithms: survey and experimental results. Int. J. Comput. Math. **79**(8), 867–888 (2002)
16. Hudaib, A., Al-Khalid, R., Suleiman, D., Itriq, M., Al-Anani, A.: A fast pattern matching algorithm with two sliding windows (TSW). J. Comput. Sci. **4**(5), 393 (2008)
17. Thathoo, R., Virmani, A., Lakshmi, S.S., Balakrishnan, N., Sekar, K.: TVSBS: a fast exact pattern matching algorithm for biological sequences. Curr. Sci. **91**(1), 47–53 (2006)
18. Kalsi, P., Peltola, H., Tarhio, J.: Comparison of exact string matching algorithms for biological sequences. In: Elloumi, M., Küng, J., Linial, M., Murphy, R.F., Schneider, K., Toma, C. (eds.) Bioinformatics Research and Development. Communications in Computer and Information Science, vol. 13, pp. 417–426. Springer, Heidelberg (2008). https://doi.org/10.1007/978-3-540-70600-7_31

19. Berry, T., Ravindran, S.: A fast string matching algorithm and experimental results. In: Proceedings of the Prague Stringology Club Workshop 1999, Collaborative Report DC-99-05, Czech Technical University, Prague, 16–26 (2001)
20. Vijayarani, S., Janani, R.: String matching algorithms for reteriving information from desktop—comparative analysis. In: 2016 International Conference on Inventive Computation Technologies (ICICT), pp. 1–6. IEEE (2016)
21. Sheik, S., Aggarwal, S.K., Poddar, A., Sathiyabhama, B., Balakrishnan, N., Sekar, K.: Analysis of string-searching algorithms on biological sequence databases. Curr. Sci. **89**(2), 368–374 (2005)
22. Al-Mayyahi, M.H.N., Hazim, N., Al-Dabbagh, S.S.M.: Fast hybrid string matching algorithm based on the quick-skip and tuned Boyer-Moore algorithms. Education **8**(6), 117–127 (2012)
23. Franek, F., Jennings, C.G., Smyth, W.F.: A simple fast hybrid pattern-matching algorithm. J. Discrete Algorithms **5**(4), 682–695 (2007)
24. Didier, G., Tichit, L.: Designing optimal-and fast-on-average pattern matching algorithms. J. Discrete Algorithms **42**, 45–60 (2017)
25. Zavadskyi, I.O.: A family of exact pattern matching algorithms with multiple adjacent search windows. In: Stringology, pp. 152–66 (2017)
26. Huang, Y., Ping, L., Pan, X., Jiang, L., Jiang, X.: A fast improved pattern matching algorithm for biological sequences. In: 2008 International Symposium on Computational Intelligence and Design 2008, pp. 375–378 (2008)
27. Kuthadi, V.M.: Detection of proficient and distinct motifs in sequence data sets using PSM. In: 2013 7th International Conference on Intelligent Systems and Control (ISCO), pp. 354–358. IEEE (2013)
28. Huang, Y., Pan, X., Gao, Y., Cai, G.: A fast pattern matching algorithm for biological sequences. In: 2008 2nd International Conference on Bioinformatics and Biomedical Engineering, pp. 608–611. IEEE (2008)
29. Prasad, J., Panicker, K.: Single pattern search implementations in a cluster computing environment. In: 4th IEEE International Conference on Digital Ecosystems and Technologies, pp. 391–396. IEEE (2010)
30. AbdulRazzaq, A.A., Nur'Aini Abdul Rashid, M.A., Abu-Hashem, A.A.H.: A new efficient hybrid exact string matching algorithm and its applications. Life Sci. J. **11**(10), 474–488 (2014)
31. Prasad, J.C., Panicker, K.: Prediction of multiple string searching algorithm performance on two Beowulf cluster configurations. J. Comput. Math. Sci. **3**(1), 19–35 (2012)
32. Klaib, A.F., Osborne, H.: Searching protein sequence database using BRBMH matching algorithm. Int. J. Comput. Sci. Netw. Secur. (IJCSNS) **8**(12), 410–414 (2008)
33. Klaib, A.F., Osborne, H.: BRQS matching algorithm for searching protein sequence databases. In: 2009 International Conference on Future Computer and Communication, pp. 223–226. IEEE (2009)
34. Cai, G., Nie, X., Huang, Y.: A fast hybrid pattern matching algorithm for biological sequences. In: 2009 2nd International Conference on Biomedical Engineering and Informatics, pp. 1–5. IEEE (2009)
35. Klaib, A.F., Osborne, H.: RSMA matching algorithm for searching biological sequences. In: 2009 International Conference on Innovations in Information Technology (IIT), pp. 195–199. IEEE (2009)
36. Smyth, W.F., Wang, S.: An adaptive hybrid pattern-matching algorithm on indeterminate strings. Int. J. Found. Comput. Sci. **20**(6), 985–1004 (2009)

37. Crochemore, M., Iliopoulos, C.S., Kociumaka, T., Radoszewski, J., Rytter, W., Waleń, T.: Covering problems for partial words and for indeterminate strings. Theoret. Comput. Sci. **698**, 25–39 (2017)
38. Lin, P.-C., Lin, Y.-D., Lai, Y.-C.: A hybrid algorithm of backward hashing and automaton tracking for virus scanning. IEEE Trans. Comput. **60**(4), 594–601 (2010)
39. Xian-feng, H., Yu-bao, Y., Lu, X.: Hybrid pattern-matching algorithm based on BM-KMP algorithm. In: 2010 3rd International Conference on Advanced Computer Theory and Engineering (ICACTE), pp. V5-310-V5-313. IEEE (2010)

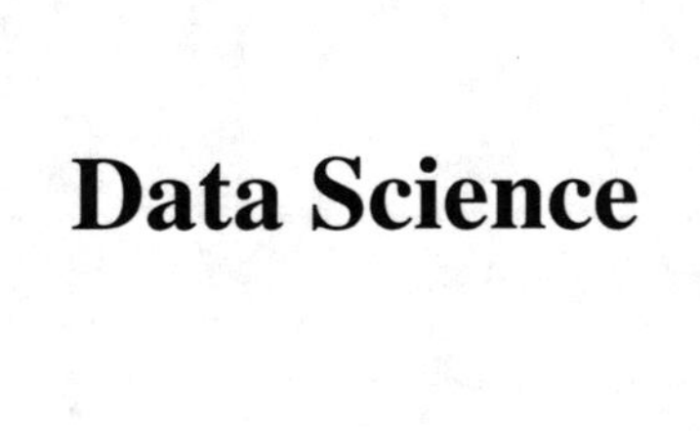

Data Science

C-SAR: Class-Specific and Adaptive Recognition for Arabic Handwritten Cheques

Ali Hamdi[1](✉), Qais Al-Nuzaili[2,5], Fuad A. Ghaleb[3], and Khaled Shaban[4]

[1] School of Computing Technologies, RMIT University, Melbourne, Australia
alihamdif@gmail.com
[2] Faculty of Engineering and Computer Science, Al-Nasser university, Sana'a, Yemen
[3] School of Computing, Faculty of Engineering, University of Technology, Johor Bahru, Malaysia
[4] Computer Science and Engineering Department, College of Engineering, Qatar University, Doha, Qatar
[5] Faculty of Engineering and Information Technology, Amran University, Sana'a, Yemen

Abstract. We propose C-SAR, a Class-specific and Adaptive Recognition algorithm for Arabic handwritten Cheques. Existing methods suffer from low accuracy due to the complex structure of Arabic script and high-dimensional datasets. In this paper, we present an adaptive algorithm that implements a class-specific classification to address these challenging issues. C-SAR trains a set of class-specific machine learning models of Support Vector Machines and Artificial Neural Networks features extracted using angular pixel distribution approach. Furthermore, we propose a class-specific taxonomy of Arabic cheque handwritten words. The proposed taxonomy divides the Arabic words into groups over three layers based on their structural characteristics. Accordingly, C-SAR performs classification on three phases, i.e., 1) similar and non-similar structures, for binary classification, 2) classes with similar structures into another two categories, and 3) class-specific models to recognize the Arabic word from the given image. We introduce benchmark experimental results of our method against previous methods on the Arabic Handwriting Database for Text Recognition. Our method outperforms the baseline methods with at least 5% accuracy having 90% average classification accuracy.

Keywords: Handwritten recognition · Image classification

1 Introduction

Computer vision and image processing methods has been utilised in various pattern recognition tasks such as image classification [1–4], few-shot learning [5, 6], object tracking [7, 8] and handwriting recognition [9–12]. Handwriting recognition is a key component of various applications such as digitizing handwritten manuscripts. Research on Arabic handwriting recognition has gained increased attention during the last two decades [13]. Many datasets have been developed to cover different types of documents written in Arabic [14–16] Arabic Handwriting Data Base for Text Recognition (AHDB) had been used for cheque literal amount recognition [17]. Existing studies present various

F. Saeed et al. (Eds.): IRICT 2021, LNDECT 127, pp. 193–208, 2022.
https://doi.org/10.1007/978-3-030-98741-1_17

methods to increase the cheque word prediction accuracy. However, it has always been a challenging recognition task due to the characteristics of the Arabic language syntax and script structure. Processing Arabic is a challenging task in handwriting recognition and Natural Language Processing. The Arabic language is written in a right-to-left script system. This system mandates to join word letters in a cursive format that has one or more components. Thus, Arabic letters are designed to be connected from one or two sides with other letters. The Arabic language has 29 letters each of which has four designs according to their position in the written word. Letters in Arabic script can be grouped based on similar shapes. These challenging characteristics make the recognition of Arabic handwritten scripts a difficult task. The main research question is how to find the best discriminative features that produce high accuracy word recognition.

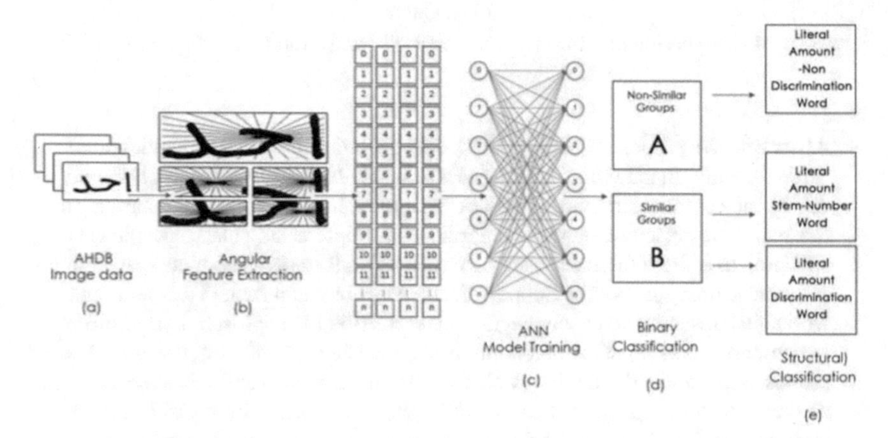

Fig. 1. The C-SAR methodology for Arabic handwritten literal amount in bank cheques.

To address this question, we revisit the baseline methods in statistical feature computing and train machine learning on class-specific approach [18]. We propose C-SAR, a Class-specific-based Adaptive Recognition Algorithm for Arabic Handwritten Cheque. We develop an angular feature extraction method that calculates the pixel distribution over different word-image regions. In this paper, we utilize the AHDB benchmark dataset of Arabic handwritten literal amounts for bank cheques. However, the dataset has more than sixty word-classes. Such a relatively high dimensional dataset leads to poor recognition accuracy. Thus, a class-specific taxonomy is proposed for the AHDB dataset based on the Arabic number syntax and structure characteristics. The proposed taxonomy facilitates the utilization of a class-specific machine learning mechanism. Specifically, we divide the dataset into groups based on the visual similarity among the Arabic letters. To train accurate machine learning models by partitioning each group into sub-groups based on a class-specific similar design. Figure 1 shows the architecture design of the proposed C-SAR, an Adaptive Recognition for Arabic Handwritten Cheques. C-SAR performs classification in three phases. First, we partition the dataset classes, according to the Arabic numbers' discriminative structural characteristics, into two main groups, i.e., similar and non-similar structures, for binary classification. Second, we group the classes with similar structures into two categories. Third, we run the class-specific models to recognize the Arabic word from the given image. This paper presents a set of contributions to build an accurate recognition system for Arabic handwritten cheque words, as follows:

1. An implementation of angular statistical feature extraction as a patch-based mechanism that offers a better understanding of the word segments and learns discriminative pixel distribution features.
2. A novel taxonomy of Arabic cheque words based on the Arabic grammar and visual structure of each word.
3. Class-specific machine learning according to the proposed taxonomy.
4. An extensive experimental work on AHDB literal amount word recognition.

The rest of this paper is organized as follows. Section 2 presents the related work. In Sect. 3, the proposed adaptive recognition algorithm is described. The results are explained in Sect. 4 and the study is concluded in Sect. 5.

2 Related Work

Pixel distribution-based approach is one of the common statistical methods which have been used in several studies for Arabic digits and text recognition. This approach can be implemented in different ways such as sliding windows or dividing the text/digit image horizontally, vertically, or using an angular concept.

Mahmoud and Olatunji [19], have investigated the pixel distribution-based features on Arabic (Indian) digits using four methods, namely angle, ring, horizontal, and vertical span methods. In the Angular method, they have used 72 and 36 features produced at 5 and 10 angle span degrees. The average recognition rates were 98.75% and 99.09% respectively using Support vector machines (SVM). The used dataset contains 21120 Arabic digit images which are divided into two parts: a training set with 75% and testing set with 25%. Arabic handwriting words recognition has been explored by Mario and Volker [20]. In their study, the pixel distribution based features were extracted using a sliding window approach from right to left on normalized images that belong to IFN/ENIT dataset. This system has achieved an 82% accuracy rate of Arabic handwriting words recognition. Farah et al. [21] used statistical features with an ANN classifier to recognize the Arabic word from the bank cheque legal amounts. The recognition accuracy rate was (74.17%) applied on a dataset of 4,800 words. The dataset was divided into two equal parts (training and testing sets).

A system for Arabic bank cheque recognition using Hidden Markov Model (HMM) has proposed also by Cheriet and Al-Ohali [22]. It has used the features from the pen trajectory that has been extracted from the (Non-touching sub-word) of the legal amount of CENPARMI database. The system recognition accuracy was 73.53%. In [15, 16] Al-Ma'adeed et al. studied the Arabic handwritten words on bank cheques using AHDB dataset. They used 4,700 handwritten words for training and testing. Hidden Markov Model (HMM) with local statistical and structural features extracted from the Arabic word bank images achieved a 45% recognition rate, while structural global features with neural network accomplished a 63% recognition rate. For Arabic handwritten word recognition, Al-Nuzaili et al. [23–25] proposed two feature extraction models called Pixel Distribution feature Model (PDM) and Perceptual Feature extraction Model(PFM). PDM is a statistical pixel distributed-based feature extraction method that combined angular, distance, horizontal, and vertical features in one vector. Angular span method alone with 30 features has achieved a 44.84% recognition rate, while the combination of all methods (PDM Model) achieved 63.35%. PFM has a structural feature extraction model. The best recognition rate that PFM has achieved was 77.39%. Both models have used Extreme Learning Machine (ELM) classifier with AHDB dataset. In [26], Al-Nuzaili presented Quadratic Angular Model (QAM) to improve the recognition rate of Arabic handwritten literal amount. QAM has extracted 120 features by dividing the word image into 4 equal parts. Then, the angular method was applied to every part to produce 30 features for every part. This model outperformed the conventional Angular method with a 59.20% recognition rate. Moreover, the combinations of QAM + PDM and QAM + PFM have archived a better recognition rate with 68.31% and 83.06%, respectively.

These exiting studies produce poor accuracy due to the characteristics of the Arabic language syntax and script structure. This paper introduces a new methodology to incorporate the state-of-art advances within a novel class-specific approach that trains a set of adapted machine learning classifiers according to the Arabic language characteristics.

3 Adaptive Recognition for Arabic Handwritten Cheques

The main problem in the Arabic cheque handwritten recognition is the low accuracy due to the high dimensionality of the datasets (i.e. 67 classes). The main objective of this research is to increase classification accuracy. In this paper, we propose an Adaptive Angular Arabic Cheque recognition algorithm. The proposed algorithm is adaptive because it performs the machine learning classification in three phases according to the Arabic cheque dataset classes groups, and angular because it uses pixel angular distribution features methods.

3.1 Angular Feature Extraction Method

There are different statistical methods to calculate the pixel distribution feature. In this paper, we employ the angular method that has been recently utilized in Arabic handwritten script recognition on the whole word image and image patches [23, 26, 27]. We combine the angular features with features from the image patches. We slice the given image into four equal non-overlapping patches. For the original image and each patch, we compute the angular features as follows. We compute centre of gravity (x_c, y_c) as in Eq. (1).

$$(x_c, y_c) = \left(\frac{\sum_{j=1}^{m} \sum_{i=1}^{n} iI[i,j]}{\sum_{j=1}^{m} \sum_{i=1}^{n} I[i,j]}, \frac{\sum_{j=1}^{m} \sum_{i=1}^{n} jI[i,j]}{\sum_{j=1}^{m} \sum_{i=1}^{n} I[i,j]} \right) \tag{1}$$

where I is a binary image of dimension $m \times n$, x_c and y_c are the x- and y- coordinates of the word COG. We then slice the word image/patch using angular lines with angles of

α degree. The number of black pixels in each slice, i.e., between every two consecutive lines, is calculated as in Eq. 2.

$$y = mx + b \tag{2}$$

where m denotes the slope of the line, b refers to the y-intercept, m equals to tan (θ) and θ is the line inclination angle. The number of black pixels in each slice is divided by the total number of black pixels in the whole word image/patch to compute angular features. The Number of Angular Features (NOAF) can be calculated as in Eq. (3).

$$NOAF = 360/\alpha \tag{3}$$

Where α refers to the angle degree between every two consecutive lines. After angular features are extracted, the feature vector is constructed. For example if our parameter value ($\alpha = 12$), then NOAF = 360/12 = 30 features.

3.2 Arabic Numbers

The grammar related to the numbers in Arabic is considered to be the most complicated thing about the language [28]. Table A1 shows the Arabic numbers, their transliteration and the Indian numbers which used in the Arabic script. The Arabic grammar for numbers 1 and 2 are different from the numbers 3 to 10. The number 1 has in the Arabic language has many different forms:

1. "وَاحِدٌ" /wạḥidu^n/ for masculine.
2. "واحدة" /wạḥdẗ/ for feminine.
3. "أحد" /ảḥd/ in eleven; "أحد عشر" /ảḥd ʿsẖr/ for masculine.
4. "إحدى" /ạḥdy̱/ in eleven; "إحدى عشرة" /ạḥdy̱ ʿsẖrẗ/ for feminine.

The number Two refers to duals and can be written in different forms:

1. "إثْنان" /ạṯẖ̊nạn/ for masculine nominative.
2. "اثْنَيْنِ" /ạṯẖạṯẖ̊naẙni/ for masculine accusative/genitive.
3. "إثْنَتانِ" /ạṯẖ̊natạni/ for feminine nominative.
4. "اثْنَتَيْنِ" /ạ ạṯẖ̊nataẙni/ for feminine accusative/genitive.
5. "اثْنَا" /ạṯẖ̊nā/ in twelve; "اثْنَا عَشَرَ" /ạṯẖ̊nā ʿasẖara/ for masculine nominative.
6. ""اثْنَي" /ạṯẖ̊naẙ/ in twelve; "اثْنَيْ عَشَرَ" /ạṯẖ̊naẙ ʿasẖara/ for masculine accusative/genitive.
7. "اثْنَتَا" /ạṯẖ̊natā/ in twelve; "اثْنَتَا عَشْرَةَ" /ạṯẖ̊natā ʿasẖ̊raẗa/ for feminine nominative.
8. "اثْنَتَي" /ạṯẖ̊nataẙ/ in twelve; "اثْنَتَيْ عَشْرَةَ" /ạṯẖ̊nataẙ ʿasẖ̊raẗa/ for feminine accusative/genitive.

For plural, the used numbers are from 3 to 10 and have two different forms according to a principle known as a reverse agreement where: "ثلاثة" /ṯẖlạṯẖẗ/ a feminine used for masculine entities such as "ثلاثة رجال" /ṯẖlạṯẖẗ rjạl/; "three men" and the masculine "ثلاث" /ṯẖlạṯẖ/ is used with feminine such as "ثلاث نساء" /ṯẖlạṯẖ nsạʾ/; "three women". This rule is generalized for the numbers 3–10 such as the number 4 "أربع" /ảrbˁ/ or "أربعة" /ảrbˁẗ/. Table A2 illustrates the numbers from 11 to19. The numbers from 20 to 99 are composed of the even tens and the earlier discussed 1–9. Table A3 shows from 20 to 90. Table A4 displays the numbers from 100 to 900 except 200 which differs where "مئتان" /mỷtạni/ for nominative and "مئتين" /mỷtyn/ for accusative/genitive.

3.3 Class-Specific Taxonomy of Arabic Cheque Words

We propose a class-specific taxonomy to train a set of machine learning models based on the above-mentioned Arabic numbering characteristics. The proposed algorithm is adaptive as it performs the machine learning classification in three phases according to the grouping of the Arabic cheque dataset classes, and angular that uses pixel angular distribution features methods. In the first phase, the classes could be grouped into two main groups, named binary, included group a and group b as stated in Table B1. In group a, the non-similar discrimination classes are grouped. While in group b, the numbers from three to ten are together. In the second phase, group a are grouped into 8 groups as shown in Table B2, and group b are grouped into 8 groups (see Table B3). The third phase is to recognize the target class. In the next subsection, we discuss the angular feature extraction method, grammar of Arabic numbers, our proposed class-specific taxonomy based on that grammar, and modelling SVM and ANN machine learning algorithms. Figure 2 shows two examples for using the proposed Adaptive Angular Arabic Cheque recognition algorithm. The two classified examples are, five /خمسة/ or class fiveb, and two thousands /ألفان/ of class twoh. In the first example fiveb, the proposed algorithm firstly classified the binary to be in groups b, secondly classified which class in groups b to and resulted the group five, and finally classified the discriminator b and return the class

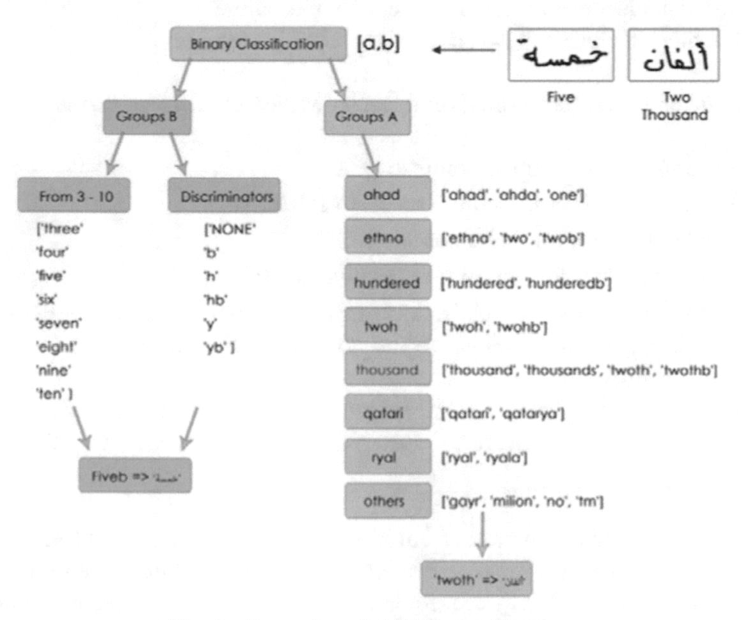

Fig. 2. Examples of C-SAR classification

fiveb. On the other hand, in the example twoh, the algorithm task 1 binary classified the example to be in group a and task 2 classified the example to be in thousand group which contains the thousand, thousands, twoth and twothb, therefore in task 3 the proposed algorithm classified it as twoth.

3.4 Machine Learning Models

The extracted angular features are used by SVM and ANN architecture to train class-specific models for each group of words according to the proposed taxonomy. The two implemented models are down-stream supervised learning tasks over the angular features representations. SVM computes the classification scores over a set of hyper-planes. It solves the classification problem by maximizing the separation between the data points. This maximum separation is achieved over iteration of learning the best hyper-plane that has largest distances to the data examples. We implement a linear version of SVM that takes a set of data points each of which is represented as multi-dimensional real vector. The linear SVM finds the maximum separating hyper-plane. The SVM is implemented to solve that optimization problem in an unconstrained set up according to the following loss function:

$$\min_{\boldsymbol{w}} \frac{1}{2}\boldsymbol{w}^T\boldsymbol{w} + C\sum_{i=1}^{l} \xi(\boldsymbol{w}; \boldsymbol{x}_i, y_i) \tag{4}$$

where w is a feature vector of a set of x and y and C denotes a penalty score greater than 0. An x point is positive if $\boldsymbol{w}^T\boldsymbol{w} > 0$ [29].

We also developed a feed-forward artificial neural network (ANN) to classify handwritten Arabic cheque words as visualized in Fig. 3. The ANN architecture has three layers. An input layer feeds the angular pixel distribution statistical features into a hidden layer. The features are fully connected to one hidden layer that calculates the network bias and weights. The final classification label is computed at an output layer. The weights of the hidden neurons are calculated based on the weights of the connected features and bias as shown in examples (z1 and z2) in Eqs. (5, 6 and 7). Equation 7 shows the computing of the prediction output (o).

$$z1 = x1^{\star}w11 + x2^{*}w12 + x3^{*}w13 + b1 \tag{5}$$

$$z2 = x1^{*}w21 + x2^{*}w22 + x3^{*}w23 + b2 \tag{6}$$

$$o = a1^{\star}w31 + a2^{\star}w32 + b3 \tag{7}$$

The implemented ANN is described by matrices of the hidden and output layers described in Eqs. (8 and 9).

$$\begin{bmatrix} x_1 \; x_2 \end{bmatrix} \begin{bmatrix} w_{11} \; w_{12} \; w_{13} \\ w_{21} \; w_{22} \; w_{23} \end{bmatrix} = \begin{bmatrix} x_1w_{11} + x_2w_{21} \\ x_1w_{12} + x_2w_{22} \\ x_1w_{13} + x_2w_{23} \end{bmatrix}' = \begin{bmatrix} h_1 \\ h_2 \\ h_3 \end{bmatrix}' \tag{8}$$

$$\begin{bmatrix} h_1 \\ h_2 \\ h_3 \end{bmatrix}' \begin{bmatrix} 1 \\ 1 \\ 1 \end{bmatrix} = h_1 + h_2 + h_3 = y \tag{9}$$

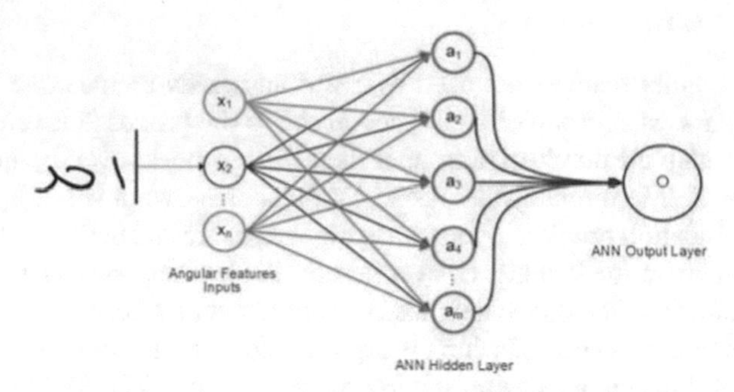

Fig. 3. The architecture of the implemented ANN.

The classification output score is calculated as the input features' element-wise dot product and a weights matrix kernel. An activation function, e.g., Rectified Linear Units (ReLU) as in Eq. 10, is then applied on layers weights before computing the final output.

$$ReLU(z) = \begin{Bmatrix} z & z > 0 \\ 0 & z <= 0 \end{Bmatrix} \tag{10}$$

Applying ReLU activation is helpful to avoid vanishing gradient. Other activation functions that can be utilised such as Sigmoid and tanh. ReLU requires fewer computational resources due to its simple mathematical operations.

4 Experiment Results

We run multiple experiments to train and test SVM and ANN on the AHDB groups according to our proposed taxonomy. The experiments follow the proposed architecture, as visualized in Fig. 1. We have implemented C-SAR on five main steps as follows:

1. Implement angular method for statistical feature extraction. We first compute the pixel distribution features of 30 slices on the whole image. Then, we divide the word image into four equal, non-overlapping patches. Each patch is used to compute the angular features. Therefore, we compute total 150 angular features; 30 of the original image and 120 of the four patches.
2. We prepare a mapping dictionary to retrieve sub-sets from the AHDB according to the proposed C-SAR taxonomy.
3. We then train SVM and ANN models for the three-layer class-specific methodology. We first train the models to learn the binary groups, i.e., a and b. Then, we train other models to learn the classification of sub-sets of each of these groups. Finally, we train the third-layer models to classify the word images classes.

4. We train various models using the different angular feature sets and class-specific taxonomy groups.
5. All models are evaluated on 10K cross-validation 70% and 30% for train and test.

Table 1 lists the cross-validation results of using different angular features sets, e.g., 30, 120 and 150 for the whole image, images patches and both, respectively. The results are shown for taxonomy level groups such as binary, group a and group b, etc. The experiment results show that the utilized ANN mostly has the best word classification accuracy over the SVM. Classifying the binary groups has 91% accuracy using the ANN. The accuracy varies from group to another. This fact highlights the significance of our proposed C-SAR taxonomy. It harnesses the similarity between each group of classes while ignoring other noisy classes. That process leads to having 99% accuracy in some models. Using the combination of the 150 features tends to have the best accuracy in most cases. However, in some cases, such as group a ethna, using only 30 angular features has the best results. Another example, using the 120 features for the four image patches have the best accuracy with multiple class-specific models. This is another benefit of training classes' models on other different feature sub-sets. We then select the best performing model of each group and use them in the final C-SAR framework.

We compare the accuracy of C-SAR with baseline models that are tested on the AHDB dataset. Table 2 lists the benchmark results and shows that C-SAR outperforms all other models. The PDM + PFM + QAM combination of models had the previous best accuracy of 85.85%. We list four different ablations of our proposed model. First, C-SAR 30 is implemented using the 30 angular features of the whole image. This version

Table 1. 10K cross-validation results using different angular features.

Level	30		120		150		Best
	SVM	ANN	SVM	ANN	SVM	ANN	Accuracy
Binary	77%	89%	74%	**91%**	80%	90%	***91%***
Groups_a	64%	84%	74%	89%	79%	**90%**	***90%***
– Groups a ahad	81%	90%	84%	90%	84%	**92%**	***92%***
– Groups a ethna	71%	**84%**	70%	79%	73%	82%	***84%***
– Groups a hundered	59%	85%	83%	**90%**	82%	89%	***90%***
– Groups a twoh	60%	83%	69%	86%	71%	**88%**	***88%***
– Groups a thousand	63%	80%	72%	80%	73%	**83%**	***83%***
– Groups a qatari	81%	92%	**99%**	**99%**	**99%**	**97%**	***99%***
– Groups a ryal	78%	90%	80%	**91%**	80%	90%	***91%***
– Groups a others	91%	91%	87%	94%	91%	**95%**	***95%***
Groups b	58%	81%	67%	86%	73%	**90%**	***90%***
Groups b discriminators	50%	75%	59%	78%	65%	**81%**	***81%***
Average Accuracy	69%	85%	77%	88%	79%	**89%**	***90%***

has 85% average accuracy. Second, C-SAR 120, of the four image patches, has improved the accuracy to 88% outperforming the baseline models. Third, C-SAR 150 combines the features of the whole image and its patches. This one has 89% average accuracy using the ANN. Finally, we list the C-SAR, on the selected model with the best accuracy in each group. C-SAR has 90% average accuracy outer performing both other versions and baseline models.

Table 2. Benchmark results.

Model	Recognition accuracy %
Quadratic Angular Model (QAM)	59.20
PDM Model	64.36
PFM Model	77.39
Combination of PDM + QAM	68.31
Combination of PDM + PFM	81.95
Combination of PFM + QAM	83.06
CFM Model Combination of PDM + PFM + QAM	85.85
C-SAR 30	85%
C-SAR 120	88%
C-SAR 150	89%
C-SAR	**90%**

5 Conclusion

We present C-SAR, a class-specific adaptive recognition algorithm for handwritten literal amount cheque word recognition. C-SAR extracts the angular features and combines them with features from the image patches. Then, such features are fed to SVM and ANN-based classifiers. C-SAR is designed on a new taxonomy of class-specific machine learning models trained on the AHDB dataset. The hypothesis behind the taxonomy is to reduce the noise and focus the training on the correlated groups of images. The results show the significance of the proposed method advancing the baseline accuracy to new state-of-the-art accuracy of 90% on average improving the baseline accuracy by around 5% on average with some classes reaching 99%. Future research should consider implementing the class-specific approach within recent Deep Learning mechanism such as Graph Convolutional Networks and attentional transformers.

Supplemental Material on the Paper "C-SAR: Class-specific and Adaptive Recognition for Arabic Handwritten Cheques".

Appendix A

Table A1. Arabic numbers

Arabic	Masculine	Transliteration	Feminine	Transliteration	Indian
1	واحِدٌ	wạḥidu^{n}	واحِدةٌ	wạḥidẗu^{n}	١
2	إثْنانِ	ạtẖnạni	إثْنانِ	ạtẖnạni	٢
3	ثَلاثَةٌ	tẖalạtẖaẗu^{n}	ثَلاثٌ	tẖalạtẖu^{n}	٣
4	أرْبَعةٌ	ạảr̊ba'ẗu^{n}	أرْبَعٌ	ạảr̊ba'u^{n}	٤
5	خَمْسةٌ	kẖam̊sẗu^{n}	خَمْسٌ	kẖam̊su^{n}	٥
6	سِتَّةٌ	sit̃ẗu^{n}	سِتٌّ	sit̃u^{n}	٦
7	سَبْعةٌ	sab̊'ẗu^{n}	سَبْعٌ	sab̊'u^{n}	٧
8	ثَمانِيةٌ	tẖamạnīẗu^{n}	ثَمانِي	tẖamạnī	٨
9	تِسْعةٌ	tis̊'ẗu^{n}	تِسْعٌ	tis̊'u^{n}	٩
10	عَشرَةٌ	'asẖraẗu^{n}	عَشرٌ	'asẖru^{n}	١٠

Table A2. Numbers from 11–19 in the Arabic language.

Arabic	Transliteration	Masculine	Transliteration	Feminine	Indian
11	ạ̉ḥada 'asẖara	أحَدَ عَشَرَ	ạịḥ̊dy 'ash̊rẗa	إحْدى عَشْرةَ	١١
12 Nominative	ạtẖ̊nạ 'asẖara	إثْنا عَشَرَ	ạtẖ̊natạ 'ash̊rẗa	إثْنَتا عَشْرةَ	١٢
12 Accusative/ Genitive	ạtẖ̊naẙ 'asẖara	إثْنَىْ عَشَرَ	ạịtẖ̊nataẙ 'ash̊rẗa	إثْنَتَيْ عَشْرةَ	١٢
13	tẖlạtẖẗa 'asẖara	ثلاثةَ عَشَرَ	tẖlạtẖa 'ash̊rẗa	ثلاثَ عَشْرةَ	١٣
14	ạảr̊ba'ẗa 'asẖara	أرْبَعةَ عَشَرَ	ạ̉r̊b'a 'ash̊rẗa	أرْبعَ عَشْرةَ	١٤
15	kẖam̊sẗa 'asẖara	خَمْسةَ عَشَرَ	kẖim̊sa 'ash̊rẗa	خِمْسَ عَشْرةَ	١٥
16	sit̃ẗa 'asẖara	سِتَّةَ عَشَرَ	sitã 'ash̊rẗa	سِتَّ عَشْرةَ	١٦
17	sab̊'ẗa 'asẖara	سَبْعةَ عَشَرَ	sib̊'a 'ash̊rẗa	سِبْعَ عَشْرةَ	١٧
18	tẖamạnyẗa 'asẖara	ثَمانيةَ عَشَرَ	tẖmạnya 'ash̊rẗa	ثمانيَ عَشْرةَ	١٨
19	tis̊'ẗa 'asẖara	تِسْعةَ عَشَرَ	tis̊'a 'ash̊rẗa	تِسْعَ عَشْرةَ	١٩

Table A3. The Arabic numbers from 20 to 90.

Arabic	Nominative Arabic word	Transliteration	Accusative/ Genitive Arabic word	Translitera-tion	Indian
20	عشرون	'sẖrwn	عشرين	'sẖryn	٢٠
30	ثلاثون	tẖlạtẖwn	ثلاثين	tẖlạtẖyn	٣٠
40	أربعون	ạ̉rb'wn	أربعين	ạ̉rb'yn	٤٠
50	خمسون	kẖmswn	خمسين	kẖmsyn	٥٠
60	ستون	Stwn	ستين	Styn	٦٠
70	سبعون	sb'wn	سبعين	sb'yn	٧٠
80	ثمانون	tẖmạnwn	ثمانين	tẖmạnyn	٨٠
90	تسعون	ts'wn	تسعين	ts'yn	٩٠

Table A4. The Arabic numbers from hundred to nine hundred except two hundred

Arabic	Arabic form 1	Transliteration	Arabic form 2	Transliteration	Indian
100	مِئة	mi̊ẗ	مائة	mạẙẗ	١٠٠
300	ثلاثُمئة	tẖlạtẖumẙẗi^{n}	ثلاثُمائة	tẖlạtẖumạẙẗi^{n}	٣٠٠
400	أرْبَعُمئة	ạ̉r̊ba'umẙẗi^{n}	أرْبَعُمائة	ạảr̊ba'umạẙẗi^{n}	٤٠٠
500	خَمْسُمئة	kẖam̊sumẙẗi^{n}	خَمسُمائة	kẖamsumạẙẗi^{n}	٥٠٠
600	سِتُّمئة	sitũmẙẗi^{n}	سِتُّمائة	sitũmạẙẗi^{n}	٦٠٠
700	سَبعُمئة	sab'umẙẗi^{n}	سَبعُمائة	sab'umạẙẗi^{n}	٧٠٠
800	ثَمانيمئة	tẖamạnymẙẗi^{n}	ثَمانيمئة	tẖamạnymẙẗi^{n}	٨٠٠
900	تِسْعُمئة	tis̊'umẙẗi^{n}	تِسْعُمائة	tis̊'umạẙẗi^{n}	٩٠٠

Appendix B

Table B1. The proposed binary grouping

a		b			
ahad	thousands	three	five	seven	nine
ahda	twoth	threeb	fifty	sevenb	nineb
one	twothb	threeh	fiftyb	sevenh	nineh
ethna	qatari	threehb	fiveb	sevenhb	ninehb
two	qatarya	thirty	fiveh	seventy	ninety
twob	ryal	thirtyb	fivehb	seventyb	ninetyb
hundered	ryala	four	six	eight	ten
hunderedb	gayr	fourb	sixb	eightb	tenb
twoh	milion	fourh	sixh	eighth	twenty
twohb	no	fourhb	sixhb	eighthb	twentyb
thousand	tm	fourty	sixty	eighty	
		fourtyb	sixtyb	eightyb	

Table B2. The non-similar discrimination groups a

Groups a							
ahad	ethna	hundered	twoh	thousand	qatari	ryal	others
ahad	ethna	hundered	twoh	thousand	qatari	ryal	gayr
ahda	two	hunderedb	twohb	thousands	qatarya	ryala	milion
one	twob			twoth			no
				twothb			tm

Table B3. The similar discrimination groups b

Groups b							
three	four	five	six	seven	eight	nine	ten
three	four	five	six	seven	eight	nine	ten
threeb	fourb	fifty	sixb	sevenb	eightb	nineb	tenb
threeh	fourh	fiftyb	sixh	sevenh	eighth	nineh	twenty
threehb	fourhb	fiveb	sixhb	sevenhb	eighthb	ninehb	twentyb
thirty	fourty	fiveh	sixty	seventy	eighty	ninety	
thirtyb	fourtyb	fivehb	sixtyb	seventyb	eightyb	ninetyb	

Table B4. The discriminators.

Discriminators					
NONE	b	h	hb	y	yb
three	threeb	hundered	hunderedb	twenty	twentyb
four	fourb	threeh	threehb	thirty	thirtyb
five	fiveb	fourh	fourhb	fourty	fourtyb
six	sixb	fiveh	fivehb	fifty	fiftyb
seven	sevenb	sixh	sixhb	sixty	sixtyb
eight	eightb	sevenh	sevenhb	seventy	seventyb
nine	nineb	eighth	eighthb	eighty	eightyb
ten	tenb	nineh	ninehb	ninety	ninetyb

Appendix C

Table C1. C-SAR using SVM and ANN on 30 Angular features of the whole image.

Level	Accuracy		Precision		Recall		f1-score	
	SVM	ANN	SVM	ANN	SVM	ANN	SVM	ANN
binary	77%	89%	77%	89%	89%	77%	74%	89%
groups_a	64%	84%	66%	84%	85%	64%	61%	84%
groups a ahad	81%	90%	82%	90%	91%	81%	81%	90%
groups a ethna	71%	84%	77%	85%	87%	71%	65%	84%
groups a hundered	59%	85%	34%	85%	86%	59%	43%	85%
groups a twoh	60%	83%	76%	83%	84%	60%	47%	83%
groups a thousand	63%	80%	63%	80%	81%	63%	59%	80%
groups a qatari	81%	92%	86%	92%	93%	81%	80%	92%
groups a ryal	78%	90%	84%	89%	90%	78%	76%	90%
groups a others	91%	91%	93%	91%	92%	92%	91%	91%
groups b	58%	81%	60%	81%	82%	58%	55%	81%
groups b discriminators	50%	75%	49%	75%	77%	50%	48%	75%

Table C2. C-SAR using SVM and ANN on 150 Angular features of the whole image.

Level	Accuracy		Precision		Recall		f1-score	
	SVM	ANN	SVM	ANN	SVM	ANN	SVM	ANN
binary	80%	90%	79%	88%	80%	90%	78%	89%
groups_a	79%	90%	80%	90%	79%	90%	79%	90%
groups a ahad	84%	92%	85%	93%	84%	92%	84%	92%
groups a ethna	73%	82%	74%	83%	74%	82%	73%	82%
groups a hundered	82%	89%	83%	90%	83%	89%	82%	89%
groups a twoh	71%	88%	71%	89%	71%	88%	71%	88%
groups a thousand	73%	83%	73%	85%	73%	83%	73%	83%
groups a qatari	99%	97%	98%	97%	98%	97%	98%	97%
groups a ryal	80%	90%	82%	91%	81%	90%	80%	91%
groups a others	91%	95%	91%	95%	91%	95%	90%	95%
groups b	73%	90%	73%	90%	73%	90%	73%	90%
groups b discriminators	65%	81%	65%	82%	65%	81%	65%	81%

Table C3. C-SAR using SVM and ANN on 120 Angular features of the whole image.

Level	Accuracy		Precision		Recall		f1-score	
	SVM	ANN	SVM	ANN	SVM	ANN	SVM	ANN
binary	74%	91%	72%	91%	74%	91%	72%	91%
groups_a	74%	89%	74%	89%	74%	89%	74%	89%
groups a ahad	84%	90%	85%	90%	84%	90%	84%	90%
groups a ethna	70%	79%	70%	80%	71%	79%	70%	79%
groups a hundered	83%	90%	85%	90%	84%	90%	84%	90%
groups a twoh	69%	86%	70%	87%	70%	86%	69%	86%
groups a thousand	72%	80%	71%	82%	71%	80%	71%	81%
groups a qatari	99%	99%	98%	99%	98%	99%	98%	99%
groups a ryal	80%	91%	82%	92%	81%	91%	80%	91%
groups a others	87%	94%	88%	95%	87%	94%	87%	94%
groups b	67%	86%	67%	86%	67%	86%	66%	86%
groups b discriminators	59%	78%	59%	80%	59%	78%	59%	78%

References

1. Hamdi, A., Kim, D.Y., Salim, F.D.: flexgrid2vec: learning efficient visual representations vectors. arXiv preprint arXiv:2007.15444 (2020)
2. Hamdi, A., et al.: Signature-graph networks. arXiv preprint arXiv:2110.11551 (2021)
3. Li, B., Li, Y., Eliceiri, K.W.: Dual-stream multiple instance learning network for whole slide image classification with self-supervised contrastive learning. In: Proceedings of the IEEE/CVF Conference on Computer Vision and Pattern Recognition (2021)
4. Rao, Y., et al.: Global filter networks for image classification. In: Advances in Neural Information Processing Systems 34 (2021)
5. Hamdi, A., Salim, F., Kim, D.Y.: GCCN: global context convolutional network. arXiv preprint arXiv:2110.11664 (2021)
6. Liu, S., Wang, Y.: Few-shot learning with online self-distillation. In: Proceedings of the IEEE/CVF International Conference on Computer Vision (2021)
7. Hamdi, A., Salim, F., Kim, D.Y.: Drotrack: high-speed drone-based object tracking under uncertainty. In: 2020 IEEE International Conference on Fuzzy Systems (FUZZ-IEEE). IEEE (2020)
8. Wang, Y., Kitani, K., Weng, X.: Joint object detection and multi-object tracking with graph neural networks. In: 2021 IEEE International Conference on Robotics and Automation (ICRA). IEEE (2021)
9. Ahlawat, S., et al.: Improved handwritten digit recognition using convolutional neural networks (CNN). Sensors **20**(12), 3344 (2020)
10. Kulkarni, S.R., Rajendran, B.: Spiking neural networks for handwritten digit recognition—supervised learning and network optimization. Neural Netw. **103**, 118–127 (2018)
11. Qiao, J., et al.: An adaptive deep Q-learning strategy for handwritten digit recognition. Neural Netw. **107**, 61–71 (2018)
12. Rabby, A.S.A., et al.: Ekushnet: using convolutional neural network for Bangla handwritten recognition. Procedia Comput. Sci. **143**, 603–610 (2018)
13. Memon, J., et al.: Handwritten optical character recognition (OCR): a comprehensive systematic literature review (SLR). IEEE Access **8**, 142642–142668 (2020)
14. Mozaffari, S., Soltanizadeh, H.: ICDAR 2009 handwritten Farsi/Arabic character recognition competition. In: 2009 10th International Conference on Document Analysis and Recognition. IEEE (2009)
15. Khayyat, M., Lam, L., Suen, C.Y.: Learning-based word spotting system for Arabic handwritten documents. Pattern Recogn. **47**(3), 1021–1030 (2014)
16. Mezghani, A., et al.: A database for Arabic handwritten text image recognition and writer identification. In: 2012 International Conference on Frontiers in Handwriting Recognition. IEEE (2012)
17. Al-Ma'adeed, S., Elliman, D., Higgins, C.A.: A data base for Arabic handwritten text recognition research. In: Proceedings Eighth International Workshop on Frontiers in Handwriting Recognition. IEEE (2002)
18. Hamdi, A., Shaban, K., Zainal, A.: CLASENTI: a class-specific sentiment analysis framework. ACM Trans. Asian Low-Resour. Lan. Inf. Process. (TALLIP) **17**(4), 1–28 (2018)
19. Mahmoud, S., Olatunji, S.O.: Handwritten Arabic numerals recognition using multi-span features & support vector machines. In: Proceedings of the 2010 10th International Conference on Information Sciences Signal Processing and their Applications (ISSPA), Kuala Lumpur, Malaysia. IEEE (2010)
20. Mario, P., Volker, M.: HMM based approach for handwritten Arabic word recognition using the IFN/ENIT- database. In: Proceedings of the Seventh International Conference on Document Analysis and Recognition, Edinburgh, Scotland. IEEE Computer Society (2003)

21. Farah, N., Souici, L., Sellami, M.: Arabic word recognition by classifiers and context. J. Comput. Sci. Technol. **20**(3), 402–410 (2005)
22. Cheriet, M., et al.: Arabic cheque processing system: issues and future trends. In: Chaudhuri, B.B. (ed.) Digital Document Processing. ACVPR, pp. 213–234. Springer, Heidelberg (2007). https://doi.org/10.1007/978-1-84628-726-8_10
23. Al-Nuzaili, Q., et al.: Pixel distribution-based features for offline Arabic handwritten word recognition. Int. J. Comput. Vis. Robot. **7**(1/2), 99–122 (2017)
24. Al-Nuzaili, Q., et al.: Feature extraction in holistic approach for Arabic handwriting recognition system: a preliminary study. In: 2012 IEEE 8th International Colloquium on Signal Processing and its Applications (CSPA). IEEE (2012)
25. Perez, C., et al.: Gender classification from face images using mutual information and feature fusion. Int. J. Optomechatronics **6**(1), 92–119 (2012)
26. Al-Nuzaili, Q., Hamdi, A., Hashim, S., Saeed, F., Khalil, M.: An enhanced quadratic angular feature extraction model for Arabic handwritten literal amount recognition. In: Saeed, F., Gazem, N., Patnaik, S., Saed Balaid, A.S., Mohammed, F. (eds.) IRICT 2017. LNDECT, vol. 5, pp. 369–377. Springer, Cham (2018). https://doi.org/10.1007/978-3-319-59427-9_40
27. Al-Nuzaili, Q., et al.: Enhanced structural perceptual feature extraction model for Arabic literal amount recognition. Int. J. Intell. Syst. Technol. Appl. **15**(3), 240–254 (2016)
28. Abboud, P.F., McCarus, E.N.: Elementary Modern Standard Arabic: Volume 1, Pronunciation and Writing; Lessons 1–30. Cambridge University Press, Cambridge (1983)
29. Keerthi, S.S., et al.: A sequential dual method for large scale multi-class linear SVMs. In: Proceedings of the 14th ACM SIGKDD International Conference on Knowledge Discovery and Data Mining (2008)

Extraction of Spatiotemporal Association Rules for Forest Fires Prediction

Mongi Boulehmi[1](✉) and Amira Ayadi[2]

[1] VPNC Laboratory, Economics and Management Sciences of Jendouba, University of Legal Sciences, University of Jendouba, Jendouba, Tunisia
mongiboulehmi@gmail.com

[2] VPNC Laboratory, National School of Computer Science ENSI Manouba, Manouba, Tunisia

Abstract. Spatiotemporal association rules extraction is an important and challenging task. It takes into the presence of the spatial and the temporal aspects. To extract this kind of association, the Support and Confidence measures can be used. But the application of only these two measures can generate hundreds to thousands of rules; many of them are redundant and/or trivial. Here we can't considered them efficient measures because they don't give good results. In order to ensure the quality of association rules In this paper we will uses the Apriori algorithm with the Support, the Confidence and the Lift measures of interest to extract relevant spatiotemporal association rules for the prediction of the forest fires in the park of Montesinho of Portugal. It is shown that the association of these three measures can be used effectively.

Keywords: Apriori algorithm · Confidence · Lift · Spatiotemporal association rules · Support

1 Introduction

With the explosion of new technologies (mobiles, sensors, etc.), large amounts of data located in space and time have become available. Associated databases are called spatiotemporal databases since each datum is described by space (a city, a neighborhood, a river, etc.) and by time (the date of an event) information. The extraction of association rules from this kind of databases is a complex problem. To face these new challenges, new processes and methods should be developed to better exploit the available data [1].

Our work is within the framework of the spatiotemporal association rule validation, which is a delicate and interesting step in the process of knowledge extraction. There are several measures of interest for the evaluation of traditional association rules, but there are no quality measures specific to spatiotemporal ones. Our research problem is the choice of the most appropriate quality measures to generate relevant spatiotemporal association rules. The support and confidence measures of interest are often efficient but insufficient to generate relevant and adequate results. It is shown, in this work, that the adding of a third measure, which is the lift, can ensure the quality by limiting the extracted association rules to more interesting ones. In this paper, we study the

F. Saeed et al. (Eds.): IRICT 2021, LNDECT 127, pp. 209–218, 2022.
https://doi.org/10.1007/978-3-030-98741-1_18

extraction of relevant spatiotemporal association rules for predicting forest fires, through the case study: the Montesinho park in Portugal [2]. The measures of interest "Support", "Confidence" and "Lift" are used in the Apriori algorithm which is implemented in a Matlab environment. It is shown that the use of the lift measure is effective and interesting spatiotemporal association rules can be obtained [3].

2 Spatiotemporal Association Rule

A spatiotemporal association rule is of the form [4]:

$$(X, t1) \rightarrow (Y, t2) \tag{1}$$

Where X and Y are sets of spatiotemporal or non-spatiotemporal predicates. The spatiotemporal association rules have the following form:

$$(P1, t1) \cap Pm, t1) \rightarrow (Q1, t2) \cap (Qn, t \tag{2}$$

Where: at least one of the predicate Pi or Qi is spatial predicate. t1 is a time (interval, date, time) during which Pi is checked. t2 is a time (interval, date, time) during which Qi is checked. Knowing that $t1 < t2$. The subsets $(P1, t1) \ldots (Pm, t1)$, $(Q2, t2)$, $(Qn, t2)$ form the spatiotemporal predicates.

3 Extraction of Spatiotemporal Association Rules Process

Figure 1 shows the spatiotemporal association rules extraction process. It starts by reading the spatiotemporal database and ends by displaying the association rules extract.

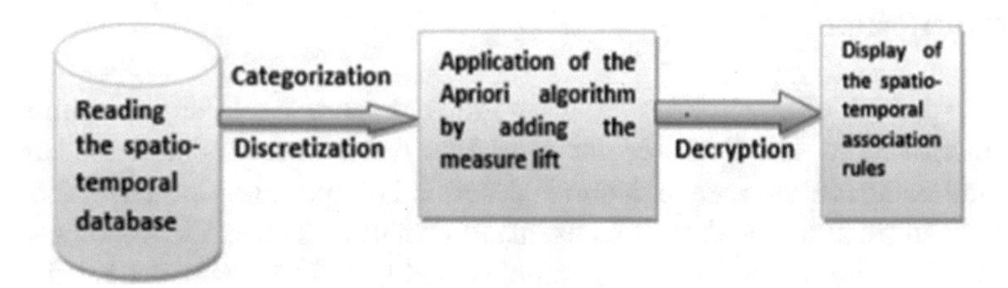

Fig. 1. Steps of the extraction of spatiotemporal association rules

3.1 Pretreatment

In our case, data is heterogeneous and complex and can not be used in its primary form. Thus, we have to deal with a complex data mining problem. Some transformations and pretreatments should be done to adapt the original data for use. We adopt, here, the categorization and the discretization.

- Categorization: Categorization consists of placing a set of objects in different categories (classes, types) according to their similarities or common criteria. It is a fundamental cognitive process in the perception and understanding of concepts and objects, in decision-making and in all forms of interaction with the environment [5].
- Discretization: Discretization makes possible to modify the characteristics of data in order to make the subsequent statistical algorithms more efficient, such as the correction of highly asymmetrical distributions [6].

3.2 Algorithm and Interest Measures Used

Once data are ready to be use, we can apply the appropriate algorithm to extract spatiotemporal association rules. It is with Khoshahval et al. [7], that we have the appearance of the first association rule extraction algorithm.

This algorithm whose pseudo code is presented in Fig. 2 is called "Apriori".

```
Apriori Algorithm Pseudocode
procedure Apriori (T, minSupport) {//T is the databaseand minSupport is the minimum support
L_1= [frequent items]:
For (k = 2;L_{k-1} !=Ø; k++) {
C_i= candidates generated from L_{k-1}
//that iscartesian product L_{k-1}* L_{k-1}and eliminating any k-1 size that is do frequent //
for each instruction t in database do {
frequent the count of all candidates in Ci that are contained in L
L_k=condidates in Ck with minSupport
} end for each
} end for
Return L_k;
}
```

Fig. 2. Apriori algorithm (http://software.ucv.ro/˜cmihaescu/ro/teaching/AIR/docs/Lab8-Apriori.pdf)

As mentioned before, the support and the confidence measures of interest are used to extract association rules. and to ensure the quality of the results, a third measure, which is the lift, is also integrated [8]:

- The support indicates the number of transactions in the database that supports the rule. It allows measuring the frequency of the association. The support is expressed as:

$$Support(X \rightarrow Y) = freq(X \cup Y) \quad (3)$$

- The Confidence is the proportion of transactions containing X that carry Y. The Confidence level is a measure of the strength of the association. The Confidence is mathematically formulated as:

$$Conf(X \rightarrow Y) = prob(Y|X) = freq(X \cup Y)/f\ req(X) \quad (4)$$

- The Lift: Confidence of the rule divided by the expected value of Confidence. Mathematically, it is given by:

$$Lift(X \rightarrow Y) = p(X \cap Y)p(X).p(Y) \quad (5)$$

3.3 Post-treatment

Once data are treated, a post-treatment phase is still necessary to get readable results. We use, in our case, decryption which consists of adapting the results in a displayable form.

4 Experimental Design

The Apriori Algorithm is implemented in a Matlab environment based on a hp machine with a Windows 7 operating system, having a 2.4 GHz Intel Core i5 processor and a 4 GB of RAM. The database is that of forest fires in Montesinho park in Portugal, collected by using the Canadian method [9], Fig. 3.

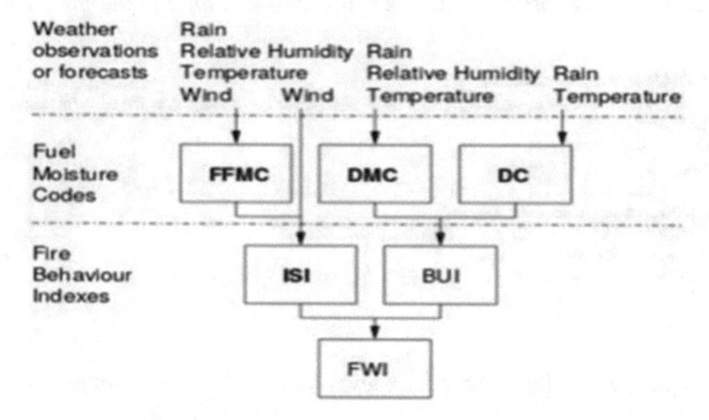

Fig. 3. The Canadian fire information system diagram (Cortez 2007)

An extract of this database is presented in Table 1.

Table 1. The Canadian fire information spatiotemporal forest fire database (http://archive.ics.uci.edu/ml/machinelearning-databases/forest-fires/)

X	Y	Month	Day	FFMC	DMC	DC	ISI	Temp	RH	Wind	Rain	Area
7	5	Mar	Fri	86.20	26.20	94.30	5.10	8.20	51.00	6.70	0.00	0.00
7	4	Oct	Tue	90.60	35.40	669.10	6.70	18.00	33.00	0.90	0.00	0.00
7	4	Oct	Sat	90.60	43.70	686.90	6.70	14.60	33.00	1.30	0.00	0.00
8	6	Mar	Fri	97.70	33.00	77.50	9.00	8.30	97.00	4.00	0.20	0.00
8	6	Mar	Sun	89.30	51.30	102.20	9.60	11.40	99.00	1.80	0.00	0.00
8	6	Aug	Sun	92.30	85.30	488.00	14.70	22.20	29.00	5.40	0.00	0.00
8	6	Aug	Mon	92.30	88.90	495.60	8.50	24.10	27.00	3.10	0.00	0.00

(*continued*)

Table 1. (*continued*)

X	Y	Month	Day	FFMC	DMC	DC	ISI	Temp	RH	Wind	Rain	Area
8	6	Aug	Mon	91.50	145.40	608.20	10.70	8.00	86.00	2.20	0.00	0.00
8	6	Sep	Tue	91.50	129.50	692.60	7.00	13.10	63.00	5.40	0.00	0.00
7	5	Sep	Sat	92.50	88.00	698.60	7.10	22.80	40.00	4.00	0.00	0.00

With: X: Coordinate of the x-axis (from 1 to 9). Y: Coordinate of the y-axis (from 1 to 9). Month: Month of the year (from January to December). Day: Day of the week (Monday to Sunday) [10]:

- FFMC: Fine Fuel Moisture Code. DMC: Duff Moisture Code.
- DC: Drought Code.
- ISI: Initial Spread Index.
- Temp: Outside temperature (in Celsius degrees).
- RH: Relative Outdoor Moisture (in %).
- Wind: Wind speed outside (in Km/h). Rain: Outside rain (in mm/mm^2).
- Area: Total burned area (in ha).

The full database can be found in (http://archive.ics.uci.edu/ml/machine-learning databases/forest-fires/), the map of the Montesinho natural park is given in [11] and the Fire Weather Index (FWI) used is structured as presented in Table 2.

Table 2. Fire Weather Index categorization (http://cwfis.cfs.nrcan.gc.ca/background/summary/fwi)

Index	Low	Moderate	High	Very high	Extreme
FFMC	0–81	81–88	88–90.5	90.5–92.4	92.5+
DMC	0–13	13–28	28–42	42–63	63+
DC	0–80	80–210	210–274	274–360	360+
ISI	0–4	4–8	8–11	11–19	19+
DUI	0–19	19–34	34–54	54.77	77+
FWI	0–5	5–14	14–21	21–33	33+

It is important to remember that our approach consists of using interest measures [12] Support and Confidence to extract association rules for the prediction of forest fires. To ensure the quality of the obtained rules, the Lift is applied. Categorization and discretization are used for the pretreatment of data while decryption is for getting readable results. In the following part, some results of the Apriori algorithm implementation on the spatiotemporal database abovementioned are given.

5 Association Rules Obtained and Interpretation

For a minimum Support of 30 and a minimum Confidence of 50, 467 association rules were obtained and could be interpreted in several ways. We present in Fig. 4 some extracted association rules where area is considered negligible if it is less than 100 m^2 [13].

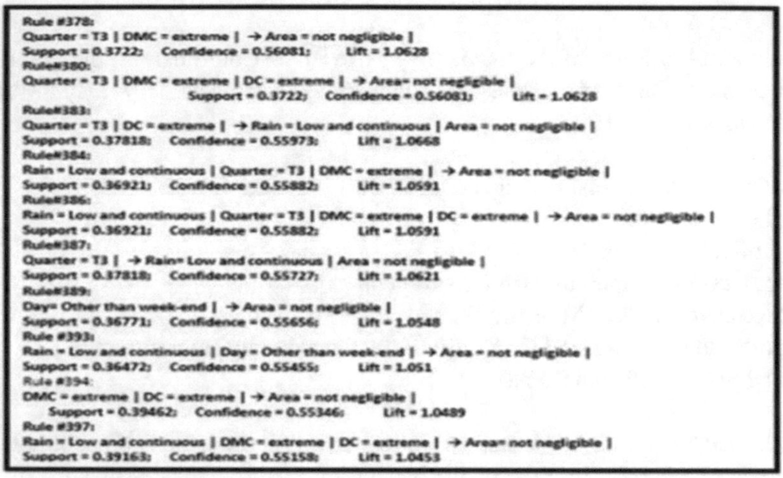

Rule #378:
Quarter = T3 | DMC = extreme | → Area = not negligible |
Support = 0.3722; Confidence = 0.56081; Lift = 1.0628
Rule#380:
Quarter = T3 | DMC = extreme | DC = extreme | → Area= not negligible |
Support = 0.3722; Confidence = 0.56081; Lift = 1.0628
Rule#383:
Quarter = T3 | DC = extreme | → Rain = Low and continuous | Area = not negligible |
Support = 0.37818; Confidence = 0.55973; Lift = 1.0668
Rule#384:
Rain = Low and continuous | Quarter = T3 | DMC = extreme | → Area = not negligible |
Support = 0.36921; Confidence = 0.55882; Lift = 1.0591
Rule#386:
Rain = Low and continuous | Quarter = T3 | DMC = extreme | DC = extreme | → Area = not negligible |
Support = 0.36921; Confidence = 0.55882; Lift = 1.0591
Rule#387:
Quarter = T3 | → Rain= Low and continuous | Area = not negligible |
Support = 0.37818; Confidence = 0.55727; Lift = 1.0621
Rule#389:
Day= Other than week-end | → Area = not negligible |
Support = 0.36771; Confidence = 0.55656; Lift = 1.0548
Rule #393:
Rain = Low and continuous | Day = Other than week-end | → Area = not negligible |
Support = 0.36472; Confidence = 0.55455; Lift = 1.051
Rule #394:
DMC = extreme | DC = extreme | → Area = not negligible |
Support = 0.39462; Confidence = 0.55346; Lift = 1.0489
Rule #397:
Rain = Low and continuous | DMC = extreme | DC = extreme | → Area= not negligible |
Support = 0.39163; Confidence = 0.55158; Lift = 1.0453

Fig. 4. Frequent motifs obtained from the database studied

For example, the extracted association rule number 69, which is considered important, can be analyzed and evaluated as follows: we can note that the northwestern region is the most affected area, and the summer season is the most appropriate for fires in the Montesinho park. The DC and DMC indexes with extreme values are also present in this significant motif [14]. These indexes accompany a light rain because of the relative increase in temperature, with negligible amounts of rain, which generates a high probability for significant areas of the park to be burned. But in this rule, we notice the absence of the area attribute, which can be explained by the fact that a small negligible area can be fired under the same atmospheric conditions as before

Rule #69

$$\textbf{\textit{Region}} = \textbf{\textit{NorthWest}}|\textbf{\textit{Quarter}} = \textbf{\textit{T3}}|\textbf{\textit{DC}} = \textbf{\textit{Extreme}}| \rightarrow \textbf{\textit{Rain}} = \textbf{\textit{lowcontinuous}}|$$

$$\textbf{\textit{DMC}} = \textbf{\textit{Extreme}}$$

$$\textbf{\textit{Support}} = \mathbf{0.30792};\ \textbf{\textit{confidence}} = \mathbf{0.98565},\ \textbf{\textit{Lift}} = \mathbf{1.3402}$$

Another notable association rule obtained is the rule number 31. It shows a strong correlation between (Rain = low and continuous), the quarter 3 which is summertime, an extreme DC and a day other than the week-end. It is important to note that for the rain, we have used the categorization shown in Table 3.

Rule #31

$$\boldsymbol{Rain = Low\ and\ continuous|Quarter = T3|Day = otherthan\ week - end \rightarrow DC = Extreme|}$$

$$\boldsymbol{Support = 0.44843; confidence = 1, Lift = 1.3143}$$

Table 3. Rain categorization 1

Low and continuous:	1_3 mm/hour
Moderate rain:	4_7 mm/hour
Heavy rain:	8 mm/hour and more

We present, in Fig. 5, the Lift measure and its impact on the number of association rules. We can note that the number of rules that have a (Li ft $\geq$ 1) is more significant than those which have a (Li ft $<$ 1). We should mention that we have to deal only with the association rules whose Lift value exceeds 1.

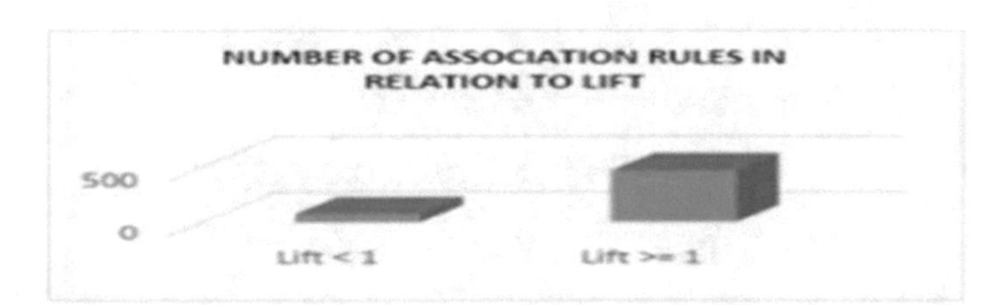

Fig. 5. Representative chart of the number of association rules according to the Lift value

We illustrate, in Fig. 6, the variation of the number of association rules according to interval 0.1 of the Lift. – We note that the majority of rules have a Lift between 1.3 and 1.4, (1.3 $\leq$ Li ft $\leq$ 1.4): which explains that the results of the rule have positively correlated with the premises of the rules.

- In the neighborhood of 1, we have almost 100 rules, which implies that they are not of interest and that the items are independent.
- But, if the Lift is less than 1, the number of rules is less important showing items that are negatively correlated.

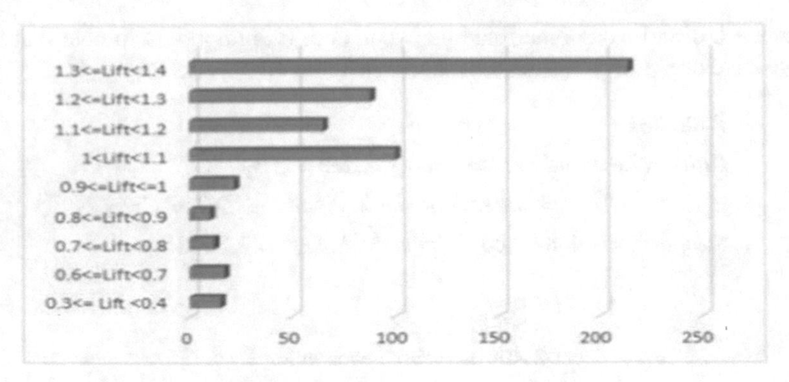

Fig. 6. Variation of the number of association rules according to interval 0.1 of the lift

Figure 7 illustrates the frequency of spatial and temporal items in spatiotemporal association rules. We can observe that forest fires in Montesinho park are probably triggered at the beginning and/or in the middle of the week of the third quarter of the year, namely June, July and August, and this is in the north-west region of the park, to ravage significant areas of it.

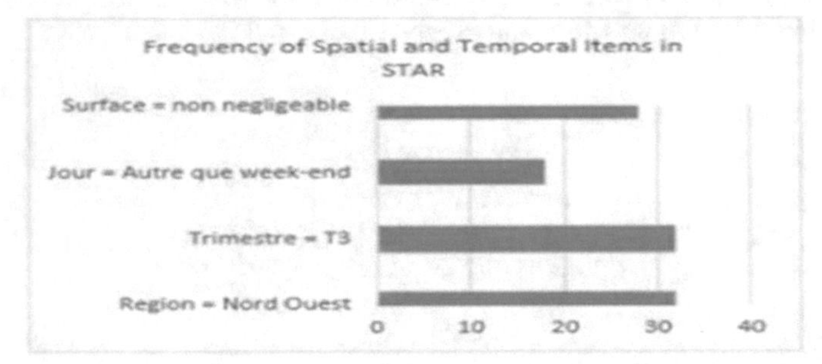

Fig. 7. Representative chart of occurrences of spatiotemporal items in spatiotemporal association rules

The frequency of appearance of the items set in the association rules is presented in Fig. 8.

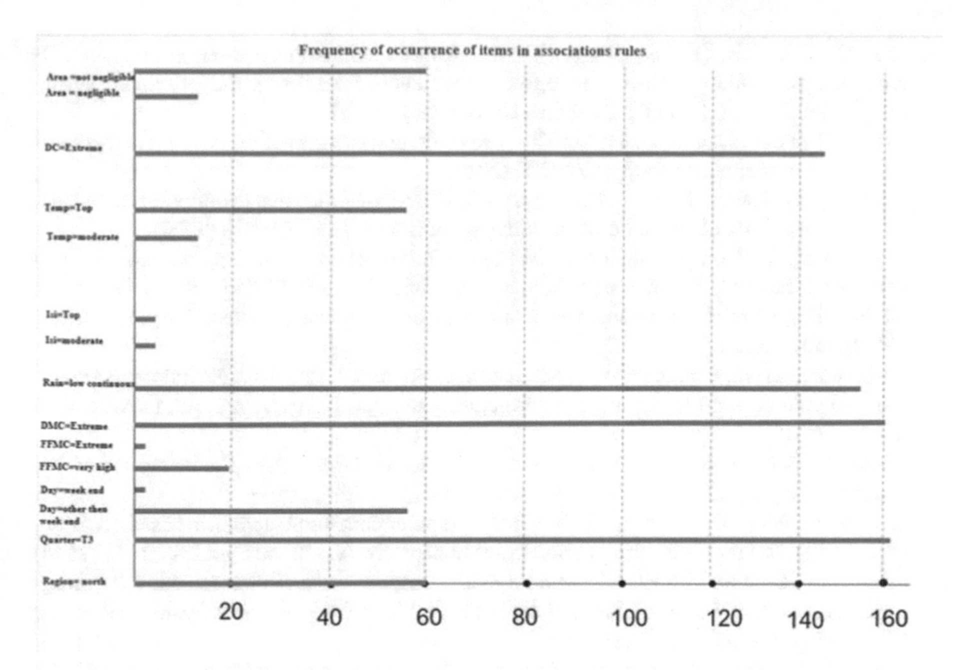

Fig. 8. Items frequency of occurrence in association rules

6 Conclusion

To sum up, in this paper, we have studied the spatiotemporal association rules extraction. Because forest fire is a natural disaster which can touch many countries in the world such as Tunisia, we have used the forest fire database in Montesinho park of Portugal as a case study to implement our approach. Discretization and categorization are done for the data pretreating. The Support, the Confidence and the Lift are applied using the Apriori algorithm in a Matlab environment. To get readable results, a decryption technique is implemented. The spatiotemporal association rules obtained confirm the validation of the approach for this kind of problem. To approve the fiability of Matlab environment we will implement Apriori alghorithm with another environment like python.

References

1. Burrough, P.A., McDonnell, R.A., Lloyd, C.D.: Principles of Geographical Information Systems. Oxford University Press, Oxford (2015)
2. Boulila, W., Farah, I.R., Hussain, A.: A novel decision support system for the interpretation of remote sensing big data. Earth Sci. Inf. **11**(1), 31–45 (2017). https://doi.org/10.1007/s12145-017-0313-7
3. Aguirre, L.A., Teixeira, B.O.S., Barbosa, B.H.G., Teixeira, A.F., Campos, M.C.M.M., Mendes, E.M.A.M.: Development of soft sensors for permanent downhole gauges in deepwater oil wells. Control Eng. Pract. **65**, 83–99 (2017)

4. Xue, C., Song, W., Qin, L., Dong, Q., Wen, X.: A spatiotemporal mining framework for abnormal association patterns in marine environments with a time series of remote sensing images. Int. J. Appl. Earth Obs. Geoinf. **38**, 105–114 (2015)
5. Brosch, T., Pourtois, G., Sander, D.: The perception and categorisation of emotional stimuli: a review. Cogn. Emotion **24**(3), 377–400 (2010)
6. Coulibaly, L., Kamsu-Foguem, B., Tangara, F.: Rule-based machine learning for knowledge discovering in weather data. Future Gener. Comput. Syst. **108**, 861–878 (2020)
7. Khoshahval, S., Farnaghi, M., Taleai, M.: Spatio-temporal pattern mining on trajectory data using arm. Int. Arch. Photogramm. Remote Sens. Spat. Inf. Sci. **42**, 395–399 (2017)
8. Grabot, B.: Rule mining in maintenance: analysing large knowledge bases. Comput. Ind. Eng. **139**, 105501 (2020)
9. Al-Kahlout, M.M., Ghaly, A.M.A., Mudawah, D.Z., Abu-Naser, S.S.: Neural network approach to predict forest fires using meteorological data. Int. J. Acad. Eng. Res. (IJAER) **4**(9), 68–72 (2020)
10. Al-Zebda, A.K., Al-Kahlout, M.M., Ghaly, A.M.A., Mudawah, D.Z.: Predicting forest fires using meteorological data: an ANN approach (2021)
11. Loia, V., Orciuoli, F., Pedrycz, W.: Towards a granular computing approach based on formal concept analysis for discovering periodicities in data. Knowl.-Based Syst. **146**, 1–11 (2018)
12. Chen, X., Lawrence Zitnick, C.: Mind's eye: a recurrent visual representation for image caption generation. In: Proceedings of the IEEE Conference on Computer Vision and Pattern Recognition, pp. 2422–2431 (2015)
13. Coulibaly, L., Kamsu-Foguem, B., Tangara, F.: Rule-based machine learning for knowledge discovering in weather data. Future Gener. Comput. Syst. **108**, 861–878 (2020)
14. Liu, Y., You, M., Zhu, J., Wang, F., Ran, R.: Integrated risk assessment for agricultural drought and flood disasters based on entropy information diffusion theory in the middle and lower reaches of the Yangtze River, China. Int. J. (2019)

Opinion Mining Using Topic Modeling: A Case Study of Firoozeh Dumas's *Funny in Farsi* in Goodreads

Muhamad Aiman Zikri Bin Muhamad Asri[1], Pantea Keikhosrokiani[1(✉)], and Moussa Pourya Asl[2]

[1] School of Computer Sciences, Universiti Sains Malaysia, 11800 Minden, Penang, Malaysia
pantea@usm.my
[2] School of Humanities, Universiti Sains Malaysia, 11800 Minden, Penang, Malaysia

Abstract. The rapid growth of the Internet and the social networking services (SNS) has allowed readers from across the globe to share their thoughts and feelings about literary works through social media platforms like Twitter, Goodreads, and Facebook, to name only a few. This study aims to perform text mining techniques—opinion mining using topic modeling—to examine the range of topics that are explored within reader reviews in social media. In pursuit of this goal, the study focuses on 844 Goodreads reviews of the Iranian diasporic writer Firoozeh Dumas's *Funny in Farsi* to analyze the variety of topics that are covered in readers' responses. As topic modelling techniques, LDA and LSA arc utilized to detect, compare and evaluate the major topics within the dataset. The optimum number of topics for both LDA and LSI is 3 with a coherence score of 0.50451438 and 0.4573542, respectively. Based on the overall performance, LDA is considered the best topic modelling method for this study.

Keywords: Opinion mining · Social media analytics · Topic modelling · Goodreads · Funny in Farsi

1 Introduction

The rapid growth of the Internet and the social networking services (SNS) has provided people around the world with a platform to express their opinions about a particular product, subject or topic. With regards to literary works and creative writings, readers from across the globe are now sharing their ideas, thoughts and feelings through social media platforms like Twitter, Goodreads, and Facebook, to name only a few. Observing and analyzing reader reviews are of great importance for publishers, booksellers and libraries for various reasons such as marketing and prize endowment. Previous studies have pointed to the impact of social networking services for product and service improvement among users [1, 2]. However, observing reader responses and analyzing the major topics of discussion, or areas of interest and dissatisfaction, from a huge number of reader reviews pose an enormous technical and methodological challenge.

F. Saeed et al. (Eds.): IRICT 2021, LNDECT 127, pp. 219–230, 2022.
https://doi.org/10.1007/978-3-030-98741-1_19

This study aims to perform text mining techniques—that is, opinion mining using topic modeling—to examine the range of topics that are explored within reader reviews in social media. In pursuit of this goal, the study focuses on the Goodreads reviews of the Iranian diasporic writer Firoozeh Dumas's *Funny in Farsi: A Memoir of Growing Up Iranian in America* to analyze the variety of topics that are covered by readers across the world. Published in 2003, the novel has drawn a lot of public and critical responses from fans and critics in form of short comments or brief reviews.

Text mining is a form of data mining where the data is extracted from a huge amount of text-based to produce a piece of meaningful information [3–6]. It is a process to transform the unstructured data format to the structured format [7] that can show clear patterns of their relationships with others. Unstructured data is raw data with no predefined data format such as text from social media, video, and audio. Structured data is in contrast with the unstructured data where the data is standardized with the predefined data format such as in a tabular form that consists of rows and columns and has inputs such as name, age, ID, etc. The structured data is used for further inspection in decision making, product planning, improvisation, etc. The text data for text mining uses natural language processing (NLP) and machine learning that allow the machine to understand and process the human language. Despite the advantages of text mining, using this technique might pose two potential difficulties that this study will seek to overcome: First, the extraction of text from users' reviews in Goodreads can be challenging because of readers' usage of various languages, text abbreviations and emotion icons (emoji). This might lead to detection of unnecessary, unrecognized, and repeated words that can reduce the accuracy of the results. Second, assigning a topic based on users' reviews is not as easy as assigning a topic from a digital-based document because it might contain a variety of text and emojis.

Therefore, in this paper, we conduct social media mining where the data is in textual form and scraped from users' reviews. Then, further analysis with the help of topic modelling tools is performed on the data to extract the major topics within the reviews. It is hoped that the study's observations on how the tools work on the text data can benefit service providers in policy and decision makings.

2 Literature Review

2.1 Social Media Mining

Social media has become a popular medium for communication in this modern day. People around the world can communicate with each other without any boundaries separating them from doing so. Social media also contains a huge amount of data that can be useful if properly analysed. For instance, they can increase the popularity of a literary work, movie or product in business. So, a new field of study has been created with a combination of big data and social media which is called social media mining. Social media mining is the process of analysing, representing, and extracting patterns of the data collected from social media [8, 9]. Facebook, Twitter, and Instagram are examples of common social media services used in social media mining to analyse the popular topic among users and draw the conclusion for various purposes.

2.2 Topic Modelling

Topic modelling is a statistical model-based technique for inferring hidden topics that exist in text documents. A series of documents that exist in raw data may consist of many hidden or undiscovered topics where each text should belong and connect between text and topic [2]. The process of classifying text to their corresponding topic is called topic modelling. There are many tools used for topic modelling; some of the famously used tools are Latent Dirichlet Allocation (LDA) [10] and Latent Semantic Indexing (LSI) [11]. In this way, a variety of topics can be extracted from a large document set in a short time thus producing a meaningful result.

Latent Semantic Analysis (LSA), also known as Latent Semantic Indexing (LSI), is a word modelling and simulation method in search of their meaning by analysing the natural text corpora representative. It is commonly used in text summarization, classification, and dimension reduction. LSA generates a document-term matrix in the corpus from the words present in the documents' paragraphs. The row represents unique words found in each paragraph while the column represents each paragraph. TF-IDF score is used within the document-term matrix to replace the raw counts. LSA also used singular value decomposition (SVD) to perform matrix decomposition that reduces the matrix number of rows [12].

Probabilistic Latent Semantic Analysis (pLSA), a novel technique proposed by Thomas Hoffman [13] is an LSA model with the probabilistic method instead of SVD to find a probabilistic model with latent topics that can generate data observe in a document-term matrix and for the analysis of two-mode and co-occurrence data. pLSA used the expectation-maximization (EM) algorithm to train the multinomial distribution. It is a method that finds the parameter likeliest estimates for a model which is unobserved latent variables dependant.

Latent Dirichlet Allocation (LDA), proposed by David M. Blei et al. [10], is a Bayesian version pLSA. It is a corpus generative probabilistic model. Dirichlet distribution is used for document-topic and word-topic distributions that make the new document generalization better than LSA and pLSA. The Dirichlet distribution is a way of sampling probability distributions of a specific type.

3 Methodology and Materials

The methodology adopted for this study is based on the Cross Industry Process for Data Mining (CRISP-DM) which is a six phases process model to represent the data science life cycle. The six phases consist of business understanding, data understanding, data preparation, modelling, evaluation, and deployment. Normally, in real-life situations, all six phases will be executed depends on the goal of our data science study. Currently, the CRISP-DM has been modified a little bit for this study where the deployment phase is eliminated.

Figure 1 shows the framework for this study that includes business understanding, data understanding, data preparation, modelling, and evaluation. For topic modelling, LDA and LSA were utilized, and the results are compared.

The data used for this study is taken from Goodreads. A number of 844 readers' reviews of the Iranian writer Firoozeh Dumas's *Funny in Farsi: A Memoir of Growing*

Up Iranian in America is extracted for the purpose of opinion mining. The memoir describes the author's move from Iran to the United States in the 1970s and the ensuing challenges of cultural encounters. In recent decades, diasporic life writings by Iranian women have attracted international attention [14, 15]. *Funny in Farsi* has likewise evoked considerable public and media responses that deserve critical examination.

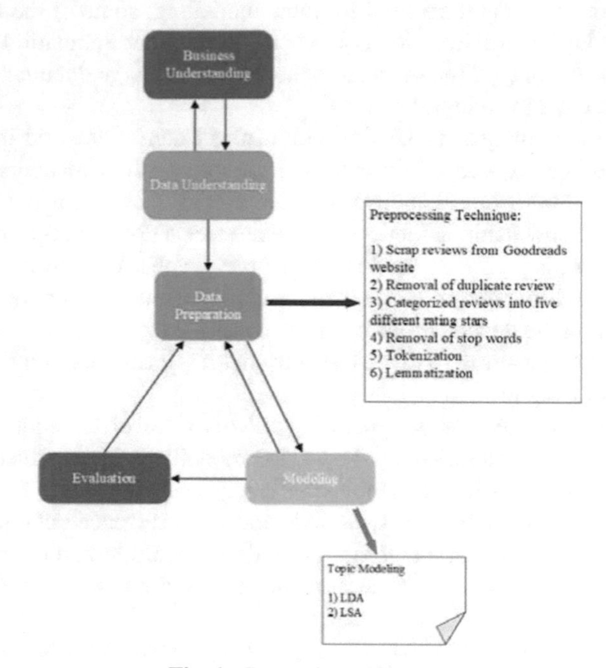

Fig. 1. Data science lifecycle

4 Results

In this study, the data was gathered from the Goodreads website based on the reviews of the novel. First, the extracted data will undergo text normalization while performing data cleaning related processes to remove any repetition and unnecessary data for producing high-quality data before the next process.

Then, topic modelling and sentiment analysis are performed to analyse and extract patterns or relations of the data which is the main purpose of this study. The following obtained results are explained below.

4.1 Text Normalization

Figure 2 shows the result of the book's rating against the number of users. Based on the data scraped from the reviews of Goodreads website for a book, Funny in Farsi: A Memoir of Growing Up Iranian in America, there was a total of 848 users' reviews but only 819 users' reviews were showed in the bar chart above as 29 of them did not rate the book. The figure above shows the number of users' reviews that were rated from 1 to 5 stars where the 4 stars form the majority of ratings (338 users) and the 1 star has the least number of users of 23 users. To conclude this bar chart, this book received a positive rating among the majority of users.

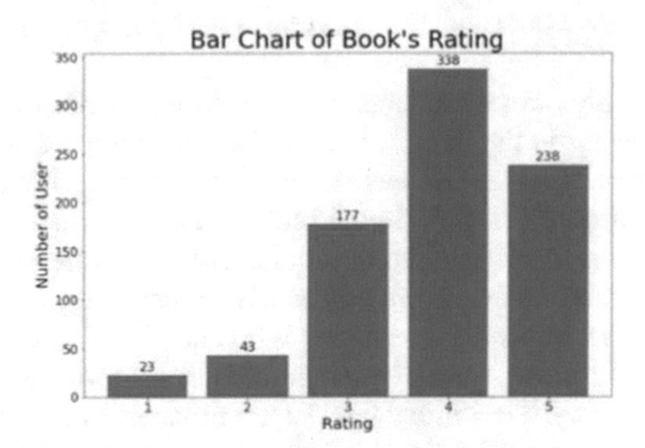

Fig. 2. Bar chart of book's rating

As for the next diagram, data cleaning was performed to remove the stop words found in the users' reviews that can reduce result accuracy for the rest of the process. Then, the lemmatization process is done to link the words that have similar meanings by grouping them, thus avoiding redundancy.

4.2 Text Visualization

Text visualization is a technique to illustrate the outcome of processes for human reading. For this section, a bar chart, Wordcloud and pie chart were used to present the results after data cleaning was executed. In this way, a better inspection can be conducted to view the pattern of the data.

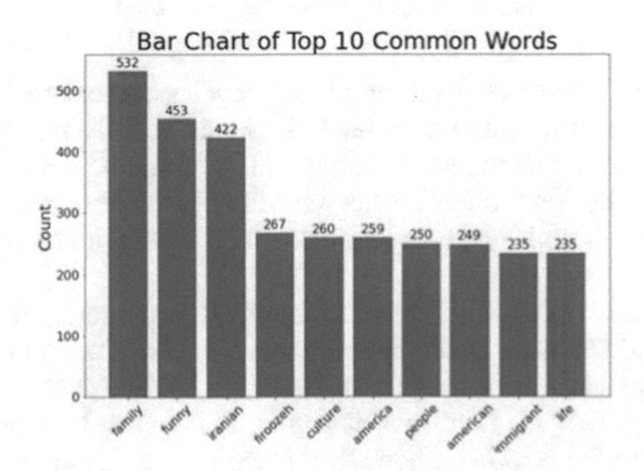

Fig. 3. Diagram of bar chart of top 10 common words

Figure 3 above shows the occurrence of common words counted from 844 reviews. The figure above shows that the word 'family', is the most frequent word presented which counted 532 times followed by 'funny' with 455 counts and 'iranian' with 422 counts. The words 'firoozeh', 'culture', 'people', 'america', 'american', 'life', and 'immigrant' have a slight count's difference when compared together and significant count's difference when compared with the top three words stated before. This bar chart also shows the relationship of these words with the storyline of the book which points out the book's theme.

Figure 4 shows a bigram words diagram where each sentence consists of two words that appeared frequently in the users' reviews. As we can see, "funny farsi" appeared with the biggest bigram font size and was indicated as the highest frequency bigram. This is also followed by "firoozeh duma", "iranian culture", and "immigrant experience". The appeared bigram in this figure is based on a collection of 100 frequent words that exist from the reviews. From this figure, we can conclude that as the bigram words' size is increased, it shows that the words' frequency is higher.

Based on the result above, most of the bigram words shown are meaningful and are related to the book's story. The "funny farsi" and "firoozeh duma" refer to the title and author of this book, respectively. This book was based on the life of an Iranian in the United States of America as an immigrant facing many challenges.

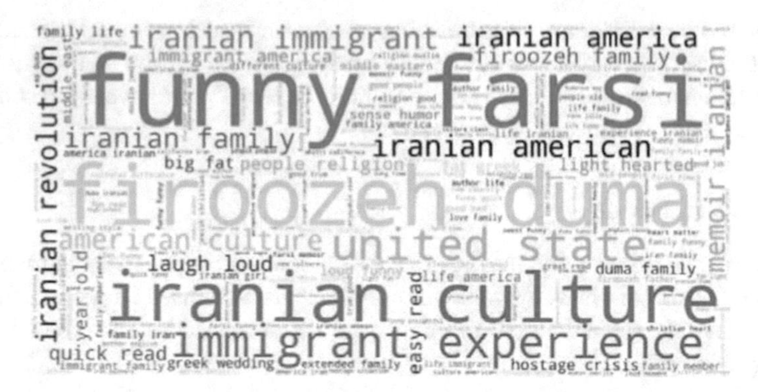

Fig. 4. Diagram of bigram wordcloud

Figure 5 shows a trigram words diagram where each sentence consists of three words frequently used by the users in their reviews. A trigram with the biggest font size is the most frequent word used by the users. As we can see from the figure above, both "big fat greek" and "fat greek wedding" are the most frequent trigram occurred in the users' reviews. The result above is gathered based on 100 trigrams processed from the users' reviews.

Based on the result of the trigram words above, all these words are meaningful. The "big fat greek" and "fat greek wedding" trigrams are related to a movie titled My Big Fat Greek Wedding whose storyline is quite similar to this book and is differentiate only by their nationality. The "religion" related trigram can be found in some reviews where they quoted it from the book as follow: "… There are good and bad people in every religion.".

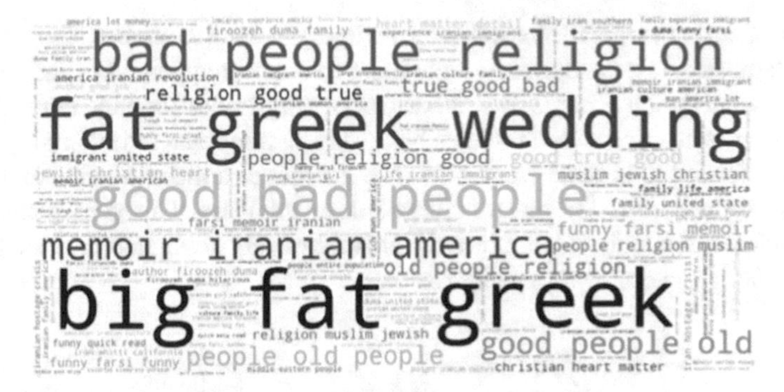

Fig. 5. Diagram of trigram wordcloud

4.3 Topic Modeling

Topic modelling is an unsupervised machine learning technique used for clustering words and similar expressions in form of a topic or more that best characterize a set of documents. This can be done using topic modelling models such as Latent Semantic Analysis (LSA) and Latent Dirichlet Allocation (LDA). The results presented below were processed and acquired using LDA.

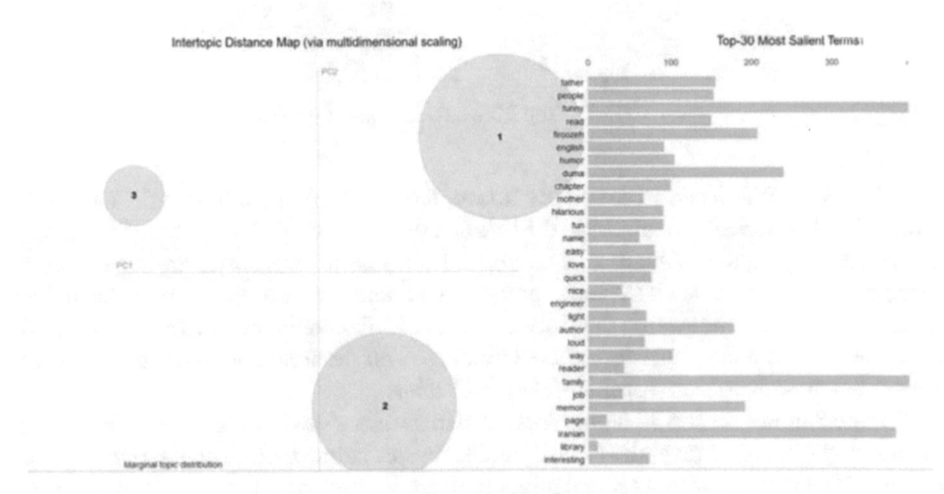

Fig. 6. Top 30 words for whole topics

Figure 6 above shows the top 30 words that regularly appeared in users' reviews with 3 bubbles of topic. This figure shows the overall result for the topic available based on the users' reviews together with their most occurrence words. As we can see from the figure above, the words such as 'funny', 'family', 'iranian', 'firoozeh' and 'duma' have occurred in the reviews with high frequency compared to others.

Figure 7 shows the top 30 words that appeared in the users' comments for topic 1. Topic 1 has the biggest bubble compared to topic 2 and topic 3. Roughly, this shows topic

1 is the most common topic discussed in the reviews. The words such as ‘funny’, ‘family’, ‘iranian’, ‘american’, and ‘duma’ are the most frequently appeared in the reviews and highlighted with the blue bar. The red bar that overlaps with the blue bar indicates the most common word used in the reviews belonging to this topic where ‘funny’, ‘family’ and ‘iranian’ have the highest frequency of occurrence as these words mainly discuss the title and some expression towards this book. In addition, the red bars that appeared in this topic have the highest cumulative words frequency compared to other topics that strongly made it a major topic among reviewers.

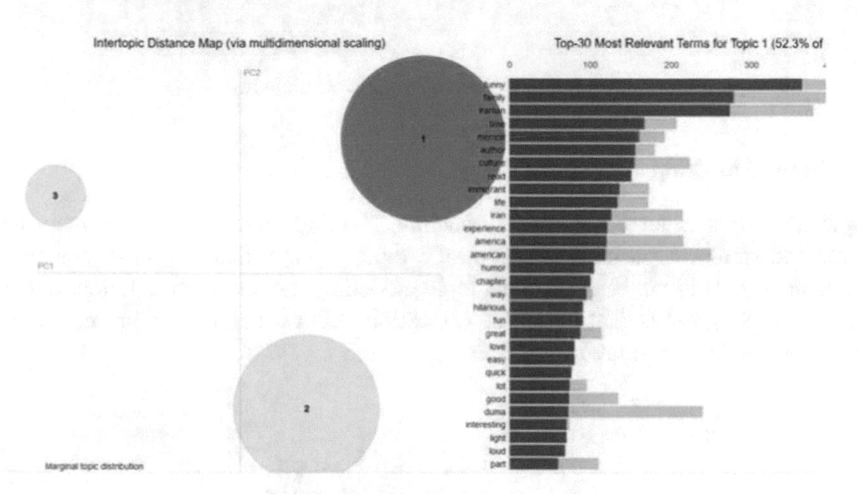

Fig. 7. Top 30 words for topic 1

From 30 words listed in the figure above, the word, ‘funny’, ‘iranian’, ‘memoir’, ‘author’ and ‘america’ are related to the title and storyline of this book where the author, an Iranian migrated to America, thus created meaningful memories in her life as a foreigner. Some words such as ‘fun’, ‘great’, ‘good’ and ‘interesting’ were related to the reviewers’ expression towards the story of this book. To conclude, this topic was mixed between the title and expression of the book based on the frequent words in the figure above, but these words are meaningful and relatable.

Figure 8 shows the top 30 words presented in the users’ reviews for topic 2. Based on the intertopic distance map, the topic 2 bubble resides below topic 1 on the right side of the line. This may show that topic 2 might have similarities with topic 1 or continuation of the latter topic but both were distanced from each other and never overlap. Mostly, the top 30 words appeared in topic 2 have similarity with the topic 1 and some of the words are different. The words appearance in topic 2 show that the users were discussing the characters and scenes of the story plot. For example, according to one of the reviewers, ‘family, ‘father’ and ‘engineer’ were the words that pointed to the author’s father who was a senior engineer and head of her family. ‘School’ is another word that pointed to a scene where the author was on her first day at elementary school in America.

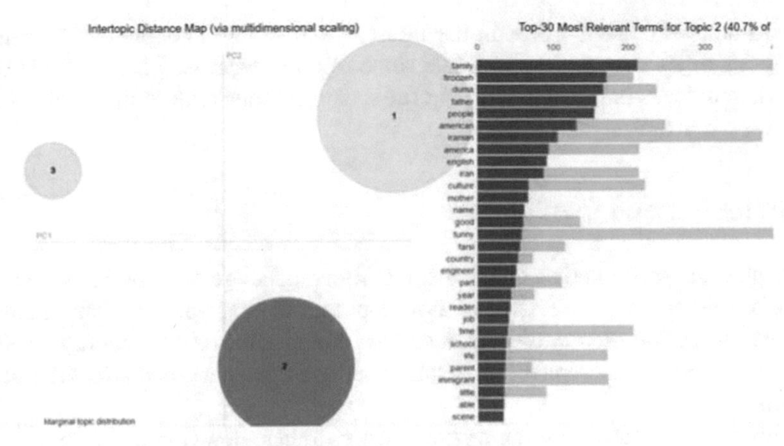

Fig. 8. Top 30 words for topic 2

In conclusion, the stated examples and the storyline of this book was relatable and connected. This topic shows how the reviewers' discussion was related to this book with the frequent words that appeared in the figure above.

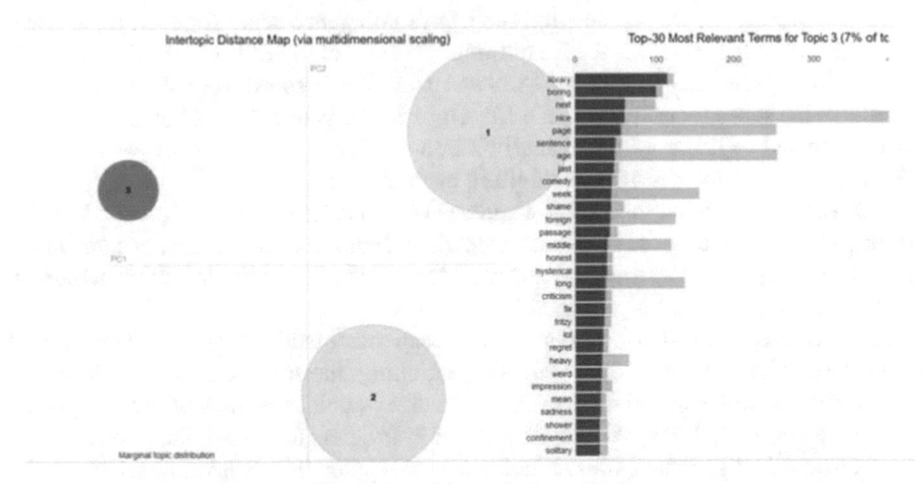

Fig. 9. Top 30 words for topic 3

Figure 9 above shows the result of the top 30 words that appeared in users' reviews for topic 3. Topic 3 has the smallest bubble compared to topics 1 and 2 which indicates it is not commonly used or high frequency of appearance in the users' reviews. Out of 30 words found based on the figure above, only a few words have higher counts highlighted in blue colour such as 'nice', 'page', 'age', 'week', etc. In this topic, some appeared words can be categorized as impression towards the story of this book were 'boring', 'nice', shame', 'regret', 'weird' and 'sadness' are words related to emotional expression. As for this topic, it shows users' expression or criticism towards this book and its story that contribute to the quality and popularity of this book.

Based on the frequent words in the figure, some reviewers expressed their thought on this book or its story as boring while some of them expressed it as nice. There was not much to discuss in this topic among the reviewers thus rank in the smallest bubble among the other topics.

5 Discussion and Conclusion

The text analysis performed on data collected from readers' reviews posted in Goodreads website has given us an overview of how topic modelling operates. The major topic discussed among 844 users was evaluated as explained in the result section. The obtained results encountered some unnecessary and repetitive data that could affect the accuracy of results.

In this study, we used the scraping method to extract reviews directly from Goodreads website for the book titled *Funny in Farsi* as our data for discovering major topics. For observing the major topic, LDA and LSI were used to test several topics from 1 to 10 and each topic was computed with a coherence score. The highest computed coherence score is indicated with the number of optimum topics as their best topic. Below is the graph of comparison between LDA and LSI to show the difference of coherence score for each topic.

Based on Fig. 10, we can see that the LDA's coherence score for each topic has a slight difference from the LSI's. The optimum number of topics for both LDA and LSI is 3 with a coherence score of 0.50451438 and 0.4573542, respectively. When measured in terms of the score for each topic, the LDA took a lead where it has a better and higher score compared to LSI even for a small difference. Based on the overall performance, LDA is considered the best topic modelling method for this study.

The analysis made on the overall results shows that the majority of users were discussing the book's author, the story backgrounds and some characters that appeared in the book. This is supported by the bar chart and bigram Wordcloud in the text visualization section and 3 topics in the topic modelling section.

Furthermore, a detailed observation has been made and weaknesses were found where the results were affected. As for the beginning, the scrapped data as a basis for this study were limited to 900 reviews and left with 844 unique reviews after 56 duplicate reviews were removed. The existing data was not sufficient to provide the best result for the whole remaining process, thus reducing the tools potential to perform analysis on the data. The stop words used in the study codes only contain the whole word while short form or abbreviation is excluded. Moreover, the data words result still contain some stop words even though the cleaning has been made. It has caused unnecessary data to accumulate and be scattered in the pool of data and affect the entire result. Some reviews contained words and sentences in languages other than English. Since this study only accepts English words, and to maintain all data in English, we performed another data cleaning to remove those words and sentences, thus reducing more of our data.

The growing popularity of the digital platforms and social network services has created an opportunity for service providers such as publishers and booksellers to understand users and readers' thoughts and expressions about a product or a literary work. By performing topic modelling analysis on the readers' responses in Goodreads to the

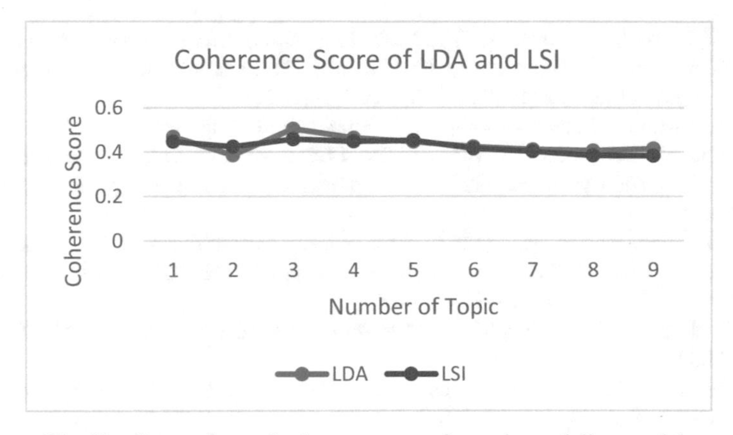

Fig. 10. Comparison of coherence score for topic modeling models

novelist Firoozeh Dumas's *Funny in Farsi*, this study highlighted major topic values shared among the public. The satisfaction and dissatisfaction come across users' mind cannot be taken for granted as it might affect their public relations. From the users' reviews, the discovered topics also draw attention to important areas for improvement and further analysis. This should trigger the decision making on satisfying the readers' needs and eliminate any flaws.

In the future, we hope that the limitations found in this study can be improved and fixed so that any unwanted fault can be reduced or gone. Data mining is a crucial and risky task because it involves analyzing data that may contain personal and government-related information where it may lead to any illegal cases such as data fraud, data breach and privacy infringement. Moreover, machine learning and natural language processing is evolving where more functions are added, and old functions are revised so that they can support many occurrence events in future.

References

1. Ghose, A., Ipeirotis, P.G.: Estimating the helpfulness and economic impact of product reviews: mining text and reviewer characteristics. IEEE Trans. Knowl. Data Eng. **23**, 1498–1512 (2011). https://doi.org/10.1109/TKDE.2010.188
2. Jeong, B., Yoon, J., Lee, J.M.: Social media mining for product planning: a product opportunity mining approach based on topic modeling and sentiment analysis. Int. J. Inf. Manag. **48**, 280–290 (2019). https://doi.org/10.1016/j.ijinfomgt.2017.09.009
3. Hashimi, H., Hafez, A., Mathkour, H.: Selection criteria for text mining approaches. Comput. Hum. Behav. **51**, 729–733 (2015). https://doi.org/10.1016/j.chb.2014.10.062
4. Jung, H., Lee, B.G.: Research trends in text mining: Semantic network and main path analysis of selected journals. Expert Syst. Appl. **162**, 113851 (2020). https://doi.org/10.1016/j.eswa.2020.113851
5. Ying, S., Keikhosrokiani, P., Asl, M.: Comparison of data analytic techniques for a spatial opinion mining in literary works: a review paper. In: Saeed, F., Mohammed, F., Al-Nahari, A. (eds.) IRICT 2020. LNDECT, vol. 72, pp. 523–535. Springer, Cham (2021). https://doi.org/10.1007/978-3-030-70713-2_49

6. Malik, E.F., Keikhosrokiani, P., Asl, M.P.: Text mining life cycle for a spatial reading of Viet Thanh Nguyen's the refugees (2017). In: 2021 International Congress of Advanced Technology and Engineering (ICOTEN), pp. 1–9 (2021)
7. IBM: Text Mining. https://www.ibm.com/cloud/learn/text-mining
8. McCourt, A.: Social Media Mining: The Effects of Big Data In the Age of Social Media. https://law.yale.edu/mfia/case-disclosed/social-media-mining-effects-big-data-age-social-media
9. Keikhosrokiani, P., Asl, M.P. (eds.): Handbook of Research on Opinion Mining and Text Analytics on Literary Works and Social Media, pp. 1–462. IGI Global, Hershey (2022). https://doi.org/10.4018/978-1-7998-9594-7
10. Blei, D.M., Ng, A.Y., Jordan, M.I.: Latent Dirichlet allocation. J. Mach. Learn Res. **3**, 993–1022 (2003)
11. Deerwester, S., Furnas, G.W., Landauer, T.K., Harshman, R.: Indexing by latent semantic analysis Scott. Kehidupan **3**, 34 (2015)
12. Xu, J.: Topic Modeling with LSA, PLSA, LDA & lda2Vec. https://medium.com/nanonets/topic-modeling-with-lsa-psla-lda-and-lda2vec-555ff65b0b05
13. Hofmann, T.: Probabilistic latent semantic indexing. In: Proceedings of the 22nd Annual International ACM SIGIR Conference on Research and Development in Information Retrieval, SIGIR 1999, pp. 50–57 (1999). https://doi.org/10.1145/312624.312649
14. Asl, M.P.: Micro-physics of discipline: spaces of the self in Middle Eastern women life writings. Int. J. Arabic-English Stud. **20** (2020). https://doi.org/10.33806/ijaes2000.20.2.12
15. Asl, M.P.: Gender, space and counter-conduct: Iranian women's heterotopic imaginations in Ramita Navai's City of Lies. Gender Place Cult. (2021). https://doi.org/10.1080/0966369X.2021.1975100

Opinion Mining Using Sentiment Analysis: A Case Study of Readers' Response on Long Litt Woon's *The Way Through the Woods* in Goodreads

Ezqil Fasha Bin Kamal Fasha[1], Pantea Keikhosrokiani[1(✉)], and Moussa Pourya Asl[2]

[1] School of Computer Sciences, Universiti Sains Malaysia, 11800 Minden, Penang, Malaysia
pantea@usm.my

[2] School of Humanities, Universiti Sains Malaysia, 11800 Minden, Penang, Malaysia

Abstract. In recent years, advancements in computer mediated technologies, such as internet, have greatly impacted disciplines like literary studies. Previous studies have shown that on-line discussion spaces have helped readers across the globe to co-construct their interpretations of a text. The increasing popularity of digital writing has prompted the book industry—that is publishers, book seller and libraries—to take close heed of readers' writings and responses in order to improve book suggestions, offer personalized book recommendations and increase their sales. The purpose of this study is to propose an analytical model to examine the dominant feeling in public's reaction to a text. To achieve this goal, the study focuses on readers' feedback in Goodreads website on Long Litt Woon's memoir *The Way Through the Woods: Of Mushrooms and Mourning* (2017). To carry out this study, this project uses a text mining technique that employs sentiment analysis using VADER and TextBlob. The results of opinion mining shows 89 positive sentiments, 5 neutral, and 28 negative sentiments using VADER whereas TextBlog results depicts 99, 5, 18 for positive, neutral, and negative sentiments respectively.

Keywords: Text analytics · Opinion mining · Sentiment analysis · Goodreads · The Way Through the Woods: On Mushrooms and Mourning

1 Introduction

In recent years, advancements in computer mediated technologies, such as internet, have greatly impacted disciplines like literary studies. Previous studies have shown that on-line discussion spaces have helped readers across the globe to co-construct their interpretations of a text. Digital writing is now a popular way for individuals not only to express and share their feelings about a text but also to find and share books of their interest. The increasing popularity of digital writing has prompted the book industry—that is publishers, book seller and libraries—to take close heed of readers' writings and

F. Saeed et al. (Eds.): IRICT 2021, LNDECT 127, pp. 231–242, 2022.
https://doi.org/10.1007/978-3-030-98741-1_20

responses in order to improve book suggestions, offer personalized book recommendations and increase their sales. However, the analysis of the huge bulk of collected data in order to assess readers' feelings towards a text requires an automated technique.

The purpose of this study is to propose an analytical model to examine the dominant feeling in public's reaction to a text. To achieve this goal, the study focuses on readers' feedback in Goodreads website on Long Litt Woon's memoir *The Way Through the Woods: Of Mushrooms and Mourning* (2017). Goodreads is an online platform that allows readers to annotate, quote, and review a book. It also helps readers to find out if a book is a good fit for you from our community's reviews. As Woon's memoir explores universal issues such as the connections between humans, nature, grief, and healing, it has growingly drawn readers' response in social media from around the world. Data is being generated at an astonishing rate and volume in today's world of internet and online services. Data analysts and scientists typically work with relational or tabular data. The data in these tabular data columns can be numerical or categorical. Text, image, audio, and video are just few of the structures that can be found in generated data. Unstructured textual data is generated by online activities such as articles, website text, blog posts, and social media posts. The textual data must be evaluated to comprehend client responses, opinions, and sentiments.

To carry out this study, the text analytics technique of Text Mining and Sentiment Analysis are used. Text mining, also known as text data mining [1, 2] or textual database knowledge discovery [3], is the means of obtaining interesting and non-trivial patterns or knowledge within unstructured text documents. Data mining or information exploration from (structured) databases can be used as an extension of this. Information processing, text analysis, information extraction, clustering, categorization, visualization, database technology, machine learning, and data mining are all forms of text mining. Sentiment is a feeling-driven attitude, idea, or judgement. Sentiment analysis, often known as opinion mining, is the study of people's feelings toward specific entities. People can upload their own content on various social media platforms, such as forums, microblogs, and online social networking sites, from the perspective of the user. From the standpoint of a researcher, many social media sites expose their application programming interfaces (APIs), allowing researchers and developers to collect and analyse data. However, there are various limitations in this form of internet data that could make sentiment analysis difficult. The first one is that because people can publish whatever they want, the quality of their opinions cannot be guaranteed. The second issue is that such internet data does not necessarily have a ground truth. A ground truth is more comparable to a label for a certain viewpoint, stating whether it is good, bad, or impartial.

2 Literature Review

2.1 Social Media and Opinion Mining

Opinion mining and text analytics are widely employed in today's culture to get insight into people's opinions, sentiments, and positions across a wide range of disciplines and fields. This information is quite useful and may be put to a variety of uses. As a result, to better understand audiences, an in-depth examination of how opinion mining and text analytics connect to social media and literature is required [4]. The role of users and readers in our information-driven society is one of the most significant changes brought about by the Internet. The rise of social media has tipped the scales in users' favor. Traditional marketing messages that were carefully orchestrated by companies are no longer binding on individuals. Social networking is the interaction between people who build, share, or exchange information and ideas in virtual communities and networks. The structure of social media data is disorganized, and it is presented in a variety of formats, including text, speech, photographs, and videos [5]. Furthermore, social media generates a huge amount of continuous real-time data, rendering conventional statistical approaches ineffective for analyzing this massive data [6]. As a result, data mining techniques may play a critical role in resolving this problem.

Data is being collected at a pace never seen before by companies through web outlets, cellular phones, and social media. SMM is the method of extracting meaningful or actionable information from vast amounts of user-generated data in the social media realm. This information can be used to enhance business intelligence, allowing businesses to offer better services and explore new opportunities. SMM is needed to make large quantities of social media driven UGC sensible and accessible. Sentiment analysis, electronic word-of-mouth (eWOM), the Web mining method, customer purchasing behaviour, and risk management are all components of SMM. These elements are analytical tools that take raw UGC and transform it into actionable data. This data will help companies increase sales by increasing customer satisfaction and advocacy, assisting in the development of successful campaigns, and facilitating customer retention.

2.2 Sentiment Analysis

Sentiment analysis is the method of analyzing consumer sentiment using natural language processing, text analysis, and statistics. Sentiment analysis is a branch of Natural Language Processing that focuses on the exploration of subjective thoughts or feelings about a topic gathered from different sources. The best companies are aware of their customers' feelings like what they're doing, how they're doing it, and what they mean. Tweets, articles, reviews, and other places where people mention your brand will reveal customer sentiment. Sentiment Analysis is the domain of using software to grasp these feelings, and it's a must-know for developers and business leaders in today's workplace [7–9].

As in many other domains, advances in deep learning have propelled sentiment analysis to the forefront of cutting-edge algorithms. To extract and categorize the sentiment of words into positive, negative, or neutral categories, we now use natural language processing, statistics, and text analysis.

To have a better understanding of sentiment analysis, one must first study the various types of sentiment analysis which are available. The primary types of sentiment analysis are further explained below.

The First Form. The polarity of an opinion is determined in ***fine-grained sentiment analysis***. It may be a straightforward binary positive/negative sentiment distinction. Dependent on the use case, this form may also go into the higher specification (for example, very positive, positive, neutral, negative, very negative) (for example, as in five-star Amazon reviews).

The Second Form. ***Emotion detection*** is a technique for detecting signals of specific emotional states in a document. In certain cases, lexicons and machine learning algorithms are used to decide what is what and why.

The Third Form. ***Aspect-based sentiment analysis*** is even more detailed and refined. Its goal is to learn what people think about a specific feature of the product. Consider the brightness of the flashlight on your smartphone. Aspect-based analysis is commonly used in product analytics to analyse how customers perceive a product and its strengths and faults.

The Fourth Form. The action is the focus of ***intent analysis***. Its aim is to figure out what kind of message intention is being conveyed. It is widely used to streamline the process in customer service systems.

There are two main types of sentiment analysis techniques. Rule-based approach is an algorithm with a clearly described definition of an opinion to classify is used in rule-based sentiment analysis. Identifying subjectivity, polarity, or the object of one's opinion is included. A simple Natural Language Processing routine is used in the rule-based approach. It entails the following operations on the database or text corpus: Parsing, Stemming, Lexicon analysis (depending on the relevant context), Part of speech tagging, and Tokenization.

The other is **Automatic Sentiment Analysis**. Although rule-based sentiment analysis is more of a toy than a serious tool, automated sentiment analysis is the real deal. It's the only method that really drills into the text and delivers. This form of sentiment analysis uses machine learning to find out the gist of the message instead of explicitly described guidelines. As a result, the operation's precision and accuracy improve dramatically, and you can process data on a variety of parameters without being too complicated. Overall, the following types of classification algorithms can be used in sentiment analysis: Naive Bayes, RNN derivatives LSTM and GRU, Support Vector Machines, and Linear Regression.

3 Methodology and Materials

Figure 1 shows the data science life cycle for this study.

The first step focuses on the business understanding which focuses on the problem statement and the goal of the study. The second step which is data collection focuses on the book reviews of *The Way Through the Woods: On Mushrooms and Mourning* by scrapping the reviews from Goodreads. Data preparation and understanding focuses on exploring the data. The next step is data preprocessing which applies data cleaning, text normalization, removal of stopwords, and lemmatization techniques. In modelling step, two sentiment analysis techniques including VADER (Valence Aware Dictionary for Sentiment Reasoning) model and TextBlob were utilized to find the positive and negative sentiments of the Goodreads reviews. Finally, evaluation step focuses on the interpretation of the results as well as comparison of the results of sentiment analysis using VADER and TextBlob.

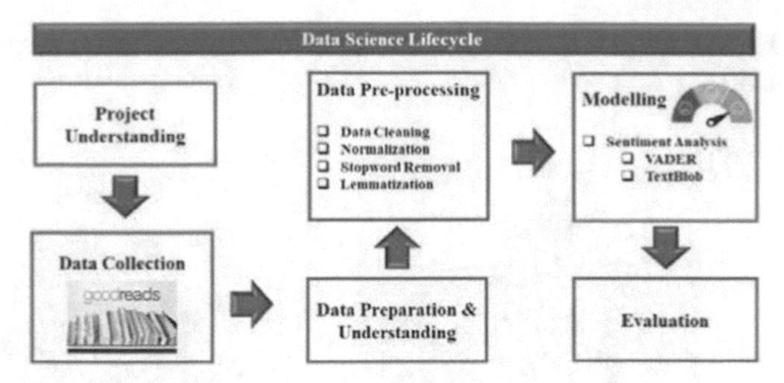

Fig. 1. The proposed framework for data science lifecycle

Python is an open-source integrated development environment (IDE) with a built-in interpreter that converts high-level programming languages into machine language that a computer can understand. Python also has a rudimentary IDE with only the most basic functionality. Several important libraries for data analytics must be installed. Some relevant libraries such as NLTK, Pandas (for data preprocessing and munging), Matplotlib (for plotting: graph, histogram, etc.), Gensim, Seaborn (for data visualization), Spacy, Numpy (holds mathematical functions), Scikit-learn (open-source learning framework for machine learning and modelling), and Pyldavisare used in this study.

The data used for this study is taken from Goodreads. A total of 122 readers' reviews of the Malaysian diasporic writer Long Litt Woon's memoir *The Way Through the Woods: Of Mushrooms and Mourning* (2017) is extracted for the purpose of opinion mining. The memoir narrates the story of two journeys: a personal journey of grief and mourning, and the outer journey into the nature. In recent decades, diasporic life writings by women writers have attracted international [10, 11]. *The Way Through the Woods* has likewise attracted enormous public and media attention that recommend the readers' responses for critical analysis.

4 Analysis and Results

4.1 Text Exploration and Visualization

The bar chart illustrated in Fig. 2 is a visualization of data regarding the number of users and the ratings of the book given by the users. The y-axis and x-axis are represented by the number of user and rating, respectively. There was a total of 122 unique user reviews for the book *The Way Through the Woods: Of Mushrooms and Mourning* (2017) by Long Litt Woon, based on data scraped from the Goodreads website, but only 116 were shown in the bar chart above since 6 of them did not provide a rating. The graph above depicts the number of user reviews that were rated on a scale from 1 to 5.

The average rating given of this book by the number of users is 3.79 which was calculated by the summation of product of the book ratings (440) divided by the total number of ratings given (116).

It is clear that the modal group of the ratings given by the number of users is a rating of 4.0 as it is the most frequent rating given by the users. There is a significant difference between the highest frequency rating given (4.0) and the lowest frequency rating given (1.0) which is 30 users.

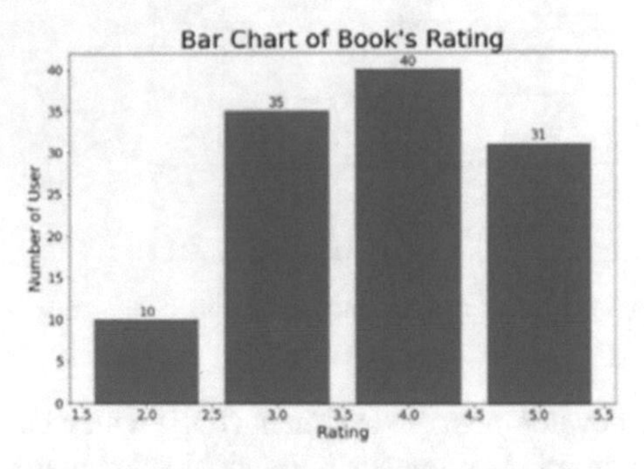

Fig. 2. Bar chart of book's rating

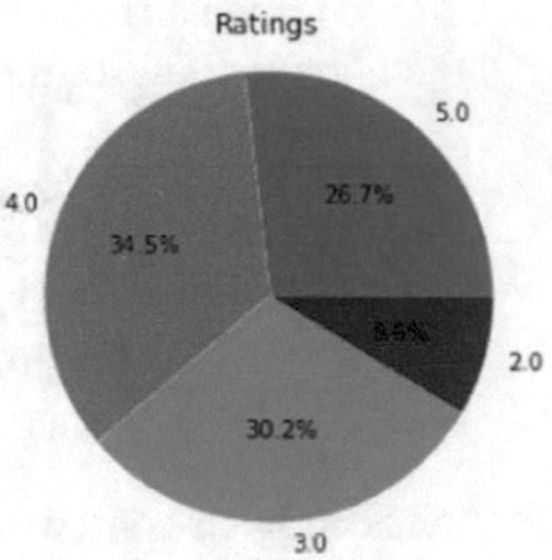

Fig. 3. Pie chart of book's rating

The pie chart in Fig. 3 shows the biggest majority of the ratings given by the users is a rating of 4.0 with 34.5%. Following that, is a rating of 3.0 with 30.2%, and a rating of 5.0 with 26.7% which leaves the rating of 2.0 being the smallest majority of the ratings given by the users. This indicates that a significant majority of the users find the book to be an above average book to read.

Figure 4 shows the visualization of data regarding the top 10 common words used by users in their reviews of the book. The y-axis and x-axis are represented by the count of words and the word itself, respectively. The top 10 common words used in the reviews are mushroom, grief, husband, life, way, woon, author, world, new, and long. The modal word of the reviews given by users is 'mushroom' as it is the most word used in the users' reviews. There is a significant difference between the most common word which is 'mushroom' and the second most common word which is 'grief' as the difference in is 179, count wise. Following the second most common word, the count decreases gradually.

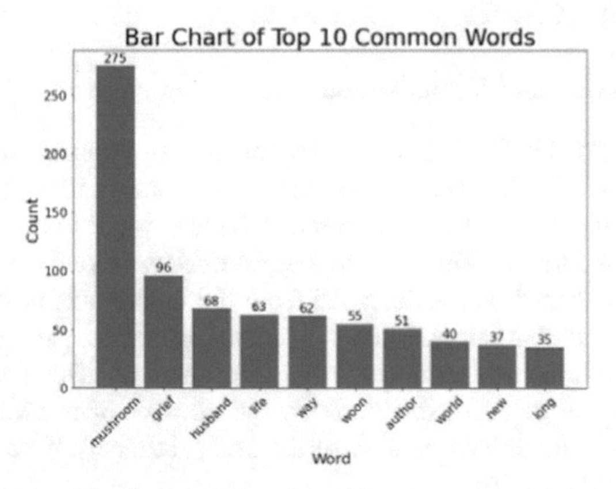

Fig. 4. Bar chart of top 10 common words

Figure 5 shows the most frequent occurring bigrams in the reviews. According to the data that has been extracted from the book reviews given by the users, 'way wood' (19), 'world mushroom' (15), 'long woon' (13), are the top 3 most frequently occurring bigrams. On the other hand, 'day husband' (2), 'foreign land' (2), and 'memoir author (2)' are the top 3 least frequently occurring bigrams. In general, these are the bigrams used in the book reviews of the users.

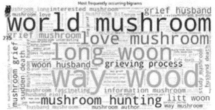

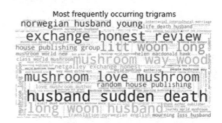

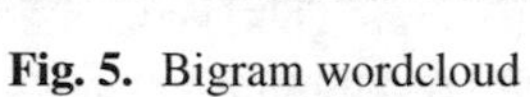
Fig. 5. Bigram wordcloud

Fig. 6. Trigram wordcloud

Figure 6 shows the most frequent occurring Trigram of the reviews. According to the data that has been extracted from the book reviews given by the users, 'husband sudden death' (4), 'exchange honest review' (3), 'long woon husband' (3), are the top 3 most frequently occurring trigrams. On the other hand, 'interest section way' (1), 'new interest section' (1), and 'mourning new interest' (1) are the top 3 least frequently occurring trigrams. In general, these are the bigrams used in the book reviews of the users.

4.2 Sentiment Analysis Results Using VADER and TextBlob

The results of the Vader algorithm and TextBlob, two Python libraries for sentiment analysis are included in this section. Machine learning algorithms can be used to classify texts in a variety of ways. Sentiment analysis is the method in which an algorithm determines whether a text is positive, negative, or unbiased based on its topic. We employ the Vader and TextBlob algorithms for this operation. Furthermore, on the text clustering side, the results were obtained using the clustering K-Means Approach, which is an unsupervised learning algorithm (meaning there are no goal labels) that allows you to identify comparable groupings or clusters of data points within your data.

To demonstrate the results, we used VADER, a lexicon and rule-based sentiment analysis tool. The sentiment score generated by the Vader algorithm ranges from -1 to 1, with -1 being the most negative and 1 being the most positive. The Way Through the Woods: Of Mushrooms and Mourning by Long Litt Woon has a total of 122 reviews. Figure 7 depicts the first five reviews out of a total of 122. We can observe from the graphic that the score has been divided into four categories: compound, negative, neutral, and positive. Positive, negative, and neutral ratings are combined to create the compound score, which is then standardized between -1 and $+1$. The text is more favorable if the compound score is nearer to $+1$. To calculate the sentence's score, VADER uses a series of rules that include punctuation, capitalization, booster words, and more to account for the impact of each sub-text on the perceived intensity of sentiment in sentence-level text.

	Score Compound	Score Negative	Score Neutral	Score Positive	Sentence
0	0.9121	0.034	0.853	0.114	The moment I heard about this book I knew I wo...
1	-0.4331	0.138	0.756	0.106	The book is about mourning and mushroom foragi...
2	0.6705	0.032	0.835	0.133	I love winning books on goodreads This book wa...
3	0.9628	0.039	0.842	0.119	35 stars I think one would need at least a pas...
4	-0.5689	0.066	0.892	0.042	The Way Through The Mushrooms If I'could retit...

Fig. 7. First 5 reviews using VADER

Figure 8 depicts the top ten positive statements from a total of 122 user reviews for Long Litt Woon's book The Way Through the Woods: Of Mushrooms and Mourning. According to the data, the positive score for 10 reviews is slightly greater than the negative score. The highest compound score is 0.9985 in review number 80. The stronger the text's positivity, the closer the compound score is to +1.

The terms "surprising" and "original" appear in the line "This is one of the most surprising and original..." in review number 103. Because it expresses a positive sentiment, these words play a vital role in deciding the sentence score.

The top 10 positive sentences are:

	Score Compound	Score Negative	Score Neutral	Score Positive	Sentence
80	0.9985	0.050	0.738	0.213	I never thought I would get so wrapped up in a...
103	0.9961	0.067	0.797	0.137	This is one of the most surprising and origina...
5	0.9955	0.023	0.775	0.202	I find I have a bit of curiosity about people ...
58	0.9952	0.060	0.758	0.182	Perhaps the most unlikely piece of nonfiction ...
16	0.9865	0.069	0.730	0.202	The Way Through the Woods is a memoir about ...
94	0.9858	0.121	0.660	0.219	Both somber and hopeful A book on grief that i...
85	0.9847	0.031	0.814	0.155	I got this book recommended by my sisterinlaw ...
87	0.9846	0.060	0.789	0.152	Applies to the Audible version Im just now ge...
89	0.9835	0.062	0.702	0.236	Cover to cover The Way Through the Woods is a ...
75	0.9817	0.106	0.691	0.204	Full disclosure I dont like mushrooms I think ...

Fig. 8. Top-10 positive sentences using VADER

The top 10 negative sentences discovered in the 122 user reviews for this book are shown in Fig. 9. Even though each of the sentences is in opposition to the positive sentences in Fig. 9, they all received a high score on neutral perspective. The positive and negative score of the sentences can be used to compare the positive and negative nature of the feeling. Each sentence's negative score is slightly greater than its positive value in the graph above. Based on the compound score, the reviews were sorted in increasing order. The lowest compound score is found on the first line of the graphic, which is line 46.

Textblob is a python module that analyses text and generates an emotion score. Textblob returns the polarity and subjectivity of a statement. The quantity of good and negative emotions in a paragraph, as well as character level sentiment, are used to

```
The top 10 negative sentences are:        Score Compound  Score Negative  Score Neutral  Score Positive  \
46              -0.9588              0.169           0.721           0.110
104             -0.9321              0.143           0.773           0.084
28              -0.9192              0.119           0.795           0.086
64              -0.8660              0.130           0.776           0.095
73              -0.8343              0.181           0.705           0.114
54              -0.7214              0.071           0.881           0.048
70              -0.7096              0.175           0.758           0.066
23              -0.7035              0.342           0.563           0.095
18              -0.6966              0.120           0.800           0.080
61              -0.6310              0.105           0.857           0.038

                                              Sentence
46   So close to a 5star book for me but falling ju...
104  Long Litt Woons book on overcoming grief throu...
28   We live in a society that regards death as a d...
64   Its not an automatic pairing really  mushrooms...
73   The book looks at the authors interest in mush...
54   When Long Litt Woons husband Eiolf unexpectedl...
70   As a Malaysian exchange student to Norway Woon...
23   Some interesting parts but overall the writing...
18   Very boring book with not much of a personal s...
61   This is an example where I misunderstood the p...
```

Fig. 9. Top-10 negative sentences using Vader algorithm

determine sentiment. All sentences with a positive sentiment are given a 1 rating, while those with a negative rating are given a −1 rating.

The text's polarity and subjectivity are determined in TextBlob. The polarity is a float with a value ranging from −1 to 1. A negative polarity score implies negative emotion, whereas a positive polarity score suggests positive emotion. Subjectivity is also a float that ranges from 0 to 1. The subjectivity of the statement is determined by its level of subjectivity. Opinion, emotion, or judgement are all examples of subjectivity.

Figure 10 depicts a list of user reviews. The number 1 sentence has a polarity of 0.215556, indicating that it has more positive sentiment, whereas the number 0 sentence has a polarity of 0.099181, indicating that the user has less positive feeling in their submitted review.

	Polarity	Subjectivity	Sentence
0	0.099181	0.484256	The moment I heard about this book I knew I wo...
1	0.215556	0.581667	The book is about mourning and mushroom foragi...
2	0.200000	0.525000	I love winning books on goodreads This book wa...
3	0.203623	0.481605	35 stars I think one would need at least a pas...
4	0.144818	0.438364	The Way Through The Mushrooms If I could retit...

Fig. 10. First 5 reviews using TextBlob algorithm

The top ten positive sentences from the 122 reviews for Long Litt Woon's book The Way Through the Woods: Of Mushrooms and Mourning are displayed in Fig. 11. Based on the polarity score, the reviews were sorted in descending order. The first line in the figure, line 91, has the greatest polarity score of 0.712121, indicating that the statement is more positive than others, while line 27 has a subjectivity value of 1.00000, indicating that the sentence mostly involves opinions rather than factual facts.

The top ten negative sentences from the 122 reviews for Long Litt Woon's book The Way Through the Woods: Of Mushrooms and Mourning are depicted in Fig. 12. Based

```
The top 10 positive sentences are:      Polarity  Subjectivity                                  Sentence
91  0.712121        0.818182  A wonderful book about the healing process of ...
62  0.616667        0.466667  This really captured the feelings of mushroom ...
93  0.612500        0.675000  Loved it A five star prediction came through f...
27  0.600000        1.000000                              A nicely written book
60  0.600000        0.733333  Perfect for the outdoor lover Nice book Read e...
26  0.577778        0.694444  Great read The author wrote a story that was i...
50  0.550000        0.700000  Heartwarming and delightful the author invites...
31  0.500000        0.600000  Do you want to fall in love with mushrooms Thi...
53  0.500000        0.500000  An interesting foray into the subculture of mu...
89  0.455833        0.820000  Cover to cover The Way Through the Woods is a ...
```

Fig. 11. Top 10 positive reviews using TextBlob

on the polarity score, the reviews were sorted in ascending order. The first line of data, line 63, has the lowest polarity score of −0.304167, indicating that the statement is more negative than others, while line 68 has a rating of 0.850000 subjectivity, indicating that the sentence mostly involves personal opinion rather than factual facts.

```
The top 10 negative sentences are:      Polarity  Subjectivity
63   -0.304167        0.216667  This was a really moving book on grief and how...
29   -0.300000        0.250000  So thankful my wife found this book for me It ...
6    -0.259896        0.498958  I went into this one hoping for more about nav...
61   -0.159821        0.326786  This is an example where I misunderstood the p...
107  -0.112500        0.242857  In the depths of my grief I had as little spar...
81   -0.109821        0.306250  The content is informative but the writingperh...
20   -0.067500        0.340000  If there is a little of the naturalist in you ...
102  -0.056111        0.539444  The premise of this book seemed so promising H...
68   -0.050000        0.850000              467 I HATE mushrooms but I loved this
46   -0.042614        0.313636  So close to a 5star book for me but falling ju...
```

Fig. 12. Top-10 negative reviews using TextBlob

5 Discussion

The text analysis done on data acquired from Goodreads users' reviews has provided us with an understanding of how topic modelling and sentiment analysis are carried out. The main topic of discussion in the 112 unique reviews out of the 159 total reviews by the users, as well as each user's sentiment, were assessed, as indicated in the results section. The gathered results come across some redundant and superfluous data, which affects the reliability of the results.

When it comes to sentiment analysis, a statement should be read in its whole before being classified as positive, negative, or neutral. The entire statement becomes a negative sentence since one or more words are labelled as negative. For instance, a sentence like "*This book was amazing, insightful, wonderful, and well-written*," with a sentiment analysis result of 626, is supposed to be a positive sentence but is incorrectly labelled as negative, which could be caused by reading a word but not the entire sentence.

Also, we utilized two distinct approaches to implement sentiment analysis. The VADER algorithm and the Textblob algorithm are those two algorithms. As we can see from the above outcomes, the VADER algorithm is used to detect the degree of positive or negative expression in the text, as well as the intensity of the emotion, in the Goodreads platform with the supplied topic. It was discovered that the top ten positive or negative statements taken from the data were assessed using Score Compound in four categories: score compound, score neutral, score negative, and score positive. On the other hand, Textblob algorithm usually outputs the polarity and subjectivity of a sentence or text. Subjectivity gauges the degree of emotional opinion and fact information in the text, as shown in the findings in Table 1.

Table 1. Comparison table: Vader algorithm and TextBlob algorithm

Sentiment analysis model	Positive	Neutral	Negative
VADER	89	5	28
TextBlob	99	5	18

6 Conclusion

By using topic modelling and sentiment analysis on reader reviews in Goodreads, this project has shown that significant topics and sentiment values have great impact on public interest. The satisfaction levels that user-readers experience should not be taken for granted because it may influence the success of a literary work. The reason for this is that digital platforms and social networks have grown so much in recent years that the book industry now has the opportunity to better understand readers' thoughts and sentiments, which may help them enhance their products and services to satisfy their customers' needs. The uncovered topics, based on user feedback, also help to focus attention on what is most vital to optimise and get better. This should prompt relevant parties to decide about how to meet the readers' needs and fix potential problems or issues.

Not to be neglected, there are a few limitations that were found throughout the course of this project that could certainly be improved and overcame. Sentiment analysis may have difficulties distinguishing unique content or humor, as it may be difficult to comprehend. With only a few sentences and a bit of text, there may not be enough context for a reliable sentiment analysis.

In a nutshell, machine learning and natural language processing are growing, with new functions and libraries being introduced along with existing functions being upgraded to handle more complex algorithms and procedures. Therefore, this implies that this project is no more than just a steppingstone in the vast number of possibilities or ways to improve in the future.

References

1. Malik, E.F., Keikhosrokiani, P., Asl, M.P.: Text mining life cycle for a spatial reading of Viet Thanh Nguyen's the refugees (2017). In: 2021 International Congress of Advanced Technology and Engineering (ICOTEN), pp. 1–9 (2021)

2. Ying, S., Keikhosrokiani, P., Asl, M.: Comparison of data analytic techniques for a spatial opinion mining in literary works: a review paper. In: Saeed, F., Mohammed, F., Al-Nahari, A. (eds.) IRICT 2020. LNDECT, vol. 72, pp. 523–535. Springer, Cham (2021). https://doi.org/10.1007/978-3-030-70713-2_49
3. Feldman, R., Dagan, I.: Knowledge discovery in textual databases (KDT). In: International Conference on Knowledge Discovery and Data Mining (KDD), pp. 112–117 (1995)
4. Keikhosrokiani, P., Asl, M.P. (eds.): Handbook of Research on Opinion Mining and Text Analytics on Literary Works and Social Media, pp. 1–462. IGI Global, Hershey (2022). https://doi.org/10.4018/978-1-7998-9594-7
5. Kavanaugh, A.L., et al.: Social media use by government: from the routine to the critical. Gov. Inf. Q. **29**, 480–491 (2012). https://doi.org/10.1016/j.giq.2012.06.002
6. Chen, H., Chiang, R.H.L., Storey, V.C.: Business intelligence and analytics: from big data to big impact. MIS Q. **36**, 1165–1188 (2018)
7. Mansour, S.: Social media analysis of user's responses to terrorism using sentiment analysis and text mining. Procedia Comput. Sci. **140**, 95–103 (2018). https://doi.org/10.1016/j.procs.2018.10.297
8. Chintalapudi, N., Battineni, G., di Canio, M., Sagaro, G.G., Amenta, F.: Text mining with sentiment analysis on seafarers' medical documents. Int. J. Inf. Manag. Data Insights **1**, 100005 (2021). https://doi.org/10.1016/j.jjimei.2020.100005
9. Daudert, T.: Exploiting textual and relationship information for fine-grained financial sentiment analysis. Knowl.-Based Syst. **230**, 107389 (2021). https://doi.org/10.1016/j.knosys.2021.107389
10. Asl, M.P.: Gender, space and counter-conduct: Iranian women's heterotopic imaginations in Ramita Navai's City of Lies. Gender Place Cult. (2021). https://doi.org/10.1080/0966369X.2021.1975100
11. Asl, M.P.: Micro-physics of discipline: spaces of the self in Middle Eastern women life writings. Int. J. Arabic-English Stud. **20** (2020). https://doi.org/10.33806/ijaes2000.20.2.12

Opinion Mining of Readers' Responses to Literary Prize Nominees on Twitter: A Case Study of Public Reaction to the Booker Prize (2018–2020)

Punetham a/p Paremeswaran[1], Pantea Keikhosrokiani[1](✉), and Moussa Pourya Asl[2]

[1] School of Computer Sciences, Universiti Sains Malaysia, 11800 Minden, Penang, Malaysia
pantea@usm.my

[2] School of Humanities, Universiti Sains Malaysia, 11800 Minden, Penang, Malaysia
moussa.pourya@usm.my

Abstract. The award of literary prizes such as the Booker Prize has a great impact on production and reception of literary works. In recent years, the Booker Prize awarding committee has faced challenges in selecting books that are more readable and popular. This study suggests that one feasible way to address this issue is to analyze readers' response and public reaction to literary works in social media. In this regard, the present study aims to develop a data analytics technique that can analyze literary readers' responses in Twitter and predict a potential prize winner. To achieve this focal goal, a Sentiment Analysis and Topic Modelling approach is designed to classify the public reactions to The Booker Prize nominees in Twitter. The data is extracted for three consecutive years of 2018, 2019 and 2020. In addition, the study utilizes Machine Learning to propose a prediction technique in selecting the best possible Booker Prize winner based on public opinion. The results reveal the main topics frequently appearing in the data as well as the positive and negative sentiments attached to them.

Keywords: Booker prize · Reader response · Opinion mining · Topic modelling · Clustering · Sentiment analysis · Twitter

1 Introduction

The award of literary prizes such as the Booker Prize has a great impact on the production and reception of literary works. The Booker Prize is a literary award that is given every year to the best novel written in English and published in the United Kingdom or Ireland. Previous studies have shown that winning the Booker Prize has an undoubted commercial impact as the publishing companies receive a quick mandate to produce and sell more copies [1, 2]. Statistical evidence confirms the impact of the Booker Prize on sales and figures of winners and shortlisted books [3]. Despite the enormously positive influence of the Booker Prize on commodifying and canonizing literary books, the prize has sparked off intense debate on how the winners are decided [4–6]. To resolve the dispute,

F. Saeed et al. (Eds.): IRICT 2021, LNDECT 127, pp. 243–257, 2022.
https://doi.org/10.1007/978-3-030-98741-1_21

the awarding committee has recently drawn up an agenda for change, aiming to select books that they deem to be readable and popular. However, no large-scale reader survey currently exists to help predict and clarify the attitudes of book readers and buyers. This study suggests that one feasible way to address this issue is to analyze readers' responses and public reactions to literary works in social media.

In recent years, participation in social networking websites such as the micro-blogging site Twitter has become commonplace. Literary enthusiasts around the world increasingly use Twitter as a platform to share their thoughts on their favorite books [7, 8]. As a result, this digital space is a potential gold mine of readers' responses and public reactions for awarding committees interested in understanding growing trends.

This study aims to develop a data analytics technique that can analyze literary readers' responses in Twitter and predict a potential prize winner. To achieve this focal goal, a Sentiment Analysis and Topic Modelling approach is designed to classify the public reactions to The Booker Prize nominees in Twitter. The data is extracted for three consecutive years of 2018, 2019 and 2020 to increase the validity of the results. Moreover, the study utilizes Machine Learning to propose a prediction technique in selecting the best possible Booker Prize winner based on public opinion.

This paper consists of 6 sections: introduction, literature review, materials & methodology, results and discussion, conclusion and references. Literature review includes sub-sections such as Topic Modelling, Sentiment Analysis and Clustering. Materials and methodology section similarly consists of sub-sections such as data science project life-cycle and implementation of tools and techniques. Results and discussion section also have sub-sections such as Topic Modelling, Sentiment Analysis and Clustering.

2 Literature Review

2.1 Topic Modelling

Topic Modelling is an unsupervised machine learning used for identifying abstract Topics that appear in a text file. Topic Modelling is usually used to analyze a text data to identify a cluster of words, that is by counting the words and grouping the words into word clusters [9, 10]. The identified words will be highlighted and used as "Topic". What makes Topic Modelling easy is that the technique does not require data training. Therefore, it is known as 'unsupervised' machine learning technique. Topic Modelling consists of two common techniques, such as Latent Semantic Analysis (LSA) and Latent Dirichlet Allocation (LDA). LDA has the capability of creating valid dictionaries and using prior knowledge to forecast topics in new collections of documents whereas LSA recovers the space's original semantic form as well as its original dimensions. The updated measurements derived from LSA research include a more accurate description of documents and queries [11, 12].

2.2 Sentiment Analysis

Sentiment analysis, also known as opinion mining, is a method of forecasting people's feelings or emotions about a person or a topic. Given the ease of access to such vast amounts of information on the internet, it becomes error-prone to manually analyze the data. As a result, methods like Sentiment Analysis are needed for automatic analysis.

Sentiment Analysis is carried out at three different levels: Document level, sentence level and feature level. In the Document level, findings are focused on feelings contained in the overall paper. Each sentence in the Sentence level is graded as positive or negative. At the Feature level, there is the possibility of a single statement expressing multiple

Table 1. Comparison of existing works for sentiment analysis

Author	Title	Technique	Result
[19]	Improved Twitter Sentiment Prediction through 'Cluster-then-Predict Model'	K-Means	The combination of supervised and unsupervised K-Means learning models enhanced sentiment prediction on Twitter
[20]	Opinion Mining on Twitter Data using Unsupervised Learning Technique	Means	As Eigen vectors are used to initialize k-means, the original and final objective function values are improved, as are the clustering effects
[21]	Clustering on Twitter: case study Twitter account of higher education institution in Indonesia	Affinity Propagation Algorithm	Higher education in Indonesia mostly utilizes Twitter to post general information, news, agenda, announcement, information to the new students, and achievement
[22]	Classification Connection of Twitter Data using K-Means Clustering	K-Means	The centroids for K-Means clustering are chosen and given. Centroids that are similar to a decent solution seem to perform the best, and using small clusters is appropriate in terms of reliability in time to iterate over all of the cluster's data points
[23]	Analysis of Twitter Data Using a Multiple-level clustering Strategy	DBSCAN	Effective at learning new things. For a small dataset, performance is surprisingly poor. Clustering time: 2 min and 9 s It is possible that large datasets would not scale well

feelings. Experimenting on twitter data, sentence level will be done because of the tweets' length restrictions [9, 13, 14].

There are 2 main sentiment analysis approaches: Lexicon-based approach and machine learning. The first makes use of lexicons or dictionaries. The semantic orientation or polarity of words or phrases in the text is used here to calculate the language orientation. The lexicon-based approach does not necessitate the handling of a vast amount of data, as a machine learning approach does. It computes the orientation of a text using a lexicon or dictionaries. Semantic Orientation (SO) is a measure of textual subjectivity and judgment that captures the polarity and power of terms or phrases. The overall sentiment orientation of the text is determined by both of these terms. Opinion lexicons can be produced manually or automatically. The manual approach to developing the opinion lexicon can be time-consuming, so it must be combined with other automated approaches [13]. Machine learning based approach consists of supervised learning method, unsupervised learning method and semi-supervised learning method [15–18]. Table 1 listed some of the related works that utilized sentiment analysis techniques.

2.3 Clustering

As an unsupervised learning approach, Clustering refers to grouping a population or set of data points into groups so that data points in the same group are analogous to other data points in the same group and dissimilar to data points in other groups. There are several types of algorithm; K means clustering, Hierarchical clustering, Fuzzy C Means, Mean shift clustering, Density based and Gaussian Mixed Models [24, 25]. K means clustering Can be generalized to any kind of data as long as it contains numerical (continuous) entities. It is better than most algorithms.

3 Materials and Methodology

Data science life cycle for this study is shown in Fig. 1 which includes data collection, topic modelling, sentiment analysis and clustering.

Tweets on shortlisted novels were extracted for an empirical analysis based on likes and dislikes. Shortlisted titles in 3 years of 2018, 2019 and 2020 were selected for data collection. As 6 shortlisted novels are announced each year, there are 18 nominees among which are some diasporic writers [29–31]. Table 2 shows shortlisted novels for Booker prize in the years of 2018, 2019 and 2020.

This work explores the latent meaning through the results of various text mining techniques and explores the sentiment of data using the best algorithm. Twitter has public's opinion on the nominees in terms of favorable and unfavorable tweets. The tool utilized in this phase is snscrape library. Snscrape is a library to be installed in Jupyter notebook and gives access to Twitter data without limitation.

Three various analyses are conducted. Firstly, topic modelling is performed in three stages. First, collecting the data to which the developed model was applied. Then, data cleaning and pre-processing such as normalization and tokenization was performed to transform unstructured data into suitable data for topical modeling. Finally, data analysis: Proposed algorithm for Topic Modelling is LDA. Through topic modelling, LDA is the

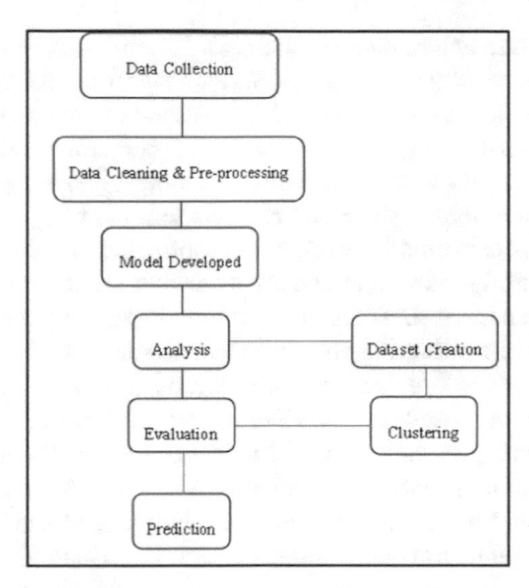

Fig. 1. The proposed data science life cycle for this study.

Table 2. Shortlisted novel of Booker prize for the year of 2018, 2019 and 2020.

Booker prize 2018	Tweets no.	Booker prize 2019	Tweets no.	Booker prize 2020	Tweets no.
– Milkman	– 990	– The testaments	– 2001	– Real life	– 2001
– Washington black	– 98	– Ducks, Newburyport	– 287	– Shuggie bain	– 183
– Everything under	– 1574	– Girl, Woman, Other	– 48	– The new wilderness	– 46
– The mars room	– 59	– An orchestra of minorities	– 39	– Burnt sugar	– 193
– The overstory	– 65	– Quichotte	– 205	– This mournable body	– 41
– The long take	– 42	– 10 min 38 s in this strange world	– 50	– The shadow king	– 135

best to analyze the public reactions as it finds the hidden themes to discover topics of discussion [26, 27]. Next wass checking the coherence score with LDA and LDA mallet to improve the quality of topic modelling analysis. Frequency of topics derived from analysis was conducted and topic with keywords was visualized.

Then, sentiment analysis was also performed to categorize opinions of people on Twitter towards tweets. First, we did pre-processing such as normalization, stemming and vectorization of data by converting unstructured text data into a structured form. For the sentiment analysis, a twitter data consisting of 1.6 million tweets utilized as training set, to test on the collected tweet datasets. Various algorithm for NLP utilized to train the training set. Logistic regression and naive bayes are the popular algorithm for NLP, supervised learning method algorithm is proposed it performs well for a wide range of text classification problems and needs a small number of training samples. Classified sentiments are reviewed into positive and negative sentiments.

Then, dataset is constructed for each of the shortlisted novels. Clustering was conducted using k-means algorithm on the dataset created. Later, both datasets were identified as imbalanced dataset, hence some methods were implemented to balance the dataset. The stages in the clustering process included balancing the dataset and computing the specific number of k for prediction. K-Means clustering algorithm was used in this phase as it is the most used unsupervised machine learning algorithm for partitioning a given data set into a set of k groups. Implementation of K-Means on Twitter data resulted in enhancement of sentiment prediction. Moreover, K-Means algorithm can be generalized to any kind of data and is simple to comprehend and perceive. Clustering centroids is used to predict to which cluster the new shortlisted novel belongs.

4 Results and Discussion

4.1 Topic Modelling

LDA model was built using Gensim implementation to establish the baseline and visualize the topics. The number of topics was set to 5 based on the coherence scores. Only 4 datasets were selected to be analyzed for topic modelling because the selected datasets have higher number of tweets. The selected datasets are 'The_testaments.csv', 'Milkman.csv', 'Everything_under.csv' and 'Real_life.csv'. The results of analysis on topic modelling are keywords of each topic with its weightage. LDAmallet implementation often gives a better quality of topics as shown in Table 3. We can identify by checking the improvement in coherence score after LDAmallet.

Table 3. Coherence score with LDA and LDAmallet algorithm

Dataset	LDA	LDAmallet
The_testaments.csv	0.5127999379950294	0.2716340140758931
Milkman.csv	0.3800795274873436	0.5442869713910351
Everything_under.csv	0.4451578345231527	0.4510800869095564
Real_life.csv	0.49166186274769863	0.42175786849926694

Analyzing The_testaments.csv dataset, the most frequent topic is 'tale' which is representative theme of 10 keywords that can be explained by words such as 'testament', 'read', 'atwood', 'tale', 'book', 'handmaid', 'margaretatwood', 'finish', 'sequel' and 'good'. Table 4 shows the topics with highest coherence scores for the book The testament.

Table 4. Keywords of each topic for the book The testaments

Topics names	Keyword
Testament	0.074 * "testament" + 0.027 * "copy" + 0.026 * "get" + 0.026 * "today" + 0.016 * "read" + 0.015 * "margaretatwood" + 0.014 * "day" + 0.014 * "go" + 0.013 * "wait" + 0.010 * "arrive"
Amazon	0.045 * "testament" + 0.017 * "institute" + 0.009 * "people" + 0.008 * "amazon" + 0.008 * "atwood" + 0.007 * "enough" + 0.007 * "ebook" + 0.006 * "available" + 0.006 * "add" + 0.006 * "tell"
Launch	0.068 * "testament" + 0.024 * "launch" + 0.015 * "atwood" + 0.012 * "handmaid" + 0.012 * "audiobook" + 0.010 * "tale" + 0.007 * "hit" + 0.007 * "call" + 0.005 * "margaret" + 0.005 * "el"
Tale	0.094 * "testament" + 0.053 * "read" + 0.029 * "atwood" + 0.026 * "tale" + 0.026 * "book" + 0.022 * "handmaid" + 0.020 * "margaretatwood" + 0.015 * "finish" + 0.013 * "sequel" + 0.012 * "good"
Order	0.028 * "testament" + 0.017 * "order" + 0.015 * "bad" + 0.011 * "amp" + 0.009 * "copy" + 0.009 * "waterstone" + 0.006 * "preorder" + 0.006 * "include" + 0.006 * "find" + 0.005 * "sign"

Table 5. Keywords of each topic for the book Milkman

Topics names	Keyword
Deliver	0.074 * "milkman" + 0.015 * "require" + 0.008 * "show" + 0.007 * "deliver" + 0.006 * "fast" + 0.006 * "great" + 0.006 * "west" + 0.006 * "fuck" + 0.005 * "ernie" + 0.005 * "new"
Milkman	0.038 * "milkman" + 0.016 * "say" + 0.013 * "want" + 0.010 * "year" + 0.010 * "milk" + 0.010 * "tell" + 0.010 * "go" + 0.010 * "new" + 0.007 * "job" + 0.007 * "eye"
Manbooker	0.091 * "milkman" + 0.023 * "shortlist" + 0.013 * "look" + 0.012 * "overstory" + 0.011 * "get" + 0.011 * "manbooker" + 0.010 * "booker" + 0.009 * "long_take" + 0.009 * "esi_edugyan" + 0.009 * "go"
Delicious	0.074 * "milkman" + 0.038 * "milk" + 0.014 * "bottle" + 0.013 * "ball" + 0.012 * "deliver" + 0.010 * "bring" + 0.009 * "get" + 0.008 * "name" + 0.007 * "put" + 0.007 * "delicious"
Work	0.035 * "milkman" + 0.016 * "good" + 0.015 * "day" + 0.011 * "see" + 0.010 * "get" + 0.010 * "know" + 0.009 * "work" + 0.009 * "make" + 0.008 * "first" + 0.008 * "people"

Analyzing the Milkman.csv dataset, the most discussed topic is topic 0 named 'Deliver' and representative theme of 10 keywords which can be explained by words such as 'milkman', 'require', 'show', 'deliver', 'fast', 'great', 'west', 'fuck', 'ernie' and 'new'. Table 5 shows the topics with highest coherence scores for the book Milkman.

Analyzing the Everything_under.csv dataset, the most discussed topic is topic 3 named ‘Sun’ and representative theme of 10 keywords which can be explained by words such as ‘sun’, ‘time’, ‘get; ‘talk’, ‘wanna’, ‘moon’, ‘need’, ‘go’, ‘tune’ and ‘come’. Table 6 shows the topics with highest coherence scores for the book Everything under.

Table 6. Keywords of each topic for the book Everything under

Topics names	Keyword
Shortlist	0.018 * “shortlist” + 0.017 * “manbooker” + 0.017 * “sun” + 0.017 * “read” + 0.015 * “overstory” + 0.014 * “make” + 0.014 * “milkman” + 0.014 * “people” + 0.011 * “long_take” + 0.010 * “see”
Control	0.030 * “sun” + 0.027 * “control” + 0.026 * “get” + 0.016 * “feel” + 0.014 * “go” + 0.014 * “day” + 0.014 * “life” + 0.011 * “love” + 0.008 * “always” + 0.008 * “let”
Time	0.078 * “control” + 0.015 * “think” + 0.015 * “god” + 0.014 * “get” + 0.011 * “time” + 0.009 * “amp” + 0.009 * “good” + 0.008 * “know” + 0.007 * “today” + 0.007 * “sun”
Sun	0.079 * “sun” + 0.024 * “time” + 0.018 * “get” + 0.016 * “talk” + 0.013 * “wanna” + 0.012 * “moon” + 0.011 * “need” + 0.011 * “go” + 0.009 * “tune” + 0.009 * “come”
People	0.029 * “sun” + 0.015 * “amp” + 0.012 * “people” + 0.010 * “take” + 0.009 * “know” + 0.008 * “make” + 0.007 * “shit” + 0.007 * “rug” + 0.007 * “give” + 0.007 * “woman”

Analyzing the Real_life.csv dataset, the most discussed topic is topic 0 named ‘Twitter’ and representative theme of 10 keywords which can be explained by words such as ‘life’, ‘real’, ‘shit’, ‘get’, ‘know’, ‘people’, ‘twitter’, ‘really’, ‘go’ and ‘bitch’. Table 7 shows the topics with highest coherence scores for the book Real life.

In Topic modelling analysis, the length of documents is important. When documents are too short, even if there are a great number of them, the LDA’s performance is likely to suffer [28]. Due to this limitation, some datasets which consist of very tiny number of tweets cannot be analyzed in Topic Modelling. The amount of the tweet must be sufficient in order to perform Topic Modelling analysis.

Table 7. Keywords of each topic for the book Real Life

Topics names	Keyword
Twitter	0.128 * "life" + 0.127 * "real" + 0.020 * "shit" + 0.016 * "get" + 0.014 * "know" + 0.014 * "people" + 0.014 * "twitter" + 0.012 * "really" + 0.012 * "go" + 0.011 * "bitch"
Logic	0.076 * "life" + 0.076 * "real" + 0.075 * "wonder" + 0.074 * "hit" + 0.073 * "logic" + 0.070 * "pre" + 0.070 * "fame" + 0.054 * "feel" + 0.005 * "light" + 0.003 * "pretty"
Feel	0.097 * "life" + 0.097 * "real" + 0.064 * "different" + 0.023 * "feel" + 0.012 * "get" + 0.011 * "people" + 0.010 * "see" + 0.009 * "good" + 0.008 * "know" + 0.008 * "look"
Relationship	0.010 * "life" + 0.010 * "real" + 0.009 * "human" + 0.008 * "leave" + 0.008 * "sex" + 0.007 * "character" + 0.007 * "video" + 0.007 * "relationship" + 0.007 * "mean" + 0.006 * "point"
Stress	0.028 * "real" + 0.027 * "life" + 0.014 * "tell" + 0.009 * "kid" + 0.009 * "play" + 0.008 * "stress" + 0.007 * "mad" + 0.006 * "sa" + 0.005 * "win" + 0.005 * "call"

4.2 Sentiment Analysis

As for classification of sentiment in NLP, Naive Bayes and Logistic regression algorithms are quite popular. Hence, these two algorithms are implemented in this study. Naive Bayes accuracy is approximately 76.85% whereas Logistic Regression archives 78.78% of accuracy. Based on the accuracy, implementation of Logistic Regression shows better results compared to Naive Bayes algorithm. Since Logistic regression is very effective on text data classification, it is tested on the extracted dataset.

The results show that words expressing positive emotions (Table 8) for Booker prize 2018, 2019 and 2020. Therefore, it can be determined that public like the novel's content and expressed positive emotions via the tweets. Words that expressed negative feelings such as 'return the overstory'. These keywords show that public want to return the novel as they dislike the novel's content.

The dataset includes only the tweets whose sentiment we need to identify. Every dataset implemented in this project consists of small number of tweets, hence it is inappropriate to split into training set and test set. A training set consisting of 1.6 million tweets, categorized into 3 sentiments, are chosen for sentiment analysis. In order to label the sentiment of a tweet, the training data has been utilized as training set.

Table 8. Sentiment analysis of Booker prize shortlisted novel datasets.

Shortlisted novel	Sentiment	Number	Tweet
The testaments	Positive	1422	– "Being able to read and write did not provide the answers to all questions. It led to other questions, and then to others." The Testaments @MargaretAtwood – "I may have hold off on 'The Song of the Lark' while I read 'The Testaments'" is probably the gayest thing I'm going to say in these @TheAdvocateMag offices today. #TheTestaments
	Negative	579	– "Why hadn't the authorities closed down the nuclear reactors before it was too late " Aunt Lydia in The Testaments by Margaret Atwood – "But it can put a lot of pressure on a person to be told they need to be strong." --Margaret Atwood, "The Testaments"
Milkman	Positive	738	– "Milk Wars", which is a DC Universe/Young Animals crossover, was such a wild ride… definitely worth checking out, especially if you like milk, Batman as a priest, Superman as a milkman and Wonder Woman breastfeeding a hand-vacuumcleaner – "The milkman delivers penguins with their chinking atonal fuss" Craig Raine #NationalPoetryDay2018
	Negative	252	– "By evening she was back in love again, though not so wholly but throughout the night she woke sometimes to feel the daylight coming like a relentless milkman up the stairs." A. Rich – "Never trust a crying women and a milkman" Irfann Khan says #Karwaan
Everything under	Positive	1082	– "All that's to come, and everything under the sun is in tune, but the sun is eclipsed by the moooon" – "If you have everything under control, you aren't moving fast enough." -Mario Andretti

(*continued*)

Table 8. (*continued*)

Shortlisted novel	Sentiment	Number	Tweet
	Negative	492	– "For the first time in my life, I've got everything under control." She just jinxed it lmao #Supergirl – "I've got everything under control", said the biggest liar
Real life	Positive	1367	– "Escobar: Paradise Lost" (2014) is the product of love of Andrea Di Stefano. Inspired by Greek tragedies, the actor turned director mixes real life characters with fiction to tell a story about good and evil. Excellent performances from Benicio Del Toro and Josh Hutcherson! – "I believe comic books are based loosely on reality -- I believe there are real life equivalents of the heroes in those books that walk the earth -- I believe your husband is one of those individuals."
	Negative	634	– "Why are you annoying on the internet but so quiet in real life?" ANXIETY BITCH THATS WHY ðŸ˜ – & now that I think about it. They did that shit in real life too

4.3 Clustering

The dataset used in this study was created based of the number of tweets and the winner of literary prize. A dataset was created for Booker prize which includes four main attributes as listed in Table 9. Logistic regression model applied to check the accuracy. In this study, K-means algorithm is selected for clustering and prediction.

Table 9. Description of dataset for clustering

Attributes	Description
Shortlisted novel	The novel shortlisted in the year of 2018, 2019 and 2020
Tweet	Number of tweets extracted based on shortlisted novel
Positive	Number of tweets classified into positive sentiment
Negative	Number of tweets classified into negative sentiment

Accuracy before (88.89%) and after (85.71%) the implementation of random oversampling method was recorded using logistic regression model. Although the accuracy is slightly decreased, but it is still quite high and acceptable. This accuracy is more meaningful as a performance metric. The Elbow method is used for computing k-means for a range of different values of k. The elbow or bend of the plot is considered to be the appropriate number of clusters. The elbow method for Booker prize in Fig. 2 shows the bend point at 2. Hence, number of clusters chosen as 2 for Booker prize clustering prediction.

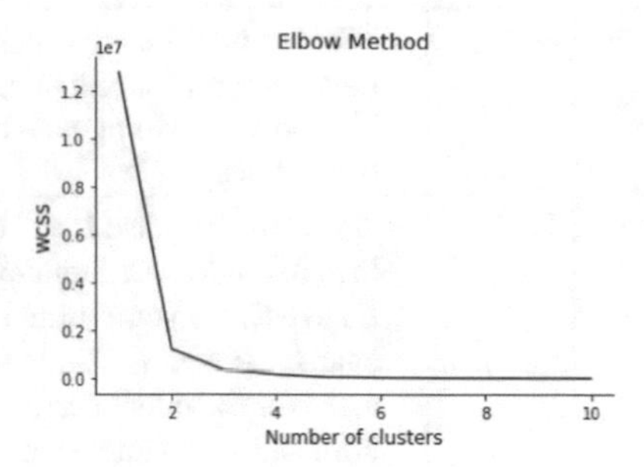

Fig. 2. Elbow method for Booker prize.

Next step is to select k centers for each cluster. Cluster centroids describe the typical new shortlisted novel for each group or cluster. Figure 3 shows that Booker prize nominees in cluster 0 have winning range of 0.142857, and losing range of 0.857143 which is higher than winning range if the nominees receive positive tweets in the range of 85.071429 and negative tweets in the range of 21.50. The Booker prize nominees in cluster 1 have winning range of 0.5 and losing range of 0.5 if the nominees receive positive tweets in the range of 1152.25 and negative tweets in the range of 489.25.

	Tweet	Positive	Neutral	Negative	Win	Lose	ClusterID
0	78.142857	57.857143	0.0	20.285714	0.142857	0.857143	0
1	2001.000000	1080.500000	0.0	920.500000	0.250000	0.750000	1

Fig. 3. Centroid of International Booker prize clusters.

Based on the results obtained from clustering using k-means clustering, we can identify that the number of positive tweets was a good predictor of the winner for literary prize. In the case presented here, juries only have to analyze the cluster centroids to know that the shortlisted novel with a higher number of positive tweets can receive the literary prize award and the shortlisted novel with the lowest number of positive tweets is least expected to win the prize. Another predictor is that in predicting the winner, negative tweets contribute less than the positive tweets.

5 Conclusion

This project aimed to predict the Booker prize winner through using readers' responses from twitter. The objective was to analyze the tweet data using Topic modelling to discover the main topics of discussion and using Sentiment analysis to classify the sentiments into positive and negative. To do this, the first task was the extraction of tweet data from twitter based on the Booker prize shortlisted novels in the years 2018, 2019 and 2020. As considering the type of tweets, snscrape library was chosen and implemented in

Jupyter notebook using python programming language to extract the tweets from 2018, 2019 and 2020. Following the extraction, analysis of public reactions to the Booker prize nominees was conducted using Topic Modelling and Sentiment Analysis. TM analysis was used to determine cluster words for a set of tweet data. SA was used to classify the sentiment of tweets into positive and negative. LDA algorithm was chosen for Topic Modelling analysis. LDAmallet algorithm was applied to check whether this algorithm gives better results. LDA algorithm gives better result compared to LDA mallet. LDA algorithm has a limitation that can only be applied on big datasets. Hence, only on 4 datasets, LDA Topic Modelling analysis has been applied. LDA algorithm with optimal number of k was applied to obtain the better quality of topics.

For Sentiment Analysis, a training dataset was utilized as a training set to classify the sentiments of tweets. In smaller datasets, splitting into training and testing set is not practical. Training set was balanced to have high number of attributes. The training set utilized in this project consisted of tweet data attributes. The training set was trained using logistic regression and naive bayes. Based on highest accuracy, logistic regression algorithm was applied on test set.

Lastly, clustering was conducted to predict the winner using the results from analysis. The dataset was created to predict the winner of Booker prize. Later, the dataset was identified as imbalanced dataset because the number of non-winners was higher than number of winners. To overcome this imbalanced dataset, random oversampling method was utilized. Then the balanced dataset was used for K-means clustering to predict the cluster of winners. The number of clusters was chosen based on the elbow method. Accuracy of dataset before implementation of random sampling method and after implementation was recorded. Although the accuracy is slightly decreased, it is still quite high and acceptable. Finally, we could analyze that positive tweets contribute more for the prediction compared to other attributes.

References

1. Roberts, G.: Prizing Literature. University of Toronto Press, Toronto (2018)
2. Squires, C.: Book marketing and the booker prize. In: Moody, N., Matthews, N. (eds.) Judging a Book By Its Cover: Fans, Publishers, Designers, and the Marketing of Fiction, pp. 71–82. Ashgate, London, Aldershot (2007)
3. Moseley, M.: On the man booker prize. Sewanee Rev. **125**(2), 296–309 (2017)
4. Asl, M.P.: Gender, space and counter-conduct: Iranian women's heterotopic imaginations in Ramita Navai's city of Lies: love, sex, death, and the search for truth in Tehran. Gender Place Cult. (2021). https://doi.org/10.1080/0966369X.2021.1975100
5. Jordison, S.: What happened? The Booker prize and concerns about process. TLS Times Literary Suppl. **6082**, 26–27 (2019)
6. Tiwari, S., Chaubey, A.K.: Politics of the man booker prize (s): the case of the white Tiger and sea of Poppies. Rupkatha J. **10**(3) (2018). https://doi.org/10.21659/rupkatha.v10n3.10
7. Al Sharaqi, L., Abbasi, I.: Twitter fiction: a new creative literary landscape. Adv. Lang. Literary Stud. **7**(4), 16–19 (2016)
8. Driscoll, B.: Twitter, literary prizes and the circulation of capital. In: Stinson, E. (ed.), pp. 103–119. Monash University Publishing (2013)

9. Ying, S.Y., Keikhosrokiani, P., Asl, M.P.: Comparison of data analytic techniques for a spatial opinion mining in literary works: a review paper. In: Saeed, F., Mohammed, F., Al-Nahari, A. (eds.) IRICT 2020. LNDECT, vol. 72, pp. 523–535. Springer, Cham (2021). https://doi.org/10.1007/978-3-030-70713-2_49
10. Keikhosrokiani, P., Asl, M.P. (eds.): Handbook of Research on Opinion Mining and Text Analytics on Literary Works and Social Media, pp. 1–462. IGI Global, Hershey (2022). https://doi.org/10.4018/978-1-7998-9594-7
11. Qomariyah, S., Iriawan, N., Fithriasari, K.: Topic modeling twitter data using latent Dirichlet allocation and latent semantic analysis. AIP Conf. Proc. **2194**(1), 020093 (2019)
12. Pirri, S., et al.: Topic modeling and user network analysis on Twitter during World Lupus Awareness Day. IJERPH Int. J. Environ. Res. Public Health **17**(15), 5440 (2020)
13. Manda, K.R.: Sentiment Analysis of Twitter Data Using Machine Learning and Deep Learning Methods, in Faculty of Computing. Blekinge Institute of Technology, Sweden (2019)
14. Malik, E.F., Keikhosrokiani, P., Asl, M.P.: Text mining life cycle for a spatial reading of Viet Thanh Nguyen's the refugees (2017). In: 2021 International Congress of Advanced Technology and Engineering (ICOTEN) (2021). https://doi.org/10.1109/ICOTEN52080.2021.9493520
15. Anjaria, M., Guddeti, R.M.R.: Influence factor based opinion mining of Twitter data using supervised learning. In: 2014 Sixth International Conference on Communication Systems and Networks (COMSNETS) (2014)
16. Mukhtar, N., Khan, M.A.: Urdu sentiment analysis using supervised machine learning approach. Int. J. Pattern Recogn. Artif. Intell. **32**(02), 1851001 (2018)
17. Hu, X., et al.: Unsupervised sentiment analysis with emotional signals. In: Proceedings of the 22nd International Conference on World Wide Web (2013)
18. Azzouza, N., et al.: A real-time Twitter sentiment analysis using an unsupervised method. In: Proceedings of the 7th International Conference on Web Intelligence, Mining and Semantics (2017)
19. Soni, R., Mathai, K.J.: Improved Twitter sentiment prediction through cluster-then-predict model. arXiv preprint arXiv:1509.02437 (2015)
20. Unnisa, M., Ameen, A., Raziuddin, S.: Opinion mining on Twitter data using unsupervised learning technique. Int. J. Comput. Appl. **148**(12), 975–8887 (2016)
21. Hamzah, A., Hidayatullah, A.F.: Clustering on Twitter: case study Twitter account of higher education institution in Indonesia. MATEC Web Conf. **154**, 03010 (2018). https://doi.org/10.1051/matecconf/201815403010
22. Patil, R., Algur, S.: Classification connection of Twitter data using k-means clustering. Int. J. Innov. Technol. Exploring Eng. **8**(6), 14–22 (2019)
23. Baralis, E., Cerquitelli, T., Chiusano, S., Grimaudo, L., Xiao, X.: Analysis of Twitter data using a multiple-level clustering strategy. In: Cuzzocrea, A., Maabout, S. (eds.) MEDI 2013. LNCS, vol. 8216, pp. 13–24. Springer, Heidelberg (2013). https://doi.org/10.1007/978-3-642-41366-7_2
24. Sadeghi Moghadam, M.R., Safari, H., Yousefi, N.: Clustering quality management models and methods: systematic literature review and text-mining analysis approach. Total Qual. Manag. Bus. Excellence **32**(3–4), 241–264 (2021)
25. Rejito, J., Atthariq, A., Abdullah, A.: Application of text mining employing k-means algorithms for clustering tweets of Tokopedia. J. Phys. Conf. Ser. **1722**(1), 012019 (2021). https://doi.org/10.1088/1742-6596/1722/1/012019
26. Annisa, R., Surjandari, I., Zulkarnain: Opinion mining on Mandalika hotel reviews using latent Dirichlet allocation. Procedia Comput. Sci. **161**, 739–746 (2019)
27. Poria, S., et al.: Sentic LDA: improving on LDA with semantic similarity for aspect-based sentiment analysis. In: 2016 IJCNN (2016)

28. Jian, T., et al.: Understanding the limiting factors of topic modeling via posterior contraction analysis, pp. 190–198. PMLR (2014)
29. Asl, M.P.: Micro-physics of discipline: spaces of the self in Middle Eastern women life writings. Int. J. Arabic-English Stud. **20** (2020). https://doi.org/10.33806/ijaes2000.20.2.12
30. Asl, M.P.: Foucauldian rituals of justice and conduct in Zainab Salbi's between two worlds. J. Contemp. Iraq Arab World **13**(2–3), 227–242 (2019). https://doi.org/10.1386/jciaw_00010_1
31. Asl, M.P.: Spaces of change: Arab women's reconfigurations of selfhood through heterotopias in Manal al-Sharif's daring to drive. KEMANUSIAAN Asian J. Humanit. **27**(2), 123–143 (2020). https://doi.org/10.21315/kajh2020.27.2.7

Dictionary-Based DGAs Variants Detection

Raja Azlina Raja Mahmood(✉), Azizol Abdullah, Masnida Hussin, and Nur Izura Udzir

Faculty of Computer Science and Information Technology, Universiti Putra Malaysia (UPM), 43400 Serdang, Malaysia
raja_azlina@upm.edu.my

Abstract. Domain Generation Algorithm (DGA) has been used by botnets to obfuscate the connections between the bot master and its bots. The recent DGAs, namely dictionary-based, or word-list DGAs are more sophisticated and difficult to detect. They have high resemblance with the legit domain names as they use a set of words from the dictionary to construct meaningful substrings. In this study, we investigate the performance of Logistic Regression, Naïve Bayes, Support Vector Machine, Decision Tree, Random Forest and Bagging Decision Tree algorithms in detecting the dictionary-based DGAs variants. A total of 21 human-engineered features were extracted from Banjori, Gozi, Matsnu, Suppobox and CharBot DGAs variants to train these machine learning models. The accuracy and area under receiver-operating characteristic curve (AUC) values of these classifiers were evaluated. Both Random Forest and Bagging Decision Tree ensemble models outperformed other classifiers in accuracy and AUC scores. Banjori, Matsnu and Gozi variants are easily detected by the classifiers, but it is difficult to distinguish Suppobox and CharBot DGAs from the benign domains. In addition, we performed feature selection based on Decision Tree classifier and determine the most important features for these variants using weighted feature importance values. The identified top features include the subdomain length mean, ratio of consecutive consonants, domain length, vowel ratio and number subdomains.

Keywords: Domain generation algorithms · Machine learning classifiers · Feature selection

1 Introduction

Bots are malware-infected computers that are remotely controlled by the command-and-control server (C&C) or bot master to perform malicious activities such as sending massive spams, phishing, performing scams or DDOS attacks. For many years, domain generation algorithms (DGAs) have been used to obfuscate the call back communication between these bots and the bot master by generating large number of pseudo-random domain names as well as changing the generated domain names frequently. The bot master registers one or few of these domains and waits for the bots to resolve the DNS queries and then establish the communication for a short period of time. These thousands of short-lived malicious domains need to be detected in timely manner to reduce the damage caused by these malwares. There are many DGAs families which can be generally

F. Saeed et al. (Eds.): IRICT 2021, LNDECT 127, pp. 258–269, 2022.
https://doi.org/10.1007/978-3-030-98741-1_22

classified into their specific generation schemes namely arithmetic-based, hash-based, word list-based or permutation-based [1]. The arithmetic-based DGAs are the most common type of DGAs, created using sequence or partial ASCII values. Hash-based DGAs use MD5 and SHA256 hash to generate the malicious domains. Dictionary-based or word list-based DGAs create domains by concatenating words from certain wordlists. Permutation-based DGAs permute initial domain names to generate malicious domains. The dictionary-based DGAs have high resemblance with the legit domain names. It uses a set of words from the dictionary to construct meaningful substrings and hence difficult to distinguish them from the benign domain names.

Detecting DGAs can be done solely based on domain name itself or based on context information such as IP addresses and query traffic patterns by the infected machines. Our study focuses on the former approach, due to lack of the network and data traffics with DGAs. In this paper, we focus on detecting dictionary-based DGAs variants using classical machine learning algorithms namely Logistic Regression, Naïve Bayes, Support Vector Machine and Decision Tree. We also implement two ensemble classifiers namely Random Forest and Bagging Decision Tree. The Banjori, Gozi, Matsnu and Suppobox dictionary-based DGAs variants are reproduced using the algorithms shared in several public DGA repositories. In this study, we also detect the newly proposed dictionary-based generated domains, the CharBot DGAs [2]. CharBot is a character-based DGA that randomly modifies two characters in well-known domains from the Alexa top domain names [3] and hence very similar to legit domains. We extract 21 features from the domain names, indicated in [4] and use them to train the machine learning models to distinguish benign and malicious domain names using labels. The performance of these classifiers, in terms of accuracy and area under the receiver operating characteristic curve (AUC) values are then discussed. Feature selection algorithms find the features that have high correlation with their respective results [5]. Feature selection enables the non-important or noisy features to be removed, hence reduces the dimensions and computational complexity during the model training as well as improving the inference accuracy. We implement Decision Tree feature importance on these extracted features for all variants and then calculate the weighted feature importance values to generalize the most important and least important features for dictionary-based DGA variants.

2 Related Works

In recent years, the increasingly popular machine learning approaches have been applied to detect DGAs variants by many researchers. In the supervised learning method, human defined features such as domain name length are manually extracted from the domain names [4, 6–9]. Many researchers proposed different combinations of features to achieve best detection results in this "featureful" method. FANCI [4] for example used 21 features meanwhile B-RF [10] used 26 features in training their respective random forest classifiers. Alternatively, the "featureless" approach relies on the learning models to automatically discover good features from the domain names during the training process. Deep neural networks models including Long Short-Term Memory (LSTM), Convolutional Neural Networks (CNN) and hybrids have been used [11–15] and they outperformed the featureful methods due to the complex and sophisticated nature of the algorithms.

The following paragraphs discuss some of the works related to DGAs detection using machine learning.

PHOENIX by Schiavoni et al. [9] used linguistic features, in particular meaningful character ratio, n-gram score and the statistical linguistic to differentiate malicious domains from normal domains. They analyzed Conficker, Torpig and Bamital DGAs, which are the early DGAs variants that exhibit a certain degree of linguistic randomness and hence can be easily distinguished from normal domains. In addition, PHOENIX fingerprints groups of domains and clusters them according to their linguistic and IP-based properties similarities. The proposed system managed to associate previously unknown DGAs into newly formed clusters and hence able to track the DGAs evolving behavior.

In 2016, Daniel Plohmann et al. provided a comprehensive survey on various domain generative malware families and variants [1]. A total of 43 DGAs been analyzed which have been categorized into four different generation schemes: arithmetic-based, hash-based, word list-based and permutation based DGAs. Their study shows that the domain randomness or the entropy of the word-list based DGAs, Gozi, Matsnu and Suppobox is significantly low than the other DGAs families. They recognize the complexity in distinguishing these DGAs variants from the legit domains.

Feature-based Automated NXDomain Classification and Intelligence (FANCI) detection system uses 21 features with random forest and SVM classifiers to detect 59 DGAs variants generated from large public DGArchive, large campus network and internal company network [4]. They performed grid search to find the optimal parameters for the classifiers. As anticipated, random forest yields high accuracy percentage at low false positive rate in comparison to SVM, in detecting both mixed DGAs and single DGA on different networks.

CharBot by [2] was proposed as an efficient black-box adversarial attack that introduces small perturbations to a set of legit domains and hence difficult to be detected. FANCI [4], B-RF [10] and LSTM.MI [11] were implemented to detect CharBot DGAs. The AUC results show the deep learning approach with score 98.89% performs better than the random forest-based methods. For the random forest methods, B-RF scores 94.67% and outperforms FANCI of score 80.46%. The authors believe this is due to the different feature sets used in both systems, which are 26 in B-RF and 21 features in FANCI.

Highnam et al. [16] proposed Bilbo, a new deep learning solution to detect dictionary-based DGAs variants, namely Matsnu, Suppobox and Gozi in real time. Bilbo is a hybrid model that processes domains names using LSTM and CNN layer in parallel. The outputs of these two architectures are then aggregated by a single-layer artificial neural network. Bilbo consistently outperforms other deep learning models in AUC, accuracy and F1 score. Bilbo was applied for several hours in live network and was reported to be able to discover at least five potential C&C networks effectively.

Kim et al. [17] performed the Recursive Feature Elimination (RFE) feature selection algorithm with Decision Tree, Random Forest and Extra-Random Forest classifiers to detect different type of malware: Trojan, Adware, Downloader and Backdoor. RFE creates a model that starts with all the features, then eliminate those with the lowest importance, checks the results and then repeats the process to create a new model. Out of 804 total features, RFE with Decision Tree selected 291, RFE with Random Forest selected 202 and RFE with Extra Random Forest selected 456 features. Performance evaluation on all features and reduced features by RFE were performed and a comparable performance was achieved even with the reduced features with difference was 3% on average,

Abawajy et al. [18] implemented few commonly filter-based feature selection methods namely Pearson, Information Gain, Anova, Chi-Square and Mutual Information to detect Android malware. The top features selected by all these methods were compared with almost all rank SMS related permissions at the top. The feature selection improves the accuracy when evaluated using Support Vector Machine, Naïve Bayes, K-Nearest Neighbours and Logistic Regression. The Naïve Bayes classifier shows significant improvement in detection results when using a subset of features as opposed to all features.

3 Methodology

3.1 Dictionary-Based DGAs

A domain name is a sequence of characters with few subdomains separated by dots, including these legit domains: irict.co, kali.tools and xn--80aaf6awgebgaa.xn--p1ai. The dictionary-based DGAs have high resemblance with the legit domains as they are composed of valid English words and hence this family variants are more difficult to detect. Moreover, the Internationalized Domain Names (IDNs) project by ICANN allows the use of domain names in few languages and scripts, such as Arabic, Chinese, Cyrillic or Devanagari which are encoded by the Unicode standard [19]. Detecting malicious domains becomes more challenging in years to come as the word corpus becomes increasingly large. In this work, we focus on detecting English-based malicious domains that are generated by five dictionary-based DGAs variants namely Banjori, Gozi, Matsnu,

Table 1. Samples of legit and malicious domain names.

Variant	Examples of domain names	Source
Alexa top domains	*vocetelecom.vc* *marketlinx.com*	https://www.alexa.com
Banjori	*xpcfestnessbiophysicalohax.com* *vlkkestnessbiophysicalohax.com*	https://data.netlab.360.com
Matsnu	*userbasesteplunchnarrowtree.com* *girlfriendjoinapplytourtransition.com*	https://github.com/andrewaeva
Gozi	*thistheimpofrtandwork.ru* *publicworklewacarrythe.ru*	https://github.com/baderj
Suppobox	*classwrite.net* *withingarden.net*	https://github.com/baderj
CharBot	*m1rkftingbank.pl* *tinnsalt.info*	[2]

Suppobox and CharBot. Table 1 shows some of the samples of both legit and malicious dictionary-based domain names used in our work.

3.2 Extracted Features

Following the work of [4], 21 features have been extracted from each domain string in this study. Each of this extracted feature is either a single scalar or vector scalars. As a result, a final feature vector of size 41 has been generated for each domain string. Thousands of these feature vectors are then used to train the respective classifiers for effective inference, resulting to efficient DGAs detection. These 21 features have been categorized into structural, linguistic, and statistical features. There are 12 structural properties and 7 linguistic properties of the domain string been considered in this work, as depicted in Table 2. Table 3 lists 2 statistical features used in this study which include n-grams. The details of these extracted features have been elaborated by the authors with FANCI codes are available on GitHub [20].

These tables contain the list of the features and the generated vector values of the respective domain strings: *vocetelecom.vc* denoted by $f(d_1)$ is a benign domain name

Table 2. 12 structural features (1–12) and 7 linguistic features (13–19).

No	Feature	$f(d_1)$	$f(d_2)$	$f(d_3)$	$f(d_4)$	$f(d_5)$	$f(d_6)$
1	Domain name length	14	30	31	24	14	16
2	Number of subdomains	1	1	1	1	1	1
3	Subdomain length mean	11	26	27	21	10	13
4	Has www prefix	0	0	0	0	0	0
5	Has valid TLD	1	1	1	1	1	1
6	Contains single-character subdomain	0	0	0	0	0	0
7	Is Exclusive prefix repetition	0	0	0	0	0	0
8	Contains TLD as subdomain	0	1	1	1	1	1
9	Ratio of digit-exclusive subdomains	0	0	0	0	0	0
10	Ratio of hexadecimal-exclusive subdomains	0	0	0	0	0	0
11	Underscore ratio	0	0	0	0	0	0
12	Contains IP address	0	0	0	0	0	0
13	Contains digits	0	0	0	0	0	1
14	Vowel ratio	0.45	0.31	0.37	0.29	0.3	0.17
15	Digit ratio	0	0	0	0	0	0.08
16	Alphabet cardinality	7	15	14	15	9	11
17	Ratio of repeated characters	0.43	0.6	3.56	0.33	0.11	0.18
18	Ratio of consecutive consonants	0	0.54	0.56	0.71	0.6	0.69
19	Ratio of consecutive digits	0	0	0	0	0	0

whereas *xpcfestnessbiophysicalohax.com* denoted by f(d_2) is a Banjori DGA, *userbasesteplunchnarrowtree.com* denoted by f(d_3) is a Matsnu variant, *thistheimpofrtandwork.ru* denoted by f(d_4) is a Gozi DGA, *classwrite.net* denoted by f(d_5) is a Suppobox DGA and *m1rkftingbank.pl* denoted by f(d_6) is a CharBot DGA.

Table 3. Statistical features.

No		Feature and vector values
20		N-Gram distribution (n = 1, 2, 3)
	f(d_1)	(0.73, 1.0, 1.57, 1, 3, 1.0, 2.0), (0.0, 1.0, 1.0, 1, 1, 1.0, 1.0), (0.0, 1.0, 1.0, 1, 1, 1.0, 1.0)
	f(d_2)	(0.77, 2.0, 1.73, 1, 4, 1.0, 2.0), (0.2, 1.0, 1.04, 1, 2, 1.0, 1.0), (0.0, 1.0, 1.0, 1, 1, 1.0, 1.0)
	f(d_3)	(1.22, 1.5, 1.93, 1, 5, 1.0, 2.0), (0.2, 1.0, 1.04, 1, 2, 1.0, 1.0), (0.0, 1.0, 1.0, 1, 1, 1.0, 1.0)
	f(d_4)	(0.61, 1.0, 1.4, 1, 3, 1.0, 2.0), (0.22, 1.0, 1.05, 1, 2, 1.0, 1.0), (0.0, 1.0, 1.0, 1, 1, 1.0, 1.0)
	f(d_5)	(0.31, 1.0, 1.11, 1, 2, 1.0, 1.0), (0.0, 1.0, 1.0, 1, 1, 1.0, 1.0), (0.0, 1.0, 1.0, 1, 1, 1.0, 1.0)
	f(d_6)	(0.39, 1.0, 1.18, 1, 2, 1.0, 1.0), (0.0, 1.0, 1.0, 1, 1, 1.0, 1.0), (0.0, 1.0, 1.0, 1, 1, 1.0, 1.0)
21		Entropy
	f(d_1)	= 2.66, f(d_2) = 3.78, f(d_3) = 3.56, f(d_4) = 3.78, f(d_5) = 3.12, f(d_6) = 3.39

3.3 Data Sets and Classifiers

We generate many DGAs using the algorithms from public DGA repositories as well as acquiring the datasets from the authors. The benign domain names taken from the Alexa site and malicious domain names are labelled accordingly. A balanced number of domains are randomly selected from both benign and DGAs databases and merged into data sets of various sizes. We prepared 5 sample datasets of various sizes and hence a total of 900 processing files were involved: 6 classifiers * 5 DGAs * 6 sample sizes * 5 sets. We then randomly split the train and test sets into 70:30 ratio. The machine learning model learns from the training data and then predict the test data.

The Python scikit-learn classifiers with default settings have been used in this experiment. No cross-validation or optimization was performed in this preliminary study. We evaluate the performance of these classifiers by calculating the average accuracy and AUC values. Accuracy is defined as $ACC = |TP| + |TN|/|population|$, where $|TP|$ is total true positives and $|TN|$ is total true negatives. Table 4 lists the parameters used in this experiment. We implemented the classical classifiers together with two ensemble models that are supported by scikit-learn package. The Bagging Decision Tree algorithm uses all the features to decide the best split, meanwhile random forest uses a random subset of features at every node to decide the best split. The experiments were performed on an Intel(R) Xeon(R) Silver 4110 CPU @ 2.10 GHz server accelerated by NVIDIA Tesla V100.

Table 4. List of parameters and values.

Parameters	Values
Balanced data sample size	10K, 20K, 30K, 40K, 50K and 60K
Number sets per sample size	5 sets (each set contains a balanced number of randomly selected benign domains and DGAs)
Train and test split	70% (train) and 30% (test)
Python scikit-learn modules	LogisticRegression(), GaussianNB(), SVC(), DecisionTreeClassifier(), RandomForestClassifier(n_estimators = 20) and BaggingClassifier(DecisionTreeClassifier(), max_samples = 0.5, max_features = 1.0, n_estimators = 20)
Performance metrics	Accuracy and area under ROC curve (AUC)

3.4 Feature Selection

The 21 extracted features resulting to 41 data dimensions that need to be computed and processed. To train 42,000 domains (or 70%) from our 60K sample data, a total of 42,000 × 41 or 1,722,000 computations needs to be performed to create a trained model. Hence, to reduce the computational complexity, we perform feature selection (FS) by calculating the feature importance values using the Decision Tree classifier model on one of the sample datasets. The feature importance values of each feature for data size from 10K to 60K of each variant were collected. For every sample size of each variant, we run the scikit-learn *compute_feature_importances()* and record the feature importance values for each vector. We collected a total of 41 vectors × 6 sample sizes × 5 DGA variants or 1,230 absolute feature importance values (ranging from value 0 to 0.499). We identified the top 5 vectors with the highest features values from each sample size, called the *top_feat* element and assigned weight value 1 to each of them. The other vectors with non-zero features values, called the *nontop_feat* elements have been assigned with weight value of 0.25. We then determine the weighted feature importance values of each vector by summing the total number of both elements for every sample size of each variant. We consider the relative importance by assigning respective weight to *top_feat* and *nontop_feat* elements, as well as the frequency of them occurring in each vector to determine the rank of each feature.

4 Results and Discussion

We evaluate the performance of the classifiers on our balanced datasets using the average accuracy and average AUC values as depicted in Table 5. For each classifier, we record the accuracy and AUC values in detecting each variant, which have 5 different sample datasets and with different sizes per sample. These collected values are then averaged and presented in Table 5. Figures 1, 2, 3, 4 and 5 depict the absolute accuracy values and AUC values taken from one sample dataset of specific size of each DGA variant to observe the performance of the classifiers. The bold values in the table show the significantly low detection rates by Naïve Bayes (NB). In general, NB only performed well on Banjori dataset but did not match well with other classifiers when predicting different variants. NB algorithm assumes all features are equally important and not related to each other and has been observed unable to detect sophisticated dictionary-based DGAs variants that may have high correlated features. The other classifiers have similar good detection results with the ensemble methods, the Random Forest (RF) and Bagging Decision Tree (BGDT) always outperformed the others as shown in Table 5.

Table 5. Summary of the classifiers' performance in terms of accuracy and AUC.

Variant	Average Accuracy Values (%) of LR, **NB**, SVM, DT, RF, BGDT	Average AUC Values of LR, **NB**, SVM, DT, RF, BGDT
Banjori	99.69, 99.92, 99.9, 99.98, 99.99, 99.97	0.9986, 0.9998, 0.9999, 0.9998, 0.9999,0.9999
Matsnu	99.4, **85.35**, 99.62, 99.45, 99.7, 99.72	0.9972, 0.9271, 0.9973, 0.9948, 0.9977, 0.9977
Gozi	99.4, **85.35**, 99.62, 99.45, 99.7, 99.72	0.9733, **0.625**, 0.9792, 0.9978, 0.9999, 0.9997
Suppobox	92.98, **61.77**,94.61, 99.76, 99.87, 99.7	0.8176, **0.6049**, 0.8479, 0.8342, 0.8644, 0.872
CharBot	81.1, **58.01**, 80.86, 79.07, 79.9, 80.47	0.8761, **0.5839**, 0.8737, 0.8233, 0.8812, 0.8899

The AUC determines the classifier's efficiency in distinguishing the classes correctly. The higher the AUC values, the better the model. An ideal classifier has AUC score of 1, which can be seen only in Fig. 1(b) when predicting Banjori DGAs. In detecting Banjori, on average, all the classifiers score above 99.6% in accuracy and score above 0.99 in AUC and hence conclude that this type of variant can be predicted easily. In detecting Matsnu and Gozi variants, all the classifiers, with the exception NB, performed well as shown in both Figs. 2 and 3. The average accuracy score for other-than-NB classifiers are above 99.4% while NB scores only 85.35% in both variants. The average AUC value for NB is significantly low when detecting Gozi variant, with 0.625 score. In detecting Suppobox and CharBot variants, NB's performance worsens with average accuracy values of 61.77% and 58% respectively (refer Figs. 4 and 5). The average NB AUC's score in detecting CharBot is around 0.58 which indicate the inability of the algorithm to correctly predict this variant, while others are performing well with score above 0.82. In general, both RF and BGDT consistently outperformed others as reflected by both of their average accuracy and AUC scores, except when detecting CharBot. Both Logistic Regression (LR) and Support Vector Machine (SVM) have higher accuracy scores than

RF and further analysis is to be carried out to fully understand the causes of it. Finally, based on the detection scores of the classifiers we can conclude that Banjori, Matsnu and Gozi variants are easy to detect by most of the classifiers in comparison to Suppobox and CharBot.

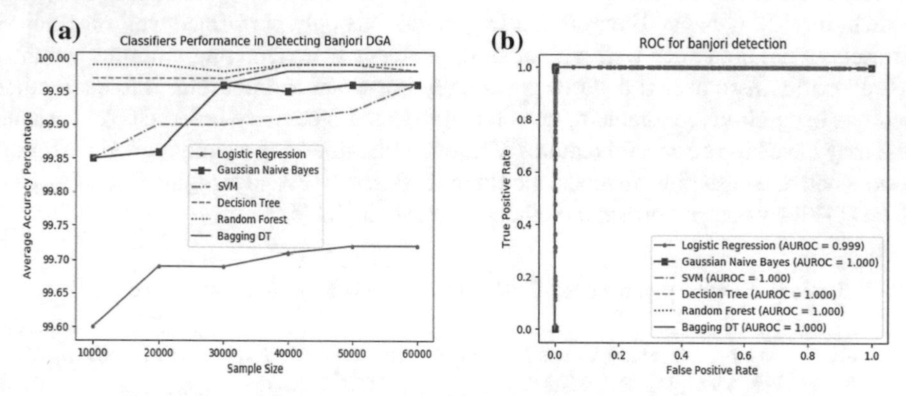

Fig. 1. (a) Average accuracy and (b) AUC results in detecting Banjori.

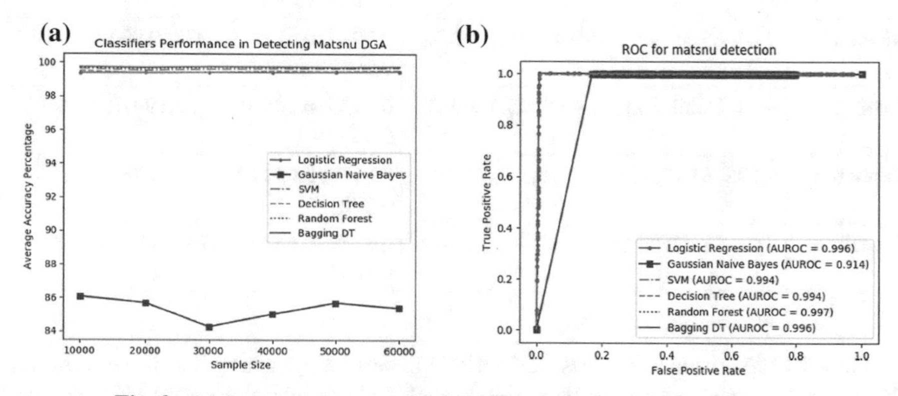

Fig. 2. (a) Average accuracy and (b) AUC results in detecting Matsnu.

Based on the weighted feature importance results shown in Fig. 6, we can conclude that the top 5 important features in detecting the dictionary-based DGA variants are as follows: (1) f3 or the subdomain length mean, (2) f18 or ratio of consecutive consonants, (3) f1 or domain length, (4) f14 or vowel ratio and (5) f2 or number subdomains. The n-gram values or f20 are not included in top 5 due to the inconsistency of the results for this sample data and further experiments are needed. It is worth noting that f3 or subdomain length mean feature has a maximum weighted value of 30 as it is listed in top 5 of each sample size in each variant, and in fact this feature has the highest absolute feature importance value for every scenario. However, these highest absolute feature importance values vary significantly from one variant to another due to the different generation algorithms, hence different resulting domain strings of each variant, as depicted in Table 1. For example, in dataset size 50K, its highest importance value

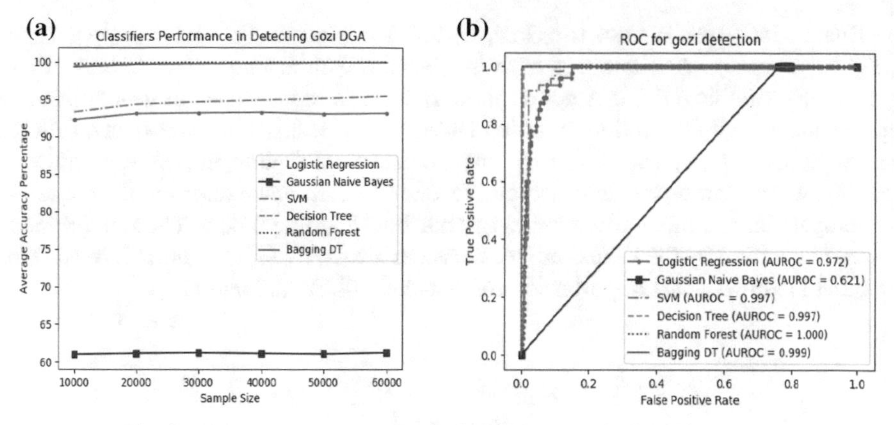

Fig. 3. (a) Average accuracy and (b) AUC results in detecting Gozi.

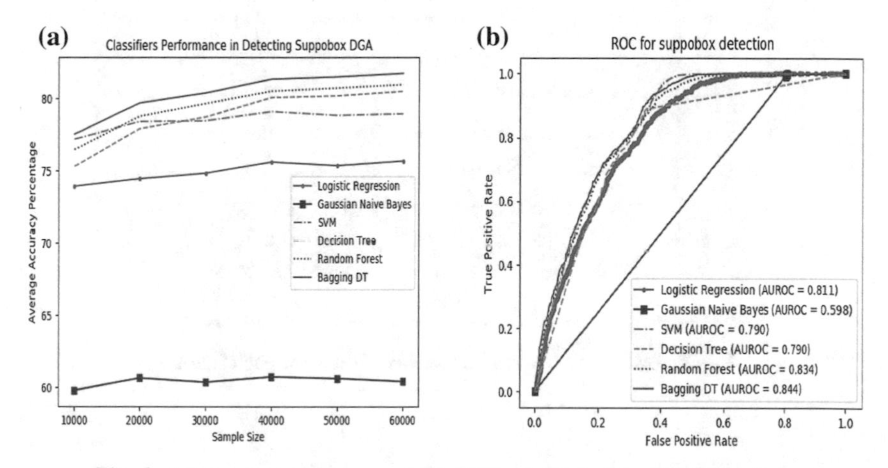

Fig. 4. (a) Average accuracy and (b) AUC results in detecting Suppobox.

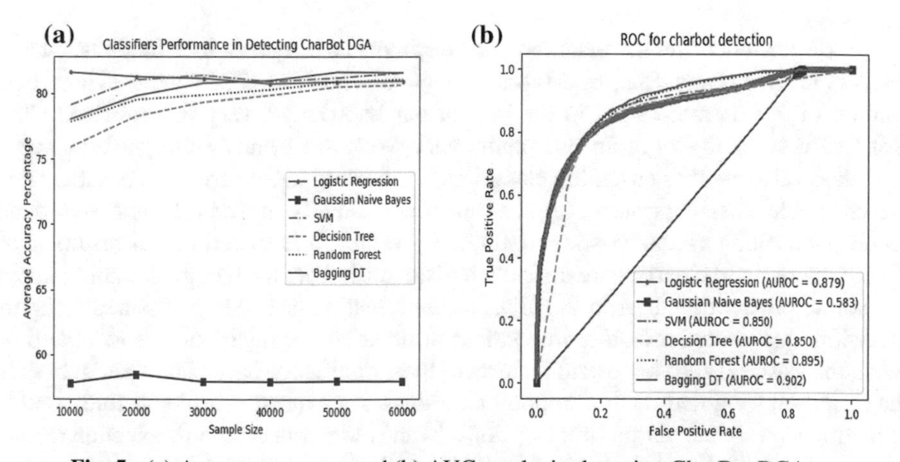

Fig. 5. (a) Average accuracy and (b) AUC results in detecting CharBot DGAs.

for Banjori is 0.499, 0.3684 for Gozi, 0.4937 for Matsnu, 0.124 for Suppobox and 0.053 for CharBot. As the range of these absolute feature importance values of each variant vary significantly, it is not accurate to include these values in generalizing the top features for all the dictionary-based DGAs variants. Instead, we assigned different weight values for features with high and low absolute feature importance values. In addition, we determine the nonimportant features, which can be removed later to reduce the computational complexity of training a machine learning model. The zero important features identified by the Decision Tree classifier are f5, f6, f7, f11 and f12. In addition, the other identified least important features include f4, f9, f10 and f19.

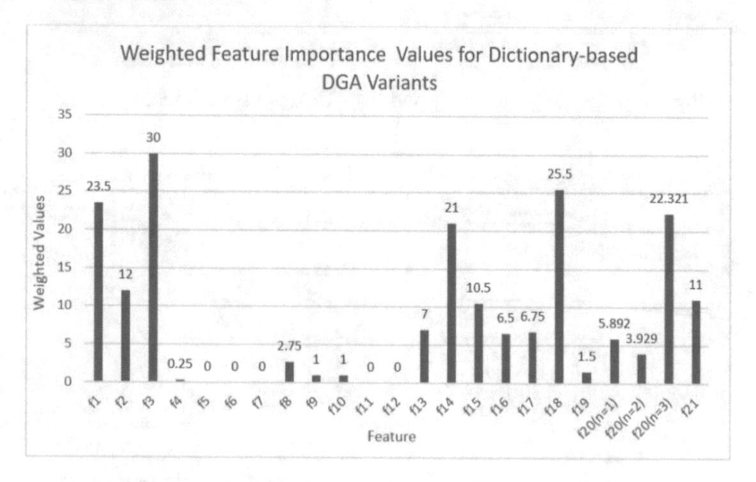

Fig. 6. Weighted feature importance values for each feature

5 Conclusion

We implemented different machine learning models to detect five dictionary-based DGAs family variants. Banjori, Matsnu, Suppobox and Gozi DGAs variants have been studied in few literatures but to the best of our knowledge, very few involved CharBot DGAs in their works. In our preliminary work, we evaluate the performance of few classical as well as ensemble classifiers in detecting these variants. As anticipated, the ensemble classifiers outperformed others consistently in accuracy and area under receiver-operating characteristic curve (AUC) values. The experimental results show that Suppobox and CharBot are difficult to distinguish from the benign domains in comparison to other variants. Additionally, feature selection has been performed using the Decision Tree classifier feature importance attribute for each variant. We identified the most, the least and zero important features of these dictionary-based DGA variants using the proposed weighted feature importance values. An extensive in-depth study will be performed to validate our preliminary findings and more robust feature selection method such as Recursive Feature Elimination (RFE) will be considered in the future.

References

1. Plohmann, D., Yakdan, K., Klatt, M., Bader, J., Gerhards-Padilla, E.: A comprehensive measurement study of domain generating malware. In: 25th Proceedings of the USENIX Conference on Security Symposium, Austin, USA, pp. 263–278 (2016)
2. Peck, J., et al.: CharBot: a simple and effective method for evading DGA classifiers. IEEE Access **7**, 91759–91771 (2019)
3. Alexa Top 1M sites. https://www.alexa.com/topsites. Accessed 13 Jan 2021
4. Schuppen, S., Teubert, D., Herrmann, P., Meyer, U.: FANCI: feature-based automated NXDomain classification and intelligence. In: 27th USENIX Security Symposium, Batimore, USA, pp. 1165–1181 (2018)
5. Dash, M., Liu, H.: Feature selection for classification. Intell. Data Anal. **1**(3), 131–156 (1997)
6. Antonakakis, M., Perdisci, R., Nadji, Y., et al.: From throw-away traffic to bots: detecting the rise of DGA-based malware. In: 21st USENIX Conference on Security Symposium, Bellevue, USA, pp. 491–506 (2012)
7. Wang, Z., Jia, Z., Zhang, B.: A detection scheme for DGA domain names based on SVM. In: International Conference on Mathematics, Modelling, Simulation and Algorithms. Atlantis Press, Chengdu (2018)
8. Li, Y., Xiong, K., Chin, T., Hu, C.: A machine learning framework for domain generation algorithm DGA-based malware detection. IEEE Access **7**, 32765–32782 (2019)
9. Schiavoni, S., Maggi, F., Cavallaro, L., Zanero, S.: Phoenix: DGA-based botnet tracking and intelligence. In: Dietrich, S. (ed.) DIMVA 2014. LNCS, vol. 8550, pp. 192–211. Springer, Cham (2014). https://doi.org/10.1007/978-3-319-08509-8_11
10. Sivaguru, R., Choudhary, C., Yu, B., Tymchenko, V., Nascimento, A., De Cock, M.: An evaluation of DGA classifiers. In: Proceedings of 2018 IEEE International Conference on Big Data, Seattle, USA, pp. 5051–5060 (2018)
11. Woodbridge, J., Anderson, H.S., Ahuja, A., Grant, D.: Predicting domain generation algorithms with long short-term memory networks. PreprintarXiv:1611.00791 (2016)
12. Saxe, J., Berlin, K.: Expose: a character-level convolutional neural network with embeddings for detecting malicious URLs, FLE paths and registry keys. Preprint arXiv:1702.08568 (2017)
13. Shaofang, Z., Lanfen, L., Yuan, J., Wang, F., Ling, Z., Cui, J.: CNN-based DGA detection with high coverage. In: IEEE International Conference on Intelligence and Security Informatics, Shenzen, China, pp. 62–67 (2019)
14. Lison, P., Mavroeidis, V.: Automatic detection of malware-generated domains with recurrent neural models. Preprint arXiv:1709.07102 (2017)
15. Yu, B., Pan, J., Hu, J., Nascimento, A., Cock, MD.: Character level based detection of dga domain names. In: International Joint Conference on Neural Networks, Rio de Janeiro, Brazil, pp. 1–8 (2018)
16. Highnam, K., Puzio, D., Luo, S., Jennings, N.R.: Real-time detection of dictionary DGA network traffic using deep learning. SN Comput. Sci. **2**(2), 1–17 (2021). https://doi.org/10.1007/s42979-021-00507-w
17. Kim, D.-W., Shin, G.-Y., Han, M.-M.: Analysis of feature importance and interpretation for malware classification. Comput. Mater. Continua **65**(3), 1891–1904 (2020)
18. Abawajy, J., Darem, A., Alhashmi, A.A.: Feature subset selection for malware detection in smart IoT platforms. Sensors **21**(4), 1374 (2021)
19. ICANN. https://www.icann.org/resources/pages/idn-2012-02-25-en. Accessed 3 June 2021
20. FANCI. https://github.com/fanci-dga-detection/fanci. Accessed 10 Feb 2021

Comparison of Unsupervised Machine Learning Analysis Using K-Means, Hierarchical Clustering, and Principal Component Analysis in Horticulture Agribusiness: Shallot and Tomato Productivity in Indonesia

Junita Juwita Siregar[1](✉) and Eka Budiarto[2]

[1] Computer Science Department, School of Computer Science, Bina Nusantara University, Jakarta 11480, Indonesia
juwita_siregar@binus.ac.id
[2] Master of Information Technology, Swiss German University, Tangerang, Indonesia
eka.budiarto@sgu.ac.id

Abstract. Horticulture agribusiness needs effective planning to boost productivity. This planning needs to be adjusted to the characteristic of the planting area. To help with grouping, clustering methods using k-means and hierarchical clustering (single link and complete link approaches) were used with case study data about shallot and tomato productivity in 33 provinces in Indonesia from 2015 to 2019. A principal component analysis was used to reduce the number of features in the transformed data. Both normalized original and transformed data were used in this study, and the results were compared. The results showed that clustering can detect general trends in productivity as well as any anomalies. The main characteristics found were high, low, and especially high average productivity as well as one case of an anomaly. Different clustering highlighted different aspects of the characteristics. The principal component analysis also provided insights into what is actually important in the productivity data. In this case, principal components highlighted the average productivity and anomaly. It is hoped that this result could be extended to more detailed data that can then be used to significantly increase productivity.

Keywords: K-Means · Principal component analysis · Horticulture productivity

1 Introduction

Horticulture needs planning to maximize productivity. This becomes increasingly important due to the population growth, giving rise to the concept of Agriculture 4.0 [1], where productivity is increased by considering the careful allocation of resources, adaption to climate change, and avoidance of food waste. In horticulture, planning should start with identifying groups within the production regions. If the groups are meaningful, then different actions or solutions can be applied according to the groups. Unfortunately, it

F. Saeed et al. (Eds.): IRICT 2021, LNDECT 127, pp. 270–282, 2022.
https://doi.org/10.1007/978-3-030-98741-1_23

is not always straightforward to make groupings, especially if the number of variables to be considered is large. One way to find the groupings is by using clustering, an unsupervised learning method that makes groups or clusters based on similarity (distance) within the data. Clustering has been used for many applications in agriculture, such as rice yield estimation from images taken by an unmanned aerial vehicle (UAV) [2], rice crop clustering over provinces [3], feasibility study of corn planting areas [4], the dynamic monitoring of wheat yield crop traits [5], and forestry harvesting productivity [6].

Previous research has examined the k-means clustering method:

Jepry et al. [17] found that k-means is used to classify the stages of maturity under ripe and overripe based on the relationship between palm oil and fruit color, where different color intensities used fuzzy classification. Kalaivani et al. [22] presented color segmentation using a tomato plant grading system with a k-means clustering algorithm. The study measured nutrient levels and health status based on leaf color, forming groups based on the matrix similarity. Ginne, M. J [19] examined tomato disease using segmentation. Tomato image samples were collected from the local market and used for further processing. The disease section was segmented into 5 different cluster processes using the k-means clustering algorithm. After all iterations, the last image was displayed in the fifth cluster. The intensity value of each centroid was a plot based on the red, green, and blue pixels for the infected part.

In this paper, a study of clustering applied to horticulture productivity was carried out, specifically for shallots and tomatoes in Indonesia, where clustering was done on the combination of both products. This approach was used to investigate whether groupings could also be done on a combination of products. Several methods in this case k-means and hierarchical clustering [20, 23], combined with principal component analysis [21] were used to identify the differences in the clustering results. The aim was to investigate the potential of using clustering to group the horticulture production areas. Using these groups, it is hoped that specific actions can be done for each group according to its characteristic in order to increase productivity.

2 Methods

2.1 Data

Data for this study included productivity information related to tomato and shallot production in 34 provinces in Indonesia from 2015 to 2019. These data were gathered from the Ministry of Agriculture, Republic of Indonesia [7]. Data for the DKI Jakarta province were removed due to not being complete (i.e., a lot of missing data). The tomato and shallot horticulture products were chosen for this study due their data completeness (i.e., no missing data). Missing data are a problem that has to be solved before the data analytics method, including the clustering method, can be executed to obtain good results. Unfortunately, the authors did not have enough information to deal with the missing data in shallot and tomato production.

2.2 Clustering Methods

Clustering is part of an unsupervised machine learning method [20]. In this study, several clustering methods were used: k-means and hierarchical clustering [20, 23]. The results of these two clustering methods were compared and analyzed. In clustering, the data are grouped based on similarities [18], which are usually measured using distances. The distances between the data points are usually computed using Euclidean distance due to its simplicity, which was also used in this study. Features are treated the same despite the scales of the numerical values of the data, and all data were normalized before the clustering process was carried out. A good cluster is one where the distances between data points within a cluster are small while distances between data points in other clusters are large. The silhouette score [8], which is usually used as a performance measure of a clustering result, is determined by measuring and comparing these distances. A good clustering will have a silhouette score near 1, which is the score used in this study.

K-means. K-means is a popular clustering method [9] that has been used in many applications, such as the analysis of average traffic speed using unmanned aerial vehicle (UAV) data [10], agriculture and crop yields such as for rice [2, 3], and air pollution [11]. The method is based on the iterative determination of centroids (the centers of the clusters), which are computed as the means of the data points in that cluster. There are several ways of defining the initial centroids, but in this study random initialization was used. The data points are then clustered according to the nearest centroid [1]. The number of clusters (usually referred as "k") to be created is determined before the method is executed. The value of k was determined using the average silhouette [18] score in this study. The k-means clustering algorithm is as follows:

1. Define k as the sum cluster you want to form. Group areas based on soil and climatic conditions according to crop needs.
2. Select the initial k centroid randomly to determine the initial cluster center and generate random numbers.
3. To calculate distance, process each piece of data for each of the centroids taken from the data value and define the value of the cluster center.
4. Choose each data centroid with the closest distance; using the results, compare and select the shortest distance between data and center clusters.
5. Determine the position of the new centroid by calculating the average value of the data located on the same centroid.
6. If the new centroid position is not the same as the old centroid go back to step 3.

Hierarchical Clustering. As stated in the name, hierarchical clustering involves clusters of clusters. A review of some methods for doing hierarchical clustering can be seen in [12]. As stated in the name, hierarchical clustering involves clusters of clusters. A review of some methods for doing hierarchical clustering can be seen in [12]. In this study, agglomerative hierarchical clustering was used, where clusters were created by combining smaller clusters, starting with each data point as a cluster. Clusters that are near or similar are combined together. There are several ways to define the distances between two clusters, such as the distance between the nearest members of the two clusters (single link) and the distance between the furthest members of the two clusters (complete link). Both single link and complete link approaches were investigated in this study.

2.3 Principal Component Analysis (PCA)

Principal component analysis (PCA) is a multivariate statistical method that extracts the weighted combinations of features (called principal components) that represent most of the variance in the data. PCA is based on the decomposition of the covariance matrix of the data into their eigenvectors and eigenvalues (see, for example, [13]). In machine learning applications, PCA has often been used to reduce the number of features used for the analysis, effectively reducing the dimension of the problem [14]. This kind of application of PCA was investigated in this study, combined with the clustering methods. In this study, PCA computation was based on non-normalized original data. The resulting principal components were then analyzed to give some additional insights.

2.4 Experimental Design

As previously mentioned, the data for this study related to shallot and tomato productivity in Indonesia for 33 provinces. The data were available on yearly basis, from 2015 to 2019. The features of the data were the yearly shallot and tomato productivity (in total, 10 features). The names of the provinces were not used to make clustering, but they were used to identify the samples. The data were represented in a matrix with 11 columns (including the names of the provinces) and 33 rows. PCA was used to extract the principal components from the original data. These principal components were used as new features (replacing the 10 original features) in the transformed data. The transformed data were also analyzed in this study. Using these original and transformed data, four kinds of experiments were carried out:

i. Clustering using k-means on original data.
ii. Clustering using hierarchical clustering (single and complete link) on original data
iii. Clustering using k-means on PCA-transformed data.
iv. Clustering using hierarchical clustering (single and complete link) on PCA transformed data.

The results of these experiments were compared and analyzed. The weights of the principal components were also analyzed to get additional insights. All the computations were done using Orange Data Mining software [15], which is free software.

3 Results and Discussion

PCA done on the non-normalized data found that 91.2% of the variance in the data could be represented by using only 2 principal components. These 2 principal components were then used as new features in the transformed data, replacing the original ones.

The principal components were weighted combinations of the original features. The distribution of the weights can be seen in Fig. 1, which shows that the first principal component was a weighted average of the original features of the data. The second principal component was more interesting, as it highlighted shallot productivity in 2019. As the clustering results demonstrate, shallot productivity in 2019 was indeed a special feature that indicated an anomaly in the data. Before determining the number of clusters to be used in k-means clustering, both on normalized original data and normalized PCA-transformed data, average silhouette scores were computed. The two highest results of these score computations are shown in Table 1.

Table 1. Average silhouette scores for different numbers of clusters using k-means with different normalized data.

Number of clusters	Normalized original data	Normalized transformed data
2	0.497	0.772
3	0.504	0.606

The complete list clustering results for both 2- and 3-cluster schemes with different methods, including hierarchical clustering, can be seen in Table 2. The plots of yearly productivity for the resulting clusters using k-means and hierarchical clustering methods can be seen in Figs. 2, 3, and 4, respectively.

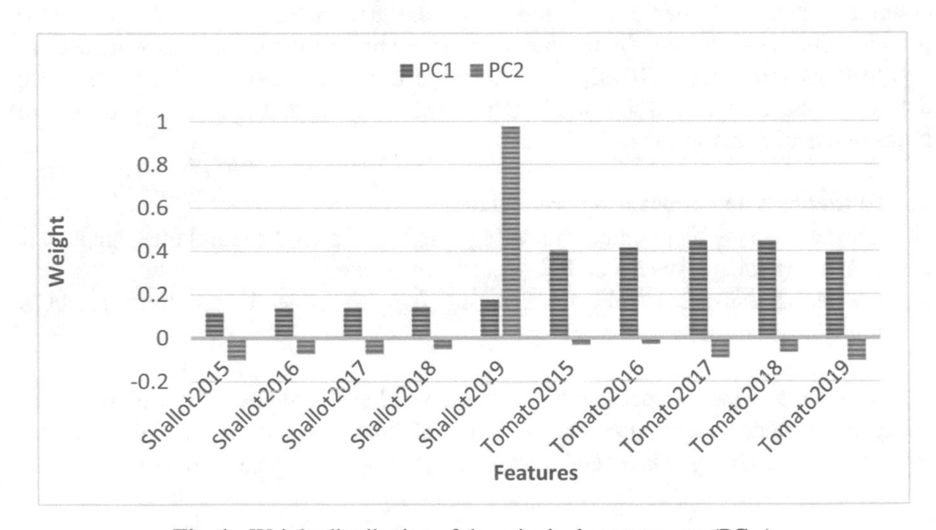

Fig. 1. Weight distribution of the principal components (PC-s).

The first principal component was a kind of weighted average of the original features, while the second one highlighted shallot productivity in 2019, corresponding to the anomaly in the data. Figure 2 shows the results of the k-means clustering. It can be seen in these plots of shallot and tomato productivity that there was a province (North Kalimantan) with abnormal behavior namely, a sudden increase in shallot productivity in 2019. The abnormal behavior was more prominent if the data were transformed using PCA, where a clustering of just 2 clusters divided the data into normal and abnormal behaviors. This corresponds well to the second principal component profile (see Fig. 1). The first principal component, which represented average productivity (also see Fig. 1), helped divide the data into 3 clusters: high and low average productivity as well as the abnormal increase in shallot productivity in 2019. Without PCA, similar clustering was also obtained using k-means. Comparing the data points in Table 2, it appears that one province, Yogyakarta, was clustered as low productivity in PCA-transformed data while this province was a member of the high productivity cluster in the original data. The silhouette score showed that this change created a better 3-group clustering (see Table 1). Further investigation also showed that Special Region of Yogyakarta contributed a negative silhouette score in the 3-cluster results for the original data, suggesting that this province might be badly clustered. For transformed data, no province had a negative silhouette score.

Unlike k-means clustering, hierarchical clustering with a single link approach identified the anomaly as a cluster in the 2-cluster scheme, even without using the PCA transformed data (see Fig. 3). In the 3-cluster scheme, the single link approach identified the clusters as low productivity, very high productivity, and an anomaly. The single link approach combines the clusters by measuring the distances between the closest members of the clusters; therefore, it is indeed likely to combine all the common data points together and leave out the outliers (in this case, the anomaly and very high productivity) as other clusters.

Table 2. Clustering results for 2- and 3-cluster-schemes with different clustering methods

	K-means				Hierarchical clustering							
					Single link				Complete link			
Province name	Original data		Transformed data		Original data		Transformed data		Original data		Transformed data	
	2	3	2	3	2	3	2	3	2	3	2	3
Aceh	H	H	N	H	N	V	N	V	H	H	N	V
North Sumatra	H	H	N	H	N	C	N	C	H	H	N	V
West Sumatra	H	H	N	H	N	V	N	V	H	H	N	V
Riau	L	L	N	L	N	C	N	C	L	L	N	L
Jambi	L	L	N	L	N	C	N	C	H	H	N	L
South Sumatra	L	L	N	L	N	C	N	C	H	H	N	L
Bengkulu	L	L	N	L	N	C	N	C	L	L	N	L

(continued)

Table 2. (*continued*)

	K-means				Hierarchical clustering							
					Single link				Complete link			
Province name	Original data		Transformed data		Original data		Transformed data		Original data		Transformed data	
	2	3	2	3	2	3	2	3	2	3	2	3
Lampung	L	L	N	L	N	C	N	C	H	H	N	L
Bangka Belitung Islands	L	L	N	L	N	C	N	C	L	L	N	L
Riau Islands	L	L	N	L	N	C	N	C	L	L	N	L
West Java	H	H	N	H	N	V	N	V	H	H	N	V
Central Java	H	H	N	H	N	C	N	C	H	H	N	V
Special Region of Yogyakarta	H	H	N	L	N	C	N	C	H	H	N	L
East Java	H	H	N	H	N	C	N	C	H	H	N	V
Banten	L	L	N	L	N	C	N	C	L	L	N	L
Bali	H	H	N	H	N	V	N	V	H	H	N	V
West Nusa Tenggara	H	H	N	H	N	C	N	C	H	H	N	V
East Nusa Tenggara	L	L	N	L	N	C	N	C	L	L	N	L
West Kalimantan	L	L	N	L	N	C	N	C	L	L	N	L
Central Kalimantan	L	L	N	L	N	C	N	C	L	L	N	L
South Kalimantan	L	L	N	L	N	C	N	C	L	L	N	L
East Kalimantan	L	L	N	L	N	C	N	C	H	H	N	L
North Kalimantan	L	A	A	A	A	A	A	A	L	A	A	A
North Sulawesi	L	L	N	L	N	C	N	C	L	L	N	L
Central Sulawesi	L	L	N	L	N	C	N	C	L	L	N	L

(*continued*)

Table 2. (*continued*)

	K-means				Hierarchical clustering							
					Single link				Complete link			
Province name	Original data		Transformed data		Original data		Transformed data		Original data		Transformed data	
	2	3	2	3	2	3	2	3	2	3	2	3
South Sulawesi	H	H	N	H	N	C	N	C	H	H	N	V
Southeast Sulawesi	L	L	N	L	N	C	N	C	L	L	N	L
Gorontalo	L	L	N	L	N	C	N	C	L	L	N	L
West Sulawesi	L	L	N	L	N	C	N	C	L	L	N	L
Maluku	L	L	N	L	N	C	N	C	L	L	N	L
North Maluku	L	L	N	L	N	C	N	C	L	L	N	L
West Papua	L	L	N	L	N	C	N	C	L	L	N	L
Papua	L	L	N	L	N	C	N	C	L	L	N	L

(L = low productivity, H = high productivity, V = very high productivity, A = abnormal, N = normal, C = common, not very high).

Figure 2 shows the yearly plots of productivity in the hierarchical clustering using the complete link approach. Using the original data, the complete link approach delivered a two-group clustering that did not register any anomalies, only high productivity and low productivity. The anomaly was only used as a cluster in the 3-cluster scheme for this approach using original data. The complete link approach combines the clusters by evaluating the distances between the most distant members of the clusters, so this approach tends to absorb outliers (in this case, the anomaly) into the bigger clusters. Interestingly, the high productivity clustering in complete link results included some provinces that were clustered as low productivity regions using other methods namely, Lampung, South Sumatra, Jambi, and East Kalimantan (see Table 2). These provinces were indeed in the overlapping regions in productivity plots in Fig. 2 and actually contributed negative silhouette scores in the 3-cluster scheme of hierarchical clustering results using the original data and complete link approach. A comparison of Table 1 and Table 3 also shows that these changes make the hierarchical clustering with a complete link worse than k-means and single link results for the same configuration (3 clusters, original data).

When PCA-transformed data were used in hierarchical clustering with a complete link, the anomaly was registered as a cluster starting in the 2-cluster scheme. This is, of course, related to the second principal component that indeed highlighted the anomaly (see Fig. 2). A comparison of Fig. 3 and Fig. 4 shows a similar grouping for the 2- and 3-cluster schemes on PCA-transformed data for hierarchical clustering using the single and complete link. Actually, the members of the very high productivity cluster in

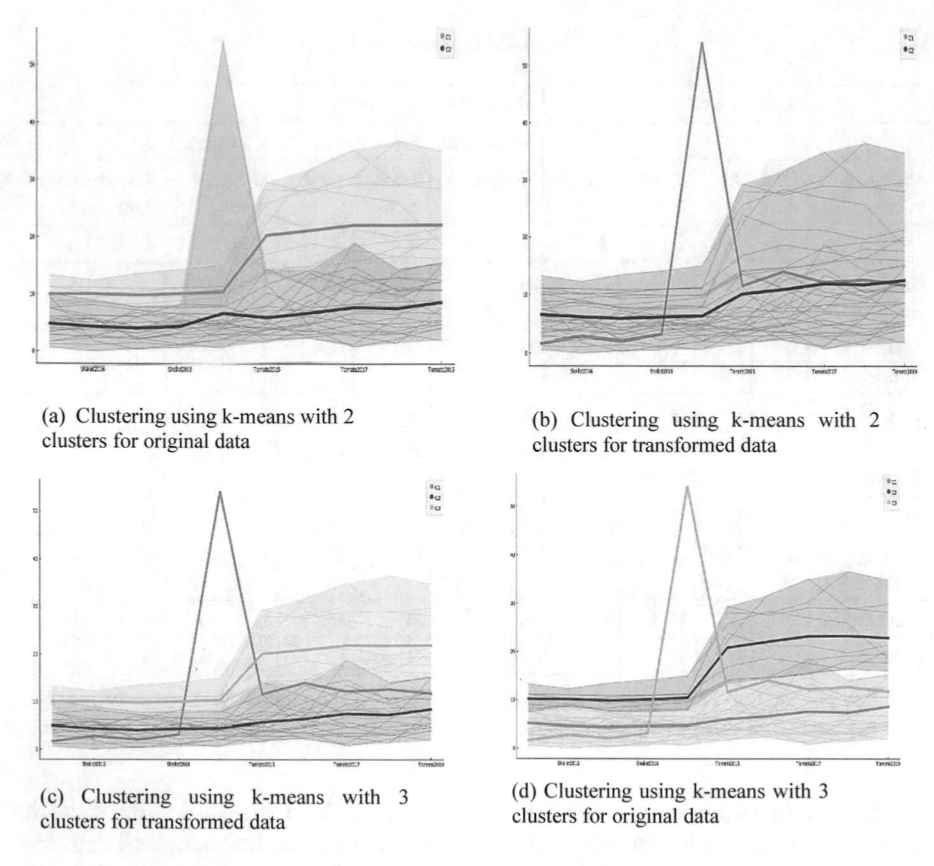

(a) Clustering using k-means with 2 clusters for original data

(b) Clustering using k-means with 2 clusters for transformed data

(c) Clustering using k-means with 3 clusters for transformed data

(d) Clustering using k-means with 3 clusters for original data

Fig. 2. Plots of productivity (y-axis) versus shallot and tomato productivity (x-axis) in 5 years (2015–2019) for normalized original data and normalized PCA-transformed data using k-means. The lines are the productivity means for each cluster.

the complete link were a bit different from the ones for the single link, but the average silhouette scores in Table 3 indicate that the changes in the complete link results actually created better clustering in this case.

In general, the silhouette score indicate that clustering is good. Nevertheless, a manual inspection of the clustering results might be beneficial. For example, the 2-scheme clustering for k-means using transformed data had the best silhouette score, but this clustering did not capture the anomaly, which might be interesting.

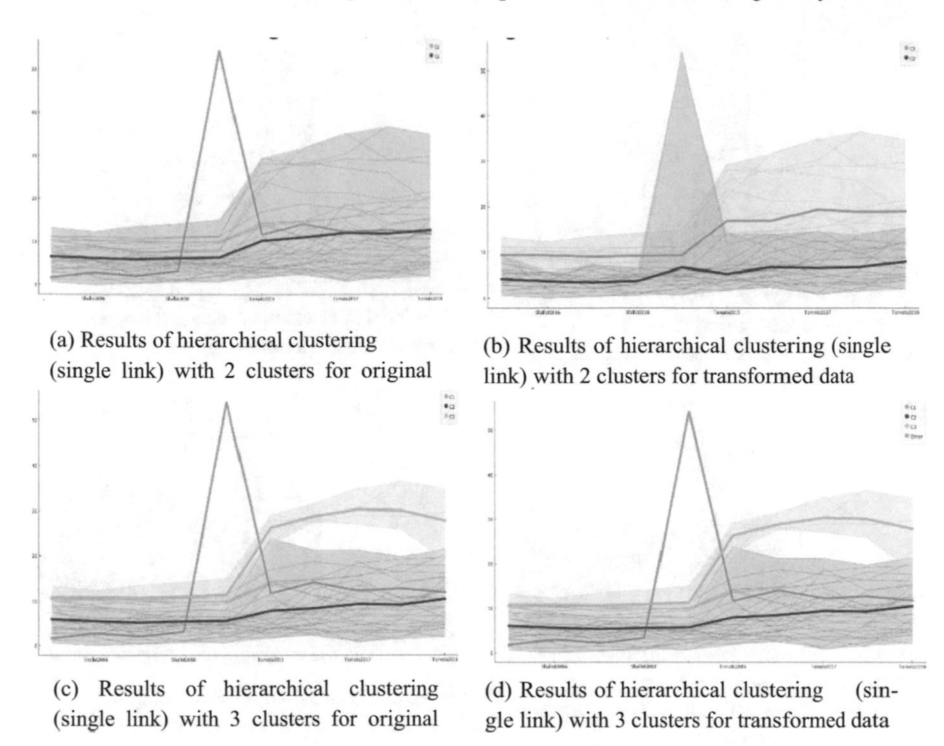

(a) Results of hierarchical clustering (single link) with 2 clusters for original

(b) Results of hierarchical clustering (single link) with 2 clusters for transformed data

(c) Results of hierarchical clustering (single link) with 3 clusters for original

(d) Results of hierarchical clustering (single link) with 3 clusters for transformed data

Fig. 3. Plots of productivity (y-axis) versus shallot and tomato productivity (x-axis) in 5 years (2015–2019) for normalized original data and normalized PCA-transformed data using hierarchical clustering with a single link approach. The lines are the means for each cluster.

Table 3. Average silhouette scores for hierarchical clustering results.

Experiment	2-cluster scheme	3-cluster scheme
Hierarchical, single link, original data	0.529	0.565
Hierarchical, single link, transformed data	0.576	0.626
Hierarchical, complete link, original data	0.372	0.398
Hierarchical, complete link, transformed data	0.576	0.633

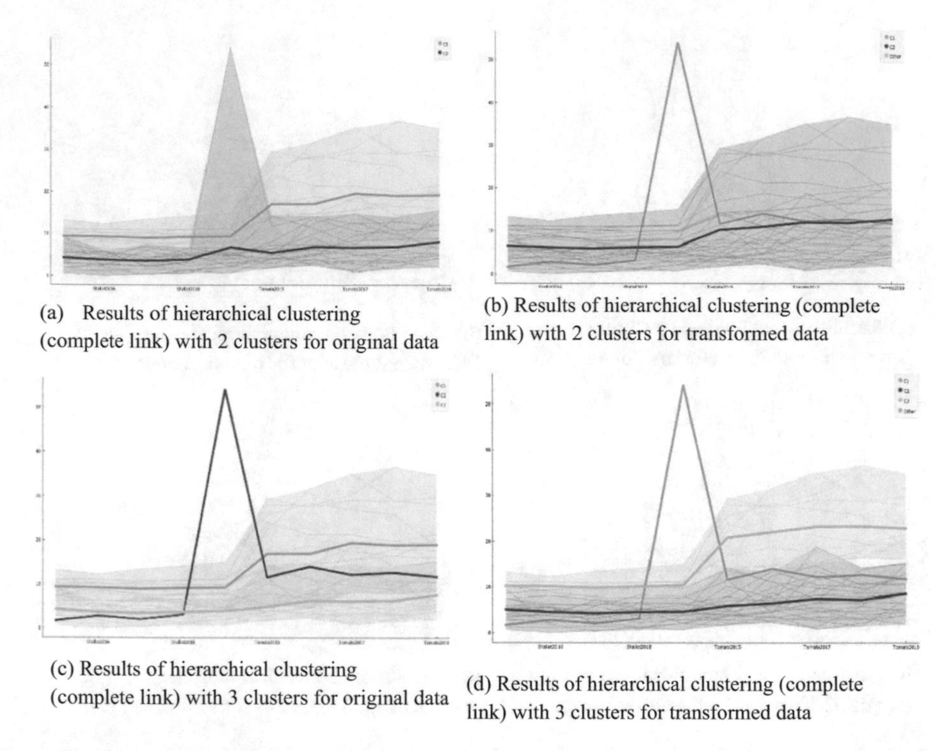

(a) Results of hierarchical clustering (complete link) with 2 clusters for original data

(b) Results of hierarchical clustering (complete link) with 2 clusters for transformed data

(c) Results of hierarchical clustering (complete link) with 3 clusters for original data

(d) Results of hierarchical clustering (complete link) with 3 clusters for transformed data

Fig. 4. Plots of productivity (y-axis) versus shallot and tomato productivity (x-axis) in 5 years (2015–2019) for normalized original data and normalized PCA-transformed data using the hierarchical clustering method with the complete link approach. The lines are the means for each cluster.

4 Conclusion

In this study, the unsupervised machine learning method using k-means and hierarchical clustering have been shown to be able to capture characteristics of the horticulture productivity data, even for a combination of products. In particular, the anomaly can be identified, as can the low and high productivity regions. Principal components can be used to further highlight interesting characteristics. Therefore, this study offers a promising way to make groupings for horticulture productivity planning.

References

1. Zhai, Z., Martínez, J.F., Beltran, V., Martínez, N.L.:Decision support systems for agriculture 4.0: Survey and challenges. Comput. Electron. Agric. **170**, 105256 (2020). https://doi.org/10.1016/J.COMPAG.2020.105256
2. Reza, M.N., Na, I.S., Baek, S.W., Lee, K.H.: Rice yield estimation based on K-means clustering with graph-cut segmentation using low-altitude UAV images. Biosyst. Eng. **177**, 109–121 (2019). https://doi.org/10.1016/j.biosystemseng.2018.09.014

3. Sudirman, Windarto, A.P., Wanto, A.: Data mining tools|rapidminer: K-means method on clustering of rice crops by province as efforts to stabilize food crops in Indonesia. IOP Conf. Ser. Mater. Sci. Eng. **420** (2018). https://doi.org/10.1088/1757-899X/420/1/012089
4. Aldino, A.A., Darwis, D., Prastowo, A.T., Sujana, C.: Implementation of K-Means algorithm for clustering corn planting feasibility area in south Lampung regency. J. Phys. Conf. Ser. **1751** (2021). https://doi.org/10.1088/1742-6596/1751/1/012038
5. Marino, S., Alvino, A.: Vegetation indices data clustering for dynamic monitoring and classification of wheat yield crop traits. Remote Sens. **13**, 1–21 (2021). https://doi.org/10.3390/rs13040541
6. Rossit, D.A., Olivera, A., Viana, C.V., Broz, D.: A Big Data approach to forestry harvesting productivity. Comput. Electron. Agric. **161**, 29–52 (2019). https://doi.org/10.1016/j.compag.2019.02.029
7. Ministry of Agriculture Republic of Indonesia 5-year agricultural data. https://www.pertanian.go.id/home/?show=page&act=view&id=61. Accessed 5 Oct 2021
8. Shahapure, K.R., Nicholas, C.: Cluster quality analysis using silhouette score. In: Proceedings of the 2020 IEEE 7th International Conference Data Science Advanced Analytics DSAA 2020, pp. 747–748 (2020). https://doi.org/10.1109/DSAA49011.2020.00096
9. Sinaga, K.P., Yang, M.S.: Unsupervised K-means clustering algorithm. IEEE Access **8**, 80716–80727 (2020). https://doi.org/10.1109/ACCESS.2020.2988796
10. Ke, R., Kim, S., Li, Z., Wang, Y.: Motion-vector clustering for traffic speed detection from UAV video. In: IEEE 1st International Smart Cities Conference ISC2 (2015). https://doi.org/10.1109/ISC2.2015.7366230
11. Govender, P., Sivakumar, V.: Application of k-means and hierarchical clustering techniques for analysis of air pollution: a review (1980–2019). Atmos. Pollut. Res. **11**, 40–56 (2020). https://doi.org/10.1016/J.APR.2019.09.009
12. Murtagh, F., Contreras, P.: Algorithms for hierarchical clustering: an overview. Wiley Interdiscip. Rev. Data Min. Knowl. Discov. **2**, 86–97 (2012). https://doi.org/10.1002/WIDM.53
13. Abdi, H., Williams, L.J.: Principal component analysis. Wiley Interdiscip. Rev. Comput. Stat. **2**, 433–459 (2010). https://doi.org/10.1002/WICS.101
14. Salem, N., Hussein, S.: Data dimensional reduction and principal components analysis. Procedia Comput. Sci. **163**, 292–299 (2019). https://doi.org/10.1016/j.procs.2019.12.111
15. Orange Data Mining - Data Mining. https://orangedatamining.com/. Accessed 8 Sep 2021
16. Ginne, M., James, T., Punitha, S.C.: Disease segmentation using K-means clustering. Int. J. Comput. Appl. (2016). https://doi.org/10.5120/ijca2016910270
17. Jafar, A., Jaafar, R., Jamil, N., Low, C.Y., Abdullah, B.: Photogrammetric grading of oil palm fresh fruit bunches. Int. J. Mech. Mechatron. Eng. (IJMME) **9**(10), 18–24 (2009)
18. Veenadhari, S., Misra, B., Singh, C.D.: Data mining techniques for predicting crop productivity – a review article. Int. J. Comput. Sci. Technol. IJCST **2**(1), 90–100 (2011)
19. Ginne, M.J.: Tomato disease segmentation using K-means clustering. Int. J. Comput. Appl. (2016). https://doi.org/10.5120/ijca201691027
20. Dabbura, I.: K-means clustering: algorithm, applications, evaluation methods, and drawbacks (2019). https://towardsdatascience.com/k-means-clustering-algorithm-applications-evaluation-methods-and-drawbacks-aa03e644b48av2021. Accessed 10 Oct (2021)
21. Klompenburga, T., Van Kassahuna, A., Catalb, C.: Crop yield prediction using machine learning: a systematic literature review. Int. J. Comput. Electron. Agric. **177** (2020). https://doi.org/10.1016/j.compag.2020.105709

22. Jolliffe, I.T., Cadima, J., Ian, T.: Jorge Cadima Secção de Matemática.: college of engineering principal component analysis: a review and recent developments (2015). https://royalsocietypublishing.org/doi/10.1098/rsta.2015.0202
23. Kalaivani, R., Murugan, S., Periasamy, A.: Identifiying the quality of tomatoes in iamage processing using Matlab. Int. J. Adv. Res. Electr. Electron. Instrum. Eng. (An ISO 3297: 2007 Certified Organization) **2**(8) (2013). http://www.ijareeie.com/upload/2013/august/4_IDENTIFYING.pdf
24. Khaur, N., Arma, Shahiwal, K., Punjab, B.: Efficient K-means clustering algorithm using ranking method. Int. J. Comput. Eng. Technol. **1**(3), 85–91 (2012)

Arabic Auto-CON: Automated Arabic Concordancer Construction from Arabic Corpus

Abdullah H. Almuntashiri[1](✉), Mohammed Al-Sarem[2,3], Omar F. Aloufi[2], Abdel-Hamid Emara[2,4], and Mhd Ammar Alsalka[5]

[1] Applied College, Najran University, Najran, Saudi Arabia
ahalmontashiri@nu.edu.sa

[2] College of Computer Science and Engineering, Taibah University, Medina 42353, Saudi Arabia
{msarem,abdemara}@taibahu.edu.sa

[3] Department of Computer Science, Saba'a Region University, Mareb, Yemen

[4] Department of Computers and Systems Engineering, Faculty of Engineering, Al-Azhar University, Cairo 11884, Egypt

[5] School of Computing, University of Leeds, Leeds 9.11f, Leeds, UK

Abstract. The use of tools and apps to understand more about a language has become popular in recent years. This technology assists the learner in gaining more knowledge about a specific language's vocabulary, collocations, grammar, etc. An example is a concordancer, which is a kind of program that can offer valuable knowledge in multiple contexts regarding the frequency of terms or word. The production of such a tool for Arabic has been limited for several years due to the complexities of the language. The purpose of this paper is therefore to create an automatic Arabic concordancer (auto-CON) with a simple GUI. The proposed method extracts information from a corpus and then provide the needed information depending on a user query. The main aim of the proposed concordance is to provide users with more information on the search word, including the concordance of the word entered, the origin of the word, the domain of each concordance, and the terms extracted from the same root word. The auto-CON tool relies on the creation of two dictionaries: the first dictionary contains all the occurrences and concordances of the word in the corpus, while the second dictionary provides the roots of the words and the words derived from those roots. Therefore, the auto-CON tool is designed to be an educational tool that could support learners of Arabic and Arabic societies. In addition, it can serve as a convenient method for people of different ages to gain more comprehensive knowledge about Arabic words and their concordances. The contribution of this tool is to develop the domain of Arabic NLP. This proposed approach was examined by user testing, in which two Arabic speakers and Arabic learners (international students) were asked to test the approach and provide feedback. The result of the user testing presented the effectiveness of the proposed method.

Keywords: Dictionary · Arabic concordancer · Word occurrence · ISRI stemmer · Tokenization

F. Saeed et al. (Eds.): IRICT 2021, LNDECT 127, pp. 283–294, 2022.
https://doi.org/10.1007/978-3-030-98741-1_24

1 Introduction

In all life fields, particularly for learning purposes, the use of a dictionary has been increased. A dictionary is an ensemble of terms/words that contain various details, for example meanings, phonetics and pronunciations in a specific language or topic ([1–4]. Dictionaries often list alphabetically sentences and words of a particular language, then translated them to another language [5]. However, the use of paper-based dictionaries has declined with technological advances, replaced by automated dictionary and other learning tools which play a role in the science and could be produced by some computer scientists. In order to help people getting a comprehensive insight of the requested word, some basic detail should be included in a dictionary. One such information is concordance which refers to a list of phrases or references that reflect on the appearance of a single term in multiple contexts [6]. With the advancement of the Natural Language Processing (NLP) domain, developing NLP-based learning tools have increased [7]. These tools can allow learners to develop a comprehensive understanding and knowledge related to the language studied. One of these tools is the concordancer, which is used to scan and retrieve the concordance of a particular word from the corpora [8]. As such learning tools are unavailable in some areas of the Arabic language, as part of a digital dictionary initiative, an automated concordance based on an Arabic corpus was constructed. This paper is aimed at presenting an automatic concordance based on the Arabic corpus (Arabic Auto-CON) which primarily extracts the Arabic words and their concordances. In addition, the proposed tool executes many other tasks, such as the determination of a word root (stem), the provision of derivative words from the same root, and the identifying of the domain of the extracted concordances from the corpora. The advantage of the proposed method is to support and deal with the complexity of the Arabic language, such as presenting the concordances from right to left and providing the roots of extracted words.

The proposed Arabic Auto-Con tool can help Arabic speakers as well as Arabic learners by preventing manual searches and therefore accelerating gaining more knowledge about the words being sought. This tool may also allow developers to better understand the occurrences of Arabic words in sentences (concordance) which leads to enrich Arabic dictionaries. The tool is publicly available on https://github.com/AbdullahHamed1/Almuntashiri_Concordancer.git.

The rest of the paper is structured as follows: The related works on existing concordnacers is given in Sect. 2. In Sect. 3, we introduce the proposed tool and how it is implemented, the used corpus, process of finding concordance, the GUI and the tool evaluation. Finally, conclusions, perspectives, and thoughts on future work are discussed in Sect. 4.

2 Related Work

Concordance is a series of phrases/sentences relating to words occurring in a context. Each concordance can be in its own textual environment [9]. Surveying literature, there is a lack of developing concordance tools (hereafter, "*concordance*" will be used) in the low-resources languages, including Arabic language. The main objective of using concordances is locating a word in the context and its presence in texts for the purpose of searching in corpora [8]. There can be several obstacles to building such tool in Arabic. One of the reasons for the lack of Arabic concordance tools is the ambiguity of the Arabic language, its complexity [10–12]. Thus, designing an Arabic concordance could be challenging task for developers. One of the most common problems faced when constructing an Arabic concordancer is the peculiarity of the Arabic script [10, 11, 13]. In addition, most of letters in an Arabic word are interlinked, which means they usually cannot be written separately.

There are several tools that were constructed for those who work with corpus linguistically like WordSmith [14], AntConc [15], arTenTen [16], aConCorde [17]. However, after examining these tools, we noted that they do not fully support Arabic script and cannot deal with diacritics as in [14]. In addition, the GUI of such tools is not appropriate for Arabic speakers. We also noted that the arTenTen tool has an issue with dealing with question mark when the text is written in Arabic.

To overcome the issues above, another tool called Ghawwas ('diver' in English) was proposed [18]. Ghawwas is an open-source tool for Arabic language processing with an Arabic/English interface. Currently, Ghawwas is compatible with many operating systems and can deal generally with texts from Arabic, English, and French. Additionally, it has many functionalities such as providing user with lists of frequency, comparing corpora, and performing pre-processing tasks, such as removing numbers and Latin characters and removing diacritics for normalizing texts. Although that, Ghawwas has no support for UTF-16 encoding.

aConCorde is a concordance platform that promotes a multi-lingual corpus, with a focus on the Arabic language. It supports an extensive variety of character encodings, including UTF-16 and ASCII [19], offers user a good set of query options, keyword, proximity, and expression. However, despite these advantages, the term/word in the sentence is shown without offering the domain of a full context or displaying Arabic roots/stems even though they have no concordances. Another limitation is that it is not capable of printing Arabic diacritics, which leads to losing meanings of Arabic words in case of unknown contexts.

3 Material and Method

In this section, we propose a novel Arabic concordance tool called Arabic Auto-CON tool to address limitations that were observed during analyzing the existing concordancers presented in the previous section. The main flow that we use during designing the proposed Arabic Auto-CON tool is shown in Fig. 1.

3.1 Arabic Auto-CON

The concordance tool that we aim to develop could assist Arabic learners and Arabic speakers to recognise concordances of words in different contexts. The implementation of this system was initially carried out as a console output, after which an interface of the desktop application for Mac OS was built. As stated earlier, the aim of this tool is to extract words and their concordances as well as other information from a corpus.

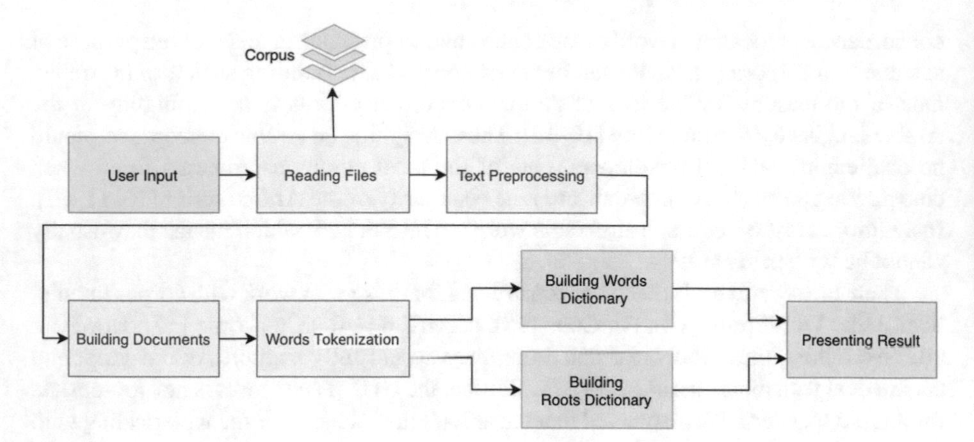

Fig. 1. An overview of the proposed tool

The building process as shown in Fig. 1 was divided into many sub-systems that are implemented and carried out separately, with each sub-system having a well-defined task. The block diagram in Fig. 2 illustrates the sub-systems; the tool will start when the user enters a word and ends with presenting the result – the concordances and other related information.

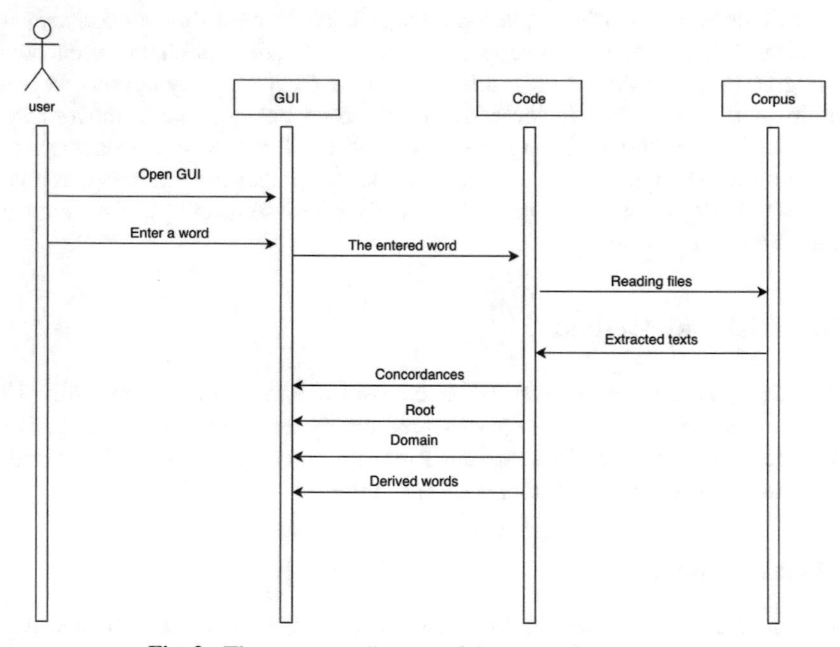

Fig. 2. The sequence diagram of the concordancer system

The proposed tool provides some text pre-processing tasks such as removal of words and expressions that are not related to the Arabic language. This sub-system is one of the most important in obtaining the correct Arabic texts without issues. Then, the extracted text is stored in temporary document storage and passed later after tokenization into to next stage. Finally, at construction stage, two types of dictionaries are built: (i) word dictionary that comprises the tokenized words, and (ii) root dictionary that contains the root of Arabic word.

3.2 Implementation Process

This section discusses and explain in detail the implementation stage of the proposed tool. This first part of this section discusses the tools that were used in building this software, including the programming language, libraries, and the Arabic corpus. The second part discusses the way of implementing the Arabic Auto-CON tool.

The Used Tools. Some tools were appended to facilitate the construction of the software, which will be discussed and explained in this section. The first tool was to find an Arabic corpus. Although many types of corpora were found, our aim was to find a monolingual corpus, i.e., a corpus containing texts in one language only. Some monolingual Arabic corpora were found on the internet, and several of these were identified and compared to choose a suitable corpus. In this work and after an extensive analysis, we decided to use Corpus of Contemporary Arabic (CCA) [20].

Stemmers. Obtaining the roots of words is a part of the main objectives of the proposed tool. Searching for existing stemmers was accomplished and several stemmers that support the Arabic language were found. The stemmers were tested and compared to each other.

Therefore, the ISRI Arabic Stemmer was chosen[1]. It is one of the NLTK[2] packages and it could be called as any library of that package. The ISRIStemmer()function was called to provide the needed roots.

3.3 Implementation of Auto-CON

To write and build the software, various programming languages were researched and compared, and Python was selected to write the automated concordancer. There were many reasons for choosing Python, the most important of which was its comprehensive standard library, which only needed to be imported. In addition, using Python allowed the programmer to dispense with auxiliary programmes. Moreover, Python is one of the most common programming languages due to its popularity and its usability [21]. Table 1 presents the needed libraries and their functions.

[1] https://www.nltk.org/_modules/nltk/stem/isri.html.

[2] https://www.nltk.org/install.html.

Table 1. The used Libraries.

The needed libraries	The names of libraries	The functions of the libraries
The libraries for reading files	Os and os.path libraries	They used in this software to read the files of the corpus
The libraries for text pre-processing	Regular expression operations library (re)	It used for text processing services
The libraries for saving words and results	The JSON library	It used in the software to save a range of data
The libraries for tokenization processes	The Natural Language Toolkit (NLTK)	It used in the software to split the sentences of texts into words and to split blocks of texts into sentences
The libraries for text coloration	The Termcolor library	It used to present the required results in different colours
The libraries for creating Graphical User Interface (GUI)	PyQt5 library	It used in the software to create a GUI

As stated earlier in Sect. 3.1, there are five main phases that Auto-CON has to perform to find the right root and concordances. Below, we present in detail how these phases were implemented:

- The *reading files* phase is considered as the first step, and it is aimed at accessing and reading the content of the CCA. It was assisted by calling *os* and *os.path* libraries, which helped to specify the paths of the corpus files. In addition, xml.etree.ElementTree library was used to parse the corpus files.
- The *text pre-processing* phase is considered the second sub-system of the software. After the capability to access the corpus files to read and extract the inside texts was verified, the texts should be prepared to extract and store the document. The meaning of preparing here is the practice of cleaning texts from some issues that could cause obstacles to the analytic processes. Several techniques of text pre-processing were done through many steps. These steps were helped by some methods of (re) library and NLTK library.
- The aim of the third sub-system is to build a list of documents to store the extracted texts, which were prepared via text pre-processing, from the corpus. This step was taken for several reasons: (i) after storing the texts in this list as sentences, they would not need to be extracted again from the corpus, (ii) the text pre-processing phase would not be applied again, and (iii) because the texts were already saved in this list, the time spent by users making queries after the first query would be decreased, as they could return to the list to continue with the next phases to obtain the final result. The list type is a set of arbitrary objects, similar to an array, and one of its main features is having more flexibility. It could be defined in the Python language by enclosing a sequence of objects, separated by commas, in square brackets ([]). The list type includes an

index and value, with each value in the list corresponding to an index number that starts with index 0. In the previous phase, each text in each file was tokenized/split into sentences. Therefore, when building this list, each file of the corpus was stored as a document in the list. Each document has an index number that started with 0 and the value that was a collection of extracted sentences and other useful information such as the file name and the domain.

- The word tokenization phase is the fourth sub-system of the entire system. Its purpose was to tokenize the stored sentences in the list into words to be used for the following stages. It is considered as one of the most important phases in this system because its results were used for several other tasks. Moreover, it was helpful to use some methods of the NLTK library to implement this phase:

  - The *WordPunctTokenizer()* function, which tokenizes any text into a series of alphabetic and non-alphabetic letters, was called. The *word_tokenize()* method was utilised, added to it the sentence that token from the list to be tokenized into words (tokens).
  - A condition was added, the *isalpha()* method, to ensure that the tokenized word was from the alphabet (string) because there are some other symbols, such as a dot and a comma. These symbols were not removed in the text pre-processing phase due to their importance in determining the meaning of the text.

- The fifth sub-system is to structure the flowed data from the previous phase in a data structure way. The meaning of the data structure is to hold some data together or to store a set of related data. The chosen type of data structure in this stage is a dictionary, which consists of key-value pairs (see Fig. 3). However, the aim of this phase is to build two dictionaries: (i) the first dictionary stored each extracted word as a key,

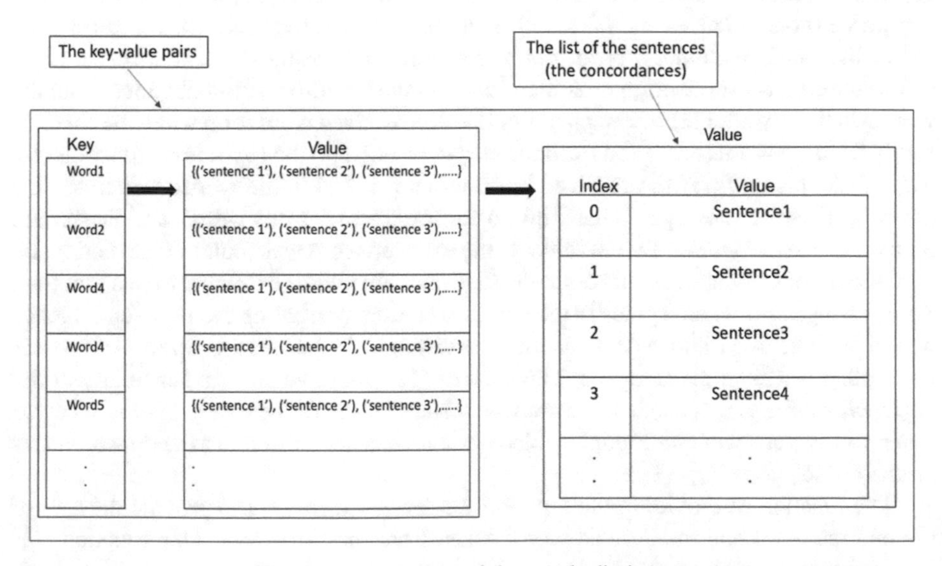

Fig. 3. The structure of the words dictionary

and the value corresponded to a list of the sentences in which the word occurred (the concordances) and (ii) the second dictionary is executed in the second iteration that aimed to store the root/stem of the extracted word as a key and the derived words of this root as a value, in which the derived words were the extracted word from the previous phase.

3.4 Finding Concordance

The dictionary included words extracted from sentences as a key and their contexts in the sentences as a value, which was stored in the created list in the building a list of documents phase. Once the sentences were tokenized into words, the root of each word and all the derived forms taken from it can be obtained. For this purpose, the ISRI Arabic stemmer is used. The purpose of stemming is to return the extracted word to its root by removing prefixes and suffixes in the word and obtaining the 'bare form'. At the last stage, the finding results are presented to the user. This phase is divided into two functions:

- o to receive the word from users and then search for it in the words dictionary to provide the concordances and the domain of each concordance (e.g. in an educational context, a sport context, etc.)
- o to provide users with the root of the received word and the derived words, which are from the same root of the entered word. These two functions will be discussed and described in detail.

In providing the concordances and the domain function, several steps were applied to achieve the required result. Firstly, the user was enabled to enter the word for which he or she wanted concordances and other information. Then, the required words are searched for in the words dictionary. Next, due to concordances being presented to users in a different form, a list of set types is identified to save the information obtained from the words dictionary after processing it. After that, the received word form would be checked if it is from the words extracted from the corpus or not, and the (if…. else) function was used to do this work. If the received word was not found in the words dictionary, the users would see a message, 'There are no concordances for this word', and they could then enter another word if they wanted. If the received word was found in the dictionary, then the list of sentences and its domains (the value) would be extracted to this function. Some changes would take place in the sentences before presenting them – each sentence would be tokenized into words in order to distinguish the word entered by the user from other words in the sentence. The *colored ()* method, which is a subsidiary of the *Termcolor* library, was used, and cyan was selected to mark the entered word, whereas other words were white-coloured or black-coloured when presenting the concordances on the console (see Fig. 4).

The function of providing the root and the derived words are to provide the root of the entered word and the derived words taken from the same root. This function was implemented in several steps. Moreover, it was done through calling the roots dictionary. Firstly, after completing the previous function, this function was called and given the

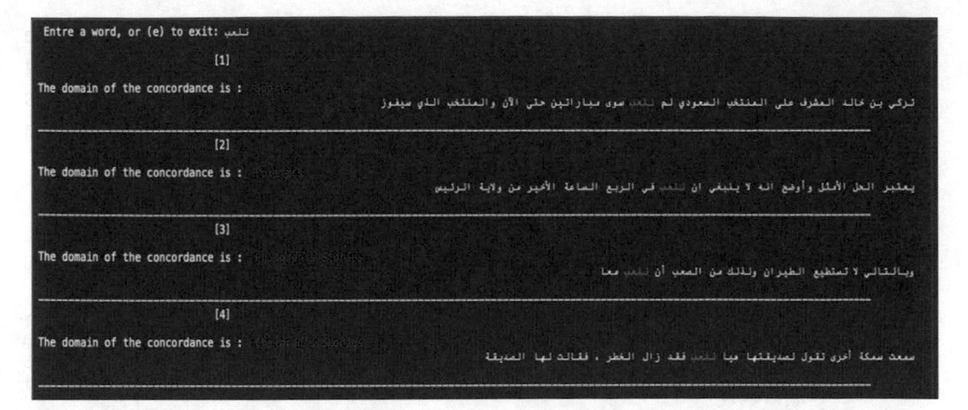

Fig. 4. The result of providing the concordances and the domain in console

entered word by the user. Secondly, the root of the words was extracted by calling the ISRIStemmer() package and using the stem() method. After that, this root would be printed to users. Then, this root was taken to check if it is from the stored roots in the roots dictionary. This step was completed by using the (if…. else) function to determine whether the root was found in the roots dictionary; if not, then the user would get a message stating that this root was not provided. Otherwise, the user would receive a list of the derived words that were already stored as a value of the root (the key).

3.5 The GUI of Auto-CON Tool

After completing the main tasks, it is suggested to create a GUI. One of the features of a GUI is its ability to adapt to Arabic and English. It was created in a simple way to be convenient for people of different ages. Moreover, the presented results can be stored in the JSON format. Currently, the GUI supported only Mac OS. Figure 5 illustrates the result of this function. The result includes the concordances of the word, the domain of each concordance, the root of the word, and the derived words from the same root. The figure presents the GUI in both languages.

3.6 The Evaluation of the Tool

The suggested tool was evaluated and tested on two distinct user groups: native Arabic speakers and Arabic learners (foreign students). The number of people who conducted testing during each iteration was restricted to a single individual from each group. In addition, nine individuals assessed the final version of the software. The evaluation process goes through three iterations as follows:

- o During the first iteration, many tasks were completed. One of these responsibilities was to provide users with concordances for the words they inputted. Following that, many helpful observations were received, which were included in the second iteration and summarized as follows:

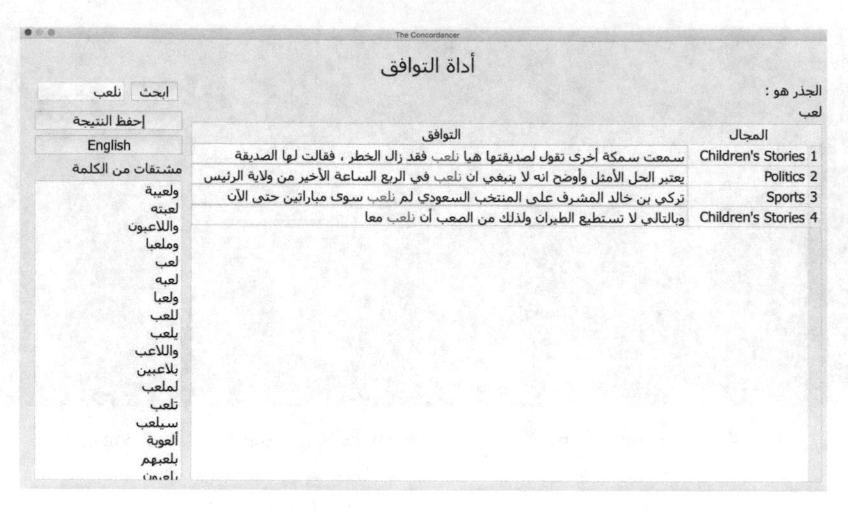

Fig. 5. The result of running the GUI

- Overall, satisfaction was very good, and the outcomes were acceptable.
- The foreign student suggested that the entered word be highlighted in a different color.
- One of the findings was that the concordances were too lengthy, so it was suggested that they be shortened.
- A helpful idea for Arabic learners was to provide the root of the entered word.

o In the second iteration, the concordance result was decreased to a maximum of 15 words based on user feedback. Additionally, the root of the word was included, which helps users know the origin of a word. Furthermore, various colors were used to enhance the results and attract people to the tool. In addition, a new characteristic was added that helps users to discover other words derived from the same root (derived words). The following is a collection of observations made by users during this iteration of the software:

- The users were satisfied with the provided results in general.
- The users found that the changes regarding the output were good.
- As the Arabic learner stated, adding the derived terms was a beneficial task.

o In the third iteration, the users' recommendations from the previous iteration were considered in the development of this tool. To simplify usage, a simple interface was developed. Due to our emphasis on Arabic, the GUI supports both Arabic and English. Each concordance now includes a general context (the domain). Users were asked to re-evaluate the system after completing the tasks in this iteration. Several helpful observations are provided in the findings, including the following:

- Satisfaction with the software was high in this iteration.

- As the Arabic learner stated, the GUI's design is simple, and the results are straightforward.

According to the Arabic speaker, adding the domain of concordances was a significant and unprecedented step in the tool, and it may aid in obtaining good knowledge of the words' occurrences in various domains.

4 Conclusion and Future Work

Although the technological development, the Arabic language has a lack of software that help its speakers and learners to effectively acquire more skills and information about the language. Therefore, in this work, we suggested an Arabic concordance tool Auto-CON that would assist Arabic communities and, particularly, non-native learners of Arabic language. In addition, the proposed tool endeavored to provide for users some relevant information, such as the stem, which is the word's root, the derivatives of the word that is derived from the same root, and the domain of the concordances. It was basically depending on an Arabic corpus that included of a set of Arabic texts. The tool automatically extracted all words and their concordances from an Arabic corpus.

The main target was to construct a concordance tool, which was completely achieved. The aim of designing the concordancer was to extract texts from an Arabic corpus and present the concordances for the word that the user entered. Moreover, the tool provides the root of the word (stem), the words that are derived from the same root and the concordances' do-mains. The Auto-CON tool provides a simple GUI that can support both Arabic and English languages. However, building this tool faced many obstacles during its phases. The main obstacle was demonstrated by the lack of Arabic resources, such as the public corpora of the Arabic language and the public stemmers of the Arabic language.

Despite the main aim and the other objectives of this tool were achieved, there were limitations on the results that need to be mentioned. The first limitation was the small number of participants who assessed the tool, i.e., nine users. Moreover, due to the inaccuracy of the stemmer, many incorrect roots were provided. In the future, we intend to improve the performance of the proposed tool by examining the impact of other stemmer techniques and prefix removal. We also aim at support corpora that have other types of formats such as TXT, HTML, JSON etc. Extend the ability of the tool to provide further information about the entered word, such as the definition of the word and focus on adding other useful lexical information that could help Arabic learners in gaining more knowledge would be worthwhile.

References

1. Abdullayevna, M.D.: Teaching vocabulary as the most important component of speech activity in a foreign language lesson. Int. J. Discourse Innov. Integr. Educ. **1**(4), 199–203 (2020)
2. Kohita, R., Yoshida, I., Kanayama, H., Nasukawa, T.: Interactive construction of user-centric dictionary for text analytics. In: Proceedings of the 58th Annual Meeting of the Association for Computational Linguistics, pp. 789–799, July 2020

3. Pratama, R.A., Suryani, A.A., Maharani, W.: Part of speech tagging for javanese language with hidden Markov model. J. Comput. Sci. Inform. Eng. (J-Cosine) **4**(1), 84–91 (2020)
4. Bergenholtz, H.: What is a Dictionary? Lexikos **22**(1), 20–30 (2012). https://doi.org/10.5788/22-1-995
5. Erali, R.: Semiological analysis of monolingual dictionaries. JournalNX **6**(10), 435–438 (2020)
6. Collins English Dictionary: Concordance definition and meaning. Collins Dictionary (2020). Accessed 15 March 2020 https://www.collinsdictionary.com/dictionary/english/dictionary
7. Wambsganss, T., Weber, F., Söllner, M.: Design and evaluation of an adaptive empathy learning tool. In: Proceedings of the 54th Hawaii International Conference on System Sciences, p. 54, January 2021
8. Kwary, D.: A corpus and a concordancer of academic journal articles. Data Brief **16**, 94–100 (2018)
9. Sinclair, J.: Corpus, Concordance, Collocation. Oxford University Press, Oxford (1991)
10. Al-Sarem, M., Saeed, F., Alsaeedi, A., Boulila, W., Al-Hadhrami, T.: Ensemble methods for instance-based Arabic language authorship attribution. IEEE **8**, 17331–17345 (2020)
11. Bahassine, S., Madani, A., Al-Sarem, M., Kissi, M.: Feature selection using an improved Chi-square for Arabic text classification. J. King Saud Univ.-Comput. Inf. Sci. **32**(2), 225–231 (2020)
12. Guellil, I., Saâdane, H., Azouaou, F., Gueni, B., Nouvel, D.: Arabic natural language processing: an overview. J. King Saud Univ. Comput. Inf. Sci. **33**, 497–507 (2019)
13. Al-Sarem, M., Cherif, W., Wahab, A.A., Emara, A.H., Kissi, M.: Combination of stylo-based features and frequency-based features for identifying the author of short Arabic text. In: Proceedings of the 12th International Conference on Intelligent Systems: Theories and Applications, pp. 1–6, October 2018
14. Yuliawati, S., Suhardijanto, T., Hidayat, R.S.: A corpus-based analysis of the terminology of the social sciences and humanities. In: IOP Conference Series: Earth and Environmental Science, vol. 175(1) (2018)
15. Anthony, L.: AntConc: design and development of a freeware corpus analysis toolkit for the technical writing classroom. In: International Professional Commu-nition Conference, pp. 729–737. IEEE, Limerick, Ireland (2005)
16. Arts, T., Belinkov, Y., Habash, N., Kilgarriff, A., Suchomel, V.: arTenTen: arabic corpus and word sketches. J. King Saud Univ. Comput. Inf. Sci. **26**(4), 357–371 (2014)
17. Roberts, A., Al-Sulaiti, L., Atwell, E.: aConCorde: towards an open-source, extendable concordancer for Arabic. Corpora **1**(1), 39–60 (2006)
18. Al-Thubaity, A., Khan, M., Al-Mazrua, M., Al-Mousa, M.: New language resources for Arabic: corpus containing more than two million words and a corpus processing tool. In: 2013 International Conference on Asian Language Processing (2013)
19. Almujaiwel, S.: A comparative evaluation of POS tagging and N-gram measures in Arabic corpus resources and tools. Int. J. Comput. Linguist. (IJCL) **11**(1), 1–17 (2020)
20. Al-Sulaiti, L., Atwell, E.: The design of a corpus of Contemporary Arabic. Int. J. Corpus Linguist. **11**(2), 135–171 (2006)
21. Srinath, K.R.: Python–the fastest growing programming language. Int. Res. J. Eng. Technol. **4**(12), 354–357 (2017)

Sentiment Analysis of Restaurants Customer Reviews on Twitter

Nouf Alharbi(✉), Ohoud Moqbel Al-Mohammadi, Raghad Abdullah Al-Rehaili, Shatha Abdulhadi Al-Rehaili, and Heba Abdullah Al-Harbi

College of Computer Science and Engineering, Taibah University, Medina 42353, Saudi Arabia
{nmoharbi,Ra.habib}@taibahu.edu.sa

Abstract. With the spread of using the Internet around the world and a huge number of social media users, social media platforms have become a popular place to share customers' opinions and experiences on a variety of services and products, such as restaurants and different consumables etc. These data can be utilized to assist in decision-making. However, collecting and managing customers' opinions on different social media platforms is a complicated and challenging task. The customers express their opinions in their colloquial language that contains spelling errors and repetition of letters, so the preprocessing stage solves these problems and enhances the quality of data to become ready to conduct sentiment polarity and calculate reputation scores. In this paper, the Saudi customers' tweets are collected for four restaurants in Madinah. The Polarity Lexicon for the Saudi dialect (PLSD) and Emoji Lexicon for Sentiment Analysis (ELSA) are developed as a core component in our system to classify the extracted tweets into positive, negative, and neutral. Next, the Net Brand Reputation (NBR) is used to derive the reputation score from the lexicon feedback. Experimental evaluation demonstrates that the results from the proposed approach were compatible with the results extracted from Foursquare, an application that measures restaurants' reputations based on customer ratings and comments.

Keywords: Polarity · Sentiment analysis · Reputation score · Lexicon · PLSD · ELSA

1 Introduction

Sentiment analysis is a field of study that analyzes and classifies opinions, sentiments from the written language to positive or negative sentiments. It is one of the foremost research areas in text mining [1]. Customer satisfaction is the level to which a customer understands that an individual or business has successfully delivered a service that meets her/his needs [2].

Today, many people communicate and exchange their opinions on varieties of topics, products, or services on the social media platforms such as Twitter. In the statistics for the year 2020, the number of Twitter users in Saudi Arabia reached 20.03 million users [3]. Customer reviews become a very important and more reliable reference for people

F. Saeed et al. (Eds.): IRICT 2021, LNDECT 127, pp. 295–308, 2022.
https://doi.org/10.1007/978-3-030-98741-1_25

and also for service providers as they can be utilized and used to increase the popularity of these service providers.

Among these fields that benefit from customer reviews is the world of restaurants. A restaurant is a workplace where people choose foods that are prepared for them against a certain amount of payment [4]. Recently, the restaurant industry has expanded significantly, and restaurants develop and produce the best quality of services in a way that competes with the global market in line with the 2030 vision of Saudi Arabia. There is a huge amount of data published about restaurants on the Twitter platform, including opinions, suggestions, or even photos that customers share on their personal accounts or also in public hashtags.

By using sentiment analysis, this big data can be utilized and can be turned into useful information which can be used to benefit both customers and business owners. The business owner's benefits can be in the form of improving the quality of the served food by identifying the level of services that are provided to the customers. Additionally, this information can help customers to find the appropriate restaurants based on their needs.

In this paper, the customer's reviews in the Arabic language about restaurants will be collected from the Twitter platform, and the sentiment analysis techniques will be applied to them. These collected reviews will serve as a guide according to the taste of customers for those who want to start such projects, which will be created according to the opinions and suggestions of customers provided through the Twitter platform. However, there is a lack of a proper Saudi dialect lexicon in the restaurant field. To tackle these issues, the proposed work has the following contributions:

- Create a Polarity Lexicon for the Saudi dialect (PLSD) and the emojis lexicon (ELSA) with positive and negative words to help categorize tweets in the restaurant field.
- The SauDiSenti lexicon [5] is combined with the PLSD lexicon in order to enrich the lexicon's vocabularies.
- Calculate sentiment analysis of customer reviews for each restaurant for the past five years.
- Calculate the reputation score of each restaurant and evaluate it during the past five years, which can be used later by business owners to improve the provided services

In this work, a customer sentiment analysis will be conducted on the data that has been extracted from the Twitter platform via the API service. Next, the extracted data will be turned into useful and concise information that benefits both the business owner and customers together. Figure 1 shows the main stages of the proposed framework, which are as follows: data collection, data preprocessing, sentiment analysis, and finally, reputation score calculation [6].

2 Related Works

Reputation systems are defined as algorithms that enable users in online communities to rate each other to create trust through reputation [7]. Reputation is the perception or belief that the individual has about something, like about a company, services, or standing of a person [8]. And it is represented by a measure of reliability that is made by gathering customer reviews and comments about something.

The reputation of the brand was calculated depending on positive and negative polarities from the classification phase by using them in the Net Brand Reputation (NBR) index as "the percentage of positive mentions minus the percentage of negative mention as follows [9]:

$$\mathbf{NBR} = \frac{Positive\ Polarity - Negative\ Polarity}{Positive\ Polarity + Negative\ Polarity} * \mathbf{100}$$

The work proposed in [10] deals with the analysis of Arabic sentiment, especially Arabic tweets, and classifies them into positive, negative, or neutral. These tweets were brought from Twitter according to the specific search keyword. They used crowdsourcing to collect a large group of tweets to create a precise tool that helps in commenting on tweets, as well as creating an API that enables the user to log in and view the tweet associated with one of the following four categories: negative, positive, neutral or not applicable. The tweets were selected based on the following criteria: each tweet consists of at least 100 characters, the hashtag in the tweet should not exceed 4, the tweet content should be freed from links, and finally, the words should not be repeated. After that, the filtered tweets were collected in a small dataset called ToBeRated to be labeled by the user from his point of view via the API interface. The tweet is displayed to him, then he labels it to (positive-negative - neutral), and the classification is saved in the database. In the processing stage, they used Rapidminer to modify the texts and extend them to all aspects of the research. In the classification, they used three classifiers combined in Rapidminer (Naive Bayes (NB), K-nearest neighbor (KNN), and support vector machines (SVM). The main contributions of this work are building a dictionary in the Jordanian dialect by turning 100 long shots among Jordanian users and building a dictionary of negative words and merging it with Rapidminer to solve the problem of equating negative words with stop words.

Another work proposed the use of a machine learning approach to analyze Arabic sentiments, specifically the Saudi dialect that related to the topic of girls' sports in Saudi Arabia [11]. The data was extracted from the Twitter platform by creating a search query using Rapidminer. In the preprocessing phase, the data were processed using the following techniques: Rapidminer Tokenizer, Stemmer (Arabic), Stemmer (light, Arabic), Filter Tokens by length, Stopwords remover (Arabic), Generate-n-Grams (Terms). Next, in the sentiment classification phase, the data were classified using three models of supervised machine learning (NB, SVM, and KNN). For validation purposes, the data with the 10-folds cross-validation method was used. Experiments were applied using Rapidminer and Text processing extension on the collected and annotated dataset that contains 1,415 positives, 2,434 negatives, and 1,634 neutral processed tweets. The results of the experiments show that the KNN with no stemming and SVM with stemming classifier outperformed the NB classifier. The main contributions of this work can be summarized into two points. First, training and processing the data set using three types of classifiers: NB, SVM, and KNN with three conditions for each one: with no stemming, with light stemming, and with stemming. Second, the replacement of tokens approach was conducted to enhance the classifiers accuracy during the learning and testing process. By replacing the Saudi dialect terms with modern terms in Standard Arabic, the results were improved, and the classifiers' accuracy was enhanced when tested on a subset of the dataset. The main limitation of this work is the manual annotation of data, and it can be improved by using crowdsourcing or a tool for semi-annotation.

The approach in [12] proposed specifically to solve the problem of a lack of annotated data for the Tunisian dialect. The Machine learning approaches result in using annotated data sets to train the classifier. A dataset for the Tunisian dialect (TSAC) was created from the comments of multiple domains such as social, education, and politics. This work was performed different experiments using several machine learning algorithms (MLP, NB, SVM) on three training sets (OCA, LABR, TSAC). The key goals of this research are to find the most suitable Tunisian Dialect that can be used as training datasets for the Tunisian dialect sentiment analysis task. The results showed that the Tunisian training corpus (TSAC) provides the best sentiment analysis performance for the Tunisian dialect. The main contributions of this work are as follows: introduce a review of the available Arabic language resources include modern standard Arabic (MSA) and dialectal, create a multi-purpose sentiment analysis training corpus in the Tunisian dialect, and assess the Tunisian dialect sentiment analysis system's performance in many different configurations.

Sentiment analysis in Sudanese dialectal tweets is proposed in [13]. The utilization of social media platforms results in building a new lexicon for the Sudanese dialect that contains 2500 tweets categorized manually to positive and negative. The Twitter API search tool was used to collect this dataset. In the preprocessing phase, the tokenization and stemming were performed using the Rapidminer tool. Additional steps in this phase, including stopwords removing and normalization, were clear with some examples of Tweet status after applying each of these steps. The classification phase has been applied in this work using three classifiers SVM, NB, and KNN. The result was illustrated in a diagram showing the difference between the output of each of these three classifiers in terms of precision, recall, accuracy, and F-measure. The results show that the SVM classifier has achieved the best recall, accuracy, and F-measure, whereas the NB has achieved the best precision score. The main contributions of this work are building the Sudanese dialect lexicon that contains 2500 tweets and assessing the Sudanese dialect sentiment analysis performance in many different classifiers. However, the limitation of this work is the reliability of the dictionary has not been tested using different specialist Arabic annotators, and this helps greatly in clarifying and confirming the accuracy of classification results.

Categorizing customer reviews into positive and negative for Surabaya restaurant was proposed in [14]. This data was obtained from the Tripadvisor website using Web-Harvy software, which is a tool that enables the collection and extraction of data from any webpage and removes punctuation and stopwords. Then the data were classified using the Waikato Environment for Knowledge Analysis (WEKA) software, one of its advantages that its ability to classify the data either with or without supervision by using the Naïve Byes (NB) algorithm and the TextBlob algorithm. When the results were obtained using NB, they compared against the one from the TextBlob. By analyzing classifiers' outcomes, it was found that the NB algorithm is more accurate than TextBlob, at a rate of 2.9%. The main contributions of this approach are the collection of 337 data samples, of which 269 were for data training and 68 were for data testing. Also, two algorithms were used to classify data, the Naive Bayes algorithm, and the TextBlob algorithm, and the results were compared against each other to identify the highest accuracy model.

Recently, the work that aims to analyze the tweets' feelings on the ATSAD dataset is proposed in [15]. The ATSAD dataset was imported from Twitter API to build a dictionary of emojis and add feelings to them from the Emojis sentiment ranking lexicon, and then use it to classify the tweets. They cleaned the Tweets by removing all metadata, non-Arabic characters, links, diacritics from the text, and duplicate tweets. They used two methods to evaluate the corpus, intrinsic by evaluating the corpus directly for accuracy and quality. To check whether the rule-based annotation (simply an emojis annotation) can be used to build a reliable corpus and use it effectively in the desired functionality. In an external evaluation, the impact of the data in the sentiment analysis field. To ensure the quality of the collected data, they used two commentators, one of whom is an expert in NLP and the other is an Arabic speaker. To annotate subsets of the corpus. The main contributions of this work are building a dictionary of emojis and classifying them from an Emojis sentiment ranking lexicon. Also, they released 8,000 tweets manually categorized and compared to human classification and pre-trained sentiment analysis models. They are also building a sentiment analysis machine learning model with the unigram features as a baseline and a complex model that uses utilizes word grams and character grams.

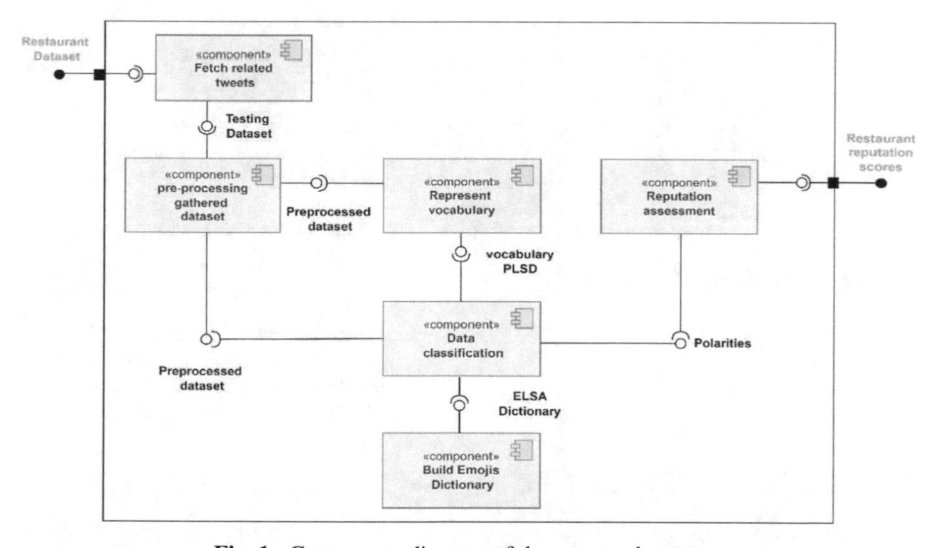

Fig. 1. Component diagram of the proposed system

3 Proposed Approach

The proposed approach consists of four main phases, which are as follows: data collection, data preprocessing, classification (sentiment analysis), and reputation score, as shown in the component diagram in Fig. 1 (Fig. 2).

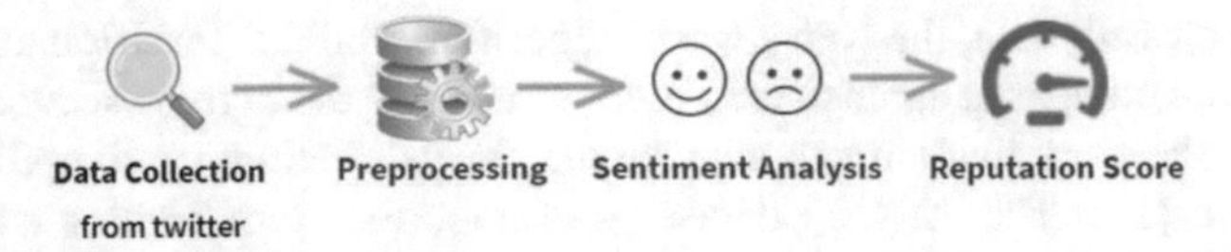

Fig. 2. The stages of the proposed framework

First, two lexicons were created, the PLSD lexicon (Polarity Lexicon for Saudi Dialect) and the ELSA lexicon (Emojis Lexicon for Sentiment Analysis). To create a lexicon of words, four main steps were followed: collecting dataset from Twitter through which used to obtain the words of the lexicon, preprocessing and filtering the collected dataset, classifying the extracted words from the previous two steps manually into positive and negative vocabularies, and finally enriching lexicon vocabularies with their synonyms.

3.1 The PLSD Lexicon Creation

# & Keywords Type	No. of results	Examples
#مطاعم_المدينة #Madina_Restaurants	5	شاورما فطوم خير رفيق لليالي الشتاء الطويلة 🎼❄️ Shawarma Fattom is a good companion for long winter nights 🎼❄️
#المطعم_جميل #The_restaurant_is_beautiful	3	فطور اليوم في المكان الجميل حمسة وتغميسة الجلسات والمكان جميل و رايق جداً الطعم شيء خرافي صراحة ❤️🤩 Breakfast today in the beautiful place that is hamsa and taghmisa, the sessions, the place is beautiful and very elegant, the taste is frankly amazing 🤩❤️
#تقييمي_للمطعم #My_review_for_the_restaurant	7	تقييمي للمطعم 10/2 سيء بصراحة. My rating for the restaurant is 2/10 honestly, it's bad.

Fig. 3. Example of search hashtags

Data Collection Phase. In this phase of lexicon creation, a dataset was collected from the Twitter platform using the API service by searching with random keywords and hashtags related to the restaurant industry in a specific period (from January 2015 until

November 2020), refer to Fig. 3 for some examples of the hashtags. The result of the collection phase was 300 unprocessed tweets. It will be processed in the next phase to obtain a group of words that indicate sentiment.

Data Preprocessing Phase. The data preprocessing phase helps to classify the data more easily and accurately, as people differ in the way of writing words through which they express their opinions. For example, some express their opinions by writing (حلوووو)/(sweeeet) while others express it by writing (حلوو)/(sweeet). In the preprocessing phase, both words are processed to be treated as one word and become "حلو"/(sweet). To prepare the data and filter the collected tweets, several preprocessing methods as in [16] were used to clean and prepare the dataset for the classification phase as follows:

1. Removing all of the diacritics marks and all non-Arabic letters and words, hashtags, mention, retweet for tweets, removing duplicate characters in words, for example (تتفقون ان هذا احسن مطعم؟)/(Do you agree that this is the best restaurant?).
2. Tokenizing the text.
3. Removing all symbols such as punctuation marks, commas, and dots, also remove numbers, selected stopwords such as the letters and words used to connect sentences and not add meaning, such as (من - إلى - على ...)/(on, to, from…)
4. Stemming the text.

The final result of the data preprocessing phase was 2937 words. These words were examined, and only those unique words that indicate feelings were selected. The total number of words after filtering becomes 300 unclassified words. These words will be classified based on their sentiment and enriched with their synonyms at the next phases.

Classification Phase. The data classification phase is the most important phase for completing the PLSD lexicon building. After selecting 300 words that indicate sentiment from the previous phase. Classification of these words is conducted manually by five annotators, into positive words expressed with the number "1" and negative words expressed with the number "−1". To expand the PLSD lexicon, these words will be later enriched with their synonyms.

Vocabulary Enrichment Phase. Linguistic enrichment is the last phase in building the PLSD lexicon. In this phase, all the 300 sentiment words extracted from the previous phases were enriched with their synonyms. At first, we decided to use the wordnet libraries to accomplish this task. However, there were no such libraries that support the Arabic language adequately, and therefore, these words were enriched manually, like all forms of the word were found in the case of masculine, feminine, singular, and plural such as (مناسب - مناسبة - مناسبين - مناسبون)/(Appropriate) through the Arabic linguistic dictionaries or by the help of the five annotators. These different forms of the words will be assigned the same labels as the original word. Additionally, the resulted lexicon is expanded by adding the vocabularies of the SauDiSenti lexicon [5]. After the enrichment phase was conducted, the total number of words reached 1372, with 637 words were classified as positive lexicons and 734 words were assigned as negative lexicons.

3.2 The ELSA Lexicon Creation

Due to the fact that the majority of Twitter users use emoji to express their opinions about restaurants, a special lexicon for emoji named Emojis Lexicon for Sentiment Analysis (ELSA) was manually created that includes about 500 emoji. In order to make the classification stage accurate, this lexicon was created manually and then categorized into positive "1" and negative "−1". To use the ELSA emojis lexicon in the classification phase, each emoji was converted to the corresponding code in the emoji library using the demojize built-in function in Python. For example, " ❤ "corresponds to it "red_heart:" Following that, all emojis within the tweet files were converted in the same way to facilitate the matching process between them and the customers' review tweets during the classification phase.

3.3 The Customers' Reviews Dataset Collection

Once the essential lexicons are created, the next step is to collect the customers' reviews dataset that will be used to assess the four restaurants' reputation scores in Madinah. Here we will present the steps that have been followed to collect the required dataset.

Data Collection Phase. The collected data is a corpus of tweets of four different restaurants. They are collected in the same way as the PLSD lexicon tweets were collected. However, in addition to using the Twitter API service, Twitter's advanced search was used to search for the four restaurants' Tweets in the specified period. These restaurants namely (Al Baik, Domino's Pizza, Maestro Pizza, and Shawarma Al Harraq Abu Siiah Restaurants). The tweets were collected for the period from January 2016 to November 2020, considering the location of the tweets, so that only the tweets that were located in Madinah and were indicated sentiment are collected (Table 1).

Table 1. Number of collected tweets for each restaurant

Restaurant name	Number of tweets
Al Baik	500
Domino's Pizza	499
Shawarma Al Haraq (Abo Siiah)	209
Maestro Pizza	292

Data Preprocessing Phase. The restaurants' data preprocessing phase is not different from the PLSD lexicon data preprocessing. The same preprocessing methods were applied to the customers' reviews dataset. The only difference in the preprocessing phase here is that we did not apply "Stemming the text" as applying this measure to the text might lead to changes in the meaning of the tweet. Often the extracted roots were wrong, and the reason for this is that the Arabic language is a multi-dialect language.

Data Classification Phase. The classification phase for the restaurants' dataset is completely dependent on the previously created PLSD and ELSA lexicons. At the same time, the words and emojis in each tweet of each restaurant will be classified as positive or negative by comparing them against the PLSD lexicon and the ELSA emojis lexicon. If the word in the tweet matches a word in the positive lexicon, it is counted as a positive word, and if it matches a word in the negative lexicon, it is counted as a negative word. The same goes for emojis with positive and negative ELSA lexicon. Otherwise, the word is considered neutral and weighted as zero. Next, if the number of positive words and emojis in the tweet, based on the PLSD and ELSA lexicons, is greater than the number of negative words and emojis in the tweet, then the classification for this tweet is positive, and it is assigned a value of "1", but if the number of positive words and positive emojis is less than negative, then this tweet will be classified as a negative tweet and a value of "−1" is assigned to it. Otherwise, the tweet is classified as neutral and assigned 0 value. For example, consider the following tweet (البيك والله عشق ايس كريم الفانيليا حق مطعم 😍💔)/(I love the vanilla ice cream from Al Baik restaurant is the best), in this tweet the word "عشق"/"love" was counted as a positive word, the emoji "😍"as a positive emoji, and "💔"as a negative one. So the sum of the positive in the tweet is "2" and the negative is "1." So, the Tweet will be classified as positive, and it will be given a value of "1".

Reputation Score Phase. The reputation score calculation process was based on the Net Brand Reputation Equation (NBR), so we calculate the reputation of all the four restaurants during five years (2016–2020), then calculate the reputation score for the restaurant as a whole.

$$NBR = \frac{Positive\ Polarity - Negative\ Polarity}{Positive\ Polarity + Negative\ Polarity} \times 100$$

Calculating the annual reputation score for each of the four restaurants and then calculating its average over the five years.

4 Experimental Results

In this section, a set of experiments were conducted to evaluate the performance of the proposed approach. First, the results of restaurants' reputation scores were compared against their reputation scores extracted from the Foursquare website [17] that evaluates restaurants globally, including Saudi Arabia. Second, the sentiment analysis outcomes were examined against a ground truth of the same dataset that is manually labeled by five different annotators to positive, negative, or neutral. Finally, the Naïve Bayes (NB) model is trained on the part of the dataset that includes the automatic sentiment labels obtained by the proposed approach to validating the quality and efficiency of the system approach to classify customers' tweets.

First Experiment: To evaluate the proposed approach, the calculated restaurants' reputation scores were compared against these restaurants' reputation scores extracted from the Foursquare website [17] that evaluates restaurants globally, including Saudi Arabia. The resulted reputation scores were almost consistent with those from Foursquare, as shown in Table 2. However, it was noticed that the scores of Al-Baik and Domino's could be slightly higher due to the high number of negative emojis used by customers to express their unbridled desire to order and eat specific meals from these restaurants. Unfortunately, these emojis result in misclassifying their tweets and labeling them as negative sentiments. For example, "💔💔💔 مشتهيه البيك حراق يمي"/"I'm craving Al Baik spicy chicken yummy 💔💔💔" Here the broken heart was used as a reference to a positive meaning in the context of the sentence, but it was calculated as negative, which led to decrease of the expected classification results. We also see another example of using the following emoji 😭in a positive sense, and it was classified as negative "اشتهيت بيتزا وعلى دومينوز ييوي 😭"/"I have a craving for pizza, to domino's DUDE! 😭😭".

Table 2. Calculated restaurants reputation scores against Foursquare scores

Restaurant name	Reputation	Foursquare
Al Baik	65.9	8.5
Domino's Pizza	56.5	7.4
Abo Siiah	68.6	9
Maestro Pizza	56.9	7.4

Figure 4 shows the average reputation scores for the four restaurants over five years. We observed a remarkable decrease in the "Abu Saiih" restaurant in 2019, where the reputation level reached 28, and after searching for the reason, it was noticed that this decrease was due to two reasons: First, customers' complaints about changing the quality of the food provided and crowding due to the smallness of the shop. Second, the emoji in this year's tweets were wrongly evaluated, as we mentioned earlier. Regarding Domino's Restaurant and Al Baik Restaurant, they are volatile, and we observe that Maestro Pizza in 2017 reached the reputation score of 80, which is the highest score obtained, but it began to decline slightly in the following years.

Second Experiment: In this study, the performance of the lexicon-based approach should be evaluated, and the correctness of sentiment analysis results needs to be examined. The performance here stands for the sentiment classification accuracy, and due to the fact that our dataset was created by us and we were unable to compare the results against other works, human annotation is considered as a good alternative. To achieve this task, five human annotators were asked to label each tweet in our dataset to one of these values (1, 0, −1). A value of "1" is given if the number of positive words and positive emojis in the tweet is more than words and emojis negative, and if the opposite happens, a value of "−1" is given. Finally, a value of "0" is given in the event of equality between them. Next, these manual annotations were considered as ground truth in our experiment. The automatic classification of the tweets resulting from our system is compared against the ground truth, and the accuracy is calculated according to the

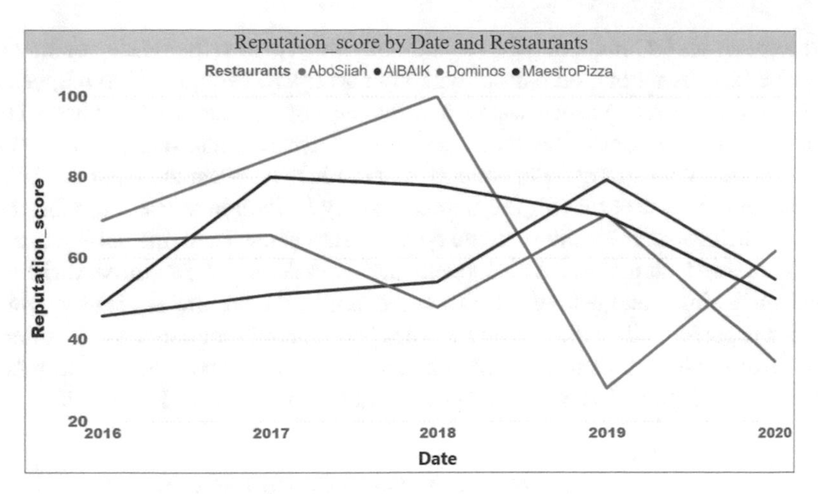

Fig. 4. Reputation scores for all restaurants over the five years

following equation.

$$Accuracy = \frac{TP + TN}{TP + TN + FP + FN} \times 100$$

Where TP refers to the true positive, TN stands for true negative, FP means the false positive, and FN refers to the false negative. A total of 1205 tweets were correctly classified by the proposed approach, and 80% accuracy was achieved compared to manual annotation references. And Fig. 5 shows the number of positive and negative words in the classified restaurants' tweets. The number of positive words in the ranked tweets is approximately three times the number of negative words.

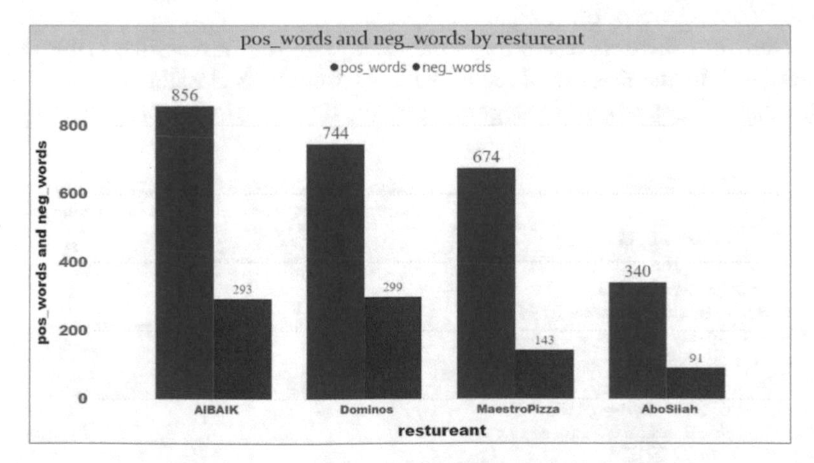

Fig. 5. Number of pos & neg words for each restaurant

Third Experiment: Conducting the second experiment proves the validity of our dataset against the human annotation dataset with high accuracy. Next, the Naïve Bayes (NB) model is applied to our dataset to assess the efficiency of the classification phase. The NB is a simple probabilistic classifier that is mainly established on the concept of applying the Bayes' theorem with strong independence assumptions between the features [18].

To conduct this experiment, the Sklearn library in Python is used to build the NB classifier. The classifier is built with the default parameters. Then, the dataset is divided into dependent (features) and independent (label) variables. Next, those variables are divided into training and testing sets. To fit the model, the training set is used while the prediction is performed on the testing set. The classification accuracy was measured, and it was relatively higher than the human annotation accuracy with 83%. The precision and recall were 79% and 76%, respectively, with low instances of FN and FP.

Table 3. The classification confusion matrix

	Predected:1	**Predected:0**	**Predected: -1**
Actual: 1	51	23	0
Actual: 0	4	59	22
Actual: -1	0	29	263

As shown in the confusion matrix in Table 3, the NB achieved promising classification results despite its simplicity. That fact is well-known in the information retrieval field as NB outperforms many sophisticated models [19]

Figure 6 below shows a sample of the results of the proposed approach compared to a sample of the results of the ground truth process.

As it turns out, there are results that are correctly rated by the classifier in the proposed approach, such as the first sample rated with -1 from both classifiers. Also, there are samples that are not properly categorized by the classifier in the proposed approach.

Tweet	**Classification resulting from the proposed approach**	**Classification resulting from ground truth method**
"اسوء مطعم البيك" **" The worst restaurant is Al Baik"**	**-1**	**-1**
" دومينوز بيتزا اطعم بيتزا 👅💗" **Domino's Pizza the best pizza 👅💗"**	**1**	**1**
" تنافست مطاعم الشاورما وتزعمها شاورما ابو صياح" **" Shawarma restaurants competed and led by Abu Sayah Shawarma"**	**0**	**1**
" الذ بيتزا في السعوديه كلها 😩💔💔💔" **"The best pizza in whole of Saudi Arabia 😩💔💔💔"**	**-1**	**1**
" الاسوأ جودة بلا منازع " **"The worst quality without a doubt"**	**1**	**-1**

Fig. 6. Samples of results

This is due to several reasons, including the difference in the way people express their opinion, as well as the difference in the local Saudi dialects that the classifier did not recognize correctly.

5 Conclusion

In this paper, we described the main phases to analyze the sentiment in the Arabic language. In our work, a lexicon-based approach was implemented to obtain the customers' tweets sentiment and calculate the reputation score for four specific restaurants in Madinah. The dataset was collected using the Twitter platform. This study was motivated by the diversity and rapid spread of restaurants today, which has led to some challenges for both customers and business owners who can benefit from the proposed system. The PLSD (Polarity Lexicon for Saudi Dialect) is an Arabic lexicon that contains a binary classification of words in the Arabic dialect into positive and negative, and the ELSA lexicon (Emojis Lexicon for Sentiment Analysis) also contains a positive and negative classification of emojis based on the classifications of 5 annotators. Our approach consists of four basic phases: the data collection phase, the preprocessing phase, the classification phase, which is conducted with the help of two lexicons (PLSD and ELSA lexicons), and finally, the reputation score phase.

References

1. Liu, B.: Sentiment Analysis and Opinion Mining. Morgan & Claypool (2012)
2. Cengiz, E.: Measuring customer satisfaction: must or not. J. Naval Sci. Eng. **6**(2), 76–88 (2010)
3. Sommerville, I.: Software Engineering," 11th ed., Addison-Wesley, 2015. Globalmediainsight.com 2020. Saudi Arabia Social Media Statistics 2020 (Infographics) - GMI Blog
4. "RESTAURANT|meaning in the Cambridge English Dictionary", Dictionary.cambridge.org. https://dictionary.cambridge.org/dictionary/english/restaurant. Accessed 7 Oct 2020
5. Al-Thubaity, A., Alqahtani, Q., Aljandal, A.: Sentiment lexicon for sentiment analysis of Saudi dialect tweets. Proc. Comput. Sci. **142**, 301–307 (2018)
6. Al-Hussaini, H., Al-Dossari, H.: A lexicon-based approach to build service provider reputation from Arabic tweets on Twitter. Int. J. Adv. Comput. Sci. Appl. **8**(4), 445–454 (2017)
7. Wikipedia: Reputation system (2020). https://en.wikipedia.org/wiki/Reputation_system 2020. Accessed 18 Oct 2020
8. Blogreputationx: What is reputation? (2020). https://blog.reputationx.com/whats-reputation. Accessed 18 Oct 2020
9. Vidya, N.A., Fanany, M.I., Budi, I.: Twitter sentiment to analyze the net brand reputation of mobile phone providers. Proce. Comput. Sci. **72**, 519–526 (2015)
10. Duwairi, R.M., Marji, R.: Sentiment analysis in Arabic tweets, p. 7 (2014)
11. Emam, A., Al-Harbi, W.: Effect of Saudi Dialect Preprocessing on Arabic Sentiment Analysis, p. 10 (2015)
12. Mdhaffar, S., Bougares, F., Estève, Y., Hadrich-Belguith, L.: Sentiment analysis of Tunisian dialects: linguistic resources and experiments. Third Arabic Natural Language Processing Workshop (WANLP), Valence, Spain, pp. 55–61, April 2017

13. Abdelhameed, H., Muñoz-Hernández, S.: Sentiment analysis of Arabic tweets in Sudanese dialect. Int. J. New Technol. Res. **5**(6) (2019)
14. Laksono, R.A., Sungkono, K.R., Sarno, R., Wahyuni, C.S.: Sentiment analysis of restaurant customer reviews on TripAdvisor using Naive bayes, p. 7 (2019)
15. Kwaik, K.A., Saad, M., Chatzikyriakidis, S., Dobnik, S., Johansson, R.: An Arabic tweets sentiment analysis dataset (ATSAD) using distant supervision and self training, p. 8 (2020)
16. Al-Twairesh, N., Al-Khalifa, H., Al-Salman, A., Al-Ohali, Y.: AraSenTi-Tweet: a corpus for Arabic sentiment analysis of Saudi tweets. Proc. Comput. Sci. **117**, 63–72 (2017)
17. Foursquare: Food Saudi Arabia (2021). https://foursquare.com/explore?ll=24.446102%2C39.662128&mode=url&q=Food . Accessed 12 April 2021
18. McCallum, A.: Graphical Models, Lecture2: Bayesian Network Representation" (PDF). Accessed 12 Apr 2021
19. Medium 2021: Intro to types of classification algorithms in Machine Learning. https://medium.com/sifium/machine-learning-types-of-classification-9497bd4f2e14. Accessed 12 April 2021

An Analysis of Students' Academic Performance Using K-Means Clustering Algorithm

Maryam Ahmad(✉), Noreen Izza Bt Arshad, and Aliza Bt Sarlan

Universiti Teknologi PETRONAS, Seri Iskandar, Malaysia
maryam_20000052@utp.edu.my

Abstract. A massive amount of data is often used to evaluate the academic performance of students in higher education. Analysis can solve this challenge through various strategies and methods. Due to the spread of the pandemic Covid-19, traditional modes of education have shifted to include online learning. This study aims to analyze the academic performance of students through data mining techniques. The objective aims to investigate the academic performance of business students at a private university in Malaysia using Educational Data Mining techniques. Students' academic performance data of a private university in Malaysia is used to analyze students' performance using demographic and academic attributes. This study used students' academic performance in the learning method to identify the patterns before and during Covid-19 using the K-Means data mining clustering technique. The results of the k-means clustering analysis showed that students were achieving higher CGPA during Covid-19 online learning compared to before Covid-19.

Keywords: Covid-19 · Educational data mining · Clustering · K-Means

1 Introduction

The number of distant education and learning methods offered in the higher education sector has risen substantially over the last decade. An individual's choice of educational delivery method is influenced by various variables [1, 2].

Coronavirus (Covid-19) has impacted the traditional education system from elementary to tertiary levels all over the world. Implementing a movement control order (MCO) in Malaysia as a preventive measure in response to the Covid-19 pandemic has hastened public acceptance of remote/distance learning. The shift to e-learning allows students and educators to mimic the traditional classroom while avoiding close contact and minimizing the danger of transmission of the virus. It is critical to establish whether greater use and availability of online teaching-learning and teaching resources and the employment of an online learning method have had a good impact on students' academic performance, as evidenced by improved learning outcomes.

The advancement of technology allows higher education institutions (HEIs) to divide large amounts of students' learning data across different learning methods and years of study. Data analytics-driven decision-making refers to the process of analyzing data to

F. Saeed et al. (Eds.): IRICT 2021, LNDECT 127, pp. 309–318, 2022.
https://doi.org/10.1007/978-3-030-98741-1_26

formulate decisions and conclusions about the current path [1]. Data mining is a process utilized for identifying hidden patterns in large data sets. Educational data mining is a field of research that uses the collected data from educational databases to improve the understanding of educational performance [3]. Evaluating students' performance is a complex issue, and the analysis can do that in various ways. Educators can use data mining to uncover the reasons behind their students' performance.

Grade Point Average (GPA) or Cumulative Grade Points Average (CGPA) is an indicator that is frequently used for the academic performance of students [4]. Several HEIs set a minimum achievable GPA that the students must maintain throughout the semesters for successful completion of their studies. Unfortunately, many students face difficulties in obtaining a high CGPA. Still, these factors could be targeted by the academic community in developing strategies to evaluate students learning and improve their academic performance by monitoring the progression of their performance [5]. Due to technological improvements and internet accessibility, education has seen a considerable transition in recent years.

This paper aims to develop a method that will allow educators and students to collect and monitor the academic performance of their students during their entire duration of studies. Being updated on their performance will allow them to help improve their teaching and learning strategies.

The paper is structured as follows: Literature Review, Methodology, Results & Analysis, and Conclusion and Future Work.

2 Literature Review

Although the researchers mainly focused on data mining for educational purposes, they also consider online education as a feasible alternative to conventional education.

2.1 Background

The learning techniques are divided into three categories: clustering, prediction, and association. The primary learning techniques are presented as Naïve Bayes, Decision Tree, etc. The techniques for prediction are linear regression, multi-linear regression, and association. Data mining is a process that collects data from various sources. It uses various techniques to extract information from the data [3].

Clustering is a process of grouping similar objects in a cluster. The objects are arranged in a different order in a cluster. It is a widely used algorithm for various applications. Some of these include data mining, pattern recognition, and machine learning. The K-Means algorithm divides the number of observations into k-clusters, where the nearest mean is the cluster with the most observations. This algorithm can be used to determine the number of clusters in each data set. Clustering analysis should choose it with the goal of achieving the best possible performance. The value of 'K' is determined using the elbow method [6]. It is a visual method to calculate the cost of training. It is usually started with $K = 2$ and then kept increasing it in each step. The goal is to reach a plateau where the K value drops dramatically. The analysis is performed using RapidMiner Studio, open-source software that provides tools for text mining, machine learning, and predictive analysis. RapidMiner is a handy tool for data analysis as it provides quick and effective data analysis.

Figure 1 explains different stages of mining information on educational data for academic decision-making.

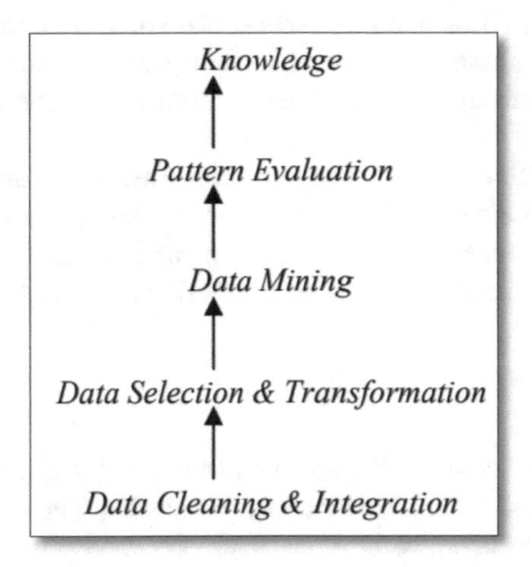

Fig. 1. Stages of data mining process [7]

2.2 Related Work

The students' performance in [8] was evaluated using various classification algorithms: naïve Bayes, random forest, decision trees, multilayer perception, and coting classifiers. The accuracy reached 80.6% for the voting algorithm using the xAPI database. Finally, [9] presented an experiment that explored the use of fuzzy rules to evaluate the students in an E-learning environment where the results showed that there is a considerable variation when compared to classical approaches.

During the pandemic, students lacked collective activities that resulted in impairing their learning. K-Means clustering was performed over a large dataset by [10] to obtain four different clusters. The study also used the learning algorithms SVM, Random Forest, Naïve Bayes, KNN, and Multilayer perception was used to determine which learning mode was most suitable for learning. The results showed 81.5% accuracy. A framework using Association rules [11] aims to benefit the participants and educators of an online learning environment. It includes rules and procedures that are designed to promote the relationship between learning and achievement.

An investigation by [12] was of the academic performance of the same students in three different online and traditional courses where it was discovered that the online. The technique produced lower grades than the traditional method. An analysis of studies conducted over 10,000 students revealed that those who studied through blended learning courses were more satisfied than those who used other learning methods [13–16]. Different learning styles must be designed to achieve optimal results in different educational environments [17]. The implementation of EDM in the previous research has become the method and tool used in analyzing available data in HEIs. It is in an interactive cycle of hypothesis formation, testing, and refinement where educators are responsible for designing, planning, building, and maintaining the educational systems.

For information discovery from databases, several algorithms and methods such as Clustering, Regression, Classification, Neural Networks, Artificial Intelligence, Decision Trees, Nearest Neighbor, Association Rules approach, and so on are employed. In addition, visualization through data mining techniques can combine the tools to envision patterns of interest [2].

This study revealed that studying students' performance before and during pandemic Covid-19 is necessary. One of the strategies used to analyze students' academic performance is based on the concept of clustering. This method aims to identify and compare students' academic performance using various attributes during their learning methods.

3 Methodology

The study aims to analyze and compare the academic performance of students using various learning methods. It uses the concept of clustering. The study is carried out using data collected from a private university. The study's objective is to identify the impact of various learning methods on the performance of undergraduate business students. The steps adopted in this research work are illustrated in Fig. 2, and further explained in the following paragraphs.

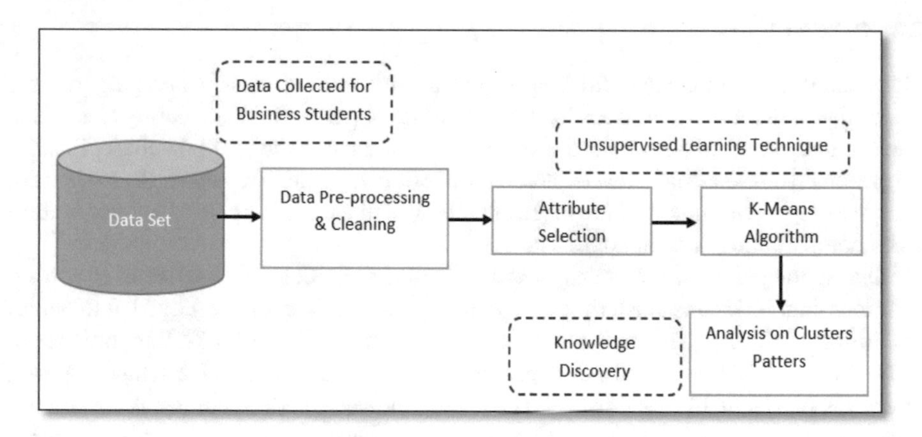

Fig. 2. Methodology adopted

The initial stage, as shown in Fig. 2, was to retrieve data from an institutional database. The data was collected from the university's repository for undergraduate business students for the year 2020. Each semester is four months of duration. Next, the data set was analyzed using the pre-processing method that helps gather essential details about the data.

1. The first step is to collect educational data.
2. The second step is where the data is pre-processing, including some being normalized.
3. The third step follows the pre-processing step, where data cleaning is carried out to remove any missing or incorrect data.
4. The fourth step is examining each attribute and its implication of which attributes should be selected for the analysis.
5. The fifth step is using the K-Means clustering algorithm to locate students with similar characteristics based on the given attributes.

The following section will explain the steps in further detail in the paragraphs that follow.

Data Set. The collected institutional was retrieved from the university's repository. A sample of 466 data sets was collected. The data set was pre-processed for missing and incorrect values. The analysis showed no missing or incorrect values obtained from the data set. This study considered various attributes for analyzing students' performance are shown in Table 1.

Table 1. Attributes selection for analysis

Attributes	Description	Selected
Student ID	ID for each student	
Student name	Name of student	
Gender	Male/Female	
Program	Business information system	√
CGPA	Cumulative grade point average	√
GPA	Grade point average	√
Student status	Pass, fail, or incomplete	√
Enrollment year	The year of studying	

Some of the irrelevant attributes were removed or not used.

Identification of 'K'. This method will aid in identifying areas where the students have a similar range of results to distinguish between their performance from good to bad. The value of 'K' was determined using the elbow method, as shown in Fig. 3. The index of k = 3 was found to be the optimal number of the cluster where the average is 0.47.

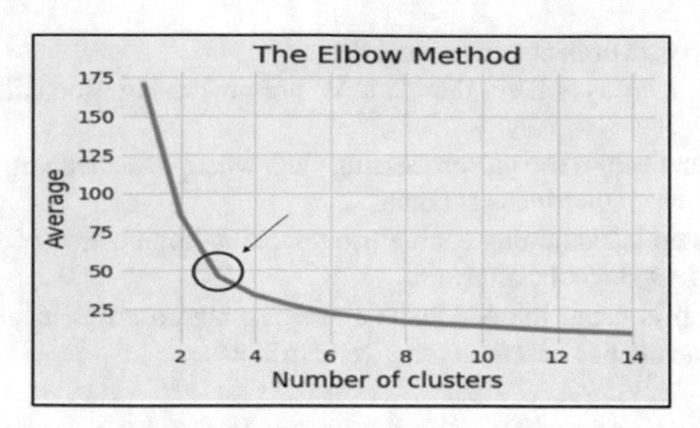

Fig. 3. Identification of elbow point

The attributes being considered to analyze the results obtained are further discussed as follows, referring to Fig. 3:

- There is a curve at k = 2 and k = 3
- K = 2 achieved a weak accuracy of 27%
- K = 3 achieved 55% of accuracy
- Hence k = 3 is considered a good number for data clustering.

The selected attributes are processed via the RapidMiner tool used for doing analysis. Refer to Fig. 4 for the arrangement of operators in the RapidMiner tool:

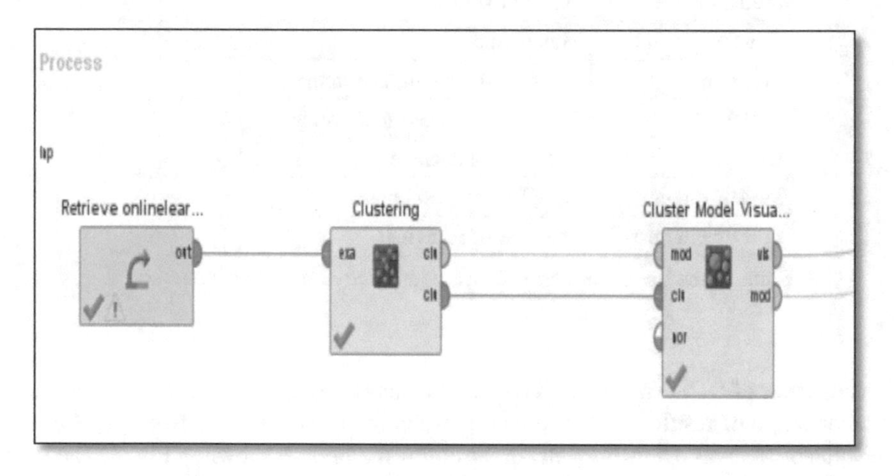

Fig. 4. Operator arrangement

The read Excel operator is used to import Excel files that have normalized data. Finally, the clustering operator is used to generate clusters based on the input data.

4 Results and Analysis

In this section, the analysis results are presented for the student's academic performance before and during the Covid-19 pandemic for the same students. The study found interesting results based on the clusters that are further discussed in the following paragraphs in each of the results. The clustering algorithm produced a model with three clusters are shown below. Clustering Analysis of students' data before Covid-19.

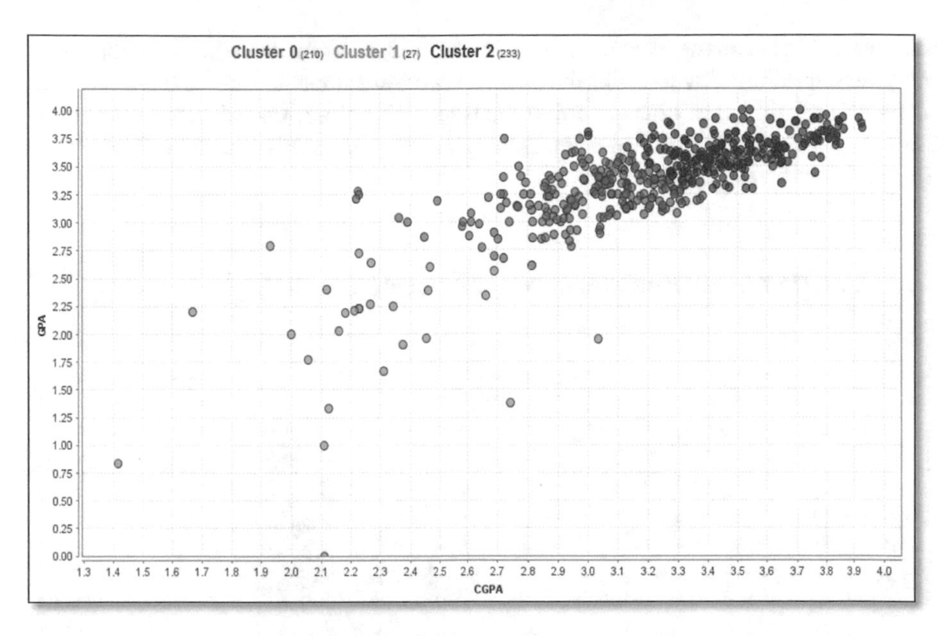

Fig. 5. Clusters plot based on CGPA and GPA of 466 students

Figure 5 above depicts a graphical representation of the distribution of the clusters for the analysis of two attributes: CGPA and GPA of the students. These two attributes were chosen to reduce the number of errors to plot the clusters easily. Table 2 presents the centroids of Fig. 5.

Table 2. Centroids of clusters of data before Covid-19

Attributes	Cluster 0	Cluster 1	Cluster 2
GPA	3.238	1.995	3.643
CGPA	3.002	2.254	3.502

Cluster 0. Based on the cluster analysis in cluster 0, it is observed that data obtained in the semester before Covid-19 for the business program students had the second-highest

data (210) among the other clusters being analyzed. Therefore, this cluster falls between 2.00 to 3.40 CGPA that indicates the student's status under this cluster is 'Pass.'

Cluster 1. Based on the cluster analysis in cluster 1, it is observed that data obtained in the semester before Covid-19 for the business program students had the least amount of data (27) the other clusters being analyzed. Therefore, this cluster falls between 1.30 to 3.10 CGPA that indicates the student's status under this cluster is 'Pass,' but the ones that are below 2.00 are at a higher risk of 'Academic Dismissal.'

Cluster 2. Based on the cluster analysis in cluster 2, it is observed that data obtained in the semester before Covid-19 for the business program students had the highest amount of data (233) the other clusters being analyzed. Therefore, this cluster falls between 3.00 to 4.00 CGPA that indicates the student's status under this cluster is 'Pass,' 'Good Standing' or 'Deans List.'

4.1 Clustering Analysis of Students' Data During Covid-19

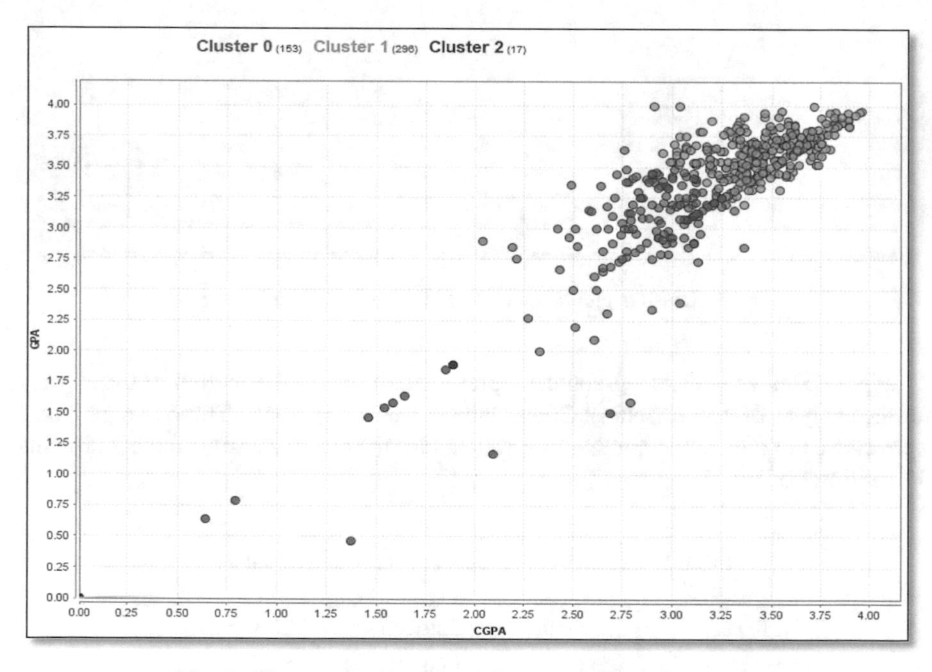

Fig. 6. Clusters plot based on CGPA and GPA of 470 students

Figure 6 above depicts a graphical representation of the distribution of the clusters to analyze two attributes: CGPA and GPA of the students. These two attributes were chosen to reduce the number of errors to plot the clusters easily. Table 3 presents the centroids of Fig. 6.

Table 3. Centroids of clusters of data during Covid-19

Attributes	Cluster 0	Cluster 1	Cluster 2
GPA	3.065	3.631	1.076
CGPA	2.897	3.471	1.254

Cluster 0. Based on the cluster analysis in cluster 0, it is observed that data obtained in the semester during Covid-19 for the business program students had the second-highest data (153) among the other clusters being analyzed. Therefore, this cluster falls between 2.00 to 3.50 CGPA that indicates the student's status under this cluster is 'Pass' or 'Good Standing.'

Cluster 1. Based on the cluster analysis in cluster 1, it is observed that data obtained in the semester during Covid-19 for the business program students had the highest amount of data (296) the other clusters being analyzed. Therefore, this cluster falls between 2.75 to 4.00 CGPA that indicates the student's status under this cluster is 'Pass,' 'Good Standing' or 'Deans List.'

Cluster 2. Based on the cluster analysis in cluster 2, it is observed that data obtained in the semester during Covid-19 for the business program students had the least amount of data (17) the other clusters being analyzed. Therefore, this cluster falls between 0.50 to 2.75 CGPA that indicates the student's status under this cluster is 'Pass,' but the ones that are below 2.00 are at a higher risk of 'Academic Dismissal.'

Based on the clustering analysis performed, the variables that were analyzed are CGPA and GPA. Comparing the highest cluster, before Covid-19, that falls under cluster 2 (233 students) and during Covid-19 falls under Cluster 1 (296 students), this shows that a higher number of students obtained better CGPA after their online learning implementation. Whereas for the least number of students in cluster 1 before Covid-19 and cluster 2 (27) during Covid-19 (17), it is observed that lower students were in the range of failing or academic dismissal after online learning was implemented.

5 Conclusion

Academic institutions worldwide are concerned about their students' academic performance, especially during the pandemic Covid-19. The hidden knowledge that may be gleaned from this data improves students' academic performance in higher education institutions. The CGPA and GPA characteristics are crucial to assess students' academic performance, as seen in the preceding study. This study analyzed the academic performance of students using a data mining algorithm. It was able to identify the consistent improvement in the students' performance. This paper presented an algorithm for determining the GPA and CGPA of undergraduate students. The algorithm is K-Means and is easily implemented. This work can be further extended using other clustering techniques like Fuzzy and DB Scan.

Furthermore, the clusters can be ranked or classified to get an enhanced students' performance analysis.

References

1. Picciano, A.G.: The evolution of big data and learning analytics in American higher education. J. Asynchronous Learn. Netw. **16**(3), 9–20 (2012)
2. Thompson, N.L., Miller, N.C., Franz, D.P.: Comparing online and face-to-face learning experiences for nontraditional students: a case study of three online teacher education candidates. Q. Rev. Distance Educ. **14**(4), 233 (2013)
3. Bakhshinategh, B., Zaiane, O.R., ElAtia, S., Ipperciel, D.: Educational data mining applications and tasks: a survey of the last 10 years. Educ. Inf. Technol. **23**(1), 537–553 (2017). https://doi.org/10.1007/s10639-017-9616-z
4. Sansgiry, S.S., Bhosle, M., Sail, K.: Factors that affect academic performance among pharmacy students. Am. J. Pharmaceut. Educ. **70**(5) (2006)
5. Oyelade, O., Oladipupo, O.O., Obagbuwa, I.C.: Application of k means clustering algorithm for prediction of students academic performance. arXiv preprint arXiv (2010)
6. Ng, A.: Clustering with the k-means algorithm. Mach. Learn. (2012)
7. Durairaj, M., Vijitha, C.: Educational data mining for student performance prediction using clustering algorithms. Int. J. Comput. Sci. Inf. Technol. **5**(4), 5987–5991 (2014)
8. Uzel, V.N., Turgut, S.S., Özel, S.A.: Prediction of students' academic success using data mining methods. In: 2018 Innovations in Intelligent Systems and Applications Conference (ASYU). IEEE (2018)
9. Wardoyo, R., Yuniarti, W.D.: Analysis of fuzzy logic modification for student assessment in e-Learning. IBID **9**(1), 29–36 (2020)
10. Lu, D.-N., Le, H.-Q., Vu, T.-H.: The factors affecting acceptance of e-learning: a machine learning algorithm approach. Educ. Sci. **10**(10), 270 (2020)
11. Bhuvaneswari, K.: Clustering based e-learning in data analytics on basis of mining prediction, vol. 9, pp. 519–524 (2020)
12. Driscoll, A., et al.: Can online courses deliver in-class results? A comparison of student performance and satisfaction in an online versus a face-to-face introductory sociology course. Teach. Sociol. **40**(4), 312–331 (2012)
13. Castle, S.R., McGuire, C.J.: An analysis of student self-assessment of online, blended, and face-to-face learning environments: implications for sustainable education delivery. Int. Educ. Stud. **3**(3), 36–40 (2010)
14. Collopy, R., Arnold, J.M.: To blend or not to blend: online-only and blended learning environments. Issues Teach. Educ. **18**(2) (2009)
15. Farley, A., Jain, A., Thomson, D.: Blended learning in finance: comparing student perceptions of lectures, tutorials and online learning environments across different year levels. Econ. Papers J. Appl. Econom. Policy **30**(1), 99–108 (2011)
16. Martínez-Caro, E., Campuzano-Bolarín, F.: Factors affecting students' satisfaction in engineering disciplines: traditional vs. blended approaches. Euro. J. Eng. Educ. **36**(5), 473–483 (2011)
17. Vasileva-Stojanovska, T., et al.: Impact of satisfaction, personality and learning style on educational outcomes in a blended learning environment. Learn. Individ. Differ. **38**, 127–135 (2015)

The Effect of Kernel Functions on Cryptocurrency Prediction Using Support Vector Machines

Nor Azizah Hitam[1(✉)], Amelia Ritahani Ismail[1], Ruhaidah Samsudin[2], and Eman H. Alkhammash[3]

[1] Department of Computer Science, International Islamic Unicersity Malaysia (IIUM), Kuala Lumpur, Malaysia
ezajaan032@gmail.com, amelia@iium.edu.my

[2] Department of Information Systems, Faculty of Computing, Universiti Teknologi Malaysia, Skudai, Johor, Malaysia
ruhaidah@utm.edu.my

[3] Department of Computer Science, College of Computers and Information Technology, Taif University, P.O. Box 11099, Taif 21944, Saudi Arabia
Eman.kms@tu.edu.sa

Abstract. Forecasting in the financial sector has proven to be a highly important area of study in the science of Computational Intelligence (CI). Furthermore, the availability of social media platforms contributes to the advancement of SVM research and the selection of SVM parameters. Using SVM kernel functions, this study examines the four kernel functions available: Linear, Radial Basis Gaussian (RBF), Polynomial, and Sigmoid kernels, for the purpose of cryptocurrency and foreign exchange market prediction. The available technical numerical data, sentiment data, and a technical indicator were used in this experimental research, which was conducted in a controlled environment. The cost and epsilon-SVM regression techniques are both being utilised, and they are both being performed across the five datasets in this study. On the basis of three performance measures, which are the MAE, MSE, and RMSE, the results have been compared and assessed. The forecasting models developed in this research are used to predict all of the outcomes. The SVM-RBF kernel forecasting model, which has outperformed other SVM-kernel models in terms of error rate generated, are presented as a conclusion to this study.

Keywords: Cryptocurrency · Computational Intelligence (CI) · Support Vector Machine (SVM) · Radial Basis Gaussian (RBF) kernel · Linear Kernel · Polynomial Kernel · Sigmoid Kernels

1 Introduction

The most rapid transformation of the Internet of Things (IoT) that is occurring around the world is known as a cryptocurrency. It is exciting to note that it also changing the way investors and traders perception towards the cryptocurrency. Social media platforms

F. Saeed et al. (Eds.): IRICT 2021, LNDECT 127, pp. 319–332, 2022.
https://doi.org/10.1007/978-3-030-98741-1_27

turn to be one of the important sources where people share their insights and predictions of the price movements [1]. This paper aims to predict the future price of the selected cryptocurrency and benchmarked datasets from Forex. The tweets on selected cryptocurrency were analyzed to assign the polarity scores of neutral, positive, and negative while the historical data were extracted from the relevant sources and merged with the sentiment data that was analyzed earlier and further experimented using SVM as a based algorithm. SVM is extensively utilized in the solution of regression and classification problems. Consequently, while utilizing the SVM to solve the highlighted issues, kernel selection is critical to ensuring that we obtain better outcomes. Choosing the right kernel function and parameters to produce a successful SVM classifier with a simple structure and a high degree of generalization [2–7] is of a paramount important. Kernel function parameters are the most central variables influencing SVM classification performance, but the technique for selecting the parameters, experimental comparison, and a broad range of search optimization are drawing many studies [8]. In their publications, [8] presented three parameter selection methods: (1) the rule of SVM generalization ability; (2) the introduction of matrix similarity measurement and the use of a kernel calibration method to determine kernel parameters; and (3) the introduction of optimization strategies. A defined kernel functions which derived from mathematical functions are used broadly in the SVM algorithm. There are different types of SVM kernel functions such as linear, polynomial, sigmoid and radial basis function (RBF). This paper, on the other hand, will concentrate on the kernel hyperparameter selection and tuning of the SVM. The scope is limited to 5 datasets and four years of sentiment and historical data.

2 Literature Review

Most time series prediction approaches have relied on traditional statistical methods. Many academics have used computational intelligence (CI) methods to improve forecast performance in financial markets. Artificial neural networks, fuzzy logics, support vector machines, and convex with various metaheuristic algorithms such as particle swarm optimization (PSO), Moth-Flame Optimization (MFO), and ant colony optimization are among the methods used (ACO). [9] stated that further research is required to improve the accuracy rate of the existing models, which is consistent with what [10] reported in their article. In addition, hybrid approaches combine many strategies and benefits of different methods to solve issues in initial feature selection, data preparation, data reduction, accuracy rate, and other areas of data science [11, 12].

[13] created the forecasting model in his work by utilizing the Gaussian radial basis function (RBF) to enhance the accuracy rate, and it was also discovered that the suggested model meets the expectations of various shareholders. Siddique et al. developed a hybrid of the OFS-SVR-TLBO model for forecasting Tata Steel stock value in [10]. [14] utilized the SVM model to evaluate the performance of five Moroccan banks' stock prices, while [15, 16] use the SVM with PSO for FTSE and Bursa Malaysia KLCI forecasting and cryptocurrency, respectively. Other hybrid techniques for commodities market, cryptocurrency, and Forex price prediction include the Qiao et al. method [17] and a convex method combining SVM with Whale Optimization Algorithm (WOA) in [18].

This paper consists of six sections. Section 2 presents the literature review. Section 3 reported the development of a forecasting models and the experiments. The nonlinear SVM, parameter selection and hyper parameter tuning are described in detail in the same section. The results and discussions of the experiments followed by the conclusions drawn from this study are presented in Sect. 4 and 5.

3 Literature Review

This section provides the SVM regression model and the kernels, followed by kernel parameter optimization techniques, and then evaluates the performance of SVM kernel parameters using a simulation experiment. This work employs the first technique of [8] in which the model employs the rule of SVM generalization ability, followed by rule determination by optimizing the kernel parameters in the SVM.

The performance of the SVM model is strongly reliant on many factors, including the value of C, the type of kernel function, kernel function parameters, and the value of ε for the ε-insensitive loss function [19]. The parameter C is used to calculate the cost of minimizing training error while also minimizing model complexity. When the value of C is low, it implies that the number of training errors is large. The kernel function parameters define the nonlinear mapping from the input space to the high-dimensional feature space [20]. The value of SVM determines the number of support vectors. It includes four kernels that may be utilized in both linear and nonlinear applications: radial B sigmoid, polynomial, and linear kernels. Non-linear regression issues are usually addressed using RBF or polynomial kernels, and they have garnered a great deal of attention from academics [15, 20–22]. In Sect. 3.1, the non-linear support vector machine model is described in depth.

3.1 Nonlinear Support Vector Machine

According to Akay et al. in [20] for nonlinear regression problems, a nonlinear mapping of the input space onto a higher dimension feature space may be utilized, and then linear regression can be conducted in the space. The nonlinear model is denoted by

$$f(x) = \langle \omega, \varphi(x) \rangle + b, \omega, x \in \Re^{d}, b \in \Re, \tag{1}$$

where

$$\begin{aligned} \overline{\omega} &= \sum_{i=1}^{\ell} (\alpha_i - \alpha_i^*) \phi(x_i), \\ \langle \omega, \varphi(x) \rangle &= \sum_{i=1}^{\ell} (\alpha_i - \alpha_i^*) \langle \phi(x_i), \phi(x) \rangle \\ &= \sum_{i=1}^{\ell} (\alpha_i - \alpha_i^*) K(x_i, x), \end{aligned} \tag{2}$$

$$\overline{b} = -\frac{1}{2}\sum_{i=1}^{\ell}(\alpha_i - \alpha_i^*)K(x_i, x_r) + K(x_i, x_s))$$

where x_r and x_s denote support vectors. It is worth noting that the dot products are using a kernel function that meets Mercer's criteria.

Equation (1) may be expressed as follow: if the term $\overline{b}$ is included in the kernel function,

$$i = 1\ell(\alpha i - \alpha i*)K(xi, x), \tag{3}$$

The radial basis function (RBF) has gotten a lot of attention recently, most commonly with a Gaussian of the form

$$K(x, x') = \exp\left(\frac{-\|x - x'\|^2}{2y^2}\right) \tag{4}$$

Where γ is the RBF's kernel's width. The Sigmoid kernel is one of the other kernel functions,

$$K(x, x') = tanh\left(\alpha x^T x' + c\right), \tag{5}$$

where α is the slope, and c is the intercept constant, and is the polynomial kernel

$$K(x, x') = tanh\left(\alpha x^T x' + c\right)^d, \tag{6}$$

where α is the slope, c is the constant term, and d is the degree of the Polynomial.

3.2 Methodology: SVM Parameter Selection and Hyperparameter Tuning

SVM parameter selection and optimization should be carried out with the goal of determining the optimum kernel parameter values (C, ε, kernel parameters) so the testing data can be predicted with minimum error values so that the testing data may be predicted with the least amount of error. One method is to use a grid search and cross-validation, and other publications [8, 20]. To construct the SVM model in this work, the package 'e1071' in the software 'R' is utilized. We used the grid-search technique to determine the best SVM parameters. According to [8], despite the fact that the grid search takes longer (because to the large number of computations), the results are more accurate and readily accessible [23]. [8] shows that the grid search method takes the values of M and N for C and γ, which the combination of M*N (C and γ). It then proceeds with the training process and estimates the accuracy rate, when the highest rate in M*N combination of (C and γ) will be considered as the optimum parameter. The grid search technique gives high accuracy rate however it rich in its computational time. For it has the independent parallel processing of each and every training in SVM algorithm, it becomes the advantage of grid search technique in the SVM algorithm. Next is the kernel parameter selection. Kernel parameters selection is performed by using the 10-fold cross validation process. The kernel parameters are then chosen. The 10-fold cross validation procedure is used to determine kernel parameters. The cross-validation procedure is well-known for being an efficient technique for choosing parameters for machine learning algorithms to prevent overfitting [24] but it is computationally costly. This will be the first step in the SVM's experimental setup, selecting the parameters that are most suitable for the SVM before constructing the forecasting model.

As stated in Sect. 3.1, this study investigated four different SVM kernels. The goal was to find the best kernel for classifying the data and to create a well-defined hyperplane for separating different sets of data. The data may be separated in each of these cases. In this case, SVM wants to soften the border in order to separate as many data as possible. Four different kernels as mentioned in the Sect. 3.1. Initially, we use four kernel functions, however, the polynomial function takes longer to train the SVM and performs worse in the pilot study than the RBF. As a result, since it has a simple structure and a high degree of generalization, the RBF function is used as the kernel function of SVMs in this research [2–4, 6, 7, 20, 25]. The grid search method was utilized to find the best RBF classifier parameters for softening the margin [3, 8, 26–28].

The optimum RBF classifier parameters are determined by adjusting the width of the SVM-RBF classifier with the parameters, constant C and epsilon, ε which governs the margin of classification. This is also signified as the hyper parameter tuning. SVM hyperparameter tuning entails defining parameters that do not change throughout the learning process. The aim of this search was to identify the optimum pair of parameters during the in-sample phase to maximize out-of-sample accuracy to the greatest extent feasible. Both parameters in R had default values of "1" for parameter C and "0.5" for parameter ε. The parameter tuning process starts with tuning of functions using the grid search method, which takes the value of parameters, the supplied parameter ranges, C and γ., in this paper, the value of the cost function, C and epsilon,ε ranges between 0–1 and will take steps of 0.1, while for cost function from 0–9 and will take the exponential steps of 2. Figure 1 depicts the constant C and epsilon, ε values used in this study, which will be tested on the 9 datasets and 2 kernel functions. The parameter C was not changed at the conclusion of our effort. Instead, it stayed constant since, after we adjusted it for the optimum sigma value for the RBF kernel, further modifying the parameter C would have resulted in a softer margin for classification, resulting in a sluggish response of the classifier (keeping the classification rate oat 1 or 0 for a long period of time). This involves a search across the hyper-parameter space, training the models, and evaluating predictions for each possible combination of hyper-parameter values in order to identify the best set of values. This is followed by the process of re-tuning the SVM parameters. The training set will be used in this tuning process, and the outcome will be the best model from the tune process. The mean absolute error (MAE), mean squared error (MSE), root mean squared error (RMSE), are used to assess, and compare the performance of the collection of parameters.

Hyper Parameter	Options
Epsilon, ε	0, 0.1, 0.2,0.3, …., 0.9, 1.0
Cost, *C*	1, 2, 4, 8, 16, …., 512

Fig. 1. Hyper parameters tuning

Figure 2 depicts the suggested approach's flowchart. The suggested method consists of nine stages. As shown in [9, 16, 18], data is first collected from appropriate sources. Using 10-fold cross-validation, the datasets are then partitioned into two independent portions, the training and testing sets. The second step is to normalize all of the data sets into SVM predictor variables such that they have a '0' zero mean and a variance of unity. This is done to prevent predictor variables with larger numeric ranges overwhelming those with lower numeric ranges in the calculation. The third step is to use 10-fold cross-validation on the training set to determine the best values of (C, ε, kernel parameters). The training data is randomly partitioned into 10 equal-sized subgroups for 10-fold cross-validation. In the fourth step, one of the 10 subsets is retrained as validation data for testing the model, while the other nine are utilized as training data. C and ε searching range have been selected as shown in Fig. 1. In step five, each value of the pair value of C and ε has been tested. The cross-validation procedure is performed ten times, with each of the ten subsets serving as the validation data precisely once. Then, 10 folds' findings were averaged to create a single estimate. Steps six and seven include selecting the double (C and ε, kernel parameters) that results in the lowest cross-validation to train the training set and produce the forecasting model. The forecasting model was used in step eight to predict the cryptocurrency and Forex price in the test subset, and it is followed by step nine, which compares and assesses the forecasting model's performance using the three-performance metrics, MAE, MSE, and RMSE.

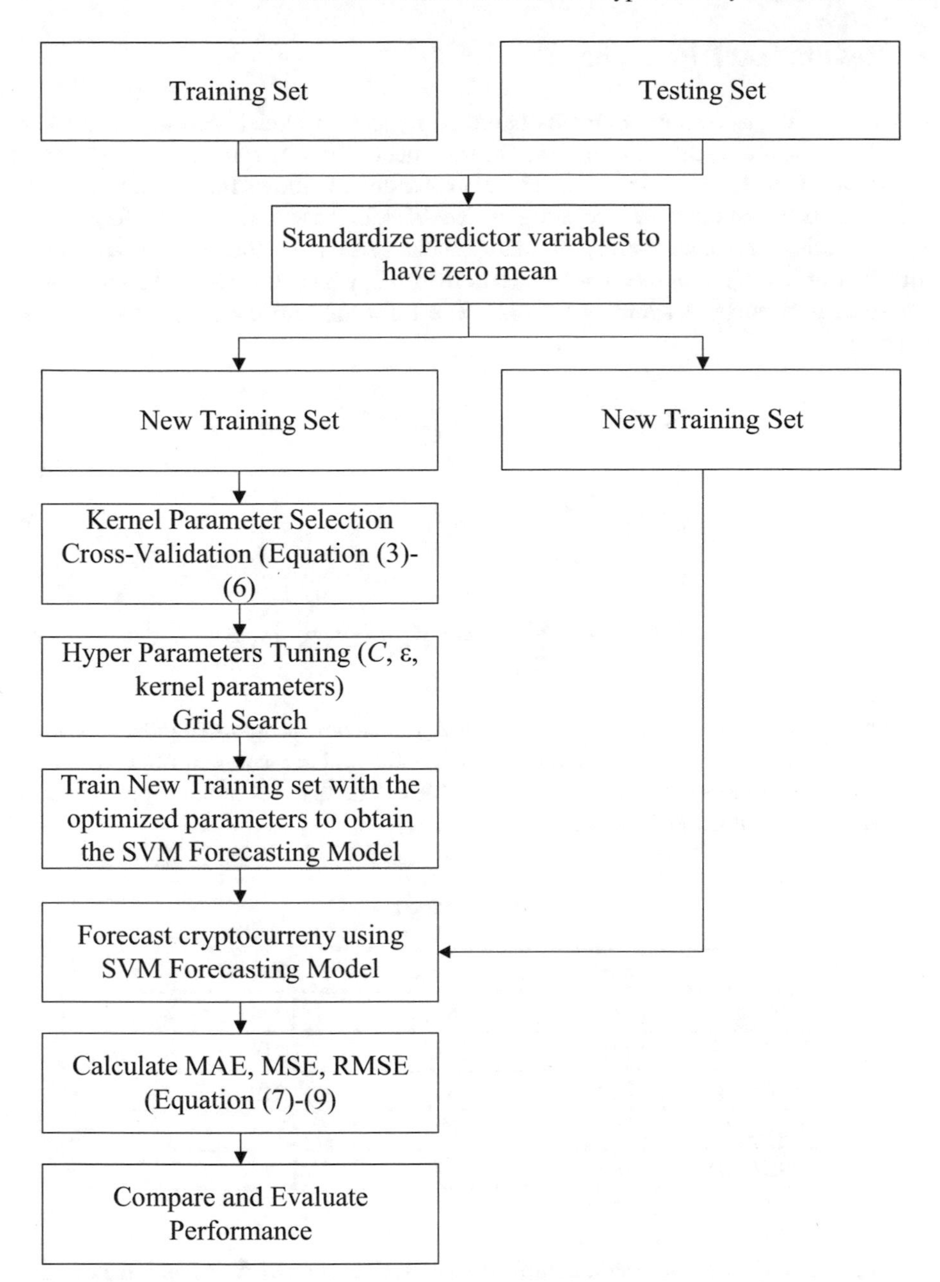

Fig. 2. Flowchart of the SVM-RBF-Kernel model for cryptocurrency forecasting

4 Results and Discussion

A set of performance measurements based on regression model accuracy metrics are used to assess the forecasting model's measurement [29]. Choosing and using a range of forecasting techniques is very beneficial to investors. It allows for comparisons to be conducted between various forecasting models. The forecasting model's performance is assessed using statistical evaluation metrics such as mean absolute error (MAE), mean square error (MSE), root mean square error (RMSE), which are among the noteworthy measures utilized by academics [29–32]. The following are the definitions of these criteria: -

$$MAE = \frac{1}{n}\sum_{i,j=1}^{n}\left|x_i - x_j\right| i, j = 1, 2, \ldots, n \tag{7}$$

$$MSE = \frac{1}{n}\sum_{i,j=1}^{n}\left(x_i - x_j\right)^2 i, j = 1, 2, \ldots, n \tag{8}$$

$$RMSE = \sqrt{\frac{1}{n}\sum_{i,j=1}^{n}\left(x_i - x_j\right)^2} i, j = 1, 2, \ldots, n \tag{9}$$

The greater the forecast accuracy, the lower the values of the three indices. Where: x_i denotes the actual values; x_j denotes the prediction values; n denotes the number of samples. We used five datasets as shown in Table 1. The features of the datasets used in this paper are depicted in Table 2.

Table 1. Datasets

Instruments	Sample size	Training set	Testing set
Bitcoin	1105	880	218
Dash	1126	880	218
Ethereum	1126	881	218
AUDUSD	783	622	154
USDCAD	781	621	153

Data normalization has been completed for all data sets, as described in Sect. 3.2. The following formula will be used to normalize all variables to the range [0,1]:

$$x = (x_{1} {-} x_{\min})/(x_{max} {-} x_{\min}) \tag{10}$$

Where x is the normalization data, $xmax$ and $xmin$ are the maximum and minimum values in the series data in that order.

Table 2. Features

No	Features	Description
1	Date	Date of the instrument on the trading day
2	Open	Opening price of the instrument on the trading day
3	High	Highest price of the instrument on the trading day
4	Low	Lowest price of the instrument on the trading day
5	Close	Closing price of the instrument on the trading day
6	Sentiment	Sentiment polarity of the instrument on the trading day
7	CCI	Technical indicator of the instrument on the trading day

The MAE, MSE, and RMSE values for all forecasting models (SVM-Linear, SVM-Radial, SVM-Polynomial, and SVM-Sigmoid, respectively) used to predict the cryptocurrency markets of Bitcoin, Dash, and Ethereum, as well as the Forex markets of AUDUSD and USDCAD, are shown in Tables 3,4,5, and 6.

The results indicate that the optimum *C* and gamma for the SVM-Linear Kernel model are 0.42 and 1, respectively, for all datasets in the SVM with a linear kernel forecasting model. The optimum *C*, gamma, and epsilon for the SVM-Basis Gaussian (RBF) kernel forecasting model are 1.0, 0.19, and 0.1, respectively. The optimal *C*, *d*, and gamma for the SVM-Polynomial kernel forecasting model are 1, 1, and 0.1, respectively, while for the SVM-Sigmoid kernel forecasting model, they are 1, 0.167, and 0.1 for *C*, gamma, and epsilon. Furthermore, nearly all MAE, MSE, and RMSE errors are lowest for SVM-RBF when compared to the other three SVM-Linear, SVM-Polynomial, and SVM-Sigmoid. Figure 3 depicts the optimum epsilon and cost factor for the SVM-RBF kernel.

Furthermore, after fitting and tuning all models, the results indicate that the SVM with RBF kernel model performs the best. Bitcoin, Dash, Ethereum, and USDCAD had the lowest MAE, MSE, and RMSE among the five datasets tested. While the AUDUSD has the lowest MAE, MSE, and RMSE. The lowest RMSE value indicates the model's ability to generate predictions that are close to the actual value. Among the SVM-kernel models, the SVM-Sigmoid model provided the least accurate results, followed by the SVM-Polynomial and SVM-Linear kernel models. This indicates that, among the models studied in this research, the SVM-RBF model is the best SVM kernel model for modelling both cryptocurrency and Forex data (Table 7).

When the optimized SVM kernel models' results are compared to the benchmark model's results, the optimized SVM models outperform all of the benchmark models. In the case of Bitcoin, the optimized SVM-RBF model with the lowest MAE, MSE, and RMSE values of 0.0261, 1.48684, and 0.0386 outperformed the best performing benchmark model. The optimized SVM-RBF model has the lowest MAE, MSE, and RMSE values for the Dash dataset, which are 1.0440, 5.7901, and 2.4063, respectively, when compared to its benchmark model, the results of which are shown in Table 6,

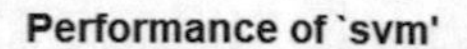

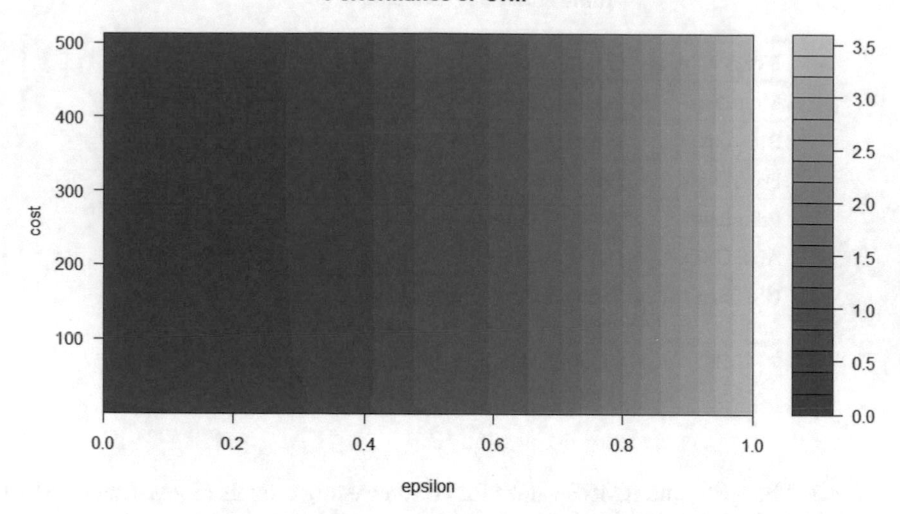

Fig. 3. Epsilon and cost factor for SVM-RBF kernel

Table 3. SVM-Linear Kernel

SVM-Linear					
Metrics	MAE	MSE	RMSE	C	γ
Bitcoin	0.2311	0.1276	0.3572	0.42	1
Dash	55.6969	58.8288	76.7000	0.42	1
Ethereum	70.5313	923.8904	96.1192	0.42	1
AUDUSD	**0.0020**	**0.00001**	**0.0025**	0.42	1
USDCAD	0.0025	0.0000	0.0033	0.42	1

Table 4. SVM-Radial Kernel

SVM-Radial Basis Gaussian (RBF)						
Metrics	MAE	MSE	RMSE	C	γ	ε
Bitcoin	**0.0261**	**1.48684**	**0.0386**	1.0	0.19	0.1
Dash	**1.0440**	**5.7901**	**2.4063**	1.0	0.19	0.1
Ethereum	**7.0236**	**11.86161**	**10.8911**	1.0	0.19	0.1
AUDUSD	0.0019	0.000006	0.0025	1.0	0.19	0.1
USDCAD	**0.0025**	**0.0000016**	**0.0032**	1.0	0.19	0.1

Table 5. SVM-Polynomial Kernel

SVM-Polynomial						
Metrics	MAE	MSE	RMSE	*C*	*d*	ε
Bitcoin	2.3090	0.1275	0.3570	1	1	0.1
Dash	56.3903	605.5746	77.8187	1	1	0.1
Ethereum	7.5450	10.3500	10.2000	1	1	0.1
AUDUSD	0.0020	0.000006	0.0025	1	1	0.1
USDCAD	0.0025	0.00001	0.0033	1	1	0.1

Table 6. SVM-Sigmoid Kernel

SVM-Sigmoid						
Metrics	MAE	MSE	RMSE	*C*	γ	ε
Bitcoin	20.080	58.710	24.231	1.0	0.167	0.1
Dash	2.114	7.568	2.751	1.0	0.167	0.1
Ethereum	14.713	31.060	17.625	1.0	0.167	0.1
AUDUSD	0.614	0.561	0.749	1.0	0.167	0.1
USDCAD	0.166	0.042	0.206	1.0	0.167	0.1

Table 7. SVM-Benchmark Models.

SVM			
Metrics	MAE	MSE	RMSE
Bitcoin	0.0291	20.1530	0.0449
Dash	30.50323	2917.1102	54.010
Ethereum	10.6959	263.2240	16.224
AUDUSD	0.0165	0.0004	0.019
USDCAD	0.0026	0.000012	0.0034

where the MAE, MSE, and RMSE are 30.50323, 2917.1102, and 54.010, respectively. The same thing is happening with Ethereum, AUDUSD, and USDCAD. Even though the SVM-Linear beats the SVM-RBF on the AUDUSD dataset, the difference is just 0.02 points. As a result, SVM-RBF is still recognized as the best prediction model in this study.

5 Conclusion

To recapitulate, the study's goal is to use the SVM and its four kernel functions to get an accurate forecast of financial instruments, namely the Bitcoin and Forex markets. This article initially presents an SVM model that uses the rule of SVM generalization ability, followed by the rule's determination by optimizing the SVM's kernel parameters. The findings show that when the optimum hyper parameters are combined with the sentiment and the technical indicator, the model produces the least amount of error, demonstrating the proposed model's generalizability. The SVM-RBF model is more predictive than the other models due to an enhanced part of the kernel function. Four kernels are used for comparison, and they are compared and assessed.

According to the final findings, SVM-RBF beat other SVM-kernel forecasting models. The variations in the prices of the instruments are also observed to be affected by the other components, which are the CCI and sentiment data. Further study in SVM with other optimization methods is required in the future to understand the role of kernels in Computational Intelligence (CI). Correspondingly, since the accuracy rate was influenced by a variety of parameters, future research will focus on constructing forecasting models that take into account a wider range of time spans and dataset types, as indicated in the introductory section.

References

1. Tandon, C., Revankar, S., Palivela, H., Parihar, S.S.: How can we predict the impact of the social media messages on the value of cryptocurrency? Insights from big data analytics," Int. J. Inf. Manag. Data Insights **1**(2), 100035 (2021)
2. Kim, K.J.: Financial time series forecasting using support vector machines. Neurocomputing **55**(1–2), 307–319 (2003)
3. Alali, A.: Application of Support Vector Machine in Predicting the Market' s Monthly Trend Direction, pp. 12–22 (2013)
4. Kazem, A., Sharifi, E., Hussain, F.K., Saberi, M., Hussain, O.K.: Support vector regression with chaos-based firefly algorithm for stock market price forecasting. Appl. Soft Comput. **13**(2), 947–958 (2013)
5. Wang, G.L.G., et al.: The performance of PSO-SVM in inflation forecasting. In: 2017 10th Int. Conf. Intell. Comput. Technol. Autom. **1**(1), 259–262 (2016)
6. Panigrahi, S.S., Reader, D.J.K.M.: Epsilon-SVR and decision tree for stock market forecasting, pp. 761–766 (2012)
7. Zhu, J.P., Zhou, L.C., Liu, C.B.: Modeling of fermentation process based on MOACO and ε-SVM. In: 2009 International Conference on Artificial Intelligence and Computational Intelligence AICI 2009, vol. 2, pp. 234–239 (2009)
8. Xiao, T., Ren, D., Lei, S., Zhang, J., Liu, X.: Based on grid-search and PSO parameter optimization for support vector machine. In: Proceedings of the World Congress on Intelligent Control Automation, vol. 2015-March, no. March, pp. 1529–1533 (2015)
9. Hitam, N.A., Ismail, A.R.: Comparative performance of machine learning algorithms for cryptocurrency forecasting. Indones. J. Electr. Eng. Comput. Sci. **11**(3), 1121–1128 (2018)
10. Siddique, M., Mohanty, S., Panda, D.: A hybrid model for forecasting of stock value of tata steel using orthogonal forward selection, support vector regression and teaching learning based optimization. Far East J. Math. Sci. **113**(1), 95–114 (2019)

11. Delimata, P., Suraj, Z.: Hybrid methods in data classification and reduction. Intell. Syst. Ref. Libr. **43**, 263–291 (2013)
12. Yang, Z., Shi, K., Wu, A., Qiu, M., Hu, Y.: A hybird method based on particle swarm optimization and moth-flame optimization. In: Proceedings - 2019 11th International Conference on Intelligent Human-Machine Systems Cybernetics IHMSC 2019, vol. 2, pp. 207–210 (2019)
13. Chen, R.: Using SVM with financial statement analysis for prediction of stocks. Analysis **7**(4), 63–72 (2007)
14. Nahil, A., Lyhyaoui, A.: Stock price prediction based on SVM : the impact of the stock market indices on the model performance, vol. 21, pp. 91–95 (2017)
15. Zhen, L.Z., Ch, Y., Muda, A.K.: Forecasting FTSE bursa Malaysia KLCI Trend with Hybrid Particle Swarm Optimization and Support Vector Machine Technique (2013)
16. Hitam, N.A., Ismail, A.R., Saeed, F.: An optimized Support Vector Machine (SVM) based on Particle Swarm Optimization (PSO) for cryptocurrency forecasting. Procedia Comput. Sci. **163**, 427–433 (2019)
17. Qiao, Y., Peng, J., Ge, L., Wang, H.: Application of PSO LS-SVM forecasting model in oil and gas production forecast. In: Proceedings of the 2017 IEEE 16th International Conference on Cognitive Informatics and Cognitive Computing (ICCI "CC" 17), pp. 470–474 (2017)
18. Hitam, N.A., Ismail, A.R., Samsudin, R., Ameerbakhsh, O.: The Influence of Sentiments in Digital Currency Prediction Using Hybrid Sentiment-based Support Vector Machine with Whale Optimization Algorithm (SVMWOA), pp. 1–7 (2021)
19. Kouziokas, G.N.: SVM kernel based on particle swarm optimized vector and Bayesian optimized SVM in atmospheric particulate matter forecasting. Appl. Soft Comput. J. **93**, 106410 (2020)
20. Akay, M.F., Abut, F., Daneshvar, S., Heil, D.: Prediction of upper body power of cross-country skiers using support vector machines. Arab. J. Sci. Eng. **40**(4), 1045–1055 (2015)
21. Lu, Y., Zhu, J., Zhang, N., Shao, Q.: A hybrid switching PSO algorithm and support vector machines for bankruptcy prediction. In: 2014 International Conference on Mechatronics Control, no. ICMC, pp. 1329–1333 (2014)
22. Shehab, M., Alshawabkah, H., Abualigah, L., AL-Madi, N.: Enhanced a hybrid moth-flame optimization algorithm using new selection schemes. Eng. Comput. **37**(4), 2931–2956 (2020). https://doi.org/10.1007/s00366-020-00971-7
23. Law, T., Shawe-Taylor, J.: Practical Bayesian support vector regression for financial time series prediction and market condition change detection. Quant. Financ. **17**(9), 1403–1416 (2017)
24. Xu, S., Chan, H.K.: Forecasting medical device demand with online search queries: a big data and machine learning approach. Proc. Manuf. **39**(2019), 32–39 (2019)
25. Lin, X., Tang, Y.: Interbank offered rate forecasting using PSO-LS-SVM. In: Proceedings - 2015 11th International Confernce on Computational Intelligent and Security CIS 2015, pp. 26–29 (2016)
26. Yeh, C.-Y., Huang, C.-W., Lee, S.-J.: A multiple-kernel support vector regression approach for stock market price forecasting. Expert Syst. Appl. **38**(3), 2177–2186 (2011)
27. Rauber, T.W., Berns, K.: Kernel multilayer perceptron. In: Proceedings - 24th SIBGRAPI Conference and Graphics, Patterns and Images, no. August, pp. 337–343 (2011)
28. Long, W., Song, L., Tian, Y.: A new graphic kernel method of stock price trend prediction based on financial news semantic and structural similarity. Expert Syst. Appl. **118**, 411–424 (2019)
29. Castoe, M.: Predicting Stock Market Price Direction with Uncertainty Using Quantile Regression Forest, no. November (2020)
30. Zeng-min, W.: Application of Support Vector Regression Method in Stock Market Forecasting, no. 3, pp. 1–4 (2010)

31. Lahmiri, S.: Minute-ahead stock price forecasting based on singular spectrum analysis and support vector regression. Appl. Math. Comput. **320**, 444–451 (2018)
32. Chanklan, R., Kaoungku, N., Suksut, K., Kerdprasop, K., Kerdprasop, N.: Runoff prediction with a combined artificial neural network and support vector regression. Int. J. Mach. Learn. Comput. **8**(1), 39–43 (2018)

Comparative Study of Service-Based Sentiment Analysis of Social Networking Sites Fanatical Contents

Salisu Garba[1](✉), Marzuk Abdullahi[2], Reem Alkhammash[3], and Maged Nasser[1]

[1] School of Computing, Faculty of Engineering, Universiti Teknologi Malaysia, 81310 UTM Skudai, Johor, Malaysia
Salisu.garba@graduate.utm.my, msnmaged2@live.utm.my
[2] School of Computer Sciences, University Sains Malaysia, 11800 USM Pulau Pinang, Malaysia
[3] English Department, University College, Taraba, Taif University, P.O. BOX 11099, Taif 21944, Saudi Arabia

Abstract. The proliferation of mobile web services (MWS) for sentiment analysis makes it hard to identify the best MWS for sentiment analysis of social networking sites' fanatical contents. This paper carries out a comparative study of service-based sentiment analysis of social networking sites' fanatical contents. This is achieved by cleaning, transformation, and reduction of fanatical contents from the publicly available social media dataset, and multiple MWS are selected for comparison using the application programming interface (API) key of the MWS. To evaluate the service-based sentiment analysis, standard measures such as accuracy, precision, recall, and f-measures of sentiment result for each MWS are used. The result shows that Dandelion SA performs better in terms of accuracy (72.5%) and recall (76.9%), while Wingify SA performs better in terms of precision (88.6%) and f-measure (75.5%), though AlchemyAPI offers the most crucial elements in analyzing sentiments such as emotion, relevance score, and sentiment type. The outcomes of this paper will benefit the sentiment analysis service developers, sentiment analysis service requesters as well as other researchers in the social media fanatical content domain.

Keywords: Sentiment analysis · Mobile web service · Social media · Fanatical contents

1 Introduction

In modern society, social networking sites (SNS) have become an integral platform for interaction between people across the world. SNS like Twitter and Facebook are widely used for sharing and accessing all sorts of content such as personal points of view, an emotion about certain topics, etc. [1]. These SNS has undoubtedly generated a massive amount of data in the form of tweets, status updates, posts, reviews, and comments which contain a lot of fanatical content. Fanatical contents are normally shared by individuals with extreme political or religious views, particularly those who advocate illegal, violent, or other extreme action [2].

F. Saeed et al. (Eds.): IRICT 2021, LNDECT 127, pp. 333–342, 2022.
https://doi.org/10.1007/978-3-030-98741-1_28

One of the global scenarios of fanaticism is about how religion has been widely blamed for violence [3]. With the rise of issues on fanaticism, there need to control the rate of users expressing or disseminating fanatical rage on SNA. It is also important to counter this kind of threat to maintaining the wellbeing of societies across the globe. As such, Natural Language Processing (NLP) techniques such as sentiment analysis are used to identify fanatical contents from the SNS to create awareness among society as it has established quite an active online presence nowadays [4]. SA deals with many challenges through NLP because it is a difficult task. It has been proven in the study made by [2], that it is extremely challenging to study the text effectively at an arbitrary level of detail as outlined in the definition, and not to forget, most of the data gathered are subjective.

A lightweight software system designed to support interoperable machine-to-machine interaction across a network with an interface described using adaptable protocols, RESTful description, smaller message formats popularly known as Mobile Web Service (MWS) are now used for SA [5, 6]. There are various choices of MWS, each has its specialty that help researchers in identifying sentiment [7]. However, not all MWS offer the same functions. Some may just allow a user to check the sentiment polarity of a text without being able to view the confidence score. Thus, in this case, it should be stressed that SA should not only aim to achieve sentiment polarity from data but also to discover the most accurate result generated by the MWS. The proliferation of MWS for sentiment analysis makes it hard to identify the best MWS for sentiment analysis of SNS fanatical contents.

Based on the existing research, not many researchers have studied MWS for SA. In rare cases, [7] compared 15 different web services specialized in sentiment analysis of three types of datasets which is from large movie dataset, Twitter dataset, and Amazon product review dataset. However, the comparative analysis of MWS for SA focused more on two datasets (movie and product review) instead of MWS for SA of fanatical contents in SNS. Knowing that SNS is widely used nowadays, the idea of extracting data from it is acceptable as it gives different accuracy results when tested in different MWS. Therefore, the focus of this research is to see how accurate each MWS is in generating sentiment results by comparing its mean square error. For the least mean square error, a value that is closer to zero will indicates a better result [8].

In this study, data is gathered from two social networking sites (Twitter and Facebook) for service-based sentiment analysis to identify fanatics-related content. multiple MWS designs for SA such as MonkeyLearn, Semantria, ParallelDots, Text2Data, etc. are selected for comparison using the application programming interface (API) key of the MWS. Standard measures such as accuracy, precision, recall, and f-measures, are used to evaluate the service-based sentiment analysis so as to find the best MWS for analyzing sentiment on social networking sites' fanatical contents.

As a contribution, this paper presents an extensive and deeper critical evaluation of the main functionalities of six SA-related MWS. This research will help in proving the best MWS in terms of giving an accurate result of SA. Moreover, it will enable other researchers to have sufficient information on the capabilities of these MWS and helps them to choose the most suitable one to be used for their specific purposes especially in analyzing sentiment related to serious issues like fanatism so as to create awareness, stimulate big techs and policymakers to control this issue from wide-spreading around the world. The remaining of the paper is organized as follows. In Sect. 2, the related works are discussed. In Sect. 3, the methodology is presented. The results and discussions are presented in Sect. 4. Finally, the conclusions and future recommendations are given in Sect. 5.

2 Related Work

This section reviews various works related to this research. These include social media fanatical content, sentiment analysis, and mobile web service.

2.1 Fanatical Contents Sentiment Analysis

Over the years, social networking sites such as Twitter, Facebook, and other discussion forums are abused by fanatics, radicals, extremists, propagandists, etc. to share and promote hate speech, offensive comments, religious ambiguity with deceptive intentions, manipulated political and social views [1]. Researchers from different domains e.g. sociology, data science, and software engineering, etc. are continually creating tools to help individuals, societies, big techs, and policymakers battle and conquer these issues of manipulation, radicalization, etc. from wide-spreading around the world [4]. Subsequently, SNS sentiment analysis and automatic detection of fanatical contents is a significant issue for peace and security. Sentiment Analysis (SA), also called Opinion Mining aims to analyze the sentiments, opinions, attitudes, and emotions of individuals towards subjects, products, individuals, organizations, and services [9–11]. SA involves the classification of sentiment text into classes such as positive, negative, and neutral.

There are numerous researches related to sentiment analysis of social networking sites' fanatical contents. For example, [6–8] highlighted the use of lexicon-based and machine learning approaches. A piece of a text message is represented as a bag of words in a lexicon-based approach. Following this representation of the message, all positive and negative words or phrases within the message are assigned to either dictionary-based sentiment values or corpus-based sentiment values. Moreover, [2, 4] experimented with models such as the unigram model, a feature-based model, and a tree kernel-based model to classify sentiment analysis on Twitter data where combining prior word polarity with their Part of Speech (POS) tags play an important role in a classification task. It's also observed that POS can be assigned to an input sequence word based on POS tag from relevant words in relevant training sequence identified using global semantic information.

2.2 Web Service-Based Sentiment Analysis

Several authors have recognized the importance of web service-based sentiment analysis [7, 8, 13, 14]. These software systems designed to support interoperable machine-to-machine interaction known as Mobile Web Service (MWS) are now used for SA and the capabilities of MWS in examining the accurate result in analyzing sentiment is the key performance indicator for determining the quality of service. According to [7], document level SA was proven as the most used feature among all levels of SA. In this features, the various task is provided including three different classifications of sentiment which is positive, negative, and neutral. Compared to the other features that mostly provide only positive and negative classes, the document level SA deals with tagging individual documents to find sentiment polarities with three different classes. Therefore, in this research, only MWS that offers document-level SA and polarity will be considered.

Several researchers have used different techniques in evaluating the capability of MWS in terms of accuracy and polarity of sentiment. For example [7, 8, 14] focus on analyzing the capabilities of MWS to classify and score various texts with regards to the sentiments in it. most of the MWS uses various categorization of SA techniques which are machine learning approach and lexicon-based approach, dictionary-based lexicon approach, and corpus-based lexicon approach. The corpus-based approach in [7, 8, 14] mainly relies on a sentiment lexicon and has statistical and semantic techniques which measure a perceived meaning of an object that led to a result of sentiment analysis. These researches focused on three different datasets which were from large movie reviews, Twitter, and Amazon product reviews.

Despite the many contributions of [1–3, 7, 8, 12–14], the comparative analysis of MWS for SA focused more on very few MWS that does not consider sentiment polarity of a text. Given that SNS like Twitter and Facebook are widely used for sharing fanatical contents by individuals (fanatics, radicals, extremists, propagandists, etc.) with extreme political or religious views, particularly those who advocate illegal, violent, or other extreme action [1, 2], there is a clear lack of focus on fanatical contents and only focused on one dataset from SNS which is Twitter, while the other two datasets are from movie and product review. Because of these shortcomings, the idea of a comparative study of service-based sentiment analysis of social networking sites' fanatical contents is very motivating and important. The focus of this research is to see how accurate each MWS is in generating sentiment results.

3 Methodology

The methodology used in conducting the comparative study of service-based sentiment analysis of social networking sites' fanatical contents comprises of four stages (data collection, data pre-processing, service-based sentiment analysis, and comparison of service-based sentiment analysis). The four stages are explained in Sect. 3.1, 3.2, 3.3, and 3.4 respectively.

3.1 Data Collection

Datasets from social networking sites (Twitter and Facebook) provide a large data for service-based sentiment analysis of fanatical contents, therefore, tweets and posts gathered from Twitter [15] and Facebook [16] are used as our benchmark data. Concerning the first collection of datasets (from Twitter), the tweets contain a lot of opinions that were expressed by different users. The second collection of datasets (from Facebook) did not show much difference from the first collection except for the longer length of sentences. Both of it contains neutral opinion as well as positive and negative opinion. However, to assess the performance of MWS, only a few documents from the whole datasets will be used. All the datasets were extracted based on the list of keywords that are associated with fanatical content.

3.2 Data Pre-processing

Pre-processing of dataset helps in preparing the raw data that has been gathered for the service-based sentiment analysis of social networking site fanatical contents. These involve text cleaning, white space removal, expanding abbreviation, stemming, stopping words removal, negation handling, etc. [3, 15, 16]. The processed dataset is further used for feature extraction to compute the polarity of the sentence which is useful in determining opinion. The RStudio provides an ability to pre-process data. Therefore, RStudio is used for cleaning, transformation, and reduction of fanatical contents from the publicly available social media dataset.

3.3 Service-Based Sentiment Analysis

Several MWS for sentiment analysis are chosen for the comparative study of service-based sentiment analysis of social networking sites' fanatical contents [7, 8, 14]. Considering that the document level SA deals with tagging individual documents to find sentiment polarities with three different classes (positive, negative, and neutral), ten MWS (DeepAI SA, AlchemyAPI, Lymbix SA, Musicmetric, Twinword SA, Semantria, ParallelDots SA, Dandelion SA, Wingify, and Sentimetrix) are selected from the programmableweb.com. Popularity, ease of use, and the maximum amount of data that each MWS can handle are used as the basis for selecting the ten MWS for sentiment analysis.

Mobile Web Service (MWS) bringing about convenience and simplicity in accessing web service through mobile devices. The sentiment analysis service provider publishes its services to the local registry. A service request is sent to the local registry. The communication between the request and the response is carried out through API. Lightweight protocols such as kXML2, kSOAP2, are adapted to overcome the significant overhead of the original SOAP implementation. Figure 1 shows the overview of MWS communication architecture. The MWS is called through the API after authentication and the dataset is parsed after which the MWS functionality is applied to obtain the SA result.

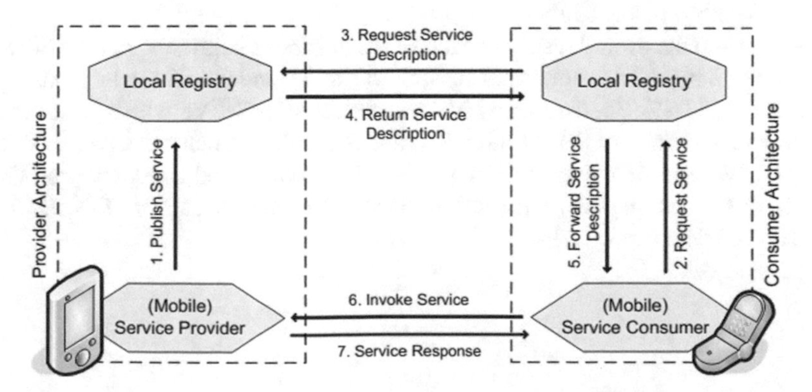

Fig. 1. Overview of MWS communication architecture.

3.4 Performance Evaluation of the Mobile Web Services

The performance of each MWS is measured by accuracy, precision, recall, and f- measure. Accuracyis the level of closeness between sentiment polarity obtained from the MWS and the actual value of the sentiment polarity, the accuracy is calculated using Eq. 1. Precision is used to measure the level of correctness of the sentiment analysis results generated by each MWS, the precision is calculated using Eq. 2. The recall is used to measure the ability of each MWS to find sentiment polarities with three different classes (positive, negative, and neutral) within the dataset, the recall is calculated using Eq. 3. F-measure is the harmonic mean or weighted average of the precision and recall. The F-measure is calculated using Eq. 4. Four classifications are used to measure the performance of each MWS. These are True Positive (TP), False Positive (FP), False Negative (FN), and True Negative (TN).

$$\text{Accuracy} = \frac{TP + TN}{TP + TN + FP + FN} \tag{1}$$

$$\text{Precision} = \frac{TP}{(TP + FP)} \tag{2}$$

$$\text{Recall} = \frac{TP}{(TP + FN)} \tag{3}$$

$$\text{F-Measure} = 2 * \frac{\text{Precision} * \text{Recall}}{\text{Precision} + \text{Recall}} \tag{4}$$

4 Results and Discussions

The performance of each MWS is obtained after experimental evaluation. The evaluation results are based on four criteria (accuracy, precision, recall, and f-measure). Table 1 presents the results of the comparative study of service-based sentiment analysis of social networking sites fanatical contents. The MWS with good accuracy are Dandelion SA, Twinword SA, AlchemyAPI, and Lymbix SA which has an accuracy of 72.5%, 69.2%, 63.4%, and 62.8% respectively.

Looking into the overall result for each MWS in Table 1 below, the MWS with a good precision are Wingify, Sentimetrix, Musicmetric, and Dandelion SA which has a precision of 88.6%, 82.4%, 75.2%, and 67.3% respectively. The MWS with a good recall are Dandelion SA, Twinword SA, Lymbix SA, and Semantria which has a recall of 76.9%, 70.5%, 68.2%, and 67.6% respectively. The MWS with good accuracy are Wingify, Dandelion SA, AlchemyAPI, and Sentimetrix which have an accuracy of 75.5%, 71.8%, 65.9%, and 65.5% respectively.

Table 1. The performance of each mobile web service for SA.

MWS	Accuracy	Precision	Recall	F-measure
DeepAI SA	0.614	0.560	0.597	0.578
AlchemyAPI	0.634	0.672	0.647	0.659
Lymbix SA	0.628	0.615	0.682	0.647
Musicmetric	0.527	0.752	0.531	0.622
Twinword SA	0.692	0.591	0.705	0.643
Semantria	0.619	0.571	0.676	0.619
ParallelDots SA	0.562	0.510	0.564	0.536
Dandelion SA	**0.725**	0.673	**0.769**	0.718
Wingify	0.591	**0.886**	0.658	**0.755**
Sentimetrix	0.571	0.824	0.543	0.655

Dandelion SA presents the highest accuracy result with 72.5%. It also computes the highest results in recall as shown in Fig. 2. Dandelion SA might seem the best MWS to classify positive text. This is because it gives the highest amount of positive sentiment among all MWS. Moreover, the amount of negative classified sentiment from Dandelion SA is the lowest. Wingify SA presents the highest precision result with 88.6%. It also computes the highest results in f-measure. Dandelion SA might seem the best MWS to classify both positive text and negative text. This is because it provided a better level of correctness in terms of positive sentiment and negative sentiments among all the MWS.

AlchemyAPI gave a comparable number for all the four criteria (accuracy, precision, recall, and f-measure) as shown in Fig. 1 and Fig. 2. It portrays a balance in terms of reviews of positive (precision and recall) and f-measures. Though it's limited when compared with other MWS such as Dandelion SA, Wingify. On average, Twinword SA, and Sentimetrix also gives a good result during testing as it appears as the second-best group of MWS (after Wingify and Dandelion SA) in terms of the four evaluation criteria. While ParallelDots SA and DeepAI SA perform slightly less than their counterpart in terms of service-based sentiment analysis of social networking sites fanatical contents.

Based on the analysis of the results, it is noticeable that all the MWS do offer a slightly higher than average result for an accurate polarity (positive, negative, or neutral) especially for service-based sentiment analysis of social networking sites fanatical contents. Contrary to what has been stated in [2, 7, 8, 14], it is proven that ParallelDots SA and Twinword SA are the most widely used MWS that classify both short and long text. While ParallelDots SA and Wingify show the best accuracy and precision respectively. However, when working with larger text, all the MWS have shown no problem in performing sentiment analysis. Despite the ironic nature of fanatical content in social networking sites, which could be regarded as very difficult to detect, it is noteworthy the fact that all the MWS can perform reasonably well. And lastly, it is essential to say that artificial intelligence-based MWS like DeepAI SA might hold the key for service-based sentiment analysis of social networking sites' fanatical contents given the trajectory of AI successes (Fig. 3).

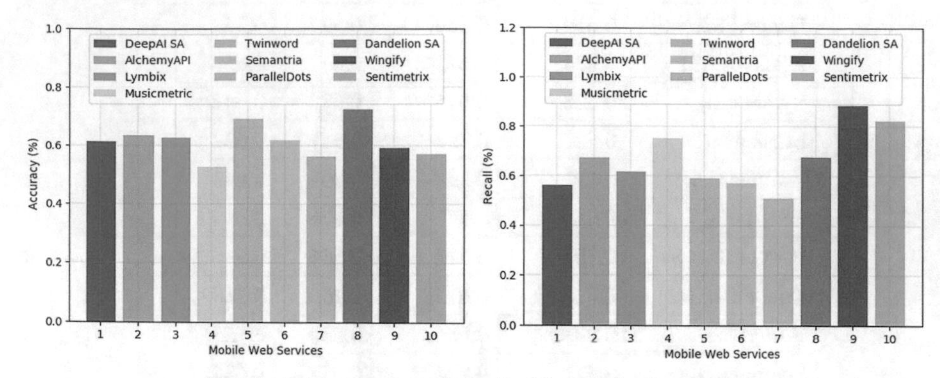

Fig. 2. The accuracy and recall of the service-based SA.

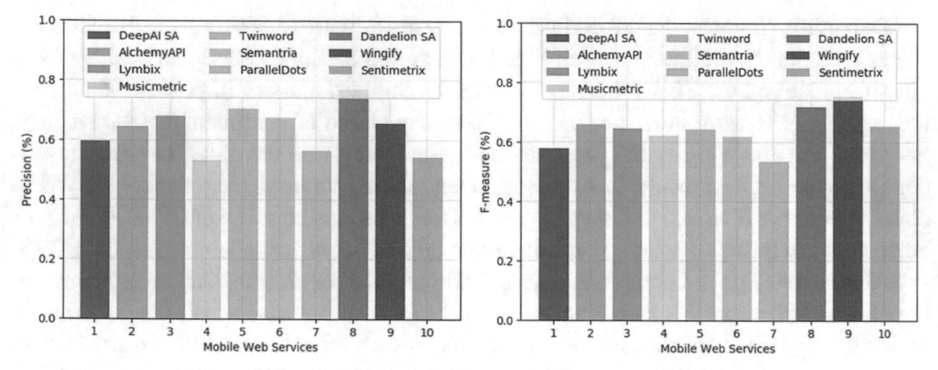

Fig. 3. The precision and f-measure of the service-based SA.

5 Conclusion and Future Work

This presented a comparative study of service-based sentiment analysis of social networking sites fanatical contents. To ease the selection of the most suitable MWS for fanatical contents sentiment analysis, ten MWS are selected for comparison using the application programming interface (API) key of the MWS, while the datasets from social networking sites (Twitter and Facebook) provide a large data for service-based sentiment analysis of fanatical contents is used as our benchmark data. Despite the ironic nature of fanatical content in social networking sites, which could be regarded as very difficult to detect, overall, the results demonstrate that Dandelion SA has the highest accuracy (72.5%) and recall (76.9%) results. While Wingify SA presents the highest precision (88.6%) and f-measure (75.5%) result. The outcomes of this paper will benefit the sentiment analysis service developers, sentiment analysis service requesters as well as other researchers in the social media fanatical content domain. The future work aims at exploiting the non-functional correlation between the MWS for sentiment analysis service developers to further improve the precision and accuracy as close to 100% as possible. Moreover, it is essential to explore artificial intelligence-based MWS like DeepAI SA which might hold the key for service-based sentiment analysis of social networking sites' fanatical contents given the trajectory of AI successes.

References

1. Adek, R.T., Bustami, Ula, M.: Systematics review on the application of social media analytics for detecting radical and extremist group. IOP Conf. Ser. Mater. Sci. Eng. **1071**(1), 012029 (2021)
2. Asif, M., Ishtiaq, A., Ahmad, H., Aljuaid, H., Shah, J.: Telematics and Informatics Sentiment analysis of extremism in social media from textual information. Telemat. Inform. **48**, 101345 (2020)
3. Karampelas, P., Bourlai, T., Surveillance, C., Wei, Y., Singh, L.: Detecting users who share extremist content on twitter. In: Karampelas, P., Bourlai, T. (eds.) Surveillance in Action, pp. 351–368. Springer, Cham (2018). https://doi.org/10.1007/978-3-319-68533-5_17
4. Kursuncu, U., et al.: Modeling islamist extremist communications on social media using contextual dimensions: Religion, ideology, and hate. In: Proceedings of the ACM Human-Computer Interaction, vol. 3, no. CSCW (2019)
5. Garba, S., Mohamad, R., Saadon, N.A.: Web service discovery approaches for dynamic mobile environment. Int. J. E-Serv. Mob. Appl. **13**(4), 16–38 (2019)
6. Garba, S., Mohamad, R., Saadon, N.A.: Search space reduction approach for self-adaptive web service discovery in dynamic mobile environment. In: Saeed, F., Mohammed, F., Gazem, N. (eds.) IRICT 2019. AISC, vol. 1073, pp. 1111–1121. Springer, Cham (2020). https://doi.org/10.1007/978-3-030-33582-3_104
7. Serrano-guerrero, J., Olivas, J.A., Romero, F.P., Herrera-viedma, E.: Sentiment analysis: a review and comparative analysis of web services. Inf. Sci. (NY) **311**, 18–38 (2015)
8. Basmmi, A.B.M.N., Abd Halim, S., Saadon, N.A.: Comparison of web services for sentiment analysis in social networking sites. In: IOP Conference Series: Materials Science and Engineering, vol. 884, no. 1, p. 12063 (2020)
9. Alam, M., Abid, F., Guangpei, C., Yunrong, L.V.: Social media sentiment analysis through parallel dilated convolutional neural network for smart city applications. Comput. Commun. **154**, 129–137 (2020)
10. Sawarn, A., Gupta, M.: Comparative analysis of bagging and boosting algorithms for sentiment analysis. Procedia Comput. Sci. **173**, 210–215 (2020)
11. Atoum, I.: A novel framework for measuring software quality-in-use based on semantic similarity and sentiment analysis of software reviews. J. King Saud. Univ. Comput. Inf. Sci. **32**(1), 113–125 (2020)
12. Ferrara, E.: Contagion dynamics of extremist propaganda in social networks. Inf. Sci. (NY) **418–419**, 1–12 (2017)
13. Khan, H.U., Peacock, D.: Possible effects of emoticon and emoji on sentiment analysis web services of work organisations. Int. J. Work Organ. Emot. **10**(2), 130–161 (2019)
14. Gao, S., Hao, J., Fu, Y.: The application and comparison of web services for sentiment analysis in tourism. In: 12th International Conference on Service Systems and Service Management (ICSSSM), pp. 1–6 (2015)
15. Pak, A., Paroubek, P.: Twitter as a corpus for sentiment analysis and opinion mining. In: Proceedings of the 7th International Conference on Language Resource Evaluation Learning 2010, pp. 1320–1326 (2010)

16. Ortigosa, A., Martín, J.M., Carro, R.M.: Sentiment analysis in Facebook and its application to e-learning. Comput. Hum. Behav. **31**(1), 527–541 (2014)

Networking and IoT

An Overview on LoRaWAN Technology Simulation Tools

Mukarram A. M. Almuhaya[1,2(✉)], Waheb A. Jabbar[1,3], Noorazliza Sulaiman[1], and A. H. A. Sulaiman[1]

[1] Faculty of Electrical and Electronic Engineering Technology, Universiti Malaysia Pahang, 26600 Pekan, Pahang, Malaysia
almohia82@yahoo.com, waheb@ieee.org

[2] Sana'a Community College (SCC), Sana'a, Republic of Yemen

[3] Centre of Software Development and Integrated Computing, University Malaysia Pahang, 26300 Gambang, Pahang, Malaysia

Abstract. Low-Power Wide Area Networks (LPWAN) technologies are playing a pivotal role in the IoT applications owing to their capability to meet the keys IoT requirements, i.e., long-range, low cost, small data volumes, massive devices number, and low energy consumption. The creation of new public and private LoRaWAN networks necessitates the use of avoiding node limits and collision prevention measures. Designers of IoT systems confront difficulty in determining the scalability of a given technology, with an emphasis on unlicensed frequency bandwidth (ISM) transmission in densely populated locations. However, picking the best simulation software might be a challenge. To provide a conceptual overview of seven LoRaWAN simulation tools, this paper outlines their key characteristics and the sorts of experiments they support. LoRaWAN simulators, resource utilization, and performance evaluation are all covered in-depth in this report. Furthermore, we classify and compare the most important simulation tools for investigating and analyzing LoRa/LoRaWAN network emulators that have been developed recently. This article will be used to help other researchers decide whether LoRaWAN simulation tool is best for their specific requirements.

Keywords: IoT · LPWAN · LoRa · LoRaWAN · LoRa simulation tools

1 Introduction

The LoRa is LPWAN technology which acquiring increasing attention from both academia and industry. To provide connectivity to a wide field of IoT devices, it is ideal for a low-power wide-area network's internet requirements(LPWAN). Chirp Spread Spectrum (CSS) modulation establishes a distinct radio layer from other types of wireless networks that use other modulations. Due to its high sensitivity, the LoRa CSS modulation allows for indoor transmissions with a range of several kilometres.[1]. To connect to the network server, the LoRaWAN device needs to be awakened and immediately transmits a packet to the network server through the gateway. This is similar to how ALOHA works [2]. The LoRaWAN systems that are spreading to various architectures

F. Saeed et al. (Eds.): IRICT 2021, LNDECT 127, pp. 345–358, 2022.
https://doi.org/10.1007/978-3-030-98741-1_29

are becoming increasingly complex, heterogeneous and pervasive. As such, it has proved difficult to research and design such systems. The lack of suitable modelling and simulation platforms to provide an end-to-end depiction of Connected IoT devices, i.e. from the basic IoT end-nodes to the cloud application and the fundamental networking infrastructure [3, 4]. Maximum node count constraints and collision avoidance algorithms are critical in the creation of new public and private LoRaWAN networks. The simulators mentioned in this article are used to model these issues. LoRaWAN techniques are equally important to model topological networks. The main challenges facing computer simulation environments are algorithms that support the positioning of gateways in combination with radio range modelling in urban environments. To assist practitioners and researchers overcome these challenges we propose this work as comparing between the commonly used LoRa/LoRaWAN simulation tools by highlighting their capabilities and features for enabling researchers to select the most suitable simulator based on their needs and programming skills. The platforms can model heterogeneous LoRa nodes (sensors, gateways, network servers, and so on) with quite well details (mobility, energy profile, scalability, and so on), diverse application logic and network connectivity models, as well. The proposed work is distinct from the existing literature, presents a comparative review of a selected seven driving LoRaWAN Simulators LoRaSim, NS3, Cupcurpon, FloRa, SimpleIoTSimulator and Mbed simulator, and gives a rundown of the most popular LoRa MAC network simulators and highlighted their most important features.

The rest of this paper is organized as follows: in Sect. 2, we exhibit an overview of the LoRa/LoRaWAN technology. Then Sect. 3 surveys the available simulation tools to analyze LoRa/LoRaWAN performance. Discussion of the comparison in Sect. 4. Finally, we conclude the article in Sect. 5.

2 LoRal/LoRaWAN

LoRa is a modulation technology patented and acquired by Semtech Corporation in 2012 for wireless communications [5]. LoRa is created to operate on a sub-GHz frequency, specifically on unlicensed bands such as 915 MHz, 868 MHz, or 433 MHz, in accordance with the regional area regulations. LoRa is a physical layer based on the Chirp Spread Spectrum (CSS) modulation, not similar to other modulations which using in other wireless networks [6]. LoRa was designed to be low-rate, low-power, and transmission with very long-range in line-of-sight or rural areas situations up to 10 or 20 km for outdoor, as a result of the higher sensitivity of LoRa CSS modulation, which enabling long distances connectivity [2]. Its low energy consumption, coupled with long-distance communication, makes LoRa be one of the potential candidates of LPWAN technologies for IoT applications [7]. As one of the most significant benefits of LoRa, the great receiver sensitivity is accompanied by an extremely wide communication connection budget. When utilizing LoRa modulation, typical values of SNR for 10 and 12 spreading factors are −20 dB and −15 dB, respectively, resulting in receiver sensitivities of −134 dBm and −129 dBm, according to the manufacturer. However, these values are only somewhat equivalent to the average sensitivity of Wi-Fi or Bluetooth receivers, which is typically in the range of 40 dBm to 80 dBm [6].

LoRaWAN networks can be generally utilized for fairly dense deployments with relaxed latency or reliability requirements. LoRaWAN offers many advantages in terms of low bit rate, power consumption, wide coverage, simplicity, and ease of management. While the LoRa modulation is proprietary, the LoRaWAN is an open standard being developed by the LoRa Alliance [8]. Each gateway in LoRaWAN networks receives messages from numerous end devices directly via a star topology. Transmitters employ TCP/IP protocols to communicate with network servers over a network connection. LoRaWAN's MAC uses Pure-ALOHA as its foundation. The LoRa specification defines three device classes that the end nodes must operate in, Class A, Class B and Class C. A LoRaWAN technology architecture defines three fundamental types of devices as follows [9]:

- End-devices (ED): These are devices that either take downlink (DL) traffic from the network server or generate uplink (UL) traffic for transmission to the gateways,
- Gateways (GW): These are the devices that demodulate LoRa communication and transmit it between the network server and the end devices in a wireless network. Wired or wireless access points link gateways to the Internet. The LoRaWAN Gateway is sophisticated, concurrently listening radio on several channels and delivering thousands of ENs simultaneously.
- Network Server (NS): The device which serves as the core backend of a LoRaWAN network, collecting traffic from all end-devices in the network and processing it on an application server

3 LoRa/LoraWAN Simulator Tools

Computer modelling and simulation is the proper method to enrich the exploration of systems performance and evaluate tactics for its functioning in imaginative or predictive approaches. A simulation model is a design that considers computing algorithms, physical and mathematical terms, and engineering formulas that summarise the behaviour and performance of a system's intangible world case studies. LoRa net-work simulation is more significant since it can be exploited without costly implementation or before the actual execution of the framework to design and evaluate a LoRa-based app. The field of LoRa offers highly specialized and freely available simulation tools. All these LoRa simulators have been developed and utilized in the literature for examining different LoRa scenarios, however, to the best of our understanding, none of the previous review studies compared in detail these simulation tools enough. Therefore, an overview of the most commonly used simulators to investigate Lo-Ra/LoRaWAN performance is presented in this section.

3.1 LoRaSim

LoRaSim has been developed based on SimPy as a discreet event simulator using Python to simulate, investigate, and analyze the LoRaWAN network scalability and collision functionality [10]. LoRaSim includes many Python scripts, the base of them are namely: loraDir.py, loraDirMulBs.py, directionalLoraIntf.py, and oneDirectional-LoraIntf.py, LoRaWAN.py, LoRaEnrgysim.py. The first script is for a lone gateway simulation, while loraDirMulBs.py is utilized to emulate several gateways (up to 24). DirectionalLoraIntf can emulate devices that are equipped with directional antennae and many networks, whereas oneDirectionalLoraIntf.py is for emulating gateways with directional antennae and many networks. A radio propagation model is implemented in LoRaSim depending on the well-known long-distance path loss model. The radio transceiver sensitivity at room temperature concerning various LoRa SFs and BWs settings is estimated. It also considers many related parameters such as the thermal noise power across, receiver bandwidth, noise figure, and SNR. Several packages are required for running LoRaSim smoothly, such as matplotlib, SimPy, and NumPy. LoRaSim offers a plots view of deployments with no graphical interface, as shown in Fig. 1. In contrast, it can show a data plot when users execute graphical code. Many improvements for LoRaSim were proposed to make it multipurpose [11–16] and support downlink due to the original version supported uplink only; thus, it can test scalability and energy consumption, and other matric performance. Many of the information is seen on the command line and exported to File-Name.dat, which can show its content data using other graphical programs such as Gnuplot, seaborn, Mplot, or others.

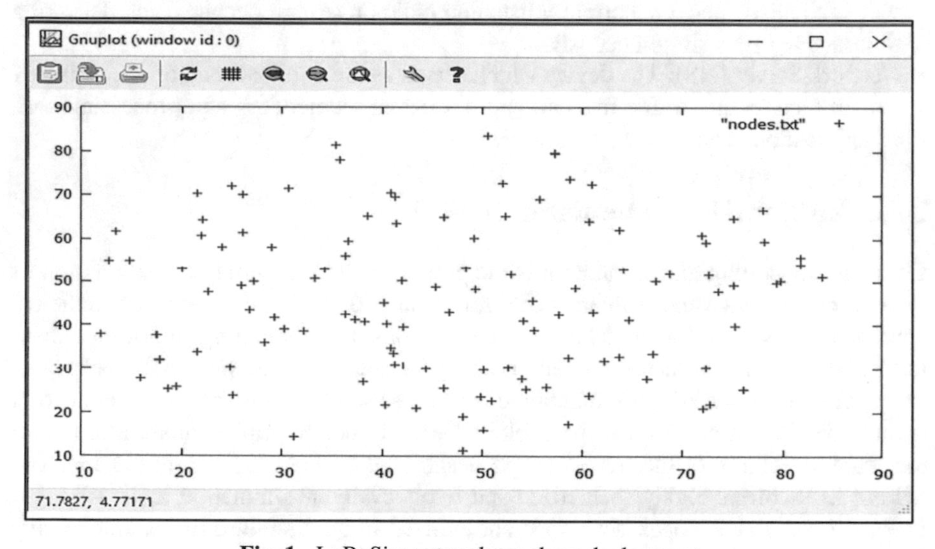

Fig. 1. LoRaSim network topology deployment

3.2 Ns-3

Ns-3 is an open-source discrete-event network simulator that was initiated in mid-2006 [17, 18] and is still under heavy development now, written by C++ and Python. The ns3 simulator supports a wide variety of protocols such as Wi-Fi, LTE, IEEE 802.15.4, SigFox, LoRa, further networks and also implements an IP networking, supports both simulation and emulation using sockets that aim to academic and research [19]. The ns-3 can be executed with pure C++, and some simulation components can be written with

Python. It is designed to be modular and can function in both graphical and command-line interfaces netanm for C++ and PyViz for Python. It also produces pcap tracks that can be used to debug. Standard software such as Wireshark [20] can be used to read trace files for network traffic analysis. The ns-3 offers a practical and well-structured setting with animation support using NetAnim, as shown in Fig. 2. A LoRaWAN Module was developed and implemented in ns-3 to provide a powerful tool for enabling the simulation of a real LoRaWAN network instead of simulating a simplified MAC protocol. This add-on module allows the research community and developers to more understanding of the behaviour of physical and MAC layers in LoRa networks. Credits to the LoRaSim that allows the users to test a network with varying SFs based on gateway feedbacks.

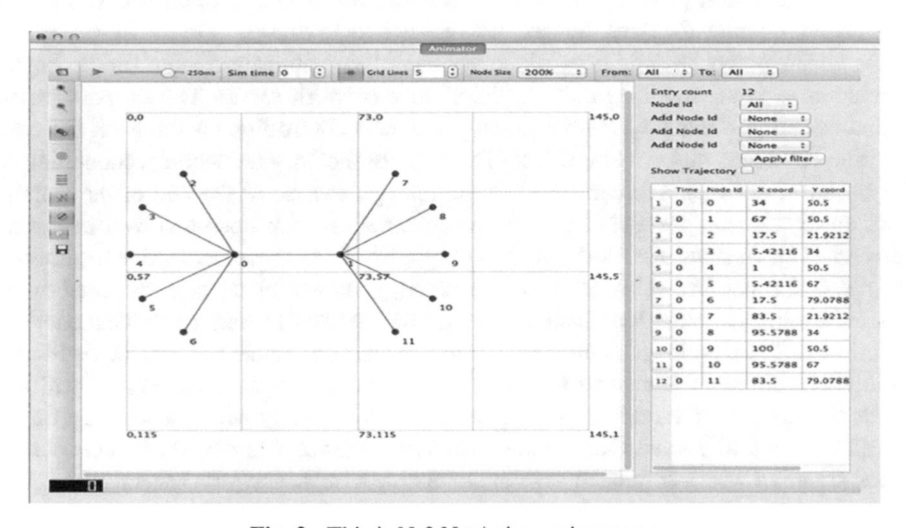

Fig. 2. This is Ns3 NetAnim environment

The LoRaWAN ns-3 module may be used to simulate LoRaWAN networks, and it is available for download here. Beyond the models created to represent different components of the network and the integrated helpers used to set them up, the ns-3 LoRaWAN module includes a packet tracker that can be used to monitor network behaviour and analyze its performance. It also includes facilities for storing the network topology in a file to debug and monitor. It also provides many scenarios as an example of simple to complex network use cases. The integrated LoRaWAN module meets the requirement of Class A devices. That means it can simulate the use cases where devices send uplinks and receive downlinks from the server. In comparison to LoRa's two other available classes (Class b and Class C), the most power-efficient end-devices is this class. To deliver a highly configurable, agile solution, the physical layer, MAC layer, and transport and use are built. Concerning the LoRaWAN-based ns-3 module's primary features, they are installation of the network server, ADR, confirmed messages and support for multi-GW. Configurability of the LoRaWAN ns-3 module proposed and allows new algorithms to be implemented on the server-side in [21]. Also, the investigational evaluation of LoRaWAN conducted by ns-3 in [22], Improving LoRa performance with CSMA [23], the power consumption model [24], scalability analysis model for significant-scale [19] and several of models in [25–29].

3.3 FloRa

Framework for LoRa (FloRa) simulator was developed to evaluate LoRa networks performance using ADR mechanism. It proved the effectiveness of ADR in increasing the PDR with improving energy efficiency. FLoRa is an end-to-end simulation framework for LoRa networks rely on the OMNeT++ network simulator and also utilizes INET system components [30]. An open-source OMNeT++ library was designed to support the experimentation process for various network protocols. FloRa code is created by C++, and it enables the development of LoRa networks that support the integration of LoRa nodes, gateways, and network server modules. Application logic can be implemented as separate modules that are linked to a network server. The network server and nodes support dynamic configuration parameters controlling via the ADR and considering collisions and capture effect. The module includes an accurate modelling of the backhaul network and can simulate multiple gateways. At the end of the simulation, energy consumption statistics can be collected in each node and over the entire network [31]. Besides, the modules of the LoRaWAN MAC protocol strive to simulate the physical layer [32]. This offers a very strong graphical interface as opposed to the other simulation applications since it is based on OMNeT++ and a graphical network description. The developed simulation module includes a sample scenario in the FLoRa simulations directory. The scenario has several features to simulate a network with ten nodes that are placed randomly in a square network topology with one gateway that is linked to a network server. Each node transmits a packet at a time based on an exponential distribution with a defined mean. For simulating a LoRa network, several parameters

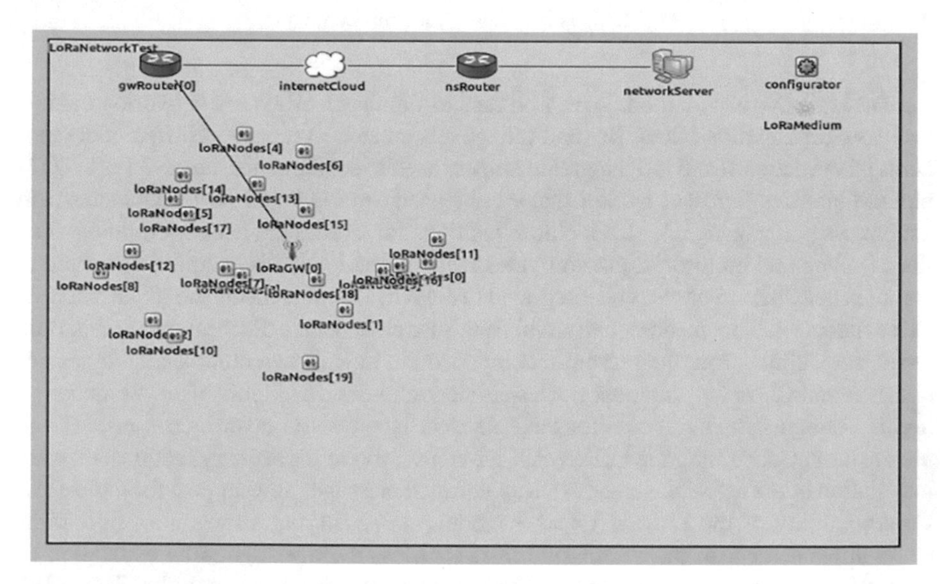

Fig. 3. FLoRa environment [30]

need to be selected, such as simulation time and warm-up period, SF, the transmission power for each LoRa end-node, backhaul network configuration, and links. The simulation statistics and tracing files are generated on completion of the run. The simulation statistics can be viewed through the OMNeT++ GUI as in Fig. 3.

3.4 CupCarbon

Carbon is an emerging framework for simulating Smart City and IoT WSNs (SCI-WSN) [33]. It aims to design, visualise, debug, and validate distributed algorithms for environment observing and data gathering. It is used to simulate various IoT application scenarios for educational and development scientific projects. In addition, to visually explain the basic concepts of WSNs, it also supports the testing of different wireless topologies, protocols, and applications. CupCarbon supports two simulation environments that enable the design of mobility scenarios (fires and gas scenarios, vehicles and UAVs, insects) and a discrete event simulation of WSNs and IoT applications. Networks can be simulated via an ergonomic and user-friendly GUI utilizing the OpenStreetMap framework to deploy sensors clearly on the map. It has a script named SenScript that enables the programming and configuration of sensor nodes individually and generates codes to be used in hardware platforms like Arduino, Raspberry Pi, and XBee. The nodes can be configured dynamically to distribute nodes into individual networks.

CupCarbon supports the calculation of energy consumption and displays it as a function of the simulation time. Such functionality permits clarification of network structure and realistic implementation before real deployments. It integrates propagation visibility with interference models and supports different communication interfaces, including, LoRa, Wi-Fi and ZigBee protocols [34]. CupCarbon is the fundamental kernel of the PERSEPTEUR ANR project aimed at developing algorithms for the accurate simulation of signal transmission in a 3D city area [35]. The ground elevation model

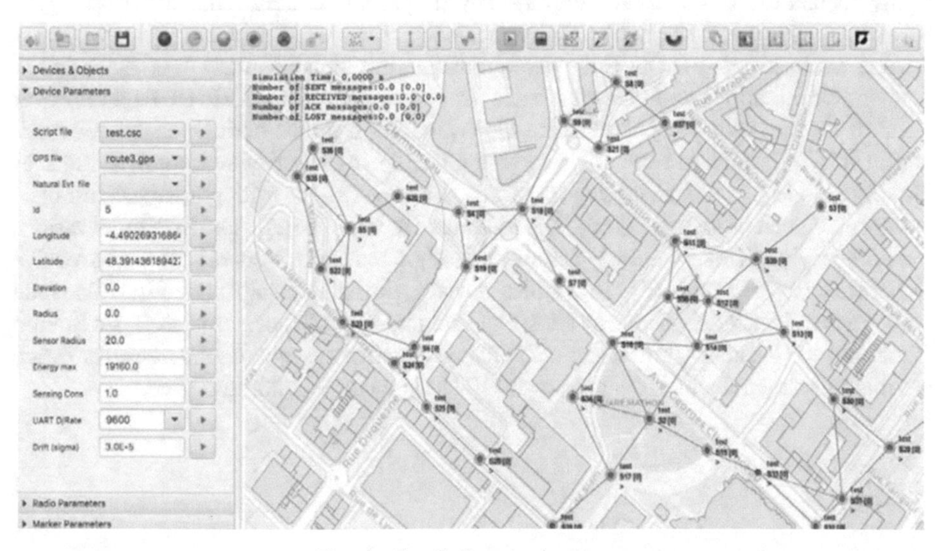

Fig. 4. CupCarbon environment

can be imported into a CupCarbon project by Google Elevation API [36]. Many recent studies were utilized CupCarbon to analyze LoRa/LoRaWAN performance [34, 37, 38]. CupCarbon offers several objects which are easy to use and easy to customize [39]. CupCarbon offers a multi-agent simulation environment that enables simulations to be conducted and events and adjustments over time to be tracked and allows the reproduction of a 3D environment consist of a floor, buildings, and different objects such as sensor nodes as illustrated in Fig. 4.

3.5 PhySimulator

PhySimulator was used as a link level assessment for LoRa, which shows that, although theoretical consideration is that spreading factors can be considered orthogonal, LoRa has a real problem with inter-spread factor collisions [5]. The objective of the PHY Simulator is to enforce LoRa's relation level. MATLAB writes PhySimulator. The purpose of the simulator shall test the reception of two LoRa transmissions interfering with various diffraction variables [40]. In particular, each spread factor output is influenced by the packet, symbol, and bit error rate that interfered with some other spread factor. The user can use this simulator to edit several parameters (change the values of the variables codes). For instance, bandwidth, payload, and maximum tests can be modified per phase, etc. Unable to alter all these factors via a graphical interface, the user must edit them directly by changing the MATLAB code. Field test and Capacity simulation of LoRaWAN in a seaport area conducted in [41], An Effective Algorithm for Vehicular Ad-Hoc Network Load Balancing in [42], smart city [43], Realistic Network Planning [44], latest update by H.Mroue called it LoRa+ [45].

3.6 SimpleIoTSimulator

Many popular IoT protocols are supported by SimpleIoTSimulator like (MQTT, MQTT-SN, MQTT Broker, HTTP/s client/server, Modbus Over TCP, BACnet/IP server, LoRa device, LoRa gateway). LoRa Device simulator part supports the Class A, B and C devices specifications and communicates produced LoRa frames (PHY Payload) over UDP to one or more associated LoRa Gateways. It promotes both Over-the-Air Activation (OTAA) and Over-the-Air Activation (ABP) for security key configuration, as illustrated in Fig. 5. When talking to certain gateways, signal strength, signal-to-noise, and channels can be specified [46]. The loading of data can be adjusted to display various sensor behaviour. LoRa Gateway is sent to a designated LoRa Network Server to receive LoRa frames (PHYPayload) from LoRa devices via UDP, encapsulated into Semtech UDP Packet Forwarder (Gateway Message Protocol-GWMP) or Semtech Basic Station (WebSockets) packets. Upon receipt of Network Server messages, downstream the frame payload is extracted and forwarded over UDP to the corresponding device.

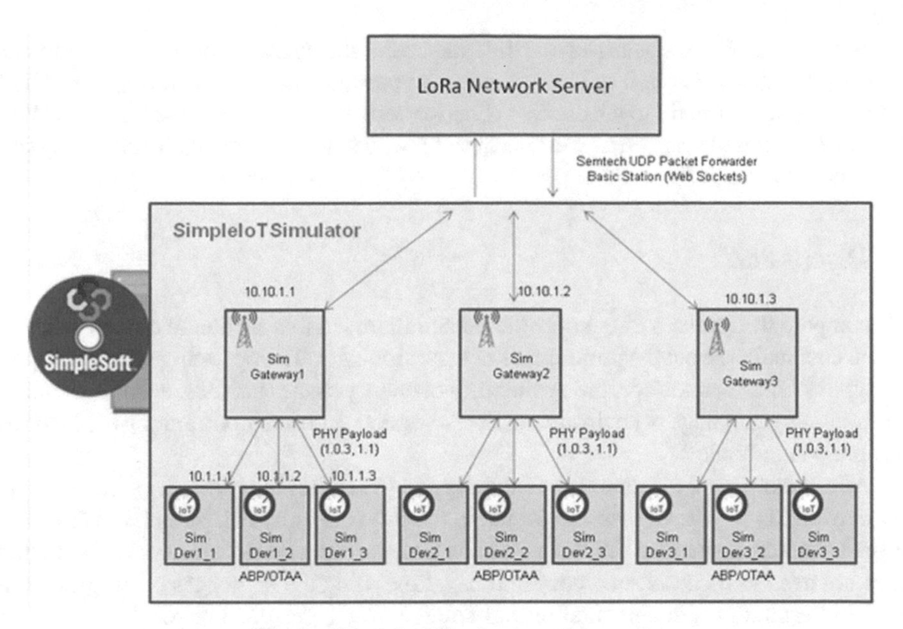

Fig. 5. SimpleIoTSimulator environment

3.7 Arm Mbed OS Simulator

The simulator is available in two versions: an online version that runs entirely within the browser and an offline version that can be used with any Mbed OS 5 project, as illustrated in Fig. 6. The online Mbed Simulator is the simplest. Running the simulator offline on any Mbed OS 5 project is also possible [47]. This makes it possible to incorporate the simulator into your development process. LoRa alliance supports this simulator. The simulator employs a bogus LoRaWAN radio driver in order to run the LoRaWAN stack.

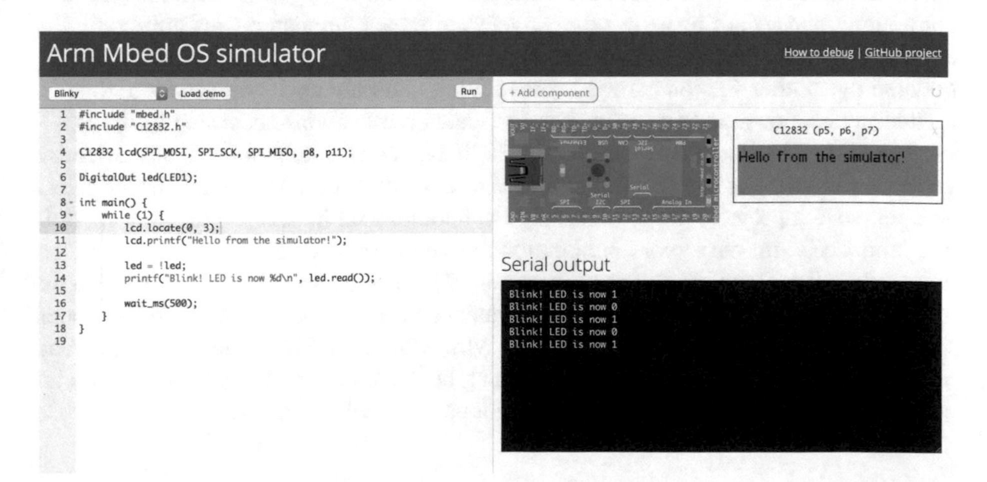

Fig. 6. Arm Mbed OS simulator

When the LoRaWAN stack tries to drive the radio, the counterfeit radio intercepts the packet. This is low enough to encrypt only the packets, data rate, and frequency. This data is then sent directly to a LoRaWAN network server that isn't actually a LoRaWAN device. This method performs well because bidirectional data, recognitions and OTAA all come together [47].

4 Discussion

We compare the features of the considered simulators in this section to come out with a useful conclusion about the preferences of each simulator. The operating system support, the type of license, interface, the availability of energy usage statistics, and the simulator programming language or environment, latest version, and update are among the feature's comparison in Table 1.

All simulators are discrete events and support the LoRaWAN protocol and can model the network as a cycle of discrete events in the time domain. This authorizes the simulators to switch to the next event if two consecutive events do not change, so the system does not need to be monitored continuously. Regarding the languages of programming used in Simulators' implementation, all simulators are designed on well-known, supportive community programming environments. This is very important as a specialist can quickly extend the capability of the simulator with the implementation of new modules as extensions for the existing simulators (e.g., enhance new network protocols, incorporation of further tools in the current environment).

In brief, Java is used for CupCarbon implementation; C++ is used for FloRa; Matlab is used for PhySimulator, Python is used for LoRaSim, and the C++ and Python implementation are used for the Ns-3 LoRaWAN module. In contrast to other simulators, CupCarbon via 2D and 3D environment, FLoRa via OMNeT++, and Ns-3 via NetAnim and PyViz have a broader graphical GUI for C++ and Python module, respectively. Whereas Only a few plots offer PhySimulator and LoRaSim, MATLAB, and Pychrom environments in that order. All of the simulators studied were published in the scientific community, and according to the official websites of each simulator: CupCurbon, FloRa, and PhySimulator have more than two related publications, but PhySimulator has been updated by another version named LoRa+. Whilst Module ns-3 includes more than 20 related publications, and LoRaSim has 11 related publications according to the SCOPUS database, the last update was in Nov 2020, but some simulator has many extended versions with different names, not included in these statistics. The ns-3 is nevertheless an open-source project with a large, large community supporting it [18]. The module ns-3 and LoRaSim have more publications in comparison to PhySimulator, CupCurbon, and FloRa. Therefore, some of the simulators provide more detailed details on the installation process and the use of the equipment on their websites. All of them are open source, and GitHub provides their codes. Whiles SimpleIoTSimulator [46] and Arm Mbed Simulator [47] are more technical using but haven't enough publication projects in spite of the Arm Mbed simulator being adopted by LoRa alliance.

Table 1. Lora simulators comparison.

Features	LoRaSim	NS-3	Flora	CupCarbon	SimpleIoTSimulator	Mbed Simulator	PHY Simulator
License type	Source is open	Source is open	Source is open	Free (education)	Not Free	Free	Free
Operating system	macOS, Linux, Windows	Linux, Windows,	Linux, Windows, macOS	macOS	Linux: RedHat, Ubuntu, CentOS	Windows.Mac os, Linux	MacOS, Windows
Installation requirements	SimPy, NumPy, matplotlib	Import all library online	OMNeT++ 6 and INET 4.3.1	Java	n/a	Online, MbedCLI Python 2.7,Git	Matlab
Type language	Python	C++, Python	C++	Java	C++	Java	MATLAB
GUI	Only plot	Yes	Yes	2D/3D with OSM	yes	Yes	Only plot
Community support	Limited	Very good	Limited	Good	limited	LoRa allaince	Good
Last update	2020	October 2020	Nov 2020	2020	2019	May 2019	2020
Last version	n/a	ns-3.32	6.0	3.8	n/a	n/a	n/a
Popularly	High	High	medium	Little	Rarely	High	High
Studies achieved by simulators	[10, 12, 14, 48–56]	[19, 21–29, 57, 58]	[30, 32]	[34, 36–39]	n/a	n/a	[41–45, 59–62]

5 Conclusions

In the networking and communication environment, simulation has proved an important tool to evaluate new solutions. However, the simulator must provide an environment similar enough to the re-created environment to produce realistic results and evaluate those solutions appropriately. There are multiple simulators on LoRaWAN, but each has different features that can be tailored to specific assessments. The paper provides a conceptual review of seven LoRaWAN simulators, LoRaSim, NS3, Cupcurpon, FloRa, SimpleIoT-Simulator and Mbed simulator. This paper provides a conceptual assessment. The only open-source emulation tools and the most popular in the academic area are LoRaSim, NS3, the Physimulator compared to the other three simulation tools, which are more techniques used. Unlike the basic implementation, the simulators provided in this work add new features to the MAC sublayer that are not available in the basic version. They have been published and are written in a variety of programming languages. To achieve this, there is no need to construct complex real-world networks or sophisticated testbeds. The results of a study that included a review of the literature and research using current simulators revealed that open-source programming environments are capable of modelling the vast majority of MAC layer mechanisms in a LoRaWAN network.

Acknowledgement. This study was supported by the Universiti Malaysia Pahang (www.ump.edu.my), Malaysia, under the Post Graduate Research Scheme PGRS200340.

References

1. Mikhaylov, K., Petäjäjärv, J., Hänninen, T.: Analysis of the capacity and scalability of the lora wide area network technology (2016)
2. Attia, T., et al.: Experimental characterization of LoRaWAN link quality. In: 2019 IEEE Global Communications Conference (GLOBECOM) (2019)
3. Salama, M., Elkhatib, Y., Blair, G.: IoTNetSim: a modelling and simulation platform for End-to-End IoT services and networking, pp. 251–261 (2019)
4. Piechowiak, M., Zwierzykowski, P.: Simulations of the MAC Layer in the LoRaWAN Networks. J. Telecommun. Inf. Technol. (2020)
5. Hornbuckle, C.A.: Fractional-N synthesized chirp generator. Google Patents (2010)
6. Semtech, SX1272/3/6/7/8: LoRa Modem Designer's Guide (2013). www.semtech.com
7. Bouguera, T., et al.: Energy consumption model for sensor nodes based on LoRa and LoRaWAN. Sensors **18**(7) (2018)
8. Augustin, A., et al.: A study of LoRa: long range & low power networks for the Internet of Things. Sensors **16**, 1466 (2016)
9. Raza, U., Kulkarni, P., Sooriyabandara, M.: Low power wide area networks: an overview. IEEE Commun. Surv. Tutor. (2017)
10. Bor, M., et al.: Do LoRa Low-Power Wide-Area Networks Scale? (2016)
11. Farooq, M.O., Pesch, D.: Poster: extended LoRaSim to simulate multiple IoT applications in a LoRaWAN. In: EWSN (2018)
12. Farooq, M., Pesch, D.: Extending LoRaSim to simulate multiple IoT applications in a LoRaWAN (2018)
13. Zorbas, D., et al.: Optimal data collection time in LoRa networks—a time-slotted approach. Sensors **21**(4), 1193 (2021)
14. Abdelfadeel, K., Farrell, T., Pesch, D.: How to make firmware updates over LoRaWAN possible (2020)
15. Zorbas, D., Kotzanikolaou, P., Pesch, D.: TS-LoRa: time-slotted LoRaWAN for the industrial Internet of Things. Comput. Commun. **153**, 1–10 (2020)
16. Abdelfadeel, K.Q., et al.: FREE—fine-grained scheduling for reliable and energy-efficient data collection in LoRaWAN. IEEE Internet Things J. **7**(1), 669–683 (2020)
17. Henderson, T.R., et al.: ns-3 project goals. In: Proceeding from the 2006 Workshop on ns-2: the IP Network Simulator (2006)
18. Simulator, N.: https://www.nsnam.org/. Accessed Nov 2020
19. Abeele, F.V.D., et al.: Scalability Analysis of Large-Scale LoRaWAN Networks in ns-3. IEEE Internet Things J. **4**(6), 2186–2198 (2017)
20. Bilalb, S.M., Othmana, M.: A performance comparison of network simulators for wireless networks. arXiv preprint arXiv:1307.4129 (2013)
21. Reynders, B., Wang, Q., Pollin, S.: A LoRaWAN module for ns-3: implementation and evaluation. In: Proceedings of the 10th Workshop on ns-3 - WNS3 2018, pp. 61–68 (2018)
22. Khan, F.H., Portmann, M.: Experimental evaluation of LoRaWAN in NS-3. In: 2018 28th International Telecommunication Networks and Applications Conference (ITNAC), pp. 453–460 (2018)
23. To, T., Duda, A.: Simulation of LoRa in NS-3: improving LoRa performance with CSMA. In: 2018 IEEE International Conference on Communications (ICC) (2018)
24. Finnegan, J., Brown, S., Farrell, R.: Modeling the energy consumption of LoRaWAN in ns-3 based on real world measurements. In: 2018 Global Information Infrastructure and Networking Symposium (GIIS) (2018)
25. Stellin, M., Sabino, S., Grilo, A.: LoRaWAN networking in mobile scenarios using a WiFi Mesh of UAV gateways. Electronics **9**(4) (2020)

26. Hariprasad, S., Deepa, T.: Improving unwavering quality and adaptability analysis of LoRaWAN. Procedia Comput. Sci. **171**, 2334–2342 (2020)
27. Finnegan, J., Farrell, R., Brown, S.: Analysis and enhancement of the LoRaWAN adaptive data rate scheme. IEEE Internet Things J. **7**(8), 7171–7180 (2020)
28. Khan, F.H., Jurdak, R., Portmann, M.: A model for reliable uplink transmissions in LoRaWAN. In: 2019 15th International Conference on Distributed Computing in Sensor Systems (Dcoss), pp. 147–156 (2019)
29. Finnegan, J., Brown, S., Farrell, R.: Evaluating the scalability of LoRaWAN gateways for class B communication in ns-3. In: 2018 IEEE Conference on Standards for Communications and Networking (IEEE CSCN) (2018)
30. Mariusz Slabicki, G.P., Di Francesco, M.: https://omnetpp.org/download-items/FLoRA.html Accessed 2020. 2017
31. site., F.o., FLoRa. 2020
32. Mariusz Slabicki, G.P., Di Francesco, M.: Adaptive Configuration of LoRa Networks for Dense IoT Deployments by OMNet++ (FLORA) simulator (2018)
33. Cupcarbon., Cupcarbon. http://cupcarbon.com. Accessed 2020
34. Lopez-Pavon, C., S. Sendra, Valenzuela-Valdés, J.F.: Evaluation of CupCarbon network simulator for wireless sensor networks. Netw. Protoc. Algorithms **10**(2), 1–27 (2018)
35. Cupcarbon. Cupcarbon User Guide (2020). https://cupcarbon.com/cupcarbon_ug.html
36. Lounis, M., et al.: 3D Environment for IoT Simulation Under CupCarbon Platform (2017)
37. Sanchez, E.B., Sadok, D.F.H.: LoRa and LoRaWAN protocol analysis using cupcarbon. In: Mata-Rivera, M.F., Zagal-Flores, R., Barria-Huidobro, C. (eds.) WITCOM 2020. CCIS, vol. 1280, pp. 352–376. Springer, Cham (2020). https://doi.org/10.1007/978-3-030-62554-2_26
38. John, A., Ananth Kumar, T., Adimoolam, M., Blessy, A.: Energy management and monitoring using iot with cupcarbon platform. In: Balusamy, B., Chilamkurti, N., Kadry, S. (eds.) Green Computing in Smart Cities: Simulation and Techniques. GET, pp. 189–206. Springer, Cham (2021). https://doi.org/10.1007/978-3-030-48141-4_10
39. Mehdi, K., et al.: CupCarbon: a multi-agent and discrete event wireless sensor network design and simulation tool (2014)
40. Croce, D., M.G., Mangione, S., Santaromita, G., Tinnirello, I. (2018). http://lora.tti.unipa.it/
41. Bardram, A.V.T., et al.: LoRaWan capacity simulation and field test in a Harbour environment. In: 2018 Third International Conference on Fog and Mobile Edge Computing (Fmec), pp. 193–198 (2018)
42. Abbas, A.H., Audah, L., Alduais, N.A.M.: An efficient load balance algorithm for vehicular ad-hoc network. In: 2018 Electrical Power, Electronics, Communications, Controls and Informatics Seminar (EECCIS) (2018)
43. Yu, F.H., Zhu, Z.M., Fan, Z.: Study on the feasibility of LoRaWAN for smart city applications. In: 2017 IEEE 13th International Conference on Wireless and Mobile Computing, Networking and Communications (Wimob), pp. 334–340 (2017)
44. Dalela, P.K., Sachdev, S., Tyagi, V.: LoRaWAN network capacity for practical network planning in India. In: 2019 Ursi Asia-Pacific Radio Science Conference (Ap-Rasc) (2019)
45. Mroue, H., et al.: LoRa+: An extension of LoRaWAN protocol to reduce infrastructure costs by improving the Quality of Service. Internet Things **9**, 100176 (2020)
46. SimpleSoft. SimpleIoTSimulator (2019). https://www.simplesoft.com/SimpleIoTSimulator.html. Accessed 23 Jun 2021
47. Lab, M. Mbed Simulator (2019). https://os.mbed.com/blog/entry/introducing-mbed-simulator/. Accessed 23 Jun 2021
48. Farooq, M.O., Pesch, D.: Evaluation of multi-gateway LoRaWAN with different data traffic models. In: 2018 IEEE 43rd Conference on Local Computer Networks (LCN) (2018)
49. Hassan, K.: Resource Management and IP Interoperability for Low Power Wide Area Networks (2020)

50. Abdelfadeel, K., Cionca, V., Pesch, D.: A Fair Adaptive Data Rate Algorithm for LoRaWAN (2018)
51. Bor, M., Roedig, U.: LoRa transmission parameter selection. In: 2017 13th International Conference on Distributed Computing in Sensor Systems (DCOSS) (2017)
52. Voigt, T., et al.: Mitigating inter-network interference in LoRa networks (2016)
53. Bor, M., King, A., Roedig, U.: Lifetime bounds of wi-fi enabled sensor nodes. Procedia Comput. Sci. **52**, 1108–1113 (2015)
54. Bor, M., Roedig, U.: OpenCL as wireless sensor network programming abstraction (2014)
55. Ta, D.-T., et al.: LoRa-MAB: a flexible simulator for decentralized learning resource allocation in IoT networks, pp. 55–62 (2019)
56. Ta, D., et al.: LoRa-MAB: toward an intelligent resource allocation approach for LoRaWAN. In: 2019 IEEE Global Communications Conference (GLOBECOM) (2019)
57. Reynders, B., et al.: Improving reliability and scalability of LoRaWANs through lightweight scheduling. IEEE Internet Things J. **5**(3), 1830–1842 (2018)
58. Magrin, D., Centenaro, M., Vangelista, L.: Performance evaluation of LoRa networks in a smart city scenario thesis. in book. (2017)
59. Tomic, I., et al.: The limits of LoRaWAN in event-triggered wireless networked control systems. In: 2018 Ukacc 12th International Conference on Control (Control), pp. 101–106 (2018)
60. Croce, D., et al.: Impact of LoRa imperfect orthogonality: analysis of link-level performance. matlab. IEEE Commun.s Lett. **22**(4), 796–799 (2018)
61. Gucciardo, M., Tinnirello, I., Garlisi, D.: Demo: a cell-level traffic generator for LoRa networks. matlab. ACM (2017)
62. Marini, R., Cerroni, W., Buratti, C.: A novel collision-aware adaptive data rate algorithm for LoRaWAN networks. IEEE Internet Things J. **8**(4), 2670–2680 (2021)

Applying a Lightweight ECC Encryption in Multi-topology Sensor Networks to Enhance Intelligent IoT Low-Cost Transportation Platforms Security Based on CoAP Constrained Protocol

Salma Ait Oussous[1](✉), Mohammed Yachou[1], Sanaa El Aidi[1], Siham Beloualid[1], Taoufiq El Harrouti[2], Abdelhadi El Allali[1], Abderrahim Bajit[1], and Ahmed Tamtoui[3]

[1] Laboratory of Advanced Systems Engineering (ISA), National School of Applied Sciences, Ibn Tofail University, Kenitra, Morocco
{salma.aitoussous,yachou.mohammed,sanaa.elaidi,siham.beloualid, abderrahim.bajit}@uit.ac.ma

[2] Department of Computer Science, Logistics and Mathematics (ILM) Engineering Science Laboratory, National School of Applied Sciences, Ibn Tofail University, Kenitra, Morocco
taoufiq.elharrouti@uit.ac.ma

[3] Laboratory of Advanced Systems, National Institute of Posts and Telecommunications, SC Department, Mohammed V University, Rabat, Morocco
tamtaoui@inpt.ac.ma

Abstract. Currently, road traffic has experienced an expansion of de- mand due to a significant increase in the vehicle fleet, which has caused an environmental nuisance due to the existing transport systems (congestion, pollution, travel time). Efforts have been made to overcome this problem, and electric mobility was one of the solutions via the insertion of the tramway in the interurban transport mode, but this mode could not be generalized on the whole network of the agglomeration for reasons of infrastructure and lack of financial means for the investment. Our work consists in proposing a mode of transport aiming at the minimization of transport cost and the optimization quality of the environment. Moreover, planning and modeling transportation systems must focus on reducing greenhouse gas emissions and promoting the deployment of emissions and renewable energy. To do this, we developed a synchronized, secure IoT platform that consists of an all-electric multimodal urban transportation network including road and streetcar networks, with a green energy source powering the charging stations. It is used to guide the MBE to take the shortest path with the maximum number of people and avoid stops as much as possible, by proposing 3 approaches to find the suitable one in terms of execution time and memory consumption. We also studied the impact of multi-topologies on the functioning of our platform, and to achieve this work, we used the CoAP protocol and a security method Elliptic Curve Cryptography ECC, the obtained results show the performance of the proposed strategy.

Keywords: Traffic vehicular parc Cost transportation IoT · Intelligent transportation · CoAP constrained IoT protocol · Star/Tree/Cluster- Tree/Mesh

F. Saeed et al. (Eds.): IRICT 2021, LNDECT 127, pp. 359–370, 2022.
https://doi.org/10.1007/978-3-030-98741-1_30

sensor network topologies · RSA-SHA256/AES-SHA256 · Elliptic Curve Cryptography ECC

1 Introduction

Given the urban expansion that Rabat-Sale has experienced, which has caused an increased demand for mobility in parallel with an increase in the number of vehicles, which has environmental nuisance due to the existing transport systems such as congestion transportation systems and pollution as well as the cost of transport [1, 2], we thought to create an intelligent and secure transportation IoT platform that will work in an existing environment such as cities without the complexity of integration with the network or other existing infrastructure. This platform is a model of an electric bus with a capacity of 50 citizens. Its role is to take the optimal path to minimize emissions of CO2, power consumption, distance traveled, and transport costs for citizens by applying 3 different approaches, and we will secure our data with ECC and also apply multi- topology sensor networks to choose the right one. The benefit of star topology is it establishes central management for network operations and makes it simple to add a new node to the network. And nodes are depending on the coordinator to transmit messages via the network [3]. For trees, multiple connected components are grouped in the shape of tree branches, it creates a natural hierarchy of parents and children because each node can only have one mutual link [4]. However, mesh doesn't have a hierarchical relationship, there is one coordinator and a set of nodes coupled where each node acts as a router, allowing other nodes to connect to it to ensure the distribution of most transmissions even when one of the connections goes down [5]. And Cluster-tree is defined in 802.15.4 standards as a simple hierarchical father-child relationship with multiple trees [6].

IoT provides an opportunity for the physical and digital worlds to interact with each other via sensors and actuators, which play a critical part in the data collection that must be recorded and processed. On the other hand, data processing can take place at the network's edge, on a remote server, or in the cloud. Moreover, the available resources, which are limited by size, energy, power, and computing capability, limit the storage and processing capabilities of an IoT device [7]. We also employed artificial intelligence AI, specifically facial recognition for detection and processing images. AI is important in IoT, and it is useful for real-time processing, as well as vice versa [8, 9]. In our platform, IoT has been used to connect camera nodes to the internet, to collect face detections data about citizens in each station to process and calculate to choose the optimal path, using different topologies to find the best one in terms of execution time and memory consumption with and without security layer.

Additionally, we focused on implementing the CoAP protocol which is an IoT web transfer protocol for communication-based on Representational State Transfer (REST) and designed for resource-constrained devices on an IP network and with limited devices in mind [10]. Furthermore, the CoAP's messages are encoded in a binary format, and its packets are simple to be processed with less energy consumption [11]. To secure CoAP, they are many secure protocols, like DTLS and IPsec [12], but to have an efficient security layer, we added lightweight ECC to study its impact on the functioning of our platform and compare it with AES-SHA256.

2 Intelligent Transport Construction and Goals

The goal of this work is to choose the optimal path by detecting the number of people's faces in each station, which is in our case a maximum of 50 people, to minimize the cost, time, and CO2 emissions applying ECC security.

Figure 1 illustrates the architecture of our platform. First, the camera nodes captured the faces of people in each station, then this data was sent to the webserver via the CoAP server. Secondly, at the webserver, we calculated the number of faces detected per station and detected the optimal path that the minibus can take, this path must have a high density of faces. Moreover, the data flowing between the nodes, the CoAP server, and the webserver must be secured to guarantee confidentiality, integrity, and availability, for this we added the ECC security layer. Then, we have studied the impact of topologies on the functioning of our platform. The images taken by the IoT camera nodes will be encrypted and sent to the CoAP server, which also sends them to the webserver where the data will be decrypted for further processing.

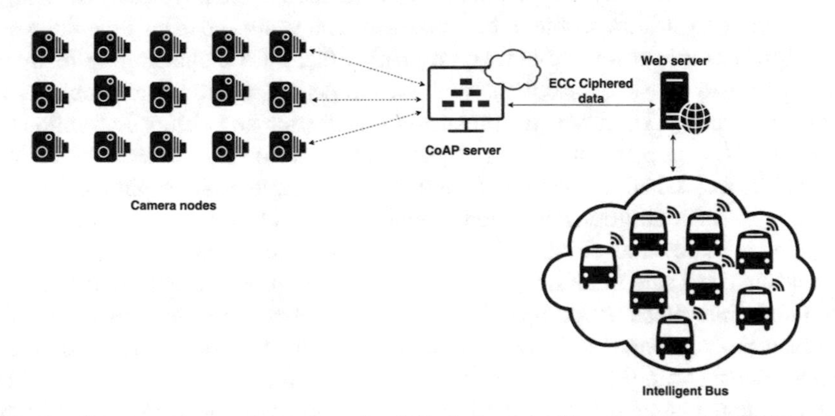

Fig. 1. Intelligent and secured transportation IoT platform Architecture based on CoAP protocol.

3 Methodology

An electric bus is supposed to transport 3 categories of people: a driver of a car VP1, driver and his companion VP2 and driver and his 2 companions VP3. The probability that a person getting into the MBE belongs to VPk, (k = 1;2;3) is pk. Our payoff is that the person getting into the MBE is a driver. An elementary probability calculation shows that: P(driver) = $p_1 + ½p_2 + 2/3p_3$.

Let N be the capacity of the MBE, so the number of cars that remained in the garages is N*P(driver) = N_v. Each car V_j (j = 1;…; N_v) travels a distance DJ during one day. Let n_s be the number of gasoline-fueled cars, and n_d the number of diesel-fueled cars ($n_s + n_d = N_v$). Assume we have a fleet of K MBEs, and each MBE makes αm rounds per day (m = 1;…; K) with a total distance traveled Dm. To cover the hole transport area, coupling between an MBE and a streetcar is realized. The role of the

MBE is to connect the population living in areas not covered by the streetcar. This allows extending the coverage of the electric mobility network. A proximity service and electric mobility via MBE will connect these areas to the tramway network. Several pick-up scenarios are considered, but the key is to provide the customer with benefits to motivate people to use this mode of transport, such as travel time, cost, comfort, and environment. This vehicular infrastructure allows the detection of several people's faces from camera nodes, to detect the monitored area and have a high density of faces; involving search and detection models of vehicular objects and human faces of AI. The communication between the MBEs and the cameras is realized via an Adhoc network that allows having direct communication between them to build an autonomous system. The route of the MBE is between source points and destination points. And our model is to describe a movement of people from k sources S_i ($1 \leq I \leq k$) that serve as pickup/load stations, to n destinations S_j ($1 \leq j \leq n$) that serve as discharge stations. However, this movement occurs through an intermediate means which is the streetcar stations ($1 \leq l \leq p$) that serve as (load/unload) transfer points.

To achieve this work with higher security, we added ECC encryption, which implements a discrete logarithm problem that existed several years ago using an elliptic curve (EC). When it comes to public-key cryptography, there are 2 challenging mathematical difficulties to consider; problems with factors decomposition, and problems with discrete logarithms [13]. ECC is the process of transferring an existing encryption technique to an EC. It implements digital signatures [14]. And its essence is to use a safe EC to execute a classical encryption technique. For example, in RSA, they were known as common modular addition and modular multiplication, but after being transferred to an EC, they are known as elliptic addition and elliptic multiplication [15]. To build it, we should choose a safe finite field to make modular addition and multiplication faster. Background finite fields are comparable for all public-key algorithms (RSA, ECC…). Researchers are interested in 2 types of finite fields, a finite field of characteristic 2, and a finite field of a big prime number. It has been proven that EC discrete logarithm problems are equally tough in mathematics for prime field and finite field of characteristic 2 whose fields are approximately equal [16]. It's hard to comprehend the calculation in the finite field of characteristic 2, which isn't addition, subtraction, multiplication, or division as we know them. There are significant distinctions between the two types of finite fields [17]. For factors, use binary code. Transform into binary integers in one mode, or choose a base from a mathematical point and utilize bases in the field to represent all factors in a finite field in another. Different of them are selected by RSA and ECC. Field factors have distinct representation methods based on different finite fields, which is relevant to all public key algorithms [18]. Many EC exists, and the secure curves that cryptography can employ should be chosen. The equation for an EC is known as the EC equation. The following is the Weierstrass equation in Descartes' coordinate system: $y^2 + a_1xy + a_3y = x^3 + a_2x^2 + a_4x + a_6$ Prime field equation: $y^2 = x^3 + ax + b$; among $4a^3 + 27b^2 \neq 0(modp)$. And the binary field equation is: $y^2 + xy = x^3 + ax^2 + b$; $(a, b \in (G_F)(2^n))$, $b \neq 0$ [19].

4 Related Works

The authors of this study [1] attempted to solve the challenge of optimizing the electric vehicle EV distribution path with various distribution centers. Then, to find EV distribution paths with high resilience, low susceptibility to uncertainty factors, and precise route-by-route schemes, the EV distribution path issue must be optimized with various distribution channels and charging facilities in mind. Based on Bertsimas' theory of robust discrete optimization, a robust EV distribution path optimization model with customizable robustness is constructed to minimize transportation time. The model is additionally solved using an up-graded three-segment genetic algorithm so that the optimal distribution scheme initially comprises all of the route-by-route data utilizing the three-segment mixed coding and decoding approach. For the EV distribution path problem with many distribution centers, this approach evaluated three challenges. The first step is to choose to identify market areas for each service center; the second is to determine each distribution center's delivery sequence; and finally, the distribution path toward the demand points and returning to the distribution centers is determined. Secondly, in this research paper [2], a novel autonomous tracking control (ATC) for intelligent electric vehicles IEVs is created using lane identification and sliding-mode control to implement precise path tracking and optimal torque distribution between the motors of IEVs. The camera first ac- quired the road image, which was then processed to extract the lane markers and determine the needed steering angle using the lateral trajectory and lateral direction tracking errors. After that, an optimal preview linear quadratic regulator (OP LQR) based on the sliding mode technique with a 2-DOF vehicle model was presented to accurately track the target path. The marking identification analysis and optimization results, as well as the traditional three controllers, are obtained and compared to prove the usefulness of the new OP LQR strategy. The lane marker identification algorithm has a high level of accuracy, according to the results. Furthermore, the suggested method allows the real path to better track the desired trajectory, and suitable differential braking torques are distributed among the four wheels. Based on these articles, we came up with the idea of creating a transportation system whose purpose is to reduce trip time by finding the most efficient route. In this article [20], the authors have created a solution that is an electric minibus, which allows detecting the optimal path that MBE will take to reduce CO2, energy consumption, time, and cost of transport, by detecting the faces of people in each station and applying two approaches, illustrated by these two algorithms.

For the first approach, the bus drives to all stations until it achieves its 50 personal capacities, then it transfers to the nearest streetcar station. For the second approach, the webserver made three tests; for citizens bigger than 50 for 3 stations maximum, or 4 stations maximum, or 5 stations maximum, using AES-SHA256 algorithm. For more details, check the document mentioned above.

Algorithm 1 The optimal path for the first approach

Require: $stations \leftarrow [S_1, S_2, ..., S_n]$
  $capacity \leftarrow 50$
  $sum \leftarrow \sum_1^n S_n$
  $N \leftarrow length(stations)$
  for $i \leftarrow 1$ **to** N **do**
    if $sum > n_{max}$ **then**
      if $S_i \neq 0 \wedge S_{i+1} \leq n_{max} \wedge capacity \leq n_{max} \wedge capacity \leq capacity - S_i$ **then**
        Move the bus to S_i
        Stay in S_i 20s
      end if
    else
      if $S_i \neq 0 \wedge S_{i+1} \neq 0$ **then**
        Move the bus to S_i
        Stay in S_i 20s
      end if
    end if
    Move the bus to S_{i+1} (5s)
  end for

Algorithm 2 The optimal path by the second approach

Require: $stations \leftarrow [S_1, S_2, ..., S_n]$
  $n_{max} \leftarrow 50$
  $capacity \leftarrow 50$
  $sum \leftarrow \sum_1^n S_n$
  $MAX \leftarrow MaxNumbers(S, 5)$
  $SUM \leftarrow sum(MAX_{1..3})$
  if $sum > capacity$ **then**
    Move the bus to S_{Max1}, S_{Max2}, S_{Max3}
  else
    if $sum(SUM, MAX_4) > capacity$ **then**
      Move the bus to S_{Max1}, S_{Max2}, S_{Max3}
    else
      if $sum(SUM, MAX_5) > capacity$ **then**
        Move the bus to S_{Max1}, S_{Max2}, S_{Max3}, S_{Max4}, S_{Max5}
      end if
    end if
  end if

5 The Proposed Approach

The goal of our proposed approach is to meet the same need as the previous ones. Well, after we get the number of people in each station, we ranked the 3 biggest numbers MAX1, MAX2, and MAX3. Then, we will apply our test. if MAX1 is greater than the capacity, it will move to the station with the largest number of people S(MAX1), if the opposite the sum of the two largest numbers will be calculated. Next, if the sum is greater than the capacity, it will move to the station with the largest number of people S(MAX1), Otherwise, the sum of the three largest numbers will be calculated. If the sum of the three largest numbers is greater than the capacity, it will move to the station with the largest number of persons S(MAX1) and S(MAX2), otherwise, it will move to the station with the largest number of persons S(MAX1) and S(MAX2) and S(MAX3).

Algorithm 3 The optimal path by the third approach

Require: $stations \leftarrow [S_1, S_2, ..., S_n]$
  $n_{max} \leftarrow 50$
  $capacity \leftarrow 50$
  $sum \leftarrow \sum_1^n S_n$
  $MAX \leftarrow MaxNumbers(S, 3)$
  $SUM \leftarrow sum(MAX_{1..3})$
  if $MAX_1 > capacity$ **then**
    Move the bus to station S_{Max1}
  else
    if $sum(SUM, MAX_2) > capacity$ **then**
      Move the bus to station S_{Max1}
    else
      if $sum(SUM, MAX_3) > capacity$ **then**
        Move the bus to station S_{Max1}, S_{Max2}
      else
        Move the bus to station S_{Max1}, S_{Max2} S_{Max3}
      end if
    end if
  end if

Figure 2 and Fig. 3 show three examples of getting the optimal path using our proposed approach. In the first case (1 station at maximum), the bus becomes full in station 4, it moves to the nearest station which is S.Tram4. In the second case (2 stations at maximum), the bus starts from station 2, moving to station 8 where it becomes full, then it will stop in S.Tram3. And for the last case (3 stations at maximum), the bus starts from station2, moving to station 4 and in station 8, it becomes full, so it moves to the nearest station which is S.Tram3.

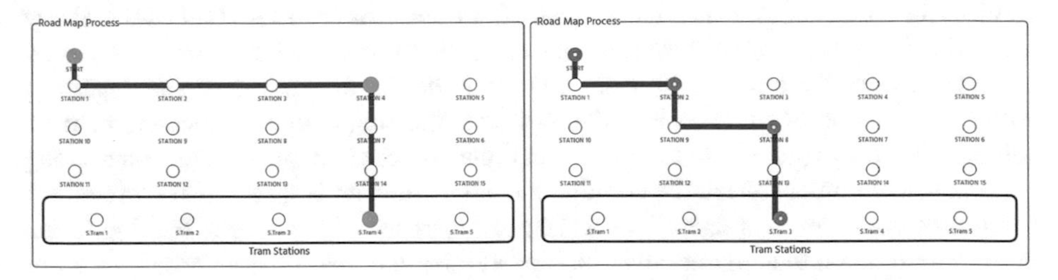

Fig. 2. Approach'3 optimal path for 1 station or 2 stations at maximum.

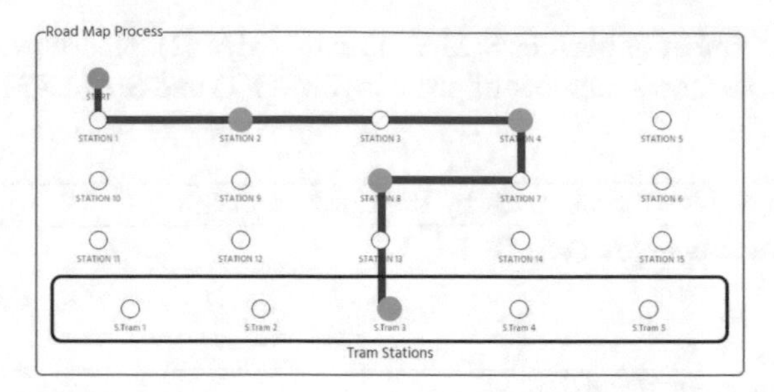

Fig. 3. Approach'3 optimal path for 3 stations at maximum.

6 Discussion and Results

The goal of this article is to apply the AES-SHA256 and ECC encryption methods on our platform, as well as to improve it according to network topologies to examine the impact of each one on the platform, taking into account that CoAP is a high constraint protocol, so it's essential to preserve the power of IoT nodes while also reducing memory usage and execution time.

The comparative outcomes of the scenario given by our platform are shown in the following figures (Fig. 4, Fig. 5). When examining the security aspect of the results, it is evident that AES-SHA256 is more expensive in terms of memory occupation and execution time, as it takes longer to execute and consumes more memory, as opposed to ECC, which is more feasible in our case as it has almost no effect on platform performance while also being a powerful encryption algorithm. Furthermore, ECC does not take a long time to process, it has excellent performance, it can quickly encrypt and decode a huge volume of data, and has low resource and memory requirements. When examining the results of each topology, it is clear that tree topology has the best memory and time performance when compared to the other topologies.

A tree topology is a hierarchical network structure in which the root node creates services for client nodes, which then transfer those services to lower-level nodes. Every level of nodes in this architecture can construct a star network with the nodes it serves. In this scenario, the tree topology structure inherits the drawbacks of star topology. Although star topology is a dependable, efficient, and simple to construct and manage solution, it is only appropriate for components that are close to one another since a long communication link between the coordinator and the end node means that more power is required to convey messages. This is the polar opposite of what we're looking for on our platform. Even though these two topologies (star and tree) do not consume a lot of memory and processing time, they are not recommended for IoT platforms, since in this research area, we need real-time responses without losing data, and if we get to choose between mesh and cluster-tree, we will choose mesh because it is based on features such as a network node remaining energy, the number of links, and the proximity between both the single node' devices or a node and the focus. This architecture can offer all of the gains of signal mode synchronization, Quality compatibility by assured segments, and the ability to build massive networks that cover vast areas.

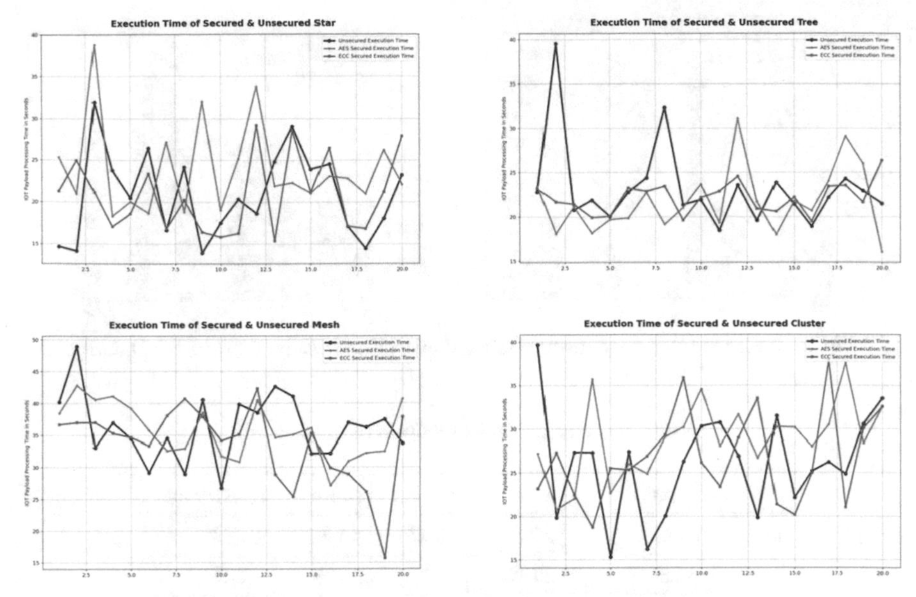

Fig. 4. Execution time unsecured and secured by topologies.

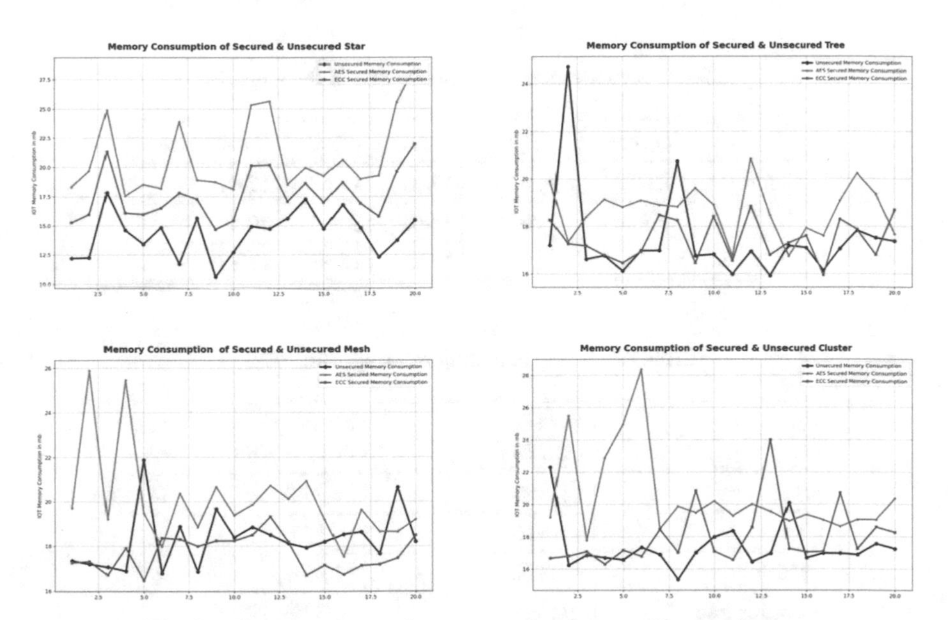

Fig. 5. Memory consumption unsecured and secured by topologies.

Moreover, according to the results shown in Fig. 6, we found that the average memory consumption by AES-SHA256 is higher and the mesh topology consumes less than the others even it takes more time because of its stronger structure. We made another test concerning the calculation of the gain of each topology by security in terms of average

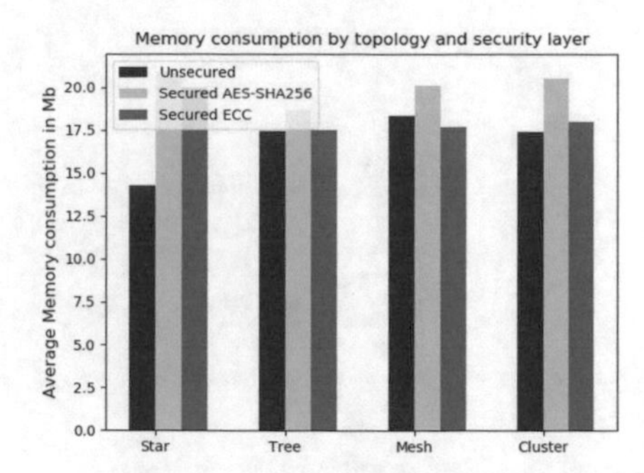

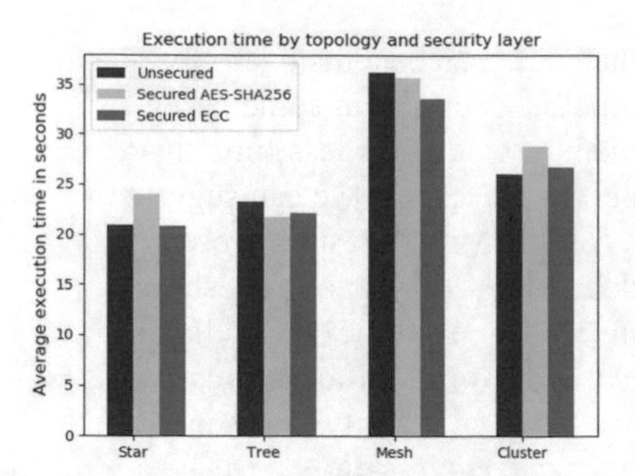

Fig. 6. Average memory consumption and execution time by topology & security.

Table 1. Average time execution of the scenario.

	Topology	Star	Tree	Mesh	Cluster tree
Time	ECC	20.78	22.15	33.48	26.74
	AES	23.93	21.73	35.69	28.84
	Unsecured	20.89	23.21	36.18	26.05

Table 2. Average memory consumption of the scenario.

	Topology	Star	Tree	Mesh	Cluster tree
Memory	ECC	19.97	17.45	17.68	17.97
	AES	20.91	18.67	20.07	20.5
	Unsecured	14.29	17.43	18.3	17.37

Table 3. ECC gain table comparing with AES.

Topology	Time ECC % AES	Memory ECC % AES
Star	12.70%	4.49%
Tree	−6.81%	6.53%
Mesh	−1.37%	11.90%
Cluster tree	9.67%	12.34%

execution time (Table1) and average memory consumption (Table 2). The results show that ECC is less consumable of time and memory, but mesh takes more time than the others. However, for memory, it doesn't consume much compared to the others. So, according to Table 3 that represents the ECC gain table compared with AES, we found that ECC had benefits over AES, it saves time as well as memory when using different topologies except in some cases, but in principle, we can say that ECC consumes less memory and takes less time than others, and since it has a high level of security and performance, then we can suggest that ECC is a good solution to secure our data.

Based on the results presented in the figures and tables mentioned before, we can deduce that the use of a mesh topology for this platform is more efficient and reliable in terms of efficiency and reliability because the connectivity of endpoints makes them extremely resilient to failures, and there may be different routes among devices in the system. For security, the setup is secure from any agreement, processing time, and memory requirement.

7 Conclusion and Perspectives

In this given work, we were able to create a secure intelligent transport IoT platform and make it more efficient and secure by using CoAP protocol with secure algorithms for encryption and decryption payloads.

The objective of this study was to apply the AES-SHA256 and ECC encryption methods on the platform, using different topologies to analyze the impact of each of them on the platform, to preserve the power of the IoT nodes, in addition to reducing their memory occupation and execution time. The results obtained assume that the security with ECC is suitable as well as the mesh topology for our platform.

In future works, we will implement another protocol which is 6lowpan with and without security layer, to study its impact on the operation of our platform to choose the best protocol, encryption algorithm, and suitable topology.

References

1. Ma, C., Hao, W., He, R., Jia, X., Pan, F., Fan, J., et al.: Distribution path robust optimization of an electric vehicle with multiple distribution centers. PLoS ONE **13**(3), e0193789 (2018). In: Xiaosong Hu, Chongqing University, CHINA (2018)
2. Zhang, X., Zhu, X.: Autonomous path tracking control of intelligent electric vehicles based on lane detection and optimal preview method. Expert Syst. Appl. **121**, 38–48 (2019)
3. Pramono, S., Putri, A.O., Warsito, E., Basuki, S.B.: Comparative analysis of star topology and multihop topology outdoor propagation based on Quality of Service (QoS) of wireless sensor network (WSN). In: 2017 IEEE International Conference on Communication, Networks, and Satellite (Comnetsat), pp. 152–157 (2017)
4. Celtek, S.A., Durdu, A., Kurnaz, E.: Design and simulation of the hierarchical tree topology based wireless drone networks. In: 2018 International Conference on Artificial Intelligence and Data Processing (IDAP), pp. 1–5 (2018)
5. Reza Permana, I.M., Abdurohman, M., Putrada, A.G.: Comparative analysis of mesh and star topologies in improving smart fire alarms. In: 2019 Fourth International Conference on Informatics and Computing (ICIC), pp. 1–5 (2019). https://doi.org/10.1109/ICIC47613.2019.8985889
6. Ouadou, M., Zytoune, O., Aboutajdine, D., El Hillali, Y., Menhaj-Rivenq, A.: Improved cluster-tree topology adapted for indoor environment in zigbee sensor network. Procedia Comput. Sci. **94**, 272–279 (2016)

7. Garg, H., Dave, M.: Securing IoT devices and securely connecting the dots using REST API and middleware. In: 2019 4th International Conference on Internet of Things: Smart Innovation and Usages (IoT-SIU), pp.1–6, Published 18 April 2019
8. Zhou, J., Wang, Y., Ota, K., Dong, M.: AAIoT: accelerating artificial intelligence in IoT systems. IEEE Wirel. Commun. Lett. **8**(3), 825–828 (2019). https://doi.org/10.1109/LWC.2019.2894703
9. Barodi, A., Bajit, A., El aidi, S., Benbrahim, M., Tamtaoui, A.: Applying real-time object shapes detection to automotive traffic roads signs. In: 2020 International Symposium on Advanced Electrical and Communication Technologies (ISAECT), Proceeding, Morocco, Kenitra, pp. 1–6 (2020)
10. Bellavista, P., Zanni, A.: Towards better scalability for IoT-cloud interactions via combined exploitation of MQTT and CoAP. In: 2016 IEEE 2nd International Forum on Research and Technologies for Society and Industry Leveraging a better tomorrow (RTSI), pp. 1–6 (2016)
11. Naik, N.: Choice of effective messaging protocols for IoT systems: MQTT, CoAP, AMQP and HTTP. In: 2017 IEEE International Systems Engineering Symposium (ISSE), pp. 1–7 (2017)
12. Kayal, P., Perros, H.: A comparison of IoT application layer protocols through a smart parking implementation. In: 2017 20th Conference on Innovations in Clouds, Internet and Networks (ICIN), Paris, pp. 331–336 (2017)
13. Majumder, S., Ray, S., Sadhukhan, D., Khan, M.K., Dasgupta, M.: ECC-CoAP: elliptic curve cryptography based constraint application protocol for Internet of Things. Wireless Pers. Commun. **116**(3), 1867–1896 (2020). https://doi.org/10.1007/s11277-020-07769-2
14. Alese, B., Philemon, E., Falaki, S.: Comparative analysis of publickey encryption schemes. Int. J. Eng. Technol. **2**(9), 1552–1568 (2012)
15. Bos, J., Kaihara, M., Kleinjung, T., Lenstra, A.K., Montgomery, P.L.: On the security of 1024-bit RSA and 160-bit Elliptic Curve Cryptography. IACR Cryptol. ePrint Arch., Vol. 2009, 389 (2009)
16. Mahto, D., Khan, D.A., Yadav, D.K.: Security analysis of elliptic curve cryptography and RSA. In: Proceedings of the World Congress on Engineering., Vol I WCE 2016, June 29 - July 1, 2016, London, U.K (2016)
17. Shantha, A., Renita, J., Edna, E.N.: Analysis and implementation of ECC algorithm in lightweight device. In: 2019 International Conference on Communication and Signal Processing (ICCSP), pp. 0305–0309 (2019)
18. Shaikh, J.R., Nenova, M., Iliev, G., Valkova-Jarvis, Z.: Analysis of standard elliptic curves for the implementation of elliptic curve cryptography in resource-constrained E-commerce applications. In: 2017 IEEE International Conference on Microwaves, Antennas, Communications and Electronic Systems (COMCAS), pp. 1–4 (2017)
19. Patel, C., Doshi, N.P.: Secure lightweight key exchange using ECC for user-gateway paradigm. In: 11th IEEE Transactions on Computers, vol.70, pp. 1789–1803. IEEE Computer Society, Los Alamitos, CA, USA (2021)
20. Yachou, M., et al.: Applying advanced IOT network topologies to enhance intelligent city transportation cost based on a constrained and secured applicative IOT CoAP protocol. In: The International Conference on Information, Communication & Cybersecurity (ICI2C 2021), (2021)

A Review on 5G Technology in IoT-Application Based on Light Fidelity (Li-Fi) Indoor Communication

Yousef Fazea[1](✉), Fathey Mohammed[2], and Abdulaziz Al-Nahari[3]

[1] Department of Computer and Information Technology, Marshall University, 1 John Marshall Drive, Huntington, WV 25755, USA
fazeaalnades@marshall.edu

[2] School of Computing, University Utara Malaysia, Kedah Darul Aman, 06010 Sintok, Malaysia
fathey.mohammed@uum.edu.my

[3] Department of Information Technology, Faculty of Business and Technology, UNITAR International University, Petaling Jaya, Malaysia
abdulaziz.yahya@unitar.my

Abstract. Representing a significant advancement over the 4G LTE network, 5G paves the door for the widespread use of IoT applications. This paper explored 5G technology in IoT applications across indoor communication employing Light fidelity (Li-Fi) technology. A comparative analysis between Wi-Fi and Li-Fi was conducted to explore the potential of 5G in IoT applications. Furthermore, by analyzing the literature related to integrating Li-Fi into the 5G and IoT-application, the issues and challenges of this integration have also been highlighted. This study illustrated that combining Li-Fi with 5G and IoT is fascinating area of study, and it might lead to further research.

Keywords: 5G · IoT · Light Fidelity · Indoor communication

1 Introduction

In recent decades, it has been demonstrated that technologies, such as smartphones, has risen rapidly and grown with time. Previous studies discovered that with the development of Fifth Generation (5G) technology into wireless network technology and the entrance of the Internet of Things (IoT), both technologies have been intriguing, but hard, issues to study [1]. Although the most intriguing study on this technology is on the 5G Technology in IoT-Application [2–5], because the main reason for the introduction of 5G is due to the IoT itself. According to an International Data Corporation (IDC) research global 5G networks will drive 70% of companies to spend $1.2 billion on communication management services [6]. In the next years, new IoT applications and business models will necessitate new performance requirements for many IoT devices, such as enormous connectivity, security, trusted wireless communication coverage, ultra-low latency, ultra-reliability, and throughput [7]. To satisfy these needs, future Long-Term Evolution (LTE) and 5G technologies are projected to introduce new networking interfaces for future IoT applications [8].

F. Saeed et al. (Eds.): IRICT 2021, LNDECT 127, pp. 371–384, 2022.
https://doi.org/10.1007/978-3-030-98741-1_31

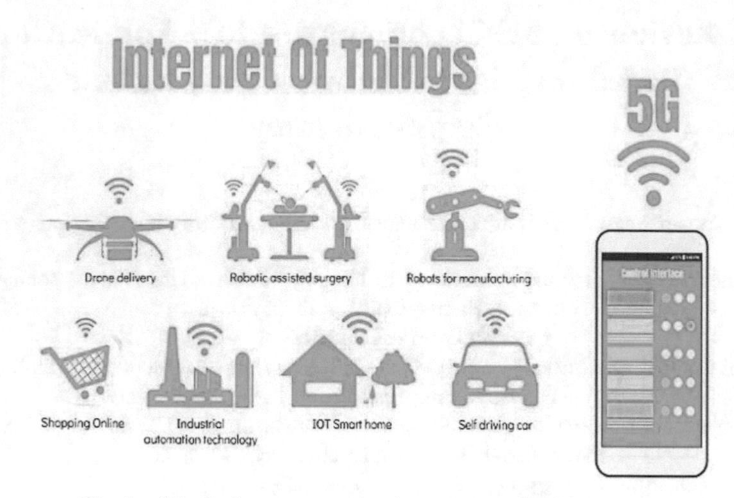

Fig. 1. 5G wireless communication relation with IoT concept

IoT in the 5G system would be a major change in future generations. It will pave the way for new intelligent services and wireless architectures [2]. As most of the sector's forthcoming services and applications will need smart cities, IoT has the potential to play the most important role in guaranteeing this [3], alongside 5G technology for the wireless infrastructure. As a result, the use of 5G network technology in IoT applications may pave the way for more advanced technologies in the coming decade. As depicted in Fig. 1, with the fast development and consideration toward smart technologies, 5G technology gives the advantage of the ability to merge with IoT services and application. As a result, there is no denying that the adoption of 5G and IoT will exist in our daily activities. Challenging of introducing these technologies to the community needs to be addressed to decrease the gap between the community and the adoption of the new technologies and precisely the different applications [9]. The requirement of applying these applications would be the high bandwidth, the accessibility and fast connectivity of the different devices with less time delay and high throughput is also a challenging task that require attention for the adoption of 5G and IoT.

This paper organized as follows; Sect. 1 presents the introduction. Section 2 presents the concept of 5G and IoT. Section 3 presents Li-Fi in 5G based on IoT. Section 4 presents the issues and challenges. Then the conclusion of the paper is presented in Sect. 5.

2 5G Concepts

The fifth generation, or 5G, wireless network of the next decade promises to make substantial improvements in service quality, such as greater throughput and reduced latency [10-12]. Although 5G is a significant advancement over its predecessor, 4G LTE technology, its deployment is difficult since it is still new and not reliable enough to be extensively used. The deployment of the upcoming 5G generation is in its early stages, with a focus on innovative radio access technology (RAT), antenna upgrades, greater frequency usage, and infrastructure development. However, the transition from 1G to

4G technologies has revealed numerous problems in the design of physical and network structures, as well as their implementation details. Despite all of the limitations of the present network, 5G has resulted in a significant advancement in cellular technology. 5G technologies require high bandwidth, which can be reached by using MIMO antenna and millimeter wave technology, and cellular networks may achieve spectrum effectiveness by allowing customers to use both licensed and unlicensed frequency bands.

2.1 5G Internet Key Features

5G offers three important features not seen in networks from the previous decade, demonstrating the advancement achieved in wireless technology since 4G. To begin, a tremendous amount of data is generated. According to the International Telecommunication Union (ITU), there are over 7.5 billion mobile devices in the globe in 2017, with the number expected to increase to 25 billion by 2020, resulting in ultra-dense networks. As a result, data volume increased explosively from 16.5 exabytes in 2014 to an expected 500 exabytes in 2020, resulting in a 30-fold growth rate [6]. Second, in order to allow highly interactive applications, rigorous Quality of Services (QoS) standards, demanding ultra-low latency and high throughput, are enforced. 5G is presently being standardized, and among other things, it covers new URLLC services. These are differentiated by the requirement to promote efficient communication, where successful data transfer can be ensured at a low failure rate while adhering to low latency limitations, such as 1 millisecond (ms) [13]. Finally, heterogeneous environments must be supported to enable interoperability of a broad range of user devices such as smartphones and tablets, QoS standards such as various latency and throughput levels for multimedia applications, network types such as IEEE 802.11 and IoT. As a result, it is apparent that 5G technology may be a step forward in the network industry.

2.2 Architecture of 5G Network

The 5G infrastructure will be built on cloud technologies, with software-defined infrastructure used in the Software Defined Radio (SDR), radio access network (Cloud RAN), and core network. Full virtualization of 5G infrastructure network operations would provide for greater control over service quality, priority, and traffic processing regulations.

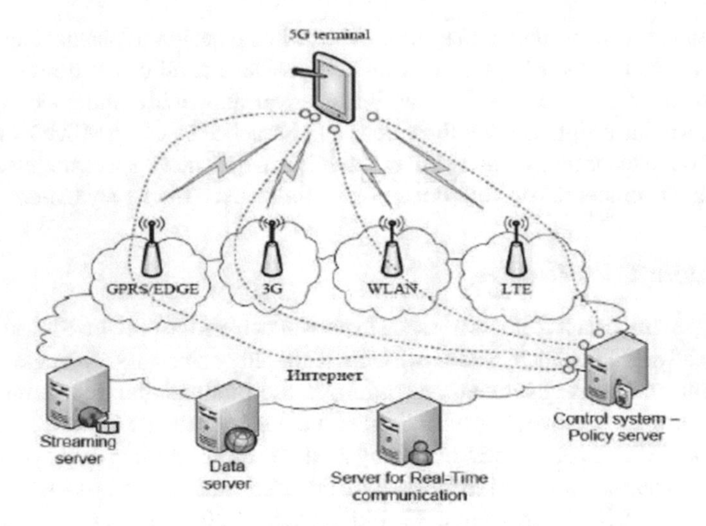

Fig. 2. 5G architecture (Source: TutorialsPoint)

According to Fig. 2, the 5G architecture consists of components that have already been utilized and are recognizable to the user. GPRS/Edge, 3G, WLAN, and LTE are among the technologies and components listed. All of this technology has already been utilized in communication, such as 1G, 2G, 3G, and 4G, and has now been merged and unified into a single 5G technology. With this cutting-edge technology, there is no dispute about the speed, performance, and other benefits of 5G technology for internet connection.

2.3 Implementation of 5G Towards User Devices

There has been much discussion regarding 5G new radio (NR) for future wireless applications such as connected and driverless cars, ultra-HD (UHD), and 3D video streaming [14, 15]. The first generation of 5G mobile networks are scheduled to be launched in the early 2020s. To enable the expansion of millimeter Wave 5G applications, the user scenario must expand beyond 5G infrastructures and eventually include personal user devices such as cellular smartphones.

As a result, the article investigated by [14] offers a unique hybrid antenna module design at millimeter-waves to accomplish spherical beam steering coverage that is structurally and systematically compatible with modern cellular devices. [14] has therefore utilized the concept of the hybrid antenna module consistently integrating two existing principles-the AiP (Antenna-in-Package) and AoD (Antenna-on-Display) to guide the primary lobe of the antenna in the end-fire and broadside direction.

As shown in Fig. 3, this approach finally benefited the majority of user devices. The implementation of devices such as smartphones may be critical, but it is one of the most important implementations for next generation smartphones. It also suggests a strong connection between IoT-applications and 5G wireless networks, with smartphones serving as ideal gateways.

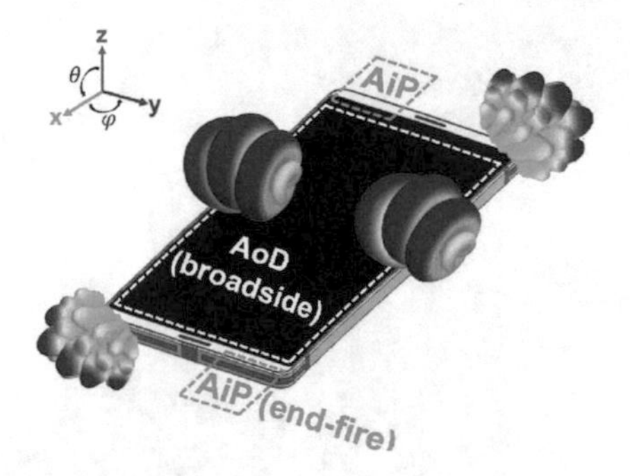

Fig. 3. Hybrid antenna module (Source: [14])

2.4 IoT as Part of 5G Network Wireless Technology

The concept and objective of 5G IoT is to link several device numbers to the similar network connectivity. Many innovative technologies of 5G wireless such as smart cities, car internet or Internet of Vehicle (IoV), smart factories, smart agriculture and smart healthcare are contributing to the IoT movement. It is expected that such a large variety of smart apps will be enabled with high-speed huge networking under the same roof as 5G wireless communication.

Furthermore, IoT should include low-cost sensors and devices, as well as low-cost installation expenditures. Concerning the IoT system, roughly 80 billion IoT devices are expected to be linked across a network, resulting in an increase in the number of connected applications. Furthermore, because the gadgets are smart and use more power, charging capacity and battery recovery should be enhanced [16]. Figure 4 shows 5G IoT network architecture scene diagram.

3 Analysis of Li-Fi in 5G Based on IoT

The Internet of Things is reshaping our daily lives by enabling a plethora of innovative apps that make use of smart and extremely diverse device settings [7]. Many studies on challenging problems for 5G and IoT, as well as critical IoT standards, have been undertaken in recent years. To meet this issue, a complete analysis with a wide variety of suggestions, as well as critical study and research, is necessary. The most intriguing study then focused on Light Fidelity (Li-Fi) wireless technology as part of the 5G and IoT integration.

3.1 Li-Fi Network Technology

According to numerous research [18-21], the wide optical band is a viable alternative for the deployment of high density and high bandwidth 5G and IoT networks. Li-Fi will make a far greater contribution to radio frequency (RF) as a signal carrier than existing technologies. It is an older technology with high data transfer speeds, human usage protection, and security [22]. Furthermore, combining lighting and communication technologies from the same source reduces infrastructure complexity and energy

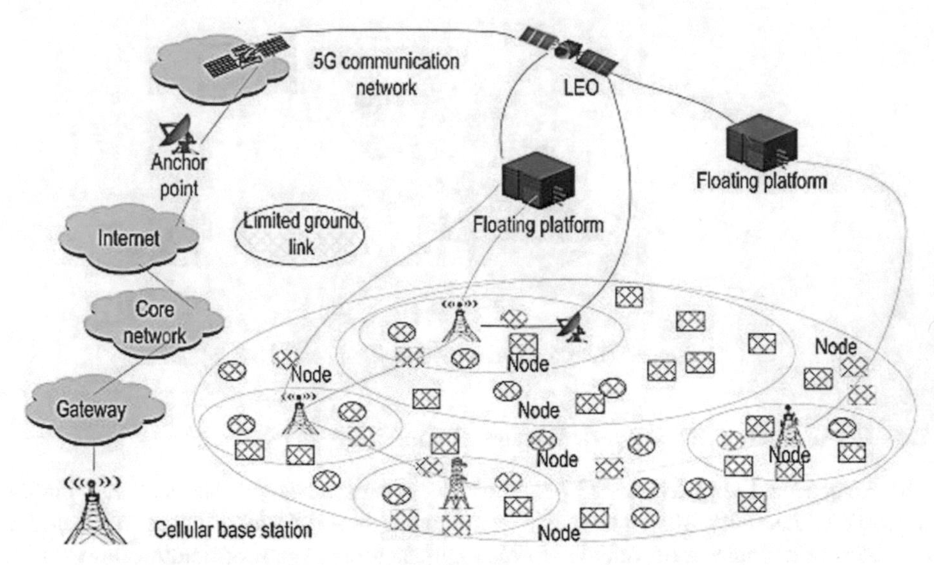

Fig. 4. The 5G IoT network architecture scene diagram (Source [17])

consumption significantly. Li-Fi technology enables new methods of transferring data at high rates and for a variety of purposes via networks. As a license-free, high-speed, bi-directional, and secure wireless communication, Li-Fi is an additional building element for fifth generation (5G) mobile networks.

Li-Fi might be one of the most efficient ways of becoming bridges towards both technologies in assuring the installation or integration of 5G and IoT-applications, such as smart house technology, that require within-indoor connectivity. Any Li-Fi attocell network may add wireless power to RF networks that are currently operating without interference. As a result, Li-Fi attocell networks may cost-effectively expand 5G cellular systems [23]. In other words, by using Li-Fi wireless technology, interference between 5G modems and any IoT-applications that require a signal to begin the job requested by the user may be avoided. Figure 5 represents the attocell in heterogenous network.

Light-Fidelity (Li-Fi) pushes visible light communication (VLC) even farther by utilizing light emitting diodes (LEDs) to comprehend fully networked wireless networks. As lights transform into Li-Fi attocells for the Internet-of-Things (IoT), 5G, and beyond, synergies are leveraged, resulting in increased wireless capability [25]. When compared to femtocell networks, the Li-Fi attocell network has the potential to achieve a 40–1800 greater area data rate. Furthermore, to attain the same efficiency as a Li-Fi attocell with Poisson Point Process (PPP) random Access Point (AP) deployment, frequency reuse of 3, and cell radius of 1 m, the highest femtocell performance will necessitate a total channel bandwidth of 600 MHz. The Li-Fi attocell network substantially increases wireless efficiency in all cases when the Li-Fi AP cell coverage is strong, and the extra theoretical throughput is between 12 and 48 Gbps for the allocated office of 400 m^2. Finally, the new wireless Li-Fi networking architecture delivers the predicted efficiency benefits from 5G, and it will provide an infrastructure for the forthcoming IoT owing to the ubiquitous usage of light emitting diodes.

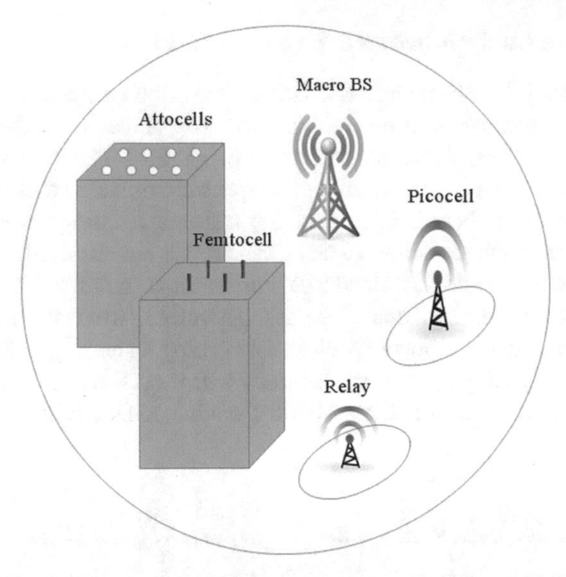

Fig. 5. The attocell in heterogenous network (Source: [24])

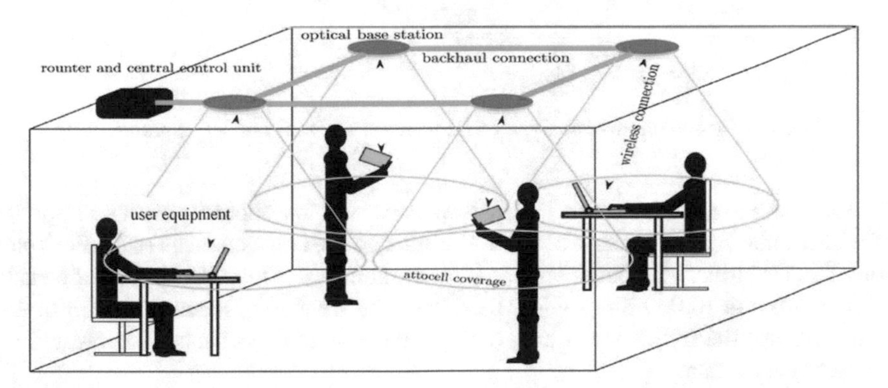

Fig. 6. The concept of Li-Fi attocell architecture within indoor communication (Source: [23])

Based on the study examined by [23], Fig. 6 depicts the concept of a Li-Fi Attocell network. The space is illuminated by a number of light fixtures that offer illumination. Because each light is powered by a Li-Fi modem or Li-Fi chip, it also serves as an optical base station or access point. The optical base stations are linked to the core network through high-speed backhaul connections. The light fixtures frequently contain an inbuilt infrared detector to relay signals from the terminals [23]. The light fixtures frequently contain an inbuilt infrared detector to relay signals from the terminals. The lighting lights are modified at fast rates.

3.2 Comparative Analysis between Wi-Fi and Li-Fi

As a VLC technology, Li-Fi has succeeded in offering effective speed in wireless communication networks. Because of its resemblance to Wi-Fi, it was given the moniker 'Li-Fi,' but instead of radio waves, it communicates using light [26]. The radio frequency band is typically located between the electromagnetic spectrum of 3 kHz and 300 GHz [18, 19]. However, because of the beneficial connection features, existing wireless technologies typically employ frequencies below 10 GHz, causing the situation to be nearly exhausted and unable to satisfy 5G and IoT standards. Furthermore, this band is closely regulated by both domestic and international agencies. Therefore, when it comes to managing high data rate transmission, optical wireless networking technologies are a good choice. According to [20], the diversity of applications will meet the requirement for high 5G technology services data rates and massive IoT device connectivity.

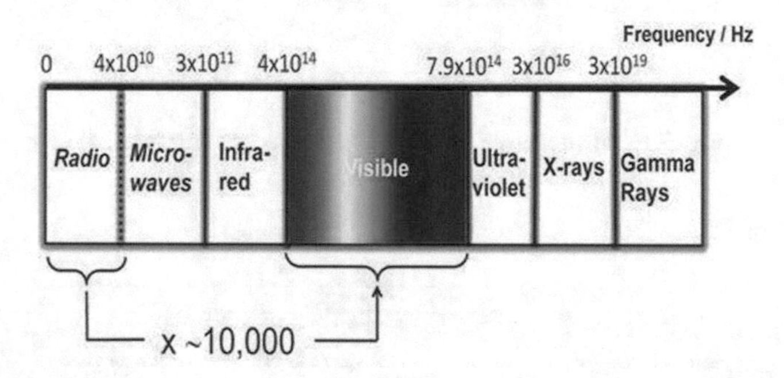

Fig. 7. The comparative analysis of frequencies for VLC and RF (Source: [27])

According to [28], based on Fig. 7, it was revealed that there were a few important differences that may offer us a better knowledge of the consequences of Li-Fi deployment. Li-Fi is built with a better and more future-proof basis than Wi-Fi since the visible light spectrum is 10,000 times wider than the radio frequency spectrum [29, 30]. As a result, because the frequency is high enough, there is a good chance of transmitting a large amount of data.

3.3 The Integration of Li-Fi Technologies into 5G and IoT

The application of Li-Fi for IoT has been the topic of the majority of recent related studies, with most early research addressing the energy-harvesting component of Li-Fi for IoT nodes or the hybrid operation of Li-Fi with RF [31]. In terms of 5G communication, service quality criteria such as data rate, latency, power use, and connection number are quite high. Furthermore, enormous connection is required for the IoT. According to [18], optical wireless networking technologies like as visible light communication, light fidelity, optical camera communication, and free space optical communication would be useful in successfully implementing 5G and IoT. Although the data rate of transmission in Li-Fi is great, the research of Li-Fi in indoor communication settings revealed that it is hard due to various issues [32]. The highlighted difficulty was the placement or orientation of the mobile device, which was stated in previous study articles [33-36] and overreliance on distance [37]. Another source of worry is accurate human motion modeling; while realistic models of human motion are available, combining them with complete channel characterization remains difficult [38]. As a result, an enabler to this problem has been researched. Demirkol et al. [39] proposed the Li-Fi approach, which is based on off-the-shelf LEDs, as an enabler for IoT in indoor environments. The article proposes LiFi4IoT, a system that, in addition to connection, provides three important functions that radio frequency (RF) IoT networks struggle to provide: The device's exact location; the ability to provide power since light can extract energy; and intrinsic protection owing to the propagation characteristics of visible light.

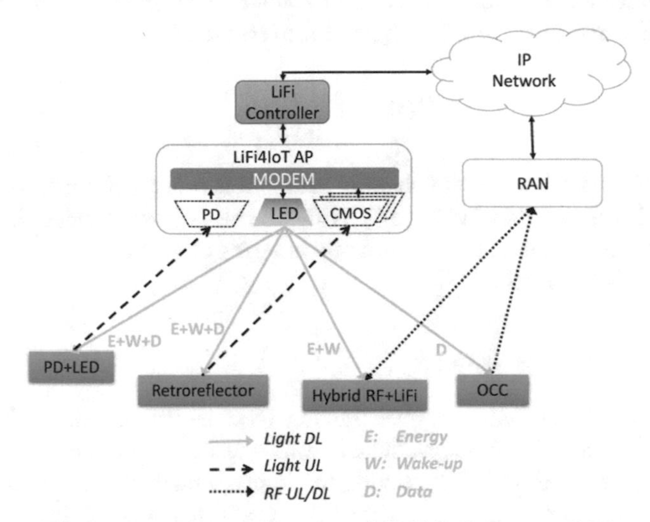

Fig. 8. The system architecture of Li-Fi4IoT (Source: [39])

Based on Fig. 8, the study [39] offers an AP solution consisting of a modulation technique that, depending on the considered uplink technologies, regulates the intensity of light of an off-the-shelf LED through the driver and optional receiver modules. The AP communicates with the LiFi4IoT devices through downlink by varying the intensity of the light. Furthermore, communication between APs is managed by a Li-Fi controller. The Li-Fi controller can communicate with the IP network and Radio Access Networks (RAN), which are required for hybrid motes that incorporate RF and Li-Fi technologies. Additional features and problems, such as the calculation and technique used to manage mobile orientation, should be examined to ensure that this enabler is operating effectively. Research papers such as [34, 40] examined an indoor VLC distribution downlink option including numerous LEDs, where a single LED supplies a single user at any given time. VLC is a developing technology that can provide illumination and communication while also increasing energy efficiency by utilizing current lighting infrastructure [41]. Next-generation wireless networks based on VLC methods promise to be much more interesting when combined with the widespread adoption of energy-efficient light emitting diodes (LEDs) as primary light emitting diodes. Spreading over VLC channels can be very directed [37], and contact is largely dependent on the availability of links to the line of sight (LOS). The depicted model ensures that the problem of mobile orientation towards the integration of Li-Fi towards 5G and IoT has opened up to various approaches and ways to assure the integration itself. The equivalent direct current (DC) channel gain is formulated as:

$$h = \frac{(\gamma + 1)A_{Rg}}{2\pi r^2} \cos^{\gamma}(\phi) \cos(\theta) \Pi\left(\frac{\theta}{\Theta}\right) \tag{1}$$

Where the LOS distance between the LED and the user is defined as r, φ is the luminosity angle, θ is the angle of incidence, $\gamma = -1/\log2(\cos(\Phi 1/2))$ is the Lambertian order, Φ 1/2 is the LED's half-power beamwidth, AR is the detection region of the receiver, and g is the gain of the optical concentrator given n2 ref/ sin2 (Θ) with *nref* being the refractive index, and Θ is the *FOV* angle of the receiver.

$$\Pi(x) \triangleq \begin{cases} 1 & |x| \leq 1 \\ 0 & |x| > 1 \end{cases} \tag{2}$$

where $\Pi(\theta/\Theta)$ indicates that the channel gain is 0 if θ is greater than Θ, or the LED is beyond the receiver field of view [34]. With the calculation provided, it is possible to verify that mobile orientation is not an issue in terms of user device consistency while connection to Li-Fi network.

4 Issues and Challenges

This study area is still available for investigation. Because the majority of the technology mentioned is still in its early stages, there is little question that there is room for further research into other methods of improving the implementation and integration of these technologies. However, because the technology is still recently created' in the network and communication fields, there is no doubt that its application might result in potentially unstable technology, leading to the problem and issue with this technology.

4.1 5G Wireless Initial Issues

Communication networks have grown fast over time and have gotten more sophisticated as network-based applications have proliferated, resulting in a large-scale and heterogeneous network architecture [6]. Because of the increasing number of users on mobile wireless networks, a reduction in cell size is necessary to enhance multi-user capacity in wireless networks [42]. 5G is a more efficient, all-in-one air interface. It has been designed with the enhanced ability to support next-generation consumer interfaces, enable new implementation models, and deliver new services. However, because it is young, it may have an unstable condition, which adds to the complexity of this work. Implementing 5G millimeter-wave (mm Wave) antenna systems within the UE, according to Junho Park et al. [14], remains one of the most challenging issues due to smartphone intrinsic features such as tight form factor, limited real-estate, and power capabilities. Wireless network transmission speed has grown more than 10,000 times in recent decades, compared to a five-fold growth in battery capacity over the same time span.

4.2 Challenges Faced by IoT

In actuality, because of their significant technological potential and community benefits, IoT technologies are currently regarded as one of the key pillars of the fourth industrial revolution [43]. Despite the fact that IoT has been studied extensively in the research area, the technology cannot avoid the problems that it faces. According to recent publications [44], IoT has been confronted with difficulties such:

- **Standards:** Technology conventions, such as network and communication protocols and data aggregation conventions, are the synthesis of information received from numerous sensors for activities such as information management, processing, and storage.
- **Integration and Reliability:** IoT is growing in a dominant manner. It incorporates numerous improvements and will ultimately evolve into a convention. This will offer substantial problems and will necessitate the development of new software and hardware to enable device connection.
- **Connectivity:** Connecting many devices would be one of the most difficult issues of the future of IoT, and this connectivity would most likely reject the existing structure and the technology connected with it.
- **Security:** The Internet of Things has raised major security issues, attracting the attention of the world's various public and private sector businesses. Adding such a large number of additional hubs to networks and the internet would give a larger venue for attackers to infiltrate the system, especially at a time when many people are experiencing the harmful effects of security flaws.

4.3 Limitation Toward Li-Fi

As a new and promising technology, Li-Fi wireless technology could not avoid the drawbacks that any new and growing technology faces. As an example, the limitations that Li-Fi may encounter, as agreed by [22, 25, 42], are as follows:

- Light does not travel through things, if an opaque item blocks the receiver, the signal is instantly turned off.
- It requires a perfect line-of-sight to receive data.
- It is a wireless short-range networking method. It is also highlighted that significant advancements have been made in data speeds, ranges, and coverage.
- In order to transfer data, the light must be on at all times. This is inefficient and may be expensive to the user.
- Interference is caused by other light sources, such as sunlight and incandescent lamps. Most modern Li-Fi devices, however, have solved this limitation since Li-Fi relies on sensing fast changes in light intensity rather than the gradually changing levels generated by natural disturbances in daylight or sunshine.

All of the difficulties and obstacles mentioned above arose as a result of this implementation and integration. With such constraints, it is also not a simple path to contribute to this article. As the issue arose, the integration of IoT and 5G technologies into the present network appeared to be unachievable, resulting in one indoor communication. However, with good Li-Fi architectural planning and component implementation, there is little question that the difficulties encountered may be resolved.

5 Conclusion

This study offered a review on 5G wireless technology in IoT-applications employing Li-Fi Indoor Communication. A brief description of the core concept of 5G, as well as its main features in comparison to its predecessor technology, and the innovative hybrid antenna module design that is utilized for user devices, has also been stated. Critical examination of Li-Fi, which is viewed as a viable option for the deployment of 5G and IoT networks due to greater data transfer than RF, which may open the door to various ways for securing the integration of the 5G and IoT technologies itself. While considering a popular technique such as LiFi4IoT, a technique that, in addition to the indoor VLC distribution downlink model with the calculation to provide consistency towards the orientation of user devices such as smartphones, is designed to address issues such as user device movement or mobile orientation that could potentially disrupt Li-Fi connections. The idea of combining Li-Fi with 5G and IoT is fascinating, and it might lead to further research and studies.

References

1. Attaran, M.: The impact of 5G on the evolution of intelligent automation and industry digitization. J. Amb. Intell. Hum. Comput. 1–17 (2021). https://doi.org/10.1007/s12652-020-02521-x
2. Chettri, L., Bera, R.: A comprehensive survey on Internet of Things (IoT) toward 5G wireless systems. IEEE Internet Things J. **7**(1), 16–32 (2019)
3. Borkar, S., Pande, H.: Application of 5G next generation network to Internet of Things. In: 2016 International Conference on Internet of Things and Applications (IOTA), pp. 443–447. IEEE (2016)
4. Hassan, N., Yau, K.-L.A., Wu, C.: Edge computing in 5G: a review. IEEE Access **7**, 127276–127289 (2019)
5. York, S., Poynter, R.: Global mobile market research in 2017. In: Theobald, A. (ed.) Mobile Research, pp. 1–14. Springer, Wiesbaden (2018). https://doi.org/10.1007/978-3-658-18903-7_1
6. (2018, 10/14/2021) 5G and IoT: the mobile broadband future of IoT," i-scoop, 06-Oct-2020. https://www.i-scoop.eu/internet-of-things-iot/5g-iot/
7. Li, S., Da Xu, L., Zhao, S.: 5G Internet of Things: A survey. J. Ind. Inf. Integr. **10**, 1–9 (2018)
8. Sutton, A.: 5G network architecture. J. Inst. Telecommun. Professionals **12**(1), 9–15 (2018)
9. Rana, A., Taneja, A., Saluja, N.: Accelerating IoT applications new wave with 5G: a review. Materials Today: Proceedings 22 April 2021 (2021)
10. Fattah, H.: 5G LTE Narrowband Internet of Things (NB-IoT). CRC Press, Boca Raton (2018)
11. Xu, L., Jurcut, A.D., Ahmadi, H.: Emerging challenges and requirements for internet of things in 5G. In: 5G-Enabled Internet of Things, pp. 29–48. CRC Press (2019)
12. Liu, L., Han, M.: Privacy and security issues in the 5g-enabled internet of things. In: 5G-Enabled Internet of Things, pp. 241–268. CRC Press (2019)

13. Sachs, J., Wikstrom, G., Dudda, T., Baldemair, R., Kittichokechai, K.: 5G radio network design for ultra-reliable low-latency communication. IEEE Network **32**(2), 24–31 (2018)
14. Park, J., Lee, S.Y., Kim, Y., Lee, J., Hong, W.: Hybrid antenna module concept for 28 GHz 5G beamsteering cellular devices. In: 2018 IEEE MTT-S International Microwave Workshop Series on 5G Hardware and System Technologies (IMWS-5G), pp. 1–3. IEEE (2018)
15. Roh, W., et al.: Millimeter-wave beamforming as an enabling technology for 5G cellular communications: theoretical feasibility and prototype results. IEEE Commun. Mag. **52**(2), 106–113 (2014)
16. Jurcut, A., Niculcea, T., Ranaweera, P., LeKhac, N.-A.: Security considerations for Internet of Things: a survey. SN Comput. Sci. **1**, 1–19 (2020)
17. Yang, D., Zhou, Y., Huang, W., Zhou, X.: 5G mobile communication convergence protocol architecture and key technologies in satellite internet of things system. Alex. Eng. J. **60**(1), 465–476 (2021)
18. Chowdhury, M.Z., Hasan, M.K., Shahjalal, M., Shin, E.B., Jang, Y.M.: Opportunities of optical spectrum for future wireless communications. In: 2019 International Conference on Artificial Intelligence in Information and Communication (ICAIIC), pp. 004–007. IEEE (2019)
19. Chowdhury, M.Z., Hossan, M.T., Islam, A., Jang, Y.M.: A comparative survey of optical wireless technologies: architectures and applications. IEEE Access **6**, 9819–9840 (2018)
20. Lu, H.-H., et al.: A 56 Gb/s PAM4 VCSEL-based LiFi transmission with two-stage injection-locked technique. IEEE Photonics J. **9**(1), 1–8 (2016)
21. Dat, P.T., Kanno, A., Inagaki, K., Umezawa, T., Yamamoto, N., Kawanishi, T.: Hybrid optical wireless-mmWave: ultra high-speed indoor communications for beyond 5G. In: IEEE INFOCOM 2019-IEEE Conference on Computer Communications Workshops (INFOCOM WKSHPS), pp. 1003–1004. IEEE (2019)
22. Albraheem, L.I., Alhudaithy, L.H., Aljaser, A.A., Aldhafian, M.R., Bahliwah, G.M.: Toward designing a Li-Fi-based hierarchical IoT architecture. IEEE Access **6**, 40811–40825 (2018)
23. Haas, H.: LiFi is a paradigm-shifting 5G technology. Rev. Phys. **3**, 26–31 (2018)
24. Gismalla, M.S., Abdullah, M.F.L.: optimization of received power and SNR for an indoor attocells network in visible light communication. Communication **14**(1), 64–69 (2019)
25. Haas, H., Yin, L., Wang, Y., Chen, C.: What is lifi? J. Lightwave Technol. **34**(6), 1533–1544 (2016)
26. Khandal, D., Jain, S.: Li-fi (light fidelity): the future technology in wireless communication. Int. J. Inf. Comput. Techn. **4**(16), 1687–1694 (2014)
27. Hussein, Y.S., Annan, A.C.: Li-Fi technology: high data transmission securely. J. Phys. Conf. Ser. **1228**(1), 012069 (2019). IOP Publishing
28. Pall, M.L.: Wi-Fi is an important threat to human health. Environ. Res. **164**, 405–416 (2018)
29. Shetty, A.: A comparative study and analysis on Li-Fi and Wi-Fi. Int. J. Comput. Appl. **150**(6), 43–48 (2016)
30. Minoli, D., Sohraby, K., Occhiogrosso, B.: IoT considerations, requirements, and architectures for smart buildings—energy optimization and next-generation building management systems. IEEE Internet Things J. **4**(1), 269–283 (2017)
31. Sharma, P.K., Jeong, Y.-S., Park, J.H.: EH-HL: effective communication model by integrated EH-WSN and hybrid LiFi/WiFi for IoT. IEEE Internet Things J. **5**(3), 1719–1726 (2018)
32. Bykhovsky, D.: Coherence time evaluation in indoor optical wireless communication channels. Sensors **20**(18), 5067 (2020)
33. Wang, J.-Y., Li, Q.-L., Zhu, J.-X., Wang, Y.: Impact of receiver's tilted angle on channel capacity in VLCs. Electron. Lett. **53**(6), 421–423 (2017)
34. Eroğlu, Y.S., Yapıcı, Y., Güvenç, I.: Impact of random receiver orientation on visible light communications channel. IEEE Trans. Commun. **67**(2), 1313–1325 (2018)

35. Soltani, M.D., Purwita, A.A., Zeng, Z., Haas, H., Safari, M.: Modeling the random orientation of mobile devices: measurement, analysis and LiFi use case. IEEE Trans. Commun. **67**(3), 2157–2172 (2018)
36. Goswami, P., Shukla, M.K.: Design of a li-fi transceiver. Wirel. Eng. Technol. **8**(04), 71 (2017)
37. Pathak, P.H., Feng, X., Hu, P., Mohapatra, P.: Visible light communication, networking, and sensing: A survey, potential and challenges. IEEE Commun. Surv. Tutor. **17**(4), 2047–2077 (2015)
38. Miramirkhani, F., Narmanlioglu, O., Uysal, M., Panayirci, E.: A mobile channel model for VLC and application to adaptive system design. IEEE Commun. Lett. **21**(5), 1035–1038 (2017)
39. Demirkol, I., Camps-Mur, D., Paradells, J., Combalia, M., Popoola, W., Haas, H.: Powering the Internet of Things through light communication. IEEE Commun. Mag. **57**(6), 107–113 (2019)
40. Luo, J., Fan, L., Li, H.: Indoor positioning systems based on visible light communication: state of the art. IEEE Commun. Surv. Tutor. **19**(4), 2871–2893 (2017)
41. Eroğlu, Y.S., Güvenç, I., Şahin, A., Yapıcı, Y., Pala, N., Yüksel, M.: Multi-element VLC networks: LED assignment, power control, and optimum combining. IEEE J. Sel. Areas Commun. **36**(1), 121–135 (2017)
42. Dinev, D.Z.: Simulation framework for realization of horizontal handover in li-fi indoor network. In: 2019 IEEE XXVIII International Scientific Conference Electronics (ET), pp. 1–4. IEEE (2019)
43. Nižetić, S., Šolić, P., González-de, D. L.-D.-I., Patrono, L.: Internet of Things (IoT): Opportunities, issues and challenges towards a smart and sustainable future. J. Clean. Prod. **274**, 122877 (2020)
44. Jindal, F., Jamar, R., Churi, P.: Future and challenges of internet of things. Int. J. Comput. Sci. Inf. Technol. (IJCSIT) **10**(2), 13–25 (2018)

Effect of Optimal Placement of Shunt Facts Devices on Transmission Network Using Firefly Algorithm for Voltage Profile Improvement and Loss Minimization

S. O. Ayanlade[1], E. I. Ogunwole[2(✉)], S. A. Salimon[3], and S. O. Ezekiel[4]

[1] Lead City University, Ibadan, Nigeria
samson.ayanlade@lcu.edu.ng
[2] Cape Peninsula University of Technology, Cape Town, South Africa
221597999@mycput.ac.za
[3] Ladoke Akintola University of Technology, Ogbomoso, Nigeria
sasalimon@lautech.edu.ng
[4] Olabisi Onabanjo University, Ago-Iwoye, Nigeria
ezekiel.sunday@oouagoiwoye.edu.ng

Abstract. Flexible alternating current transmission systems (FACTS) are power electronics-based static controllers which control the transmission network parameters to improve system performance. They are used to solve various power system problems which include; voltage stability, voltage deviation and power losses. However, these devices need to be optimized to achieve desired results. This paper presents the application of firefly algorithm (FA) to optimize Static Var Compensator (SVC) and Static Synchronous Compensator (STATCOM) for voltage profile improvement and power loss minimization on IEEE 14 bus system. The results showed that the active and reactive power losses were minimized by 8.7 and 10.1%, respectively with FA optimized SVC and 10.7 and 14.7%, respectively with FA optimized STATCOM. Therefore, the optimal allocation of SVC and STATCOM improve the performance of the network which indicates the effectiveness of FA in optimizing SVC and STATCOM.

Keywords: FACTS · STATCOM · SVC · FA · Voltage magnitude · Power loss

1 Introduction

Electrical power is conveyed from generating station to load through an extensive transmission and distribution networks. Nowadays, as population and industrialization are increasing exponentially, so also the power demanded. This results in an increase in losses on the transmission network and consequently poor voltage profile, which is due to shortage of reactive power. Voltage profile deviation and insufficient reactive power in a transmission system usually lead to total system collapse and consequently, disruption of power to the consumers and high economic loss for manufacturing industries [1].

F. Saeed et al. (Eds.): IRICT 2021, LNDECT 127, pp. 385–396, 2022.
https://doi.org/10.1007/978-3-030-98741-1_32

There are two ways to solve these problems; firstly, the expansion of the existing transmission network and secondly, the use of traditional procedures such as placement of capacitor bank and FACTS devices. The first method is ineffective, tedious, challenging and very expensive. The second method, which is simpler and the most comfortable, entails compensating the reactive power in the network. It is inexpensive than to construct or expand the transmission network [2].

The advancement of technology in power electronics brought about FACTS devices, and they are power electronics based. According to IEEE, FACTS controllers are power electronics-based static controllers that enhance the controllability of the network. They have been effectively utilized on transmission network for power flow control, loss reduction, voltage regulation, transient stability enhancement, and system oscillation mitigation by regulating their parameters. Also, FACTS devices can control various network parameters to improve the network performance [3]. They also help in the reduction of overloading of the lines and minimization of the I^2R losses in the network when utilized to integrate the transfer capability of the system from sending end to receiving end [4].

To serve the primary purpose of these FACTS devices on the transmission network, they must be appropriately placed in the best position referred to as the optimal position. Their performances depend mostly on their appropriate placement on the network. Quite a lot of methods have been used to solve FACTS controllers optimal placement problems on transmission networks [5].

These methods include evolutionary programming (EP), particle swarm optimization (PSO), cuckoo search algorithm (CSA), genetic algorithm (GA), biogeography based optimization (BBO), simulated annealing (SA), chaotic ant swarm optimization (CASO), firefly algorithm (FA) etc. [6]. Also, majority of the works carried out in this field of study only consider the optimal placement of a single type of FACTS controllers in improving the performance of the network but do not seek to compare the effects of different types of FACTS controllers on transmission networks. This paper therefore, utilized FA for optimal allocation of SVC and STATCOM to compare their effectiveness in reducing voltage magnitude deviations and power losses in transmission networks. Matlab programme was used to perform the simulations on IEEE 14-bus network.

2 STATCOM Structure and Operation Mode

It is a switching converter static VAR generator that is parallel-connected which could either absorb or generate reactive power through different kinds of switching operations within the converter, without the use of any energy storages [7]. Reactive power in the transmission system, could be effectively compensated by the optimal placement of this controller. Reactive power is generated or absorbed from the network to improve the efficiency and reliability of the network [8]. The configuration of STATCOM is shown in Fig. 1. It comprises voltage source converter (VSC), a dc capacitor, and a coupling transformer. The DC voltage in the configuration is converted to 3-phase output voltages with appropriate frequency, amplitude, and phase by the VSC electronic part [9].

The reactive power exchange between the power network and the device is regulated by varying the 3-phase voltage magnitude, V_{vsc}, of the converter. When V_{vsc} of the converter is greater than V_{ac} (i.e. $V_{vsc} > V_{ac}$), the STATCOM injects reactive power to the system. Otherwise, if V_{vsc} is lesser than V_{ac} (i.e. $V_{vsc} < V_{ac}$), reactive power is absorbed from the network. Also, if V_{vsc} and V_{ac} are equal in magnitudes (i.e. $V_{vsc} = V_{ac}$), the STATCOM is in standby mode. The power flow equations for STATCOM controller are given in Eqs. 1–4.

$$P_m = P_{sh} + \sum_{j=1}^{N} |V_m||V_j||Y_{mj}|\cos(\theta_{mj} - \delta_{mj}) \tag{1}$$

$$Q_m = Q_{sh} + \sum_{j=1}^{N} |V_m||V_j||Y_{mj}|sin(\theta_{mj} - \delta_{mj}) \tag{2}$$

$$P_{sh} = G_{sh}|V_m|^2 - |V_m||V_{sh}||Y_{sh}|cos(\theta_{msh} - \delta_{sh}) \tag{3}$$

$$Q_{sh} = B_{sh}|V_m|^2 - |V_m||V_{sh}||Y_{sh}|sin(\theta_{msh} - \delta_{sh}) \tag{4}$$

where, $V_m\angle\theta_m$ = voltage at bus m, $V_{sh}\angle\theta_{sh}$ = injected shunt voltage, Q_m, P_m and Q_{sh}, P_{sh} are the reactive and active powers at bus m and STATCOM, respectively, G_{sh}, Y_{sh} and B_{sh} are the STATCOM conductance, admittance and susceptance, respectively, $Y_{mj}\angle\delta_{mj}$ = admittance between buses m and j, N = bus number at bus m.

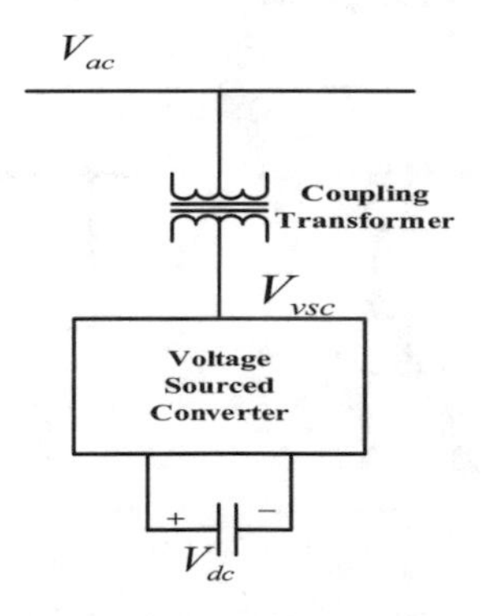

Fig. 1. STATCOM basic structure

3 SVC Structure and Operation Mode

SVC is a parallel-connected FACTS controller type, which comprises a series thyristor-switched-reactor (TSR), which absorbs reactive power and thyristor-switched-capacitor (TSC), which injects reactive power to the system at the required time of need. It also comprises various filters to filter harmonics out of the system. Figure 2 shows a typical configuration of SVC connected in a transmission network. SVC works on the basic principle of controlling shunt susceptance. Generally, SVC is subdivided into two viz;

fixed-capacitor thyristor-controlled reactor (FC-TCR) and thyristor-switched capacitor thyristor-controlled reactor (TSC-TCR).

In this paper, TSC-TCR was adopted because of its flexibility and very low rating of the reactor that generates fewer harmonics that can easily be mitigated with the help of a filter. The SVC voltage control equations can be expressed as:

$$V = V_{ref} + X_s\left(-B_{c,\max} < B < B_{1,\max}\right) \tag{5}$$

$$V = \frac{I}{B_{c,\max}} \quad \text{(for inductive SVC)} \tag{6}$$

$$V = \frac{I}{B_{1,\max}} \quad \text{(for capacitive SVC)} \tag{7}$$

where, V and V_{ref} are the positive sequence and reference voltages respectively, $B_{c,max}$ and $B_{1,max}$ = maximum capacitive and inductive susceptance, respectively, I = reactive current, X_s = droop/slope reactance.

The slope values are required to avoid hitting limit for little bus voltage variation and they are in 0.02–0.05 p.u. range. Just like STATCOM, SVC equations were also incorporated into the Newton Raphson power flow algorithm for modification, and the results of both shunt FACTS devices are compared and presented.

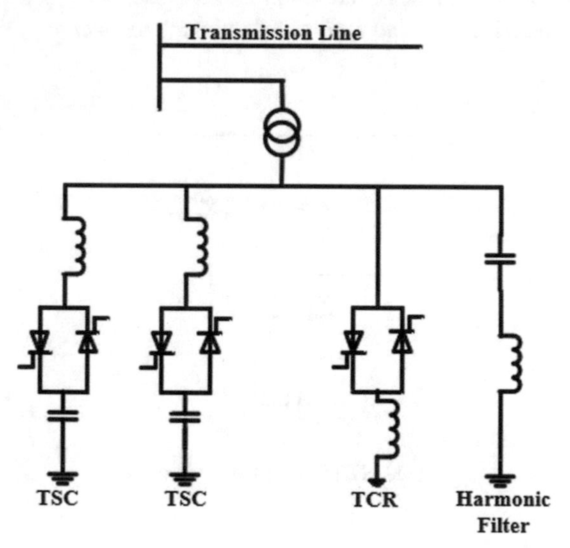

Fig. 2. Typical configuration of SVC.

4 Problem Formulation

4.1 Load Flow Analysis

Newton Raphson load flow method has proved to be most successful, due to their strong convergence characteristics, as a reliable solution to real-life transmission systems. Therefore, Newton Raphson power flow solution technique was adopted to solve the non-linear load flow algebraic steady state equations of the transmission network. SVC and STATCOM equations were integrated into the Newton Raphson power flow algorithm.

4.2 Objective Function

FACTS device placement in transmission network minimizes network power losses, subjected to voltage constraints. Minimization of the transmission active power loss is the objective function, which is expressed mathematically as in Eq. 8:

$$Min\ P_{loss} = \sum_{i=1}^{n} G_i(V_i^2 + V_j^2 - 2V_iV_j \cos\delta_{ij}) \tag{8}$$

Subjected to the constraints as follows:

Equality Constraints. The balanced power flow equations that are expressed as Eq. 9 and Eq. 10, below [10]:

$$P_{Gi} - P_{Di} = P_i(V, \delta) \tag{9}$$

$$Q_{Gi} - Q_{Di} = Q_i(V, \delta) \tag{10}$$

Inequality Constraints. These are voltage and reactive power generation limits imposed on load (PQ) constraints on the network generator (PV) buses and STATCOM as given in Eqs. 11 and 12

$$V_{\min}^i \le V_i \le V_{\max}^i \tag{11}$$

$$Q_{Gi}^{\min} \le Q_{Gi} \le Q_{Gi}^{\max} \tag{12}$$

4.3 Firefly Algorithm

FA is a nature-based algorithm developed by Yang to solve continuous optimization problems. It is an algorithm for solving optimization problems especially in power system [11].

It was developed on three rules.

1. Artificial fireflies are unisex.
2. Attractiveness depends on flashing brightness of the fireflies and it is inversely proportional to the distance from the other firefly. As the most attractive firefly is the brightest one, it attracts the neighboring fireflies and if there is no brighter one, it moves randomly [12].
3. The flashing light brightness is the objective function to be optimized. The intensity of light is dependent on the objective function magnitude for problem maximization.

Using FA, the intensity of light and brightness represent the objective function, and attraction and movement towards the brightest firefly resemble reaching an optimal solution. The factors that affect the algorithm are discussed below:

Attractiveness. The firefly attractiveness is a function of its brightness and is given in Eq. 13.

$$\beta_{(r)} = \beta_o e^{-yr^2} \tag{13}$$

where, $\beta_o =$ firefly attractiveness value at $r = 0$, $\gamma =$ media light absorption coefficient.

Distance. The distance r_i between two fireflies i^{th} and j^{th} located at x_i and x_j, respectively, is given as

$$r_{ij} = \left\| x_i - x_j \right\| = \sqrt{\sum_{k=1}^{d} \left(x_i, k - x_j, k\right)^2} \tag{14}$$

Movement. A firefly i^{th} is attracted to a more attractive firefly j^{th} as in Eq. 15.

$$x_i^{t+1} = x_i^t + \beta_o e^{-yr_{ij}^2}\left(x_j^t - x_i^t\right) + \alpha(rand - 0.5) \tag{15}$$

where, $t =$ current iteration number, $x_i =$ less bright firefly, $x_j =$ brighter firefly location, $\alpha =$ randomization parameter, γ is the absorption coefficient.

In Eq. 15, above, the second term is as a result of relative attraction, and the third term is a randomization parameter which is usually selected to be in the range 0–1 and *rand* is a number generated randomly between 0–1. γ parameter is used to introduce the attractiveness variation and it is between the range of 0.01–10. The algorithm approaches the global optima when $n \to \infty$, and the iteration number exceeded one but in reality, it converges rapidly [13].

The algorithm compares the new firefly attractiveness position with the previous value. When a higher attractiveness value is produced by the new position, the firefly moves to a new position; else, the firefly remains in the previous position. FA termination criterion is dependent on a predefined fitness value. The random movement of the brightest firefly is given in Eq. 16 [14]:

$$x_i^{t+1} = x_i^t + \alpha\varepsilon_i \tag{16}$$

$$\varepsilon_i = (rand - 0.5) \tag{17}$$

The optimal solution is obtained by maximizing light intensity, I_m, function. The function is obtained by transforming the power loss function of Eq. 8, and the voltage constraints of Eq. 11, to function in Eq. 18.

$$Max.I_m = \frac{1}{1 + \Phi} \tag{18}$$

where,

$$\Phi = P_{loss} + \sum_{i \in \Psi} \left(V_i - V_i^{\lim it} \right)^2 \tag{19}$$

$$V_i^{\lim it} = \begin{cases} V_i^{\min} & if\ V_i < V_i^{\min} \\ V_i^{\max} & if\ V_i > V_i^{\max} \\ V_i & otherwise. \end{cases} \tag{20}$$

It is to be noted that, within the load flow technique, the limits of reactive power generated are varied and needed not to be controlled via the intensity function. By using Eq. 18, each firefly intensity is calculated from the randomly generated firefly population. Depending on the intensity of light, each of the fireflies moves to the optimal solution by Eq. 15, and the iteration continues until convergence is achieved. Figure 3 illustrates the flowchart for the proposed method.

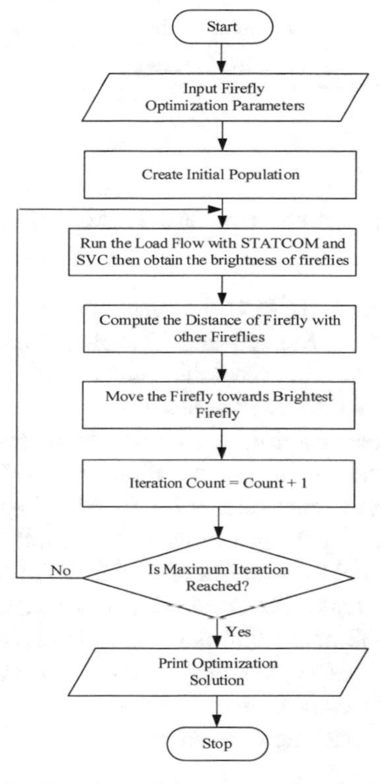

Fig. 3. Flowchart of the proposed methodology

5 Results and Discussion

The method was applied to IEEE 14-bus system and the results discussed under three sub-sections. The results were presented in line with voltage profile improvement, active and reactive loss minimizations. Table 1 shows the limits for the control, dependent variables and range for the FA parameters. The optimal location of STATCOM and SVC as determined using FA was bus 9 and the optimal size was 9.54 MVAr.

Table 1. Optimal values of FA parameters

		Min	Max
Power system variable	Voltage Magnitude (p.u)	0.95	1.05
	Q_{STAT} (MVar)	−50	
Firefly algorithm parameters	Randomness (α)	0.0	0.2
	Attractiveness (β)	0.4	1.0
	Absorption (γ)	0.1	1.0
	No. of Dimension (d)	0.0	0.2
	Population Size	3.0	0.0
	No. of Iterations	–	200

5.1 Voltage Profile Improvement with Firefly Algorithm Placed SVC and STATCOM

The effect of optimal SVC and STATCOM placements using FA, on the system voltage profile is presented in Table 2. Buses 7 and 13 violated upper voltage limit but were reduced to values which lie within acceptable voltage limits when 9.54 MVAr of SVC and STATCOM controllers were placed at bus 9.

The incorporation of these controllers with FA eliminates voltage limit violation at any of the buses and also, there is further overall network voltage profile enhancement. With the incorporation of SVC controller at bus 9, the voltages at buses 7 and 13 were minimized to 1.04 and 1.035 p.u., respectively which fall within acceptable voltage limits compared to their initial magnitudes of 1.068 and 1.067 p.u., respectively. Also, when STATCOM controller was incorporated at bus 9, the voltages at buses 7 and 13 were minimized to 1.043 and 1.038 p.u., respectively which also fall within the acceptable voltage limits. This implies that STATCOM proved superior in improving the network voltage profile compared to SVC. However, the incorporation of these controllers resulted in improved network voltage profile and stable network operation and performance.

Table 2. Voltage comparison of IEEE 14 Bus

Bus no	Base case	SVC (FA Placed)	STATCOM (FA Placed)
	Vm (p.u.)	Vm (p.u.)	Vm (p.u.)
1	1.060	1.060	1.060
2	1.045	1.048	1.046
3	0.960	0.982	0.985
4	0.969	0.978	0.981
5	0.963	0.978	0.981
6	1.020	1.012	1.015
7	**1.068**	**1.040**	**1.043**
8	0.990	0.972	0.975
9	1.027	1.026	1.029
10	1.033	1.031	1.034
11	1.030	1.025	1.028
12	1.033	1.026	1.029
13	**1.067**	**1.035**	**1.038**
14	1.047	1.044	1.047

5.2 Effect of Firefly Algorithm Placed SVC and STATCOM on Active Power Loss

Figure 4 illustrates an obvious comparison of the performance of both FACTS devices for the target objective of active loss reduction. It can be seen clearly that all the transmission lines recorded loss minimizations when SVC and STATCOM controllers were located with FA. Nevertheless, loss minimization differs for the two controllers. It is obvious that loss minimizations in the lines with FA placed STATCOM supersede that with FA placed SVC.

The base case total loss was 6.251 MW but was minimized to 5.707 and 5.581 MW when SVC and STATCOM were optimally placed, respectively. The reduction of 0.544 and 0.670 MW corresponding to 8.7 and 10.1%, respectively were achieved when SVC and STATCOM were optimized with FA. With FA placed STATCOM, the total active power loss was significantly reduced when compared with FA placed SVC. Notwithstanding, with the optimal locations of these two controllers, the total active loss was minimized.

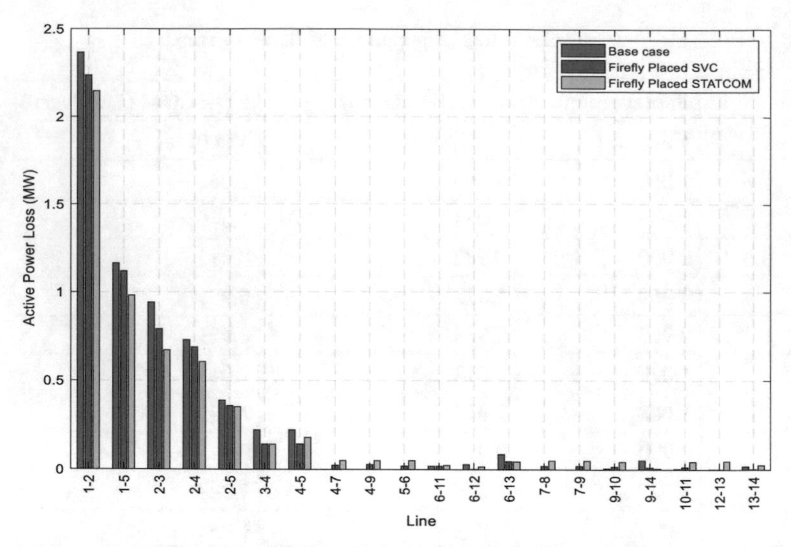

Fig. 4. Active loss minimization of the three cases

5.3 Effect of Firefly Algorithm Placed SVC and STATCOM on Reactive Power Loss

Figure 5 illustrates an obvious comparison of the performance of both FACTS devices for the target objective of reactive loss reduction. The total reactive loss as well as the total active loss reductions are depicted in Fig. 6 to better appreciate the performance of FA for SVC and STATCOM optimizations. The reactive power loss, which was 14.256 MVAr without the controllers, was minimized to 12.818 and 12.156 MVAr when SVC and STATCOM were optimally allocated, respectively using FA. There is an achievement

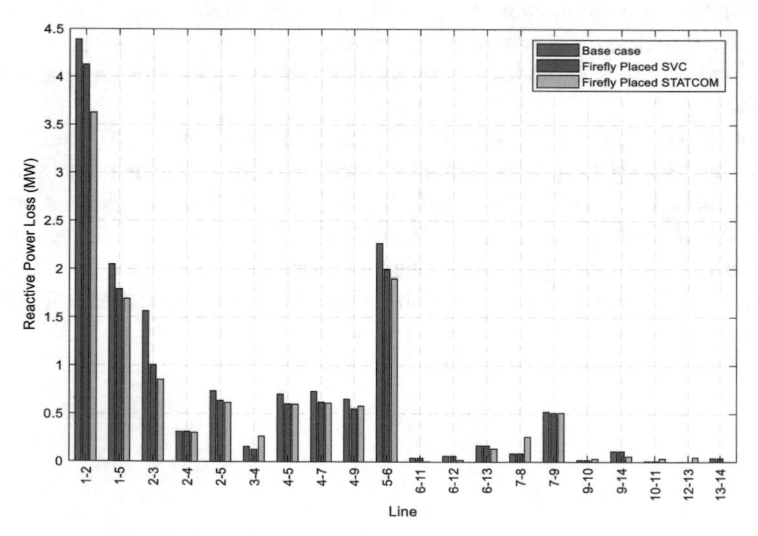

Fig. 5. Reactive power minimization for all three cases

of 1.438 and 2.100 MVAr total reduction corresponding to 10.1 and 14.7%, respectively. Also, FA placed STATCOM gave better results when compared with FA placed SVC. However, optimal placements of both controllers result in an optimal achievement of the desired objectives.

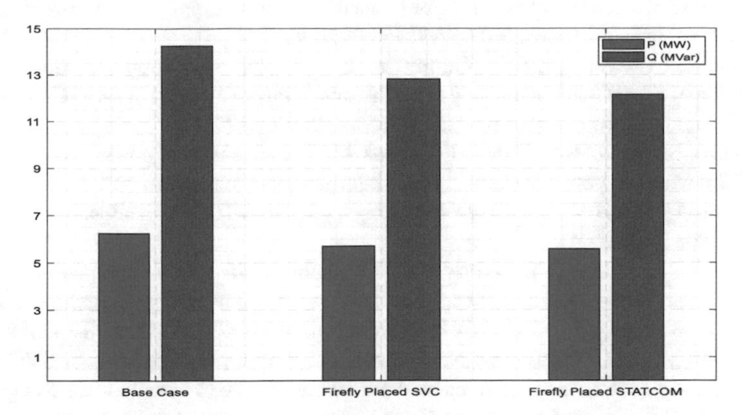

Fig. 6. Total real and reactive power reduction for all three cases

6 Conclusion

The use of FA for optimal location of shunt FACTS devices has been presented. It was observed that optimal size and placement of STATCOM and SVC controllers improved the network voltage profile and simultaneously reduced the active and reactive power losses. However, STATCOM performed better than SVC in both voltage profile improvement and loss minimizations. Hence, this work demonstrated the efficacy of FA to optimally place SVC and STATCOM on transmission network.

Contribution. The contribution of this paper is the establishment of the superiority of optimal allocation of STATCOM over SVC in reducing power losses and enhancing the transmission network voltage profile.

References

1. Damor, K.G., Patel, D.M., Agrawal, V., Patel, H.G.: Comparison of different fact devices. Int. J. Sci. Eng. **1**(1), 372–375 (2014). https://doi.org/10.1109/APCC.2016.7581484
2. Ayanlade, S.O., Komolafe, O.A., Adejumobi, I.O., Jimoh, A.: Distribution system power loss minimization based on network structural characteristics of network. In: 1st Faculty of Engineering and Environmental Sciences Conference Proceedings, pp. 849–861, Uniosun, Osogbo, Nigeria (2020)
3. Ayanlade, S.O., Komolafe, O.A.: Distribution system voltage profile improvement based on network structural characteristics of network. In: 2019 OAU Faculty of Technology Conference (OAU TekCONF 2019) Proceedings, pp. 75–80, OAU, Ile-Ife, Nigeria (2019)

4. Manoj, R.H., Kavita, S.G., Jogi, V.: Voltage regulation of STATCOM using flexible PI control. In: 2017 2nd International Conference on Communication and Electronic Systems (ICCES) 2017 Proceedings, pp. 128–133 (2017). https://doi.org/10.1109/CESYS.2017.8321248
5. Adewolu, B.O., Saha, A.K.: Performance evaluation of FACTS placement methods for available transfer capability enhancement in a deregulated power networks. In: 2020 International SAUPEC/RobMech/PRASA Conference Proceedings, pp. 1–6 (2020). https://doi.org/10.1109/SAUPEC/RobMech/PRASA48453.2020.9041146
6. Okelola, M.O., Ayanlade, S.O., Ogunwole, E.I.: Particle swarm optimization for optimal allocation of STATCOM on transmission network. J. Phys. Conf. Ser., CMVIT **1880**(012035), 1–7 (2021). https://doi.org/10.1088/1742-6596/1880/1/012035
7. Chirantan, S., Swain, S.C., Panda, P.C., Jena, R.: Enhancement of power profiles by various FACTS devices in power system. In: 2nd International Conference on Communication and Electronic Systems (ICCES) 2017 Proceedings, pp. 896–901 (2018). https://doi.org/10.1109/CESYS.2017.8321212
8. Tamboli, A.S., Jadhav, H.T.: Hybrid STATCOM for reactive power compensation. In: 2018 International Conference on Current Trends Towards Converging Technologies (ICCTCT 2018) Proceedings, pp. 1–5 (2018). https://doi.org/10.1109/ICCTCT.2018.8550889
9. Ceaki, O., Vatu, R., Golovanov, N., Porumb, R., Seritan, G.: Analysis of SVC influence on the power quality for grid-connected PV plants. In: 2014 International Symposium on Fundamental Electrical Engineering, (ISFEE) 2014 Proceedings, pp. 1–5 (2015). https://doi.org/10.1109/ISFEE.2014.7050604
10. Laifa, A., Boudour, M.: Optimal placement and parameter settings of unified power flow controller device using a perturbed particle swarm optimization. In: 2010 IEEE International Energy Conference Proceeding, pp. 205–210 (2010). https://doi.org/10.1109/ENERGYCON.2010.5771677
11. Wang, J., Liu, G., Song, W.W.: Firefly algorithm with proportional adjustment strategy. In: Hacid, H., Sheng, Q.Z., Yoshida, T., Sarkheyli, A., Zhou, R. (eds.) QUAT 2018. LNCS, vol. 11235, pp. 78–93. Springer, Cham (2019). https://doi.org/10.1007/978-3-030-19143-6_6
12. Xing, B., Gao, W.-J.: Innovative Computational Intelligence: A Rough Guide to 134 Clever Algorithms. Springer, Cham (2014). https://doi.org/10.1007/978-3-319-03404-1
13. Yang, X.S., He, X.: Firefly algorithm: recent advances and applications. Int. J. Swarm Intell. **1**(1), 36 (2013). https://doi.org/10.1504/ijsi.2013.055801
14. Selvarasu, R., Kalavathi, M.S., Rajan, C.C.A.: SVC placement for voltage constrained loss minimization using self-adaptive firefly algorithm. Arch. Electr. Eng. **62**(4), 649–661 (2013). https://doi.org/10.2478/aee-2013-0051

Efficient and Secure Topology Discovery in SDN: Review

Olomi Isaiah Aladesote(✉) and Azizol Abdullah

Faculty of Computer Science and Information Technology, Universiti Putra Malaysia, Seri Kembangan, Selangor, Malaysia
gs57427@student.upm.edu.my

Abstract. Effective and efficient management of the Software-Defined networks (SDN) requires that the controller has the current or detailed information on the network, and its topology. The controller achieves topology discovery in SDN when an appropriate channel; that permits all network devices and communication channels between links to be recognized by it, such that the controller connects with the forwarding elements positioned at a higher level using OpenFlow channels. The use of OpenFlow Discovery Protocol (OFDP) that leverages on the Link Layer Discovery Protocol (LLDP) packet for link topology discovery has shown to be inefficient and insecure. LLDP is vulnerable to attacks (Flooding, Replay, and Poisoning) due to the lack of packet authentication, the absence of integrity check, and the reuse of static packets. Many researchers have proffered state-of-the-art solutions to an efficient and secure topology discovery. Therefore, this study provides an overview of the Architecture and topology discovery in SDN. In addition, this study also discusses the state-of-the-researches that provided solutions to an efficient and secured topology discovery. Also, the study suggests challenges and future directions.

Keywords: SDN · Topology discovery · OFDP · Topology discovery attacks · LLDP

1 Introduction

SDN helps to address the defeat of visibility of network devices (routers, switches) which is achieved by installing a monitoring system in the traditional network [1], and it is a state-of-the-art computer networking strategy that seeks to fix the shortcomings of traditional networking. In modern data networks, it is a novel method for programming the switches used [2]. It is an evolving network standard that separates the data layer from the control layer; this makes it better at solving practical problems than traditional networks [3–7]. SDN is the recent network notion that simplifies the management of the network through the implementation of logically centralized controller, known as the brain of the network or network operating system that interacts via the southbound interface with the data layer and also via the northbound interface with the application layer [8, 9].

F. Saeed et al. (Eds.): IRICT 2021, LNDECT 127, pp. 397–412, 2022.
https://doi.org/10.1007/978-3-030-98741-1_33

SDN transition to a highly scalable and centralized network management design conforms to the increasingly high networks occurring in large data centers today [10, 11]. Instead of attempting to force application-specific forwarding into outdated systems that are inappropriate for the task, SDN allows developers to direct the flow of traffic through programming an open software-based controller. Network administrator(s) can set up network services and assign virtual resources to one centralized location to direct the network infrastructure in real-time mode.

In SDN, a logically centralized controller plays an important role. One of the functions of the controller is to conduct a correct, secure, and almost real-time discovery of topology that offers a current view of the network [12]. The Discovery of a switch, the link, and host are three sections in topology management and their results in global view in SDN [13, 14]. In switch discovery, information about the switch is obtained when a connection is established between an OpenFlow switch and an OpenFlow enabled controller; link discovery enables the controller to have the knowledge and information of all the devices in the network, coupled with links through which information is exchanged [15]. The identification of hosts provides the controller with valuable information used in network management roles [16].

OFDP is used in discovery links in legacy networks before it is adopted for the same purpose in SDN. OFDP leverages LLDP to perform link topology discovery in SDN, however, it is susceptible to attacks such as poison, replay, and flooding attacks [17, 18], due to lack of SDN standardization and authentication techniques [19]. The risks associated with the current link topology discovery have prompted researchers to propose effective, secure, and reliable link discovery methods.

The main contribution in this review work, therefore are to present a background knowledge of SDN, including the topology discovery; to provide a comprehensive review of an efficient and secure link topology discovery, and to provide challenges and future directions. To achieve this, we carefully select the required articles in this domain by excluding the unsuitable ones by critically studying the titles, abstract, full text and the year of publication.

The remainder of the paper is as follows: the second section introduces SDN architecture. Section 3 presents the topology discovery in SDN, the state-of-the-art researches are presented in 4. Section 5 discusses challenges and future directions, and the conclusion in Sect. 6.

2 Overview of SDN Architecture

SDN is a networking concept that alters the existing architecture of a conventional network by removing the control modules from the switch or router and positioning them on a central location, called the controller [20]. The principles of separating the two planes (the control layer from the data layer) through a Southbound API are the result of the numerous plane separation efforts made by academia and researchers in the following researches on Open signaling [21], Active Networking [22], RADIUS [23], Orchestration [24], SANE [25], ForCES [26], 4D [27], Ethane [28]. There are three layers or planes to categorize the SDN architecture: infrastructure, control, and application [29, 30]. Besides the layers in SDN, there exist many application program interfaces (APIs): northbound and southbound [31]. We introduce the three layers or planes of SDN architecture [32] with the interfaces here.

2.1 Infrastructure Layer

The infrastructure layer, referred to as the data plane [33], is made up of network equipment such as switch/router, used explicitly for forwarding packets, coupled with other network elements that are SDN-enabled [34, 35]. In logic, each network element stands for all or part of the resources of the physical network [36]. It is an OpenFlow-based switch that contains a flow table. The flow table majorly stores flow entries, but the packets are processed based on the matched flow entry. Its role is to relay packets based on the instructions or policies issued by the controller [37, 38].

2.2 Control Layer

The control layer is also called the controller, and the brain of the network helps establish network devices and enables data and control planes communication via southbound API [39]. It is logically centralized to interpret the specifications from the application layer to the data layer. The functions of the control layer include management of topology, the configuration of the network, policy implementation, the discovery of links, entry of the flow table, among others [33]. The SDN controller's task is to monitor the network as a whole.

2.3 Application Layer

An application plane contains SDN applications, which are programs that clearly and systematically communicate through a northbound interface [40]. The application layer consists of an application or more, with each having complete influence over SDN controllers exposed to a collection of resources [41].

2.4 Southbound API

Southbound interfaces are APIs that allow interaction between the data layer and the control layer using OpenFlow protocol [33, 34]. That is, OpenFlow is a protocol that defines how OpenFlow-enabled switches communicate with one or more control servers. An OpenFlow controller places flow entries in switches by an OpenFlow controller so that these OpenFlow switches can redirect traffic based on such flow entries [35]. OpenFlow is a protocol specification that defines how OpenFlow switches and OpenFlow controllers communicate [42].

2.5 Northbound API

It is the API that exists in-between the control layer and the application layer. It permits communication between the two layers and offers a network abstraction interface to both applications and management systems on top of SDN architecture [43].

3 Topology Discovery in SDN

Discovering the topology of the network is one of the important processes for the SDN to function efficiently. In this process, the controller must have current or detailed information about the network, including its topology, to function as a centralized controller and handle data plane forwarding requests [44]. The controller achieves topology discovery in SDN when an appropriate channel; that permits all network devices and communication channels between links to be recognized by it, such that the controller connects with the forwarding elements positioned at a higher level using OpenFlow channels. The forwarding elements at the higher level further connect with both forwarding elements at the lower level and forwarding elements with Access Point (AP) using links between switches. Network applications such as load-balancing, routing, etc., and services largely depend on an up-to-date and overall view of the network to function efficiently [45]. SDN accomplishes network topology in three ways: Switch discovery, host discovery, and link discovery [46].

3.1 Switch Discovery

An OpenFlow switch initiates a session with the SDN controller through the handshake. During the initiation, the switch sends information on its identity, characteristics, active ports, and support functions via the exchange of "Features Request/Reply" messages to the controller. The controller then uses a periodic Echo (Request / Reply message) mechanism to keep the node in good working order. An OF switch can send out Port-Status messages to alert the controller when a state port changes. TCP communication is used for switch discovery and can be protected with Transport Layer Security (TLS) [47].

3.2 Host Discovery

The approach to the host discovery is centered on the principle that whenever there is a table-miss, packet_in messages are sent to the controller. Thus, when a host sends traffic to the switch because there are no flow rules yet installed for the incoming flow, the switch transmits the first packet as a packet in message to the controller, and this enables the controller to discover the host. The host discovery is done with the help of traffic provided by the hosts and this affects its mobility and the identification of hosts provides the controller with valuable information that can be used in network management roles before traffic is generated. To discover hosts on the network, different controllers use different host tracking applications [48].

3.3 Link Discovery

Links are discovered with the use of OFDP. The link discovery enables the controller to have the knowledge and information of all the devices in the network, coupled with links through which information is exchanged [15]. Different controller platforms utilize separate link discovery services to discover network links.

4 State-of-the-Art Studies in Link Discovery Topology

It is worth noting that OFDP uses LLDP packets to accomplish SDN topology discovery. However, the OFDP is inefficient, and LLDP is insecure due to the inability of the controller to identify genuine LLDP control messages, reuse static packets, and its failure to determine the source authentication of LLDP packets. OFDP is a distributed protocol that most SDN controllers use as a core protocol for discovering network topology, such that each port on each switch receives its own LLDP packet from the SDN controller; It means that during an OFDP discovery round, a controller must send the same number of packet-out messages as the number of ports in the network.

Numerous authors have presented several state-of-the-art studies to improve the efficiency of protocol. Authors in [49, 50] amended the existing topology discovery method to improve the efficiency and reduce the control load of a controller. The de facto standard of the topology discovery is adjusted to form OFDPv2 with similar performance with OFDP by sending an LLDP frame per switch, which leads to a reduction in the number of LLDP messages. Furthermore, a switch sends (broadcasts) the LLDP packet to all of its active ports. It leads to a decrease in controller load and outstanding performance. Researchers in [51, 52] presented sOFTDP, a Secure and Efficient Topology Discovery Protocol, to resolve the reliability and scalability issue of OFDP. The bidirectional forwarding detection (BFD) technique helps to detect link topology asynchronously and notify the controller; packets are encrypted with hash values to prevent spoofing attacks and controller fingerprinting. Nevertheless, the study has not been assessed in larger testbeds and cannot reliably detect fabricated links.

To successfully manage topology discovery in SDN, Tarnaras et al. [53] introduced a ForCES-based structure that automatically discovers network topology. In this work, the neighbors update their flow tables when the controller and the switch exchange LLDP packet. The controller polls the topology information regularly and calculates the learning time. As a result, there is a reduction in controller load and network resource utilization. However, ForCES lacks open implementation, which leads to its rejection. The authors in [54] designed SD-TDP to address the lack of a topology discovery process based on layer two approaches. SD-TDP, an enhancement to OFDP, allows only a few switches to send information to the controller. A TDP – Request permits the information exchange during the interaction between the father node (FN) and active nodes (AN). AN sends messages to the closest or nearest node via active ports. All TDP messages of each AN in the network are taken by FN. After which, the controller can acquire the FN topology structure and create the entire network topology. The state is changed to AN whenever network changes occur and FN does not have AN connection. It enhances the performance of topology discovery in SDN by reducing the number of messages and discovery time. However, it does not address LLDP based security threats.

Hong et al. [55] introduced a defense mechanism tagged TopoGuard, that focuses on securing flaws in the OpenFlow controller's host monitoring and communication discovery services when the security of topology discovery became a serious concern. It keeps track of the host identity and the authorized user to ensure smooth operation. When the controller's identity and the host's identity don't fit, the machine creates a new profile and checks LLDP packets for network topology poisoning attacks using the incoming port information. It adds a keyed-hash-based message authentication code

(HMAC) to LLDP packets to improve their authenticity and helps in preventing poison attacks. Nevertheless, the research failed to analyze the effect of the link spoofing attack on routing, and also it is not free from replay attacks. Nguyen & Yoo [56] prevent the link spoofing attack orchestrated by injecting a fabricated LLDP packet into the network by adding a controller-based authenticator TLV into the packet. The HMAC approach helps determine the packet originality in the network. However, the study does not include the development of the preventive measures of the attacks.

Alharbi et al. [57] enhance TopoGuard (Hong et al., 2015) by proposing a technique to tackle the security challenges in OFDP caused by a deficiency of LLDP packets validation that exposes packets to falsification. The study uses a cryptographic Message Authentication Code (HMAC) method to validate the genuineness of LLDP packets. The HMAC, with a dynamic key, is used to determine (calculate) the MAC code, which prevents both replay and poison attacks. The technique makes it difficult for attackers to launch an effective attack, as it is tough to compute the MAC value owing to the difficulties in determining or guessing the key.

Rojas et al. [58] propose the Tree exploration discovery protocol (TEDP), a mechanism that allows switches to discover network topology automatically. The controller sends only one probe frame, which floods the network instead of neighbouring switches to send and receive messages. Two forms of TEDP: TEDP-S and TEDP-H, create a direct route throughout the discovery process with no additional messages. TEDP approach is different from LLDP, as it launches a probe frame by distributing routing information in the network and discovering the network topology at the same time. Nevertheless, the network may experience a delay during network discovery in a large data centre.

The existing approaches to preventing link fabrication attacks suffered from time delays, and also the creation of fake links by attackers drastically affect the network performance. The authors proposed ESLD [59] to address the stated challenges by sending LLDP packets to all ports except those attached to the hosts. It involves three stages (port classification, LLDP packets sending, and link detection). A time-marked HMAC (tHMAC) verification technique is used to prevent link fabrication attacks. For the SDN to function optimally, there is a need to secure both the network topology and the data layer against any form of attack. To achieve this, Sphinx [60] is introduced to detect any attack from compromised hosts and switches in the network topology and the forwarding plane, such as poison. It creates a flow graph for each type of traffic and regularly updates the network. It scans the networks for abnormal traffic and triggers a warning if found. To improve the performance of an SDN controller by reducing its traffic, SHTD [61] adopts the concept of assigning resources to the data plane to cater for the absence of an integrated method for discovering links between switches and provision of control plane fault recovery without involvement of SDN Controller. Topology is discovered by sending a top request message from the controller. This multicast message propagation uses nodes that have non-discovered, leaf, v-leaf, or core features. Controlled components and autonomic managers help the system recover from port failure.

Similarly, lm-OFDP [62], an improvement on OFDP, formulates rules for the discovery process, as it alters the switch response to LLDP packets from other switches to enhance the topology discovery protocol. The receiving switch returns the LLDP packet to the sending switch rather than sending the LLDP packet as a packet-in message to the controller. The sending switch directly sends the packet to the controller as a packet-in message to establish a bidirectional link between the sending and the receiving switches. It can only protect against link fabrication attacks while also reducing controller load. However, it is not a secured system as it is vulnerable to flooding attacks. This study proposes a Lightweight Automatic Discovery [63] to strengthen the inefficiency of OFDP and work on the unsuitability of LLDP for SDN. The controller randomly chooses a core switch and forwards the packet-out message to it. The LLDP message is then sent from the core switch to its nearby switches, who subsequently pass it to their neighbours, and so on. Every switch must forward the received LLDP message as a packet-in to the controller. The OpenFlow protocol is combined with a meter table to prevent flooding. However, it takes a longer time to discover the links between switches. It is vulnerable to attacks, as attacks can occur before introducing the block-ports.

Authors in [64] introduced TILAK, a token-based prevention technique that would handle both authentication and integrity checks on LLDP packets. The packets are legitimate if they hold authentic tokens upon verification since SDN controllers have no security approach to safeguard network topology information. Also, the port of transmission is on the eligible port table. Nevertheless, this is a need for a secure and efficient link discovery protocol to address collaborating LLDP attacks. The drawbacks in [51, 55, 56, 58] motivated authors in [65] to propose a secure and lightweight approach to link discovery protocol aimed to avoid, identify, and reduce the security risks of LLDP, which are poison, replay, and flooding attacks. Their work uses an eligible port checklist to prevent attacks, and packets are received only from ports found in the port checklist for processing. In this way, it has a better performance in overhead. However, at the initial iteration, that is, at network start-up, all ports in each switch are eligible; as a result, the network is vulnerable to attacks as the controller cannot prevent packets from any of the ports.

The limitation found in [65] prompted Chou et al. [66] to prevent attackers from exploiting the insecure nature of OFDP to perform various degrees of attacks. The study analyzes the time difference between round-trip times of each Link Layer Discovery Protocol, finds the correlation between links in the network and determines whether there is an attack or not. A match of generated verification keys with details of the packets_in messages received by the controller and comparing the number of received packets with the number of fabricated LLDP packets help determine an attack. However, blocking a port that sends more LLDP packets without further investigation can cause the removal of a legible port from the transmission.

To further improve bandwidth consumption and remove unnecessary fields in the LLDP packet, the study proposes OFDPx [67], an extended OFDP that uses a 14-byte packet format. The study splits the network view into many paths, and a packet probe is responsible for detecting links in the same path. There is a reduction in the number of packets used for the discovery and effective use of bandwidth resources. However, the discovery time may be high as OFDP is used to resolve faulty links.

Baidya & Hewett [68] explore a link validation approach to securing the network topology discovery. Their work addressed security threats associated with compromised hosts and switches by generating a table to store all active links, ports, and switches. Any link whose properties show that its port is either a host port or connects to two different switches is an illegal link. Nevertheless, the routing approach is unsuitable for tree & fat topologies, and attackers can forge LLDP packets. Chang et al. [69] propose a delegation function approach that uses LLDP-enabled switches to transmit and receive LLDP frames between neighbouring switches and report links back to the topology manager in the controller. The study is to reduce the resources required and to prevent resource conflicts between topology discovery and rerouting. It reduces the CPU utilization, traffic load, and also the number of packets for the discovery.

Authors in [70] propose an ICLF to determine links between OpenFlow switches and legacy switches in a hybrid SDN. In this study, the controller sends a single packet_out to the legacy switch, and in turn, transmits it within the network to determine bidirectional links. However, the controller is insecure, which makes the network vulnerable to attacks. The summary of the approaches to Efficient and Secure Link Topology Discovery is presented in Table 1.

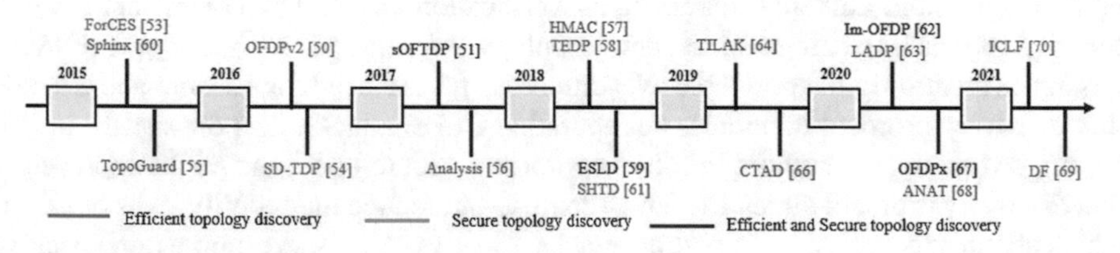

Fig. 1. Timeline for the development of Topology Discovery in SDN

Table 1. Comparison of approaches to Efficient and Secure Link Topology Discovery

Reference	Packet used	Technique proposed	Merits	Limitation
Pakzad et al. [49]	LLDP packet	OFDPv2	Two modified versions are better than OFDP in terms of the reduction in CPU overload and control traffic	It operates regularly; this can lead to needless discovery traffic, and it is unreliable when applied in a large network environment
Azzouni et al. [51]	LLDP packet	sOFTDP	It reduces CPU utilization and learning time, and the study can detect and prevent spoofing attacks and controller fingerprinting	The study has not been assessed in larger testbeds and cannot reliably detect fabricated links

(*continued*)

Table 1. (*continued*)

Reference	Packet used	Technique proposed	Merits	Limitation
Tarnaras et al. [53]	LLDP packet	ForCES	It helps in resources utilization and effectively carries out topology discovery	Lacks open implementation, which leads to its rejection and the LLDP exchange time is not considered
Ochoa-Aday et al. [54]	LLDP packet	SD-TDP	It enhances the performance of topology discovery in SDN by reducing the number of messages and discovery time	It does not address the LLDP-based security threats
Hong et al. [55]	LLDP packet	TopoGuard	The prototype is effective to prevent poison attacks with minimal overhead	It is unreliable and susceptible to replay attacks since it employs a static key with no nonce
Nguyen & Yoo [56]	LLDP packet	OFDP	The study proves or establishes that link discovery is vulnerable to attacks	The study does not include the development of the preventive measures of the attacks
Alharbi et al. [57]	LLDP packet	OFDP	Difficult for attackers to initiate an effective Poison and replay attack, and it carries out the impact evaluation on routing	It causes time delay and leads to increased overhead
Rojas et al. [58]	TEDP frame	TEDP	There is a reduction in CPU usage and the amount of bandwidth used	In a large data centre, there is the probability that the network will experience a delay while discovering topology

(*continued*)

Table 1. (*continued*)

Reference	Packet used	Technique proposed	Merits	Limitation
Zhao et al. [59]	LLDP packet	ESLD	Reduction of packet-out messages and can prevent link fabrication attacks	A Port classification stage of ESLD requires a significant number of messages, and there is an increase in CPU usage
Dhawan et al. [60]	LLDP packet	Sphinx	Able to detect abnormal behaviour in network topology and data plane	It has a single point of failure
Ochoa-Aday et al. [61]	LLDP packet	SHTD	It allows network devices to recover from port failure with less overhead	It cannot recover from network failure
Gu et al. [62]	LLDP packet	Im-OFDP	Reduction in controller load	It is susceptible to other attacks like flooding
Jia et al. [63]	LADP frame	OFDP	Efficient and reduces the controller load with no modification to OFDP	It takes a long time to discover the links between switches and is vulnerable to attacks, as attacks can occur if a compromised host links to a switch before the block-ports list installation
Nehra et al. [64]	LLDP packet	TILAK	It shows that all controllers under review are vulnerable to one attack or the other	Ineffective in handling packet integrity and it consumes bandwidth
Nehra et al. [65]	SLDP frame	OFDP	It performs well in terms of overhead	At the initial iteration, the network is vulnerable to attacks and its efficiency need to be improved upon

(*continued*)

Table 1. *(continued)*

Reference	Packet used	Technique proposed	Merits	Limitation
Chou et al. [66]	CTAD LLDP format	OFDP	It has the capacity to detect abnormal packets	Blocking a port that sends more LLDP packets without further investigation can cause the removal of a legible port from the transmission
Tong et al. [67]	Ethernet frame	OFDPx	There is a reduction in the number of the packet used and effective use of bandwidth resources	The discovery time may be high as OFDP is used to resolve faulty links
Baidya & Hewett [68]	LLDP frame	OFDP	It can detect poisoning attacks from compromised hosts and switches	It is not a secure system as it can only prevent poisoning attacks, and attackers can forge LLDP packets
Chang et al. [69]	LLDP packet	OFDP	Reduction in both the discovery time and messages used	The study fails to secure the topology discovery
Hussain et al. [70]	ICLF	ICLF	Capable of discovering links in a hybrid SDN and there is a reduction in packet_in messages	It does not perform well when there is an increase in the number of legacy switches in an Atlanta Topology

5 Challenges and Future Directions

Figure 1 depicts the progress made in the topology discovery in SDN over the past seven years. Despite the significant progress made in pursuit of an efficient and secure link topology discovery in SDN, several questions remain unanswered:

5.1 Standard Evaluation Metrics

The articles [50, 53], [72], [56, 59, 67, 69, 70] work on an efficient topology discovery, the following researchers [55-57, 60, 63, 64, 66, 68] focus on a secure topology discovery while [51, 57, 60] work on both efficient and secure topology discovery. These studies use some of the following parameters to measure the performance of their work: number of packet_out and packet_in messages sent and received by the SDN controller, CPU utilization, learning time, mode of operation, bandwidth consumption, control location for the discovery and discovery time. However, standard assessment criteria for measuring the performance of efficient and secure topology discovery are needed, as this will aid in evaluating the quality of research in this area.

5.2 Need for Standardized Protocol

Efficient link discovery begins with the use of OFDP, in which the controller encapsulates packet_in message with LLDP packet such that the controller sends packets to all switch ports. It results in sending numerous packets to discover links between switches. Some researchers [50, 55, 60, 61, 64, 67–69, 71] made minor modifications to enhance and improve OFDP, by sending a packet_in message to the SDN switch with an instruction to forward the packet into its ports. Other studies [51, 53, 56, 59],{Formatting Citation} use a different protocol for the discovery. Each one creates a research gap that necessitates additional investigation. Therefore, a standardized link discovery protocol is required.

5.3 Secured Cryptography Development

The link topology uses cryptography techniques such as HMAC, hash values, tHMAC, MD5, etc., and a token-based approach to preventing attackers from carrying out malicious acts during the operation. It is worthy of note that the use of these cryptography techniques has been ineffective in preventing attacks during the topology discovery [66], and no other approach has guaranteed a secure system; without the assumption that one or more of the following (the controller, switch, or host) is free from attacks. However, there is the need for algorithms that will guarantee a secure system in topology discovery.

5.4 Hybrid Parameters Formation

All the researchers use one or both nodes (the controller, switch) to hold the control logic. However, none of these researchers has conducted a single experiment employing the above parameters to determine the optimum node. Therefore, more research is required to develop a secure link topology discovery that identifies which node is the best to hold the control logic.

6 Conclusion

We present a detailed analysis of the recent cutting-edge techniques for effective and secure link topology discovery in SDN. We examine the packets, protocol/technique, security technique, and controller used, all of which are important to the current study. Each study is spotlighted, and the benefits and drawbacks of each are weighed. Also, we provide performance evaluation metrics used in existing studies and also state future research works. This survey paper can be useful for beginners and researchers who want to conduct a new and additional study in link discovery topology. Beginners and researchers who desire to conduct a new or further study in topology discovery may find this survey article interesting.

References

1. Mishra, S., AlShehri, M.A.R.: Software defined networking: research issues, challenges and opportunities. Indian J. Sci. Technol. **10**(29), 1–9 (2017)
2. Nisar, K., Welch, R., Hassan, R., Sodhro, A.H., Pirbhulal, S.: A Survey on the Architecture, Application, and Security of Software Defined Networking. Internet of Things, 100289 (2020)
3. Yang, C.T., Chen, S.T., Liu, J.C., Su, Y.W., Puthal, D., Ranjan, R.: A predictive load balancing technique for Software Defined Networked Cloud Services. Computing **101**(3), 211–235 (2019)
4. Zhang, H., Cai, Z., Liu, Q., Xiao, Q., Li, Y., Cheang, C.F.: A survey on security-aware measurement in SDN. Secur. Commun. Networks (2018)
5. François, J., Festor, O., Dolberg, L., Engel, T.: Network security through Software Defined Networking: a survey. In: 14th Proceedings of the Conference of Principles, Systems and Applications of IP Telecommunication (IPTComm), vol. 4, pp. 1–8 (2014)
6. Kreutz, D., Yu, J., Ramos, F.M.V., Esteves-Verissimo, P.: Anchor: logically centralized security for software-defined networks. ACM Transactions on Privacy and Security 22(2), 2019
7. Alsaeedi, M., Mohamad, M.M., AlRoubaiey, A.A.: Toward adaptive and scalable OpenFlow-SDN flow control: a survey. IEEE Access **7**, 107346–107379 (2019)
8. Cox, J.H., et al.: Advancing software-defined networks: a survey. IEEE Access **5**, 25487–25526 (2017)
9. Shaghaghi, A., Kaafar, M.A., Buyya, R., Jha, S.: Software-Defined Network (SDN) data plane security: issues, solutions, and future directions. In: Handbook of Computer Networks and Cyber Security: Principles and Paradigms, pp. 341–387 (2019)
10. Kim, H., Feamster, N.: Improving network management with software defined networking. IEEE Commun. Mag. **51**(2), 114–119 (2013)
11. AlShammari, W.M., Alenazi, M.J.F.: BL-Hybrid: a graph-theoretic approach to improving software-defined networking-based data center network performance. Trans. Emer. Telecommun. Technol. **32**(1), 1–20 (2021)
12. Li, W., Meng, W., Kwok, L.F.: A survey on openflow-based software defined networks: security challenges and countermeasures. J. Netw. Comput. Appl. **68**, 126–139 (2016)
13. Blial, O., Ben Mamoun, M., Benaini, B.: An overview on SDN architectures with multiple controllers. J. Comput. Networks Commun. (2016)
14. Marin, E., Bucciol, N., Conti, M.: An in-depth look into SDN topology discovery mechanisms: Novel attacks and practical countermeasures. In: Proceedings of the ACM Conference on Computer and Communications Security, pp. 1101–1114 (2019)
15. Phemius, K.: DISCO: Distributed Multi-domain SDN Controllers. https://hal.archives-ouvertes.fr/hal-00854899v2/document. Accessed 13 Feb 2021
16. Manzanares-Lopez, P., Muñoz-Gea, J. P., Delicado-Martinez, F.M., Malgosa-Sanahuja, J., De La Cruz, A.F.: Host discovery solution: An enhancement of topology discovery in OpenFlow based SDN networks. In. Proceedings of the 13th International Joint Conference on e-Business and Telecommunications, vol. 1, pp. 80–88 (2016)
17. Toufga, S., Abdellatif, S., Owezarski, P., Villemur, T.: OpenFlow based topology discovery service in software defined vehicular networks: limitations and future approaches. In: IEEE Vehicular Networking Conference (VNC), 1–4 (2019)
18. Huang, X., Shi, P., Liu, Y., Xu, F.: Towards trusted and efficient SDN topology discovery: a lightweight topology verification scheme. Comput. Networks **170**, 107119 (2020)
19. Li, D., Wang, X., Gu, Y.: A model to detect faked link in software defined network. In: 2018 3rd International Conference on Computational Modeling, Simulation and Applied Mathematics 310(CMSAM), pp. 109–114 (2018)

20. Paliwal, M., Shrimankar, D., Tembhurne, O.: Controllers in SDN: a review report. IEEE Access **6**, 36256–36270 (2018)
21. Campbell, A.T., Katzela, I., Miki, K., Vicente, J.: Open signaling for ATM, internet and mobile networks (OPENSIG'98)". Comput. Commun. Rev. **29**(1), 97–107 (1999)
22. Xia, W., Wen, Y., Foh, C.H., Niyato, D., Xie, H.: A survey on software-defined networking. IEEE Commun. Surv. Tutor. **17**(1), 27–51 (2015)
23. Trotsek, D.: 済無No title no title. J. Chem. Inf. Model. **110**(9), 1689–1699 (2017)
24. Rotsos, C., et al.: Network service orchestration standardization: a technology survey. Comput. Stand. Interf. **54**, 203–215 (2017)
25. Casado, M., et al.: SANE: a protection architecture for enterprise networks. In: 15th USENIX Security Symposium, pp. 137–151 (2006)
26. Breu, F., Guggenbichler, S., Wollmann, D.J.: Forwarding and Control Element Separation (ForCES) Protocol Specification, pp. 1–124 (2008). http://medcontent.metapress.com/index/A65RM03P4874243N.pdf. Accessed 17 Aug 2020
27. Greenberg, A., et al.: IMSLP25164-PMLP56458-Steibelt_-_Rondos_and_Sonatinas. In: ACM SIGCOMM Computer Communication Review, vol. 35, no. 5, pp. 41–54 (2005)
28. Casado, M., Freedman, M.J., Pettit, J., Luo, J., McKeown, N., Shenker, S.: Ethane: taking control of the enterprise. In: ACM SIGCOMM Computer Communication Review, pp. 1–12 (2007)
29. Paliwal, M., Shrimankar, D., Tembhurne, O.: Controllers in SDN: a review report. IEEE Access **1**(6), 36256–36270 (2018)
30. Khairi, M.H.H., Ariffin, S.H.S., Latiff, N.M.A., Abdullah, A.S., Hassan, H.K.: A review of anomaly detection techniques and Distributed Denial of Service (DDoS) on Software Defined Network (SDN). Technol. Appl. Sci. Res. **8**(2), 2724–2730 (2018)
31. Bera, S., Misra, S., Vasilakos, A.V.: Software-defined networking for Internet of Things: a survey. IEEE Internet Things J. **4**(6), 1994–2008 (2017)
32. Open Networking Foundation: Software-Defined Networking: The New Norm for Networks [White Paper], pp. 1–12 (2012). https://www.opennetworking.org. Accessed 06 Apr 2020
33. Zhang, Y., Cui, L., Wang, W., Zhang, Y.: A survey on software defined networking with multiple controllers. J. Comput. Networks Comput. Appl. **103**, 101–118 (2018)
34. Kreutz, D., Ramos, F.M.V.P., Verissimo, E., Rothenberg, C.E., Azodolmolky, S.D.S., Uhlig, S.: Software-defined networking: a comprehensive survey. Proc. IEEE **103**(1), 14–76 (2015)
35. Rawat, D.B., Reddy, S.R.: Software defined networking architecture, security and energy efficiency: a survey. IEEE Commun. Surv. Tutor. **19**(1), 325–346 (2017)
36. Fan, Z., Xiao, Y., Nayak, A., Tan, C.: An improved network security situation assessment approach in software defined networks. Peer-to-Peer Network. Appl. **12**(2), 295–309 (2017). https://doi.org/10.1007/s12083-017-0604-2
37. Lin, C.H., Li, C.Y., Wang, K.: Setting malicious flow entries against SDN operations: attacks and countermeasures. In: IEEE Conference on Dependable and Secure Computing (DSC), pp. 1–8 (2019)
38. Isyaku, B., MohdZahid, M.S., BteKamat, M., AbuBakar, K., Ghaleb, F.A.: Software defined networking flow table management of OpenFlow switches performance and security challenges: a survey. Future Internet **12**(9), 147 (2020)
39. Jo, H., Nam, J., S. Shin, J.: NOSArmor: Building a Secure Network Operating System. Security and Communination Networks
40. Prajapati, A., Sakadasariya, A., Patel, J.: Software defined network: Future of networking. In: Proceedings of the 2nd International Conference on Inventive Systems and Control, (ICISC), pp. 1351–1354 (2018)
41. Open Networking Foundation (ONF). https://www.opennetworking.org/wp-content/uploads/2014/11/TR_SDN-ARCH-1.0-Overview-12012016.04.pdf. Accessed 11 Feb 2019

42. Goransson, P., Black, C., Culver, T.: Software defined networks: a comprehensive approach **53**(9) (2017)
43. Tijare, P.V., Vasudevan, D.: The northbound APIs of software defined networks. Int. J. Eng. Sci. Res. Technol. **5**, 501–513 (2019)
44. Tarnaras, G., Athanasiou, F., Denazis, S.: Efficient topology discovery algorithm for software-defined networks. IET Networks **6**(6), 157–161 (2017)
45. Ochoa Aday, L., Cervelló Pastor C., Fernández Fernández, A.: Current Trends of Topology Discovery in OpenFlow-based Software Defined Networks, 1–6 (2015)
46. Nehra, A., Tripathi, M., Gaur, D.M.S.: Global view in SDN, pp. 303–306 (2017)
47. Nehra, A.: Architectural improvements for architectural improvements for secure SDN topology discovery, Ph.D. thesis (2019)
48. Khan, S., Gani, A., Abdul Wahab, A.W., Guizani, M., Khan, D.M.K.: Topology discovery in software defined networks: threats, taxonomy, and state-of-the-art. IEEE Commun. Surv. Tutor. **19**(1), 303–324 (2017)
49. Pakzad, F., Portmann, M., Tan, W.L., Indulska, J.: Efficient topology discovery in software defined networks. In: 8th International Conference Signal Processing Communination Systems ICSPCS 2014
50. Pakzad, F., Portmann, M., Tan, W.L., Indulska, J.: Efficient topology discovery in OpenFlow-based Software Defined Networks. Comput. Commun. **77**, 52–61 (2016)
51. Azzouni, A. Boutaba, R., Trang, N.T.M., Pujolle, G.: sOFTDP: secure and efficient topology discovery protocol for SDN. In: IEEE/IFIP Network Operations and Management Symposium: Cognitive Management in a Cyber World, NOMS, pp. 1–6 (2018)
52. Azzouni, A. Trang, N. T. M., Boutaba, R., Pujolle, G.: Limitations of openflow topology discovery protocol. In: 16th Annual Mediterranean Ad Hoc Networking Workshop, Med-Hoc-Net, pp. 9–11 (2017)
53. Tarnaras, G., Haleplidis, E., Denazis, S.: SDN and ForCES based optimal network topology discovery. In: 1st IEEE Conference on Network Softwarization: Software-Defined Infrastructures for Networks, Clouds, IoT and Services, NETSOFT 2015 (2015)
54. Ochoa-Aday, L., Cervelló-Pastor, C., Fernández-Fernández, A.: Discovering the network topology: an efficient approach for SDN. ADCAIJ Adv. Distrib. Comput. Artif. Intell. J. **5**(2), 101–108 (2016)
55. Hong, S., Xu, L., Wang, H., Gu, G.: Poisoning network visibility in software-defined networks: new attacks and countermeasures. In: 2015 Network and Distributed System Security (NDSS) Symposium, pp. 8–11 (2015)
56. Nguyen T.H., Yoo, M.: Analysis of link discovery service attacks in SDN controller. In: International Conference on Information Networking, pp. 259–261 (2017)
57. Alharbi, T., Portmann, M., Pakzad, F.: "The (In)Security of topology discovery in openflow-based software defined network. Int. J. Network Secur. Appl. **10**(3), 01–16 (2018)
58. Rojas, E., Alvarez-Horcajo, J., Martinez-Yelmo, I., Carral, J.A., Arco, J.M.: TEDP: an enhanced topology discovery service for software-defined networking. IEEE Commun. Lett. **22**(8), 1540–1543 (2018)
59. Zhao, X., Yao, L., Wu, G.: ESLD: an efficient and secure link discovery scheme for software-defined networking. Int. J. Commun Syst **31**(10), 1–18 (2018)
60. Dhawan, M., Poddar, R. Mahajan, K., Mann, V.: SPHINX: detecting security attacks in software-defined networks, pp. 8–11(2015)
61. Ochoa-Aday, L., Cervello-Pastor, C., Fernandez-Fernandez, A.: Self-healing topology discovery protocol for software-defined networks. IEEE Commun. Lett. **22**(5), 1070–1073 (2018)
62. Gu, Y., Li, D.. Yu, J.: Im-OFDP: an improved OpenFlow-based topology discovery protocol for software defined network, pp. 628–630 (2020)

63. Jia, Y., Xu, L., Yang, Y., Zhang, X.: Lightweight automatic discovery protocol for OpenFlow-based software defined networking. IEEE Communun. Lett. **24**(2), 312–315 (2020)
64. Nehra, A., Tripathi, M., Gaur, M.S., Battula, R.B., Lal, C.: TILAK: a token-based prevention approach for topology discovery threats in SDN. Int. J. Commun. Syst. **32**(17), 1–26 (2019)
65. Nehra, A., Tripathi, M., Gaur, M.S., Battula, R.B., Lal, C.: SLDP: a secure and lightweight link discovery protocol for software defined networking. Comput. Netw. **150**, 102–116 (2019)
66. Chou, L.D., et al.: Behavior anomaly detection in sdn control plane: a case study of topology discovery attacks. In: 10th International Conference on ICT Convergence: ICT Convergence Leading the Autonomous Future, pp. 357–362 (2019)
67. Tong, H., Li, X., Shi, Z., Tian, Y.: A novel and efficient link discovery mechanism in SDN, pp. 357–362(2019)
68. Baidya, S.S., Hewett, R.: Link discovery attacks in software-defined networks: topology poisoning and impact analysis. J. Commun. **15**(8), 596–606 (2020)
69. Chang, Y.C., Lin, H.T., Chu, H.M., Wang, P.C.: Efficient topology discovery for software-defined networks. IEEE Trans. Netw. Serv. Manage. **18**(2), 1375–1388 (2021)
70. Hussain, M.W., Reddy, K.H.M., Rodrigues, J.J.P.C., Roy, D.S.: An indirect controller-legacy switch forwarding scheme for link discovery in hybrid SDN. IEEE Syst. J. **15**(2), 3142–3149 (2021)
71. Azzouni, A., Boutaba, R., Trang, N.T.M., Pujolle, G.: SOFTDP: secure and efficient OpenFlow topology discovery protocol. In: IEEE/IFIP Network Operations and Management Symposium: Cognitive Management in a Cyber World, pp. 1–7 (2018)

The Good, the Bad, and the Ugly: Review on the Social Impacts of Unmanned Aerial Vehicles (UAVs)

Mohammed Yaqot and Brenno Menezes(✉)

Division of Engineering Management and Decision Sciences, College of Science and Engineering, Hamad Bin Khalifa University, Doha, Qatar Foundation, Qatar
bmenezes@hbku.edu.qa

Abstract. Cutting-edge technologies in drones or unmanned aerial vehicles (UAVs) have the potential to transform and disrupt businesses and economic sectors. UAV technology can reconfigure the design and operation of services, resulting in improved productivity expansion and economic growth. Multiple studies extol the potential social, economic, and environmental tradeoffs of this technology by outlining processes that could be optimized along the value chain. However, the picture does not have to be completely positive. Although UAVs have the power to transform and significantly enhance our society, there are still certain socio-techno-economic consequences associated with the way this technology is applied. This paper presents an overview of recent trends in researching, developing, and deploying (RD&D) the most extensively UAVs applications usage towards drones as a service (DaaS). These themes will be discussed in threefold method: the 'Good UAVs' explores how these technological tools can promote our societies; the 'Bad UAVs' discusses a more nuanced view of the potential negative externalities generated by drones. Finally, the 'Ugly UAVs' investigates the possible risks generated by commercial drones. All themes have been briefly exemplified in the agriculture industry. The level of automation linked with the human factor in-, on-, and out-the loop of cyber-physical systems should be given more research attention, emphasizing and capturing inner social perspectives of commercial UAVs. Deploying new technologies should be based on the quality and value of the job itself to create a new class of human workers who can be evolved and are not just be valuable but be valued.

Keywords: UAVs · Drones · Data · Social · Human-machine · Technology

1 Introduction

The current trend in academia and industries towards exploring, researching, developing, testing, and deploying novel apparatuses and operations in engineering management within the so-called precision engineering is revolutionizing industrial sectors. The transformations in every working environment are accelerating at a never-before-seen pace and scale. This fast shift has put labor markets off-kilter and produced a very volatile

F. Saeed et al. (Eds.): IRICT 2021, LNDECT 127, pp. 413–422, 2022.
https://doi.org/10.1007/978-3-030-98741-1_34

business environment in which competitive advantages are becoming more transitory. Evolving market disruptions facilitate new ways of getting work done by emerging societies' collective intelligence, where a talented workforce overtakes capital as a critical driver of corporate success. Population growth rate, technological advancement, increasing over-choice, and state-of-the-art working environment are some key structural and cyclical trends driving societies' transformation.

Globally, the population is rapidly aging while birth rates are declining [1]. In the technological society, employers are having a more challenging time finding employees with the necessary skills. Organizations will need to better tap underutilized talent pools like all the workers, glass ceiling, women, minorities, migrants, and people with disabilities. The fourth industrial revolution, or what is known as Industry 4.0 (I4), is evolving at an unprecedented pace, lowering barriers and boosting transparency at all levels. Individuals are also finding it increasingly difficult to maintain their skills up to date, which results in a growing bifurcation in the workforce between those with in-demand skills and those without them. The technological revolution's impact on work has started with the rise of automation, robotics, and artificial intelligence to the emergence of new business models like the sharing economy, circular economy, crowdsourcing of expertise in a freelancing fashion, and on-demand employment. Over time, multiple jobs and several career waves are in constant need of new skills. The employer-employee relationship is changing dramatically, where most individuals now concentrate on career security (relying on up-to-date knowledge) rather than long-term positions in the working environment. This entails gaining the required skills and competencies to advance their independence from their employer. Organizations are using big data and supply chain strategies in their human resource functions, which has made recruiting and retention more complex. The demand for real-time insights into workforce practices and work requirements leads organizations to seek new ways to increase efficiency and boost productivity.

This paper is a continued discussion opened by Yaqot et al. [2] and Yaqot and Menezes [3] on UAVs applications from a socio-techno-economic perspective as an efficient manpower replacement tool in engineering disciplines. In the current case, we are emphasizing more the agriculture industry. Agricultural processes are still considered labor-intensive duties, where its level of automation is considered low compared to other industries. In such a field, artificial intelligence (AI) has the potential to be manifested as the intelligent diversion and automation of processes with human in-on-out of the loop of cyber-physical systems (CPS) for enhanced modeling to improve operational efficiencies. Agricultural communities and industries need to have a strategic view on continuous improvement techniques through executing easier, better, faster, and cheaper plans to maintain and further improve competitive operational excellence. Current debates indicate that investments in UAVs capabilities will remodel vast operational processes under social pillar principles, resulting in a process system re-engineering [2]. Agricultural UAVs can enhance processes' economies of scale coupled with eco-friendly applications, but the social consequences are still controversial.

In this paper, the discussions on UAVs are explored in a threefold method. Initially, we present the "Good" aspects as the potential vast benefits of UAVs and how likely it increases as AI is on constant refinement, leading societies into a new era of enormous prosperity. In the "Bad", we show the negative side of UAVs and their drawbacks with arisen societal anxieties. In the "Ugly", it presents why UAVs are not considered destructive because of their misuse; rather, they become ugly by the fact that it would obliterate many human jobs and cause major social disruption in the first place, as well as to its overlooked hazardous risks. Automation is inevitable due to its economic advantages, but privacy, regulations, and technical issues are still in the development stage. This argument aims to address how these three aspects of the same phenomena (UAVs technology) with distinct objectives can be joined in a successful pathway for society.

2 The UAV Era

Drone or UAV is an ambiguous term that refers to any unmanned vehicle, irrespective of its operating medium (land, sea, or air). Therefore, it is quite often referred to as drones, despite the fact that the terminology used to describe drones and autonomous systems might be perplexing at first. The literature has referred to UAVs as remotely piloted aircraft, remotely piloted vehicles, unmanned aircraft, remote sensor platforms, pilotless aircraft, and robot planes, where UAV is a remotely piloted vehicle controlled from a ground control station. In 2005, the Federal Aviation Administration (FAA) adopted the idiom "unmanned aircraft system" (UAS) to refer to the whole integrated operation system environment, which encompasses the air vehicle, the ground-based control station, and the communication modules, as seen in Fig. 1 [4]. The commercial UAVs are being customized with new functionalities added in a vast scope of niche domains due to the upgrowth and integration of inexpensive technologies. Massive customization of UAV applications on a large scale is now viable, and human societies are becoming more interlinked and intelligent due to technological advancements. The human-machine relationship in the division of work is always becoming vague and redefined in all disciplines [5, 6]. The applications of UAS technology in the Industry 4.0 mandate have boomed as a pre-necessity of evolving to the next generations of the so-called Society 5.0.

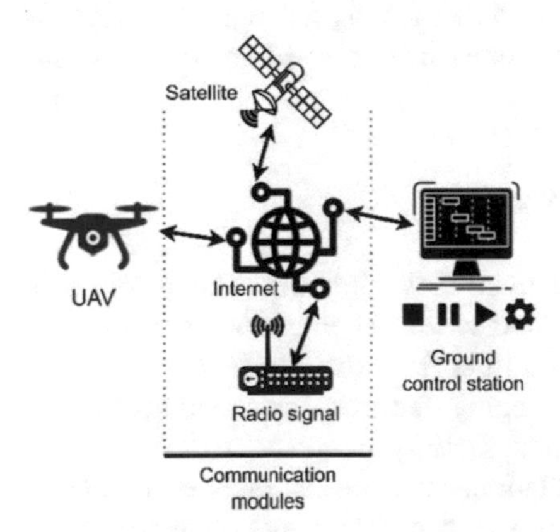

Fig.1. Typical UAS architecture.

3 The Good of UAVs

In contrast to the past, the contemporary era is characterized by a focus on connection, quality, quantity, dynamic changes, and service values. Service science has both tangible and intangible elements, and the interaction between them is active in the exchange fusion and value creation. Drones are cracking massive boundaries in the way businesses operate. With sophisticated airborne sensors and add-on technologies, it precisely allows many enterprises to see, sense, move, and transform the physical world [7]. The resulted forms of big data can be analyzed and processed using machine learning and artificial intelligence to create several applications, also known as data analytics (DA). DA techniques ensure super-fast optimized decisions to maximize efficiency, minimize cost, and, at the same time, promote safety, since UAV applications are industry agnostic with specialization occurring using different robust sensors and DA techniques (descriptive, detective, predictive, and prescriptive). With these DA techniques in an automated fashion, some sort of cognitive analytics can be reached to promote adaptive and learning processes [8].

For example, multifunctional agriculture is a broad concept encompassing agricultural productivity, sustainable resource management, and socioeconomic viability [9]. As a labor-intensive industry and having lower levels of automation when compared to other industries, a new stage of this industry, towards the so-called precision agriculture, aims to substantially increase the production of arable crop yields. By 2050, global population growth is expected to exceed 9.7 billion people, 27% higher than in 2020, and meeting food demand is crucial [10]. In this stage, farmers are still seeking innovative methods to save costs and maximize yields. By using UAVs, they can capture data faster, perform precise monitoring, boost production, optimize efficiency, and automate unnecessary activities. For example, large-scale acres can be sighted and utilized autonomously using agriculture UAV in an extremely fast timescale, resulting in accurate control resource management, e.g., water, spraying, fertilizers, and pesticides. As a result, it is an eco-friendly tool where soil contamination is decreased since fewer herbicides are consumed. Furthermore, heavy fossil-fueled machinery does not create soil compaction. It is also worth mentioning that agroecological farming is becoming more feasible because of fewer emissions resulteding from low-altitude flights and effective spraying technologies [3].

4 The Bad of UAVs

When it comes to commercial UAVs appraisal, social communities can be split into two groups: enthusiasts or adversaries. As numerous sectors are altered by drones, social views and behaviors, resulting from their impact on our everyday lives, change. The advent of UAVs is challenging traditional conceptions in some interconnected dimensions of stability, technical security, personal privacy, data ownership, shared liability, and administrative regulation. This conflict creates significant barriers to its inclusion into present public and private companies, as well as personal use [11]. The arisen societal anxieties of UAVs can be categorized into three main domains; social, technical, and systemic, in which each can be seen as an issue, obstacle, or barrier [12]. Social issues are oriented on fear the new. It refers to anything a person inwardly comprehends, which may or may not be built on fact and might even be driven by public media, common understanding, cluelessness, or deception. On the other hand, technological issues refer to the technical and procedural competencies (human-machine interaction) that stymie UAVs' evolution is influenced by contemporary expertise in the context of technology. At the same time, people are negatively affected by the emotionless estimated vision of where technological advances may go. Furthermore, it encompasses factors such as safety, security, reliability, technological capability, trustworthiness, and fast scalability. Finally, the systemic challenges that point to all issues linked with building up system solutions, are unparalleled in UAVs development speed for its integration into the standard airspace aviation system and requirements.

These three domains (social, technical, and systemic) can be plotted within the triangle of the "good", "bad", and "ugly" on the implications of the UAV in society, as seen in Fig. 2. Starting from the base of the triangle, in the orthogonal projection of the "good", there is nothing rather than the human (H), where, a) its replacement by any technology, b) the desired requirement of systematic procedures, and c) any sort of robustness from the merge of social, technical, and systemic aspects, are not mandatory. This stage belonged to pre-industrial periods, although agricultural civilizations such as the pre-Colombian ones (Inca, Azteca, Maya) applied techniques to agriculture in a systematic way, in which the societal structure had been defined. After such time in humankind's history, in the industrial societies, demands of requirements of management of systems and cascade of workloads denoted that the human was controlling the decisions to carry out actions in the progress of the processes. This stage is known as human-in-the-loop (HITL), also named human-centric-automation.

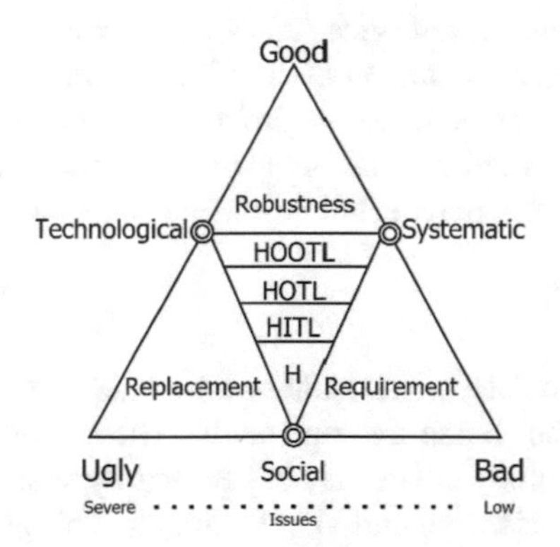

Fig.2. Threefold social impact of UAVs.

Moving up inside the triangle in Fig. 2, from the basis of the social ground, there was the period of history when started the requirements of systematic procedures and advances in technology by the evolution of industry (from the mechanical and electrical powers to the digital processing). In this era, the idea of human-on-the-loop (HOTL) was initiated from when human beings have taken decisions based on information of the systems. Today, as an aftermath of the so-called smart industry of the I4 mandate, the spread of the human-out-of-the-loop (HOOTL) cycle brings the state-of-the-art of a fully automated decision-making environment without human intervention. In such a place, the pace and path of the human-machine interaction push the robustness to the targeted level of performance to be matched when starts the non-human cognition of the artificial intelligence and advanced analytics techniques.

As an assessment of a field where UAV technologies are transforming the human-related work, Yaqot and Menezes [3] analyze the application of such mechanical, electrical, digital, and smart novelties in the agriculture industry. With radical new technologies and working techniques, the digital transformation of farms is reshaping the agriculture face and revolutionizing production, but this comes at social consequences due to the current operating limitations. Digitizing key labor-intensive routine tasks in agriculture will evoke a new set of social externalities for both farmers and farmworkers. For example, UAVs displaces farmworkers from time-consuming, tedious cultivation activities (e.g., fertilizing, spraying, monitoring, inspection, etc.). In addition, employing agriculture drones will gradually force farmers to raise automation investments and make it difficult for them to find enough skilled workers in such technologies. Farming has always been seen as a risky working environment, with low-profit margins and more frequently volatile inconsistent yields, such as rivalry for water and land, labor shortages, low wages, harsh conditions, labor justice, inadequate infrastructure, and rising environmental regulations to an already onerous agenda [2]. However, there are direct jobs for people who design, operate, extract, and maintain agricultural UAV applications. In addition, sometimes, complete new industries may be built on the applications throughput, e.g., pre-production, production, and post-production farming activities. By aligning business vision with digital strategies, complexities are simplified by integrating all agriculture's entities and conceivable cloud computing models like infrastructure as a service (IaaS), software as a service (SaaS), platform as a service (PaaS), and data as a service (DaaS) to run a digital ecosystem into a single hub anything as a service (XaaS), which in this case can be so-called drones as a service (DaaS). Nevertheless, the forgotten part is the indirect effect of labor-saving inventions since organizations can do more with less to expand and maybe add new large-scale processes.

5 The Ugly of UAVs

With the rise of UAV in society, what could best be described as ugly is that people will not just be unemployed but being unemployable. The reason for this ugly scenario is that the wealth that technology creates is not necessarily shared with all workers, especially the labor-intensive of the so-called blue-collars. This is known as sociotechnical change. Such a situation can be proved when the income of most families stays flat or in decline as the economy grows and the inflation rate is accumulated [13]. Even if the unemployment rate remains low, automation may exacerbate economic inequality, especially in the United States, which currently has an inequality higher than in most other developed countries. However, since governments decide how a society confronts disruptions, technology is not destiny, which worries people on all sides of the argument regarding risks and the future of work.

According to a recent widely referenced analysis [14], robotics will overtake 47% of United States jobs due to technological automation capabilities in the next one or two decades. However, it did not attempt to determine the actual extent of automation or its overall impact on employment. It also does not imply that new employment would occur immediately (time gap) or would be placed in an exact location (geographic gap), nor will it pay the same wage (skills gap) as the ones that were lost or replaced (Fig. 2). As a result, the need for human work has not gone away.

Furthermore, the increased usage of UAVs has raised public concern and debate, particularly over privacy and safety issues. Therefore, a detailed literature review [15] of commercial UAVs spanning 2010 to 2015 is carried to investigate societal, governance, privacy, and ethical dimensions of their usage, driven by a techno-ethical framework which is the study of technology influence on ethical and moral values of societies. The findings imply that, while commercial UAVs may help improve livelihood and boost efficiency, more attention must be made to unforeseen repercussions and potential negative consequences in order to encourage commercial UAVs' ethical use. While the agriculture industry has begun a radical transformation in the last fifteen years, agriculture evolved from a labor-intensive industry to mechanized and robotic-intensive production systems spanning the previous century. During this shift there was a constant labor outflow from agriculture, primarily from standardized tasks within the production processes. In today's stage of the industrial evolution applied to engineering and society, which is based on cost-effective methods facilitated by AI, UAVs can now be used to perform non-standardized tasks (e.g., weed control, crop protection, etc.) formerly assigned for human workers at a faster and more efficient pace. Consequently, automation in agriculture is no longer restricted to standardized tasks within production systems [16]. Even though the robotic ecology has significant ethical, legal, and social implications, UAVs will drastically collaborate with humans rather than eliminate them in many agriculture instances.

6 Discussion

As the debate continues, scholars, labor entities, theoreticians, and practitioners involved in any discussion on the advantages of new technology should include the quality and value of the job itself. A new class of human workers can be developed who are not just be valuable but be valued if we can use technological advancement to make them more skilled, productive, and more efficient. The most cutting-edge technology on current markets will eventually become standard and inexpensive tools, implying that the true power and potential lie with the people who work (blue-collars) and, more specifically, agriculture workers. Robotics involving UAVs are significantly faster, efficient, precise, and accurate in capturing, processing, analyzing, and extracting data compared to powerless human capabilities. In robotics and integrated cyber-physical systems, a shift in human-factor involvement from in-the-loop to on-the-loop to out-of-the-loop can be observed, which is also widely noticeable in recent Internet of Things (IoT) applications. Because of the rising amount of data from numerous sources that should be processed, integrated, and then interpreted into decision-making, the transition from (in-on-out) of the loop has exponentially evolved from a complete human interaction (H) to the human-in-the-loop (HITL), a type of a human-centric-automation engine, which denotes that the human had the control or decision required to carry out an action in the system. In the further state, a human-on-the-loop (HOTL) represented human decisions relying on information gathered from the system. That, with the rise of the widespread information and computing technologies (ICT) of the new century of Industry 4.0, yielded the human-out-of-the-loop (HOOTL) within the autonomy of the processes (without human intervention) in the decision-making environment (Fig. 3).

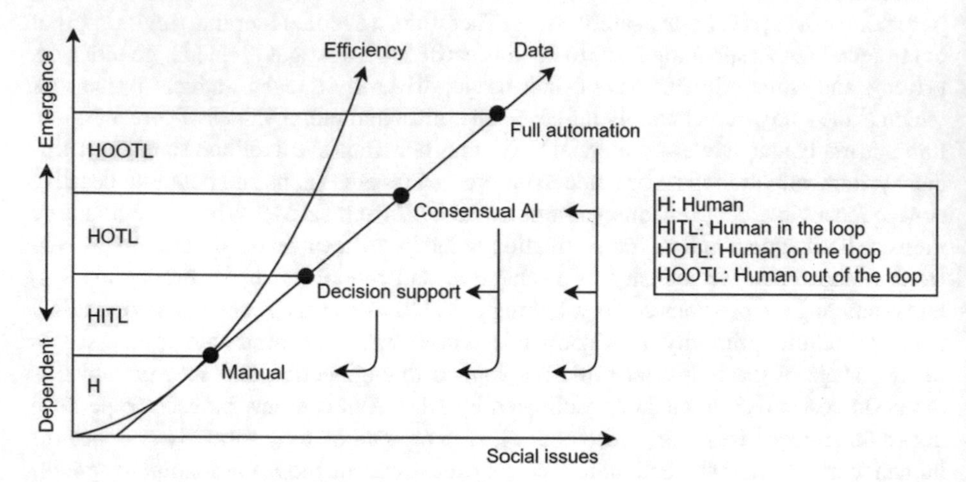

Fig. 3. Human-machine interaction and levels

Due to the extreme potential for rapid deployment and high return on investment, the use of UAVs has become a hot topic in the business sector. However, UAVs are a novel technology, and further research is needed to leverage positive societal impact on our daily lives. Instead of prohibiting physical usage due to safety concerns, a new set of systematic policies and regulations should have a broader social viewpoint.

From laboratory-level to mature industries, advanced manufacturing production systems are evolving to identify, design, and evaluate new opportunities in the way forward of research, development, and deployment (RD&D) stages [17]. The three parameters have been broken further to some key features and then evaluated based on the RD&D stage, requirement, and whether good, bad, or ugly (Table 1).

Table 1. UAVs social impacts

	Commercial UAVs impact	RD&D stage	Req. [a]	Type
Social	Replacement	Research	↑↑☻	Ugly
	Awareness	Research	↑↑☻	Bad
	Trust	Research	↑↑☻	Ugly
	Skills	Research	↑↑☻	Bad
	Privacy	Research	↑↑☻	Ugly
	Social safety	Research	↑↑☻	Bad
	Job security	Research	↑↑☻	Ugly
	Ethical use	Research	↑↑☻	Ugly
	Harassment	Research	↑↑☻	Bad
Technical	Safety	Development	↑☻	Bad
	Privacy	Development	↑☻	Ugly
	Ownership	Development	↑☻	Ugly
	Malfunctions	Development	↑☻	Bad
	Security	Development	↑☻	Bad
	Task-time	Deployment	↔	Good
	Accuracy	Deployment	↔	Good
	Efficiency	Deployment	↔	Good
Systematic	Business model	Research - Development	↑↑	Bad
	Operating system	Research - Development	↑↑	Bad
	Liability	Development	↑↑☻	Bad
	Regulation	Research - Development	↑↑☻	Bad

[a] Note: requitements, ↔: stable; ↑: demanded; ↑↑: highly demanded; ☻human risk

7 Conclusion and Future Work

The expansion of smart mobile applications, wireless communication systems, and internet infrastructure has greatly influenced trade and development in a globalized knowledge-based society. The interaction between information and communication technologies and human-machine aspects are critical for revolutionizing businesses, job creation, e-commerce, and socio-economic growth. Governments are required to foster productive and inclusive use of UAVs by providing the necessary physical infrastructure, policy, institutional, legal, ethical, and socio-technical frameworks to create trust and thereby more productive use of UAV applications in the agribusiness industry, among others. Data analytics via drones as a service may aid in the conservation of biodiversity and ecosystems by providing farmers with information on sustainable and precise farming practices as well as new market avenues.

By the reduced literature on UAVs, we cannot provide in-depth coverage of certain application domains. The agriculture industry is exemplified from a strategic business point of view due to its low level of automation and towards the digital ecosystem. The development and deployment of UAVs in numerous fields are the subjects of intense controversy, from where we focus on their societal implications. Finally, this work foresees further investigation to involve needed socio-technical systems and level of automation linked with human factor in-, on-, and out-the-loop of CPS studies through scholarly research focusing on capturing inner perspectives on UAVs regulation. As such, surveys need to be undertaken to gather practical procedures from UAVs specialists. Furthermore, an inherent quantitative approach on the impact of UAVs as complementarity versus substitution of human workers is required.

References

1. World-Bank Homepage, World Population Prospects: 2019 Revision, World Bank Open Data (2021)
2. Yaqot, M., Menezes, B.C., Al-Ansari, T.: Unmanned aerial vehicles in precision agriculture towards circular economy: a process system engineering (PSE) assessment, pp. 1559–1565. Computer Aided Process Engineering, Istanbul (2021)
3. Yaqot, M., Menezes, B.C.: Unmanned aerial vehicle (UAV) in precision agriculture: business information technology towards farming as a service. In: 1st International Conference on Emerging Smart Technologies and Applications, pp. 1–7. IEEE, Sanaa (2021)
4. Elias, B.: Unmanned aircraft operations in domestic airspace: US policy perspectives and the regulatory landscape, pp. 1–29 Congressional Research Service (2016)
5. Doyle Kent, M., Kopacek, P.: Do we need synchronization of the human and robotics to make industry 5.0 a success story? In: Durakbasa, N.M., Gençyılmaz, M.G. (eds.) ISPR 2020. LNME, pp. 302–311. Springer, Cham (2021). https://doi.org/10.1007/978-3-030-62784-3_25
6. Jarrahi, M.H.: Artificial intelligence and the future of work: Human-AI symbiosis in organizational decision making. Bus. Horizons **61**(4), 577–586 (2018)
7. Maghazei, O., Netland, T.: Drones in manufacturing: exploring opportunities for research and practice. J. Manuf. Technol. Manag. **31**(6), 1237–1259 (2019)
8. Menezes, B.C., Kelly, J.D., Leal, A.G., Le Roux, G.C.: Predictive, prescriptive and detective analytics for smart manufacturing in the information age. IFAC-Papers Online **52**(1), 568–573 (2019)
9. Li, K., et al.: Field management practices drive ecosystem multifunctionality in a smallholder-dominated agricultural system. Agr. Ecosyst. Environ. **313**, 107389 (2021)
10. UN. http://www.ncbi.nlm.nih.gov/pubmed/12283219. Accessed 20 Aug 2021
11. Rao, B., Gopi, A.G., Maione, R.: The societal impact of commercial drones. Technol. Soc. **45**, 83–90 (2016)
12. Kraus, J., Kleczatský, A., Hulínská, Š: Social, technological, and systemic issues of spreading the use of drones. Transp. Res. Procedia **51**, 3–10 (2020)
13. Charalampidis, N.: The U.S. Labor income share and automation shocks. Econ. Inq. **58**(1), 294–318 (2020)
14. Frey, C.B., Osborne, M.A.: The future of employment: how susceptible are jobs to computerisation? Technol. Forecast. Soc. Chang. **114**, 254–280 (2017)
15. Luppicini, R., So, A.: A technoethical review of commercial drone use in the context of governance, ethics, and privacy. Technol. Soc. **46**, 109–119 (2016)
16. Marinoudi, V., Sørensen, C.G., Pearson, S., Bochtis, D.: Robotics and labour in agriculture. A context consideration. Biosyst. Eng. **184**, 111–121 (2019)
17. Menezes, B.C., Kelly, J.D., Leal, A.G.: Identification and design of industry 4.0 opportunities in manufacturing: examples from mature industries to laboratory level systems. IFAC-PapersOnline **52**(13), 2494–2500 (2019)

Big Data Analytics for Large Scale Wireless Body Area Networks; Challenges, and Applications

Haider Rasheed Abdulshaheed[1], Haider Hadi Abbas[2], Ehsan Qahtan Ahmed[3], and Israa Al-Barazanchi[1,4](✉)

[1] Computer Engineering Techniques Department, Baghdad College of Economic Sciences University, Baghdad, Iraq
haider252004@yahoo.com

[2] Computer Technology Engineering Department, Al-Mansour University College (MUC), Baghdad, Iraq
haider.hadi@muc.edu.iq

[3] Department of Computer Science, AL Nahrain University, Baghdad, Iraq
Ehsan.qahtan@nahrainuniv.edu.iq

[4] College of Computing and Informatics, Universiti Tenaga Nasional (UNITEN), Kajang, Malaysia
Israa44444@gmail.com

Abstract. With the development of technology and connectivity, it is has become easier to gather data regarding a necessity, and use that to analyze, observe and provide solutions to day-to-day problems. The development of science and technology has brought immense benefit and comfort to human society allowing us to venture further with ease. The same applies to Wireless Body Area Network (WBAN), the system that measures the medical parameters of a human subject to treat his or her ailments. The data gathered from various patients can be collected and provided to the medical authority and doctors accordingly. This is used to generate patterns from a definitive source and provide clarity of the patient's disease and/or any condition to the doctors. However, doing that for many patients and hospital records requires an immense amount of time and people. This is where big data analytics comes into play, a cloud based analytics technology that scans extraordinarily large amounts of data, identifies similarities and differences, and observes the patterns to help doctors solve their patients' diseases or conditions. Using this technology prevents unnecessary deaths of patients. This paper will explain the implementation process of big data analytics in large scale WBAN, the difficulties and challenges that may occur, and its applications and benefits.

Keywords: Big data analytics · Large scale WBAN · Cloud · Wireless sensor network

F. Saeed et al. (Eds.): IRICT 2021, LNDECT 127, pp. 423–434, 2022.
https://doi.org/10.1007/978-3-030-98741-1_35

1 Introduction

Big data analytics is a business and commercially based analytical tool, based on the existing methods of analyzation and with upgraded automation and cloud systems. It is made to handle huge amounts of data, technically in terabytes and petabytes, and produce accurate human-like, or better, analyzation results. The paper focuses on explaining the methods and practices of both big data analytics and large scale WBAN individually, and then the implementation process of big data in WBAN. The common challenges, benefits, and the application of both the methods are discussed in detail with respect to the implementation process. The process of implementing big data analytics in the healthcare stream is simple and can be carried out using different methods. The first steps would be the initialization of both big data analytics and WBAN separately, with a big data analytics cloud system being set up correspondingly with the WBAN system. Each of the systems has its own methods of action and usage, and each of them are to be carefully designed depending on the end consumer. With the initialization completed, the WBAN is connected to the cloud system through basic to high security measures and encryption process depending on the sensitivity of the raw data. Once the primary implementation is carried out, the overall processing is monitored and possible chances of errors in the functioning of the system, analytical and pattern prediction errors, internal network errors, and failure of sensor units. With this setup achieved, doctors and the hospital management can then communicate with the patient either directly via the internet or via private mobile apps to ensure the patient's health condition improves. The sensor measurements are constantly fed into the system, and possible critical health conditions are easily predicted even before they occur. The methodology will be further elaborated in depth in the following topics, [1, 2].

2 Big Data Analytics

Big Data Analytics simply refers to the analyzation of huge amounts of data in batches or clusters. The idea was introduced to reduce human work and errors and reduce the time consumption while increasing the accuracy of the analyzation results. Big data analytics is a cloud based technology and, by means of the internet, companies can directly upload their data records and process all the information of the analysis in no time. In recent years, big data was brought into the healthcare field to improve treatment methodologies and assisted living systems. Through the internet, all the data collected from the WBAN installed on the patient is fed to the cloud system, where the analyzation process is carried out by software frameworks and AI systems. This technique makes it faster and easier to learn about a patient's condition and treat him or her appropriately and it also allows doctors to constantly check on their patients. The advantages of this are faster and cheaper analytics, plus easily and remotely accessible information which is reliable and accurate. The disadvantages are that traditional data analysts have lost their jobs, also security attacks might sabotage the workflow and cause some vulnerabilities in the system. Figure 1 shows the Big Data Analytics System [3, 4].

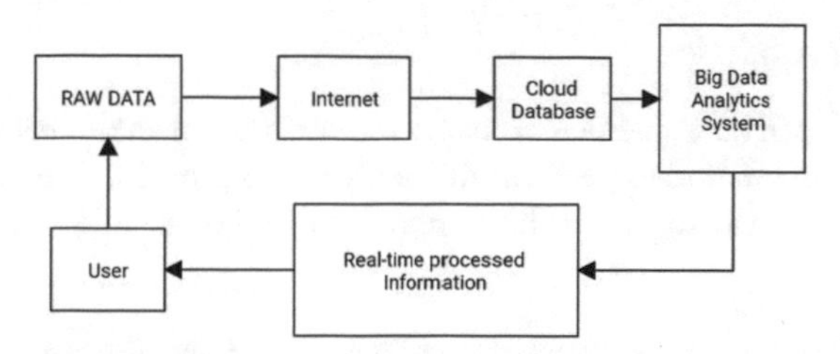

Fig. 1. Big data analytics system

2.1 Characteristics of Big Data Analytics

There are various characteristics that determine the type and usability of a big data analytics system, explained as follows. Each of these characteristics may or may not influence each other, depending on its magnitude [5–7].

- **Velocity:** Velocity refers to the continuous flow of data fed to the cloud base, and the amount of data that can be processed at one time with respect to the rate of data flow. his is providing a clarity of how much data and how fast the data is being processed by the system. Since, data flows from various resources and aspects, and different priority levels are provided for various sources, it is necessary to learn of this characteristic to fully use the analytics system.
- **Volume:** Volume refers to the immense amount of data that are to be processed and stored. This only requires an efficient cloud storage system. There is nothing much to improvise here, except for a proper backup system, which will be managed by the cloud storage system. Through this, the raw data, and processed data, from WBAN, is collected by doctors and hospital authorities for further usage.
- **Variety:** Variety refers to the different sets of data, and how the system should be able to distinguish them and process each data as defined by the user. This will widely vary depending on the field in which big data analytics is used. For WBAN, the variety of data may come from the heartbeat sensor, breathing levels, blood pressure and so on, depending on the patient.
- **Veracity/Value:** Veracity or value refers to the quality of the data received. Some data might become corrupted and provide different values than the original data, some data might contain values that are too high or low, and the analysation process might suffer and provide inaccurate results. For WBAN, this is solved by providing higher/lower limits for data received, and by consistent maintenance of the whole WBAN system and the physical sensors.
- **Volatility:** This refers to the validity of the data, or the time period after which the data is rendered useless. This is for data that are constantly changing or data that has already expired and cannot be processed, or in case the data can be processed the end analysation will be fruitless due to the volatility of the data. This characteristic is very important in terms of WBAN, since some factors might have short volatility and some factors might have to be read for longer times.

2.2 Methods of Analytics

Big data analytics can be implemented using many different analytical methods, either a singular or a hybrid method to perform the analyzation process. The methods, and their advantages and disadvantages will be explained in relation to WBAN and healthcare systems [8–13].

Data Mining: Data mining is the purpose of examining and observing patterns in unorganized data. The process works by comparing various random data and discovering the pattern; therefore data mining is the most used and preferred analytical method, because of its straightforward method and accuracy.

Data Management: Data management is a sub process of the analytics system, and can subsequently with other analytical methods, allowing users to view their processed data and records. The data management system makes it easier to store data, process data, and organize and manage all the raw data and information making things easier for both the user and the system. There are no considerable pros or cons for this system.

In-memory Analytics: In In-memory analytics, the entire raw data is stored in the Random Access Memory (RAM), which acts as a temporary memory. In-memory analytics is preferred for faster analysation process; 'In-Memory' refers to 64 bit architecture with RAM, meaning the time taken for the system to read and write from the hard storage is greatly reduced since the entire user data and database and the processed information is stored on the RAM drives.

Predictive Analysis: Predictive Analysis refers to the analytical method of predicting the future trends and statistics. With the basic analytics carried out with data mining, text analytics or machine learning, the resultant information is used to identify patterns and predict and create future information about the field from which the raw data was collected.

Machine Learning: Machine Learning is a significant big field, but when used with big data, the whole process of analytics and producing benefiting results is greatly improved. Machine Learning is the process of studying algorithms, statistics, and analytics instead of coded instructions, and providing the system the power to process information through patterns, references, and pre-existing data. This is like an Artificial Intelligence (AI) system, and the analysation process is more effective in terms of quality result.

Deep Learning: Deep Learning is like machine learning, but better and it has a broader range of operations. Deep learning is a system that reads raw data, identifies, and recognizes the different patterns that appear over the raw data and making it as collective memory and proceeds with that to identify even more patterns, and by doing so the system can make human-like predictions and analyzations. This type of analytical method is often necessary for fields like healthcare where it may help prevent medical deaths.

Hadoop: Hadoop is an open source distributed processing framework which can be used to produce some of the many methods described above, or to generate a new set of systems and collectible information that can perform analyzations, pattern recognitions and predictions, without needing to correlate to other analytical methods. Any part of the system or framework being developed or used, can be modified and certain versions of the variables can be made into constants and vice versa [17] (Table 1).

Table 1. Comparison of various big data analytical methods

Method	Environment of use	Advantages	Disadvantages
Data mining	Finance, Intelligence, Healthcare, Telecommunications, Ecommerce, etc....	1. Predicting future trends 2. Decision making 3. Predicting user habits	1. Privacy/security issues may occur 2. Predicted results might not be accurate every time
Data management	Used in every field requiring huge to massive data organization	1. Easily accessible data modules 2. Specialized/customized tools for data organizations	Software interface must be customized depending on the field of use and the overall amount of data storage
In-memory analytics	Big data analytical systems that require high end processing power	High speed processing of information and faster data transfer between the systems	Only preferred in systems requiring high speed data processing
Predictive analysis	Assessing risk factors, healthcare, sales Forecasting, crisis management and fraud detection	Powerful decision making, adaptive nature and better accuracy	Requires supervision for prediction regarding WBAN and patient's health conditions and other critical assets
Machine learning	Used in place of Artificial Intelligence, in critical fields	Better analysis and higher quality over time of usage	Higher error susceptibility and chances of procedural mistakes, requires human supervision at times
Deep learning	Used for deep pattern identification and accurate prediction methods	Easier pattern identification and accurate predictions	Requires more time for initialization and complex technical work
Hadoop	Backend software framework for big data analytics system	Depending on the developers and the field of use, advantages and disadvantages vary. Easier to adapt existing system in concern with existing and future problems	

3 Large Scale WBAN

A Wireless Body Area Network is a network of sensors placed in various parts of the patient's body, to sense and track parameters and remotely transfer this information to the relevant medical professional to process further. While Large Scale WBAN refers to the system that interconnects a huge number of patients' WBAN systems with the hospital management, and the regularization and database management of all those data, a basic WBAN consists of sensor nodes, gateway nodes and internet connectivity. The sensor nodes consist of sensors attached to various parts of the human body, to measure medical parameters and capsules/containers that inject certain medical fluids necessary to improve the patient's condition the sensor nodes transfer the measured data to the gateway nodes. The gateway node is a device that can interact with these data and transfer them accordingly and organized, through the internet to the concerned medical authority or system. The gateway node may or may not encrypt data multiple times before transferring them, depending on the amount of security needed to be implemented, this is in the case of high level targets whose medical information is to be kept extremely confidential and secure [18]. The second method is the Emergency Traffic, here when a sensor reading goes higher or lower than the threshold's medical standard, the emergency protocol is initiated, the nearest medical authority is informed about the patient's whereabouts, and the rest of the medical procedures are carried out from there on. The third method would be On-Demand Traffic. Figure 2 represents a simple loop diagram of the system.

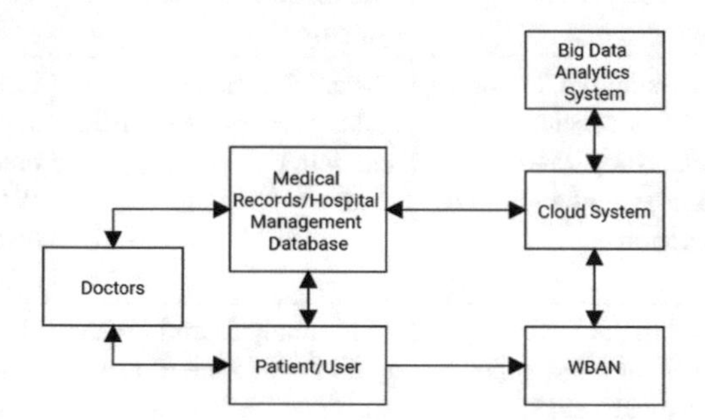

Fig. 2. Large scale WBAN with big data analytics

3.1 Routing Protocols

A routing protocol is a method by which routers or nodes communicate and transfer data to and from nodes. The routing protocols will help a network by directing and redirecting data traffic, for smoother networking, reliability, and energy efficiency. The commonly used routing protocols for WBAN are listed below. A WBAN may use one or more routing protocols depending on the patient's conditions and medical standards.

Posture Based Routing: Posture based (or position based) routing protocol is specified by the positions of the sensors in the human body, and the distance between them.

Depending on the day to day activities performed, the distance between the sensors varies, for example with exercise. With these changes in the distance, the nodes are specified to direct traffic to the nearest neighbouring node at that time instance. In the diagram below (Fig. 3), the node in the left hand is quite far from the gateway node, hence it pairs with the nearby node which reroutes the data traffic back to the gateway node path [19].

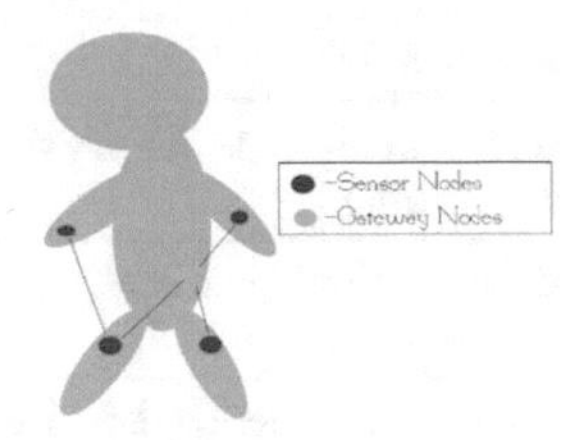

Fig. 3. Posture based routing

Temperature Based Routing: Temperature based routing is opted for nodes that may become overheated. When a sensor or any node is made to handle data traffic continuously, the node may overheat and the neighbouring nodes will redirect the data traffic through cooler nodes, to protect the sensor and gateway nodes from heat damage.

Cross Layer Routing: Cross layer routing is the integration or hybridization of different routing protocols depending on the need. Using cross layering to integrate multiple protocol methods makes the WBAN system more dynamic and provides more comfort for the patient. This method also allows prioritization of certain nodes over others, helping medical professionals to focus on critical areas.

Cluster Based Routing: Cluster based routing works on forming clusters which will have a cluster head that connects to other cluster heads and direct traffic henceforth. Figure 4 below explains the cluster based routing protocol method. Here, nodes N2, N4 and N5 are cluster heads, and through these the sensor data from other sensors are routed to the other nodes or the modem.

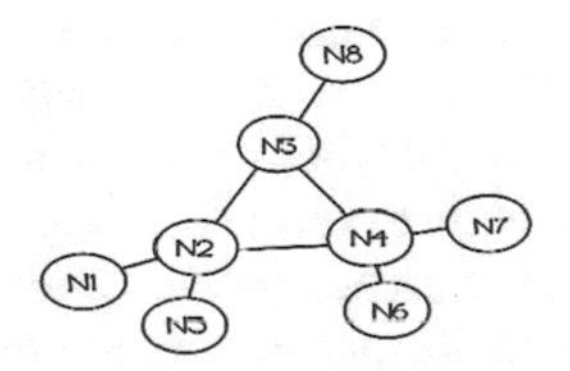

Fig. 4. Cluster based routing

QOS Based Routing: Quality of Service (QOS) based routing uses data traffic methods, such that the delivered data to the end user is of high quality. The data here will be re-routed less so that the quality is maintained, and in terms of long distance nodes the data is routed through multiple neighbour nodes to maintain the quality (Table 2).

Table 2. WBAN routing protocols

Routing protocols	Environment of use
Posture based routing	Used for athletics, special physical training, and for some medical testing
Temperature based routing	Used for monitoring critical sensor points that may become overheated
Cross layer routing	Used for events where hybridization of routing methods is required
Cluster based routing	Used for events requiring usage of several sensor units, or requiring multiple sensors with varying data traffic from time to time
QOS based routing	Used for events requiring higher data quality and data consistency

3.2 Applications

There are various fields of applications for a WBAN or large scale WBAN, some are listed below and it is explained how WBAN plays a vital role in those fields. The WBAN is mainly used for medical diagnostics and physical testing [2022] however, major applications are: General Purposes; Medical Diagnostics; Military Purposes; Assisted Living.

4 Implementing Big Data Analytics for Large Scale WBAN

The implementation process is quite simple; the basic WBAN transfers data and alerts to the hospital database, medical records, doctors, and the emergency medical team, while the big data analytics system performs statistics and analytics from the received raw data. The implementation of the big data analytics system is processed by transferring the raw data from the WBAN sensors directly to the cloud system, and the big data analytics will process the raw data and provide analytics and the different methods of analytics used, and the hospital management and doctors are able to use this information to treat their patients more effectively. Automating the analyzation of medical parameters saves time and lives, and big data is commonly used for many different sets of patients depending on their medical conditions [23] (Fig. 5).

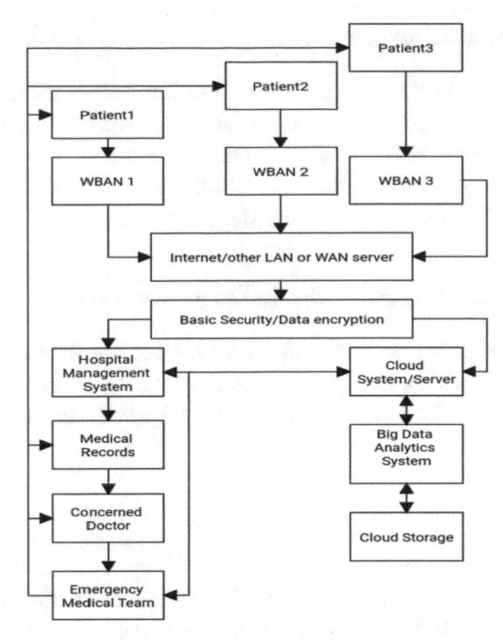

Fig. 5. Implementation of big data analytics in large scale WBAN

The large scale WBAN consists of thousands of patients with various diseases and health conditions. The testing purposes, all the diseases, conditions, and physical test protocols must be categorized and organized in the cloud storage, enabling easy access for and to patients, doctors, athletes, hospital management, students, and medical researchers/scientists. With the various active categories, it is easier for the analytical system to process certain categories and make accurate predictions by studying the different variations observed from within a category. This makes the big data analytics system more robust and reliable in the healthcare field.

4.1 Benefits of Big Data Analytics in WBAN

There are various benefits of implementing big data analytics in WBAN, the list below provides WBAN-specific big data system benefits [24].

1. Provides analysis and almost accurate predictions concerning the patient's health condition
2. Provides better digital support and flexibility, when compared with the basic WBAN
3. Helps in identifying risks and failures in the WBAN system.
4. Cost effective and higher performance when compared with other methods.
5. Provides better control over user data, easier access and data organizing tools and storage.
6. Online storage with remote accessibility.
7. Provides powerful predictive methods, helping in better treatment of patients and optimized physical testing.

4.2 Implementation Challenges

There are a variety of challenges concerning the implementation process of big data analytics in large scale WBAN. Possible challenges in the implementation process and the internal challenges in WBAN which reflect the results of the analytical system are: Security and privacy issues; Inter-operability; Sensor Validation; Data Consistency; Network/Signal Interference; Sensor Data Management.

4.3 Application of Big data Analytics in Large Scale WBAN

There are numerous numbers of basic applications for big data in WBAN and hybrid technologies and applications, but the most used applications are Remote Patient Monitoring; Rehabilitation; Biofeedback; Special Forces/Sport Training and Remote Assisted Living [25, 26].

5 Conclusion

With the advancement of science in every field, implementation of one system over another and hybridization has become very common and immensely helpful. The concept of WBAN and automation has revolutionized the healthcare industry and provides remote and automated care with its technologies and big data which allows analysing of various results, in turn developing new ways of treatment. Both big data analytics and WBAN are strong players and implementing big data in large scale WBAN has reduced the overall burden on, and the time consumption of, both patients and medical professionals.

References

1. Rawat, D.B., Bhattacharya, S.: Wireless Body Area Network for Healthcare Applications. Data Analytics in Medicine [Internet]. IGI Global 2002–17. http://dx.doi.org/10.4018/978-1-7998-1204-3.ch100
2. Thumati, B.T., Siva Subramania, H., Shastri, R., Kalyana Kumar, K., Hessner, N., Villa, V., et al.: Large-scale data integration for facilities analytics: challenges and opportunities. In: 2020 IEEE International Conference on Big Data (Big Data) [Internet]. IEEE, 2020 December 10. http://dx.doi.org/10.1109/bigdata50022.2020.9378440
3. Awad, T., Mohamed, W., Abdellatif, M.M.: IoTIwC: IoT industrial wireless controller. In: Hassanien, A.E., Darwish, A. (eds.) Machine Learning and Big Data Analytics Paradigms: Analysis, Applications and Challenges. SBD, vol. 77, pp. 565–581. Springer, Cham (2021). https://doi.org/10.1007/978-3-030-59338-4_27
4. Sahu, N.K., Patnaik, M., Snigdh, I.: Data Analytics and Its Applications in Brief. Advances in Data Mining and Database Management [Internet]. IGI Global; 2021;115–25. http://dx.doi.org/10.4018/978-1-7998-6673-2.ch008
5. Arya, A., Pathania, S., Kaushal, C.: Cloud-based wireless body area network for healthcare monitoring system. In: Advances in Computer Science and Information Technology (ACSIT) Print ISSN: 2393–9907; Online ISSN: 2393–9915; Volume 2, Number 8; April-June, 2015 pp. 1–5

6. Barazanchi, I.Al., Abdulshaheed, H.R., Shawkat, S.A., Binti, S.R.: Identification key scheme to enhance network performance in wireless body area network. Period. Eng. Nat. Sci. **7**, 895–906 (2019)
7. Sethi, D., Anand, J.: Big data and WBAN: prediction and analysis of the patient health condition in a remote area. Eng. Appl. Sci. Res. **46**(3), 248–255 (2019)
8. Anand, J., Sethi, D.: Comparative analysis of energy efficient routing in WBAN. In: 2017 3rd International Conference on Computational Intelligence & Communication Technology (CICT): 9–10 February 2017, Ghaziabad, India. USA, pp. 1–6. IEEE (2017)
9. Barazanchi, I.Al., Abdulshaheed, H.R., Safiah, M., Sidek, B.: Innovative technologies of wireless sensor network: the applications of WBAN system and environment. Sustain. Eng. Innov. **1**, 98–105 (2020)
10. Ha, I.: Even energy consumption and back side routing: an improved routing protocol for effective data transmission in wireless body area networks. Int. J. Distrib. Sens. Netw. **12**(7), 1–11 (2016). https://doi.org/10.1177/1550147716657932
11. Barazanchi, I.Al.: An analysis of the requirements for efficient protocols in WBAN. J. Telecommun. Electron. Comput. Eng. **6**, 43 (2014)
12. Barakah, D.M.; Ammad-uddin, M.: A survey of challenges and applications of wireless body area network (WBAN) and role of a virtual doctor server in existing architecture. In: 2012 Third International Conference on Intelligent Systems, Modelling and Simulation (ISMS), pp. 214,219, 8–10 February 2012. https://doi.org/10.1109/ISMS.2012.108
13. Xu, G., Wu, Q., Daneshmand, M., Liu, Y., Wang, M.: A data privacy protective mechanism for wireless body area networks. In: Wireless Communication Mobile Computing, 24 November 2015. https://doi.org/10.1002/wcm.2649
14. Ullah, F., Islam, I.U., Abdullah, A.H., Khan, A.: Future of big data and deep learning for wireless body area networks. In: Deep Learning: Convergence to Big Data Analytics. Springer Briefs in Computer Science SCS, pp. 53–77. Springer, Singapore (2019). https://doi.org/10.1007/978-981-13-3459-7_5
15. Shibghatullah, A., Barazanchi, I.Al.: A survey on Central Control Unit (CCU) in WBAN. In: International Symposium Research Innovation Sustainability 2014 (ISoRIS 2014) 15–16 October 2014, Malacca, Malaysia 14, 15–16 (2014)
16. Acharjya, D.P., Kauser Ahmed, P.: A survey on big data analytics: challenges, open research issues and tools. Int. J. Adv. Comput. Sci. Appl. **7**(2) (2016)
17. Bangash, J., Abdullah, H., Anisi, H., Khan, A.W.: A survey of routing protocols in wireless body sensor networks.. Sensors **14**, 1322–1357 (2014). https://doi.org/10.3390/s140101322. www.mdpi.com/journal/sensors
18. Barazanchi, I.Al., Abdulshaheed, H.R., Safiah, M., Sidek, B.: A survey: issues and challenges of communication technologies in WBAN. Sustain. Eng. Innov. **1**, 84–97 (2020)
19. Lin, R., Ye, Z., Wang, H., Wu, B.: Chronic diseases and health monitoring big data: a survey. IEEE Rev, Biomed. Eng. **PP**(99), 1–1 (2018). https://doi.org/10.1109/RBME.2018.2829704
20. Du, Y., Hu, F., Wang, L., Wang, F.: Framework and challenges for Wireless body area networks based on big data. In: IEEE International Conference on Digital Signal Processing (DSP), July 2015. https://doi.org/10.1109/ICDSP.2015.7251922
21. Barazanchi, I.Al, Sahy, S.A., Jaaz, Z.A.: Traffic management with deployment of Li-Fi technology traffic management with deployment of Li-Fi technology. J. Phys. Conf. Ser. 1804 (2021)
22. Al-Barazanchi, I., Jaaz, Z.A., Abbas, H.H., Abdulshaheed, H.R.: Practical application of IOT and its implications on the existing software. In: 2020 7th International Conference on Electrical Engineering Computer Science Informatics (EECSI), Yogyakarta, Indones, pp. 10–14 (2020). https://doi.org/10.23919/EECSI50503.2020.9251302

23. Quwaider, M., Jararweh, Y.: An efficient big data collection in Body Area Networks. In: 5th International Conference on Information and Communication Systems (ICICS), Jordan April 2014. https://doi.org/10.1109/IACS.2014.6841986
24. Abdulshaheed, H.R., Yaseen, Z.T., Salman, A.M., Al_Barazanchi, I.: An evaluation study of WiMAX and WiFi on vehicular ad-hoc networks (VANETs). IOP Conf. Ser. Mater. Sci. Eng. Pap. **3**, 1–7 (2020)
25. Oleiwi, S.S., Mohammed, G.N., AlBarazanchi, I.: Mitigation of packet loss with end-to-end delay in wireless body area network applications. Int. J. Electr. Comput. Eng. (IJECE) **12**(1), 460–470 (2022)
26. Barazanchi, I.A., Aborujilah, A., Hashim, W., Alkahtani, A.A.: Design and implementation of WBAN smart system connection to control covide19 patients remotely. Period. Eng. Nat. Sci. **9**(4), 977–998 (2021)

A Review of the Role of Latency in Multi-controller Placement in Software-Defined-Wide Area Networks

Cindy Ujan[1(✉)], Mohd Murtadha Mohamad[1], and Anisah Kasim[2]

[1] Universiti Teknologi Malaysia (UTM), 81310 Johor, Malaysia
ujan.cindy@graduate.utm.my

[2] Universiti Teknikal Malaysia Melaka (UTeM), 76100 Melaka, Malaysia

Abstract. Software-Defined Networking (SDN) is a computer network technology that physically separates the traditional switch architecture's control and data planes into two separate systems enabling the configuration of SDN compliant devices to become centralised and independent via the SDN controller. Essentially, the separation simplifies an administrator's task of managing a computer network and is cost-effective due to purchasing inexpensive switches with low processing power. Networks are then dynamically scalable as they can be partitioned into multiple data planes and controllers with policies that can be synchronised across the board. However, researchers have discovered that, in SDN, the location of these controllers impacts a network's performance capabilities and furthermore, the control plane provides fault management and performance in SDN. Therefore, knowing where to deploy and how many controllers are needed is fundamental. This paper surveys the recent literature on this ongoing issue known as the Controller Placement Problem (CPP), its application to the Wide Area Network (WAN), and the role latency plays in it.

Keywords: Software-Defined Networking · Controller Placement Problem · Wide Area Network · Latency

1 Introduction

The purpose of a traditional Wide Area Network (WAN) is to bridge an organisation's remote branch offices to its corporate headquarters and allow its authorised users and employees access to its data and applications over the legacy, and costly Multiprotocol Label Switching (MPLS) links. Thus, depending on the organisation's business needs, the traditional WAN may hinder its agility and growth—particularly with distributed configuration, whereby every router and switch stores its configuration locally. Furthermore, any policy change would require each network device to be accessed individually to implement the change needed. Therefore, depending on the number of network devices that must be reconfigured, the reconfiguration can be a tedious and time-consuming task. Some of the biggest known challenges of WANs are related to performance, complexity, and cost. However, the Software Defined-Wide Area Network (SD-WAN) can change

F. Saeed et al. (Eds.): IRICT 2021, LNDECT 127, pp. 435–445, 2022.
https://doi.org/10.1007/978-3-030-98741-1_36

the way WANs are deployed and managed. For example, when implemented as an overlay technology to an existing topology, SD-WAN is more beneficial over the legacy MPLS as it can leverage the local broadband Internet and 5G/LTE connectivity at the remote branch locations. Furthermore, by centralising control, organisations can expect better performance and operational simplicity as well as cost-effectiveness. Saving cost is essential since unnecessary spending drains business' profits, and SD-WAN solves this by enabling the option to choose the desired hardware and software based on necessary specifications and protocol requirements.

1.1 Software-Defined Networking (SDN)

Software-Defined Networking (SDN) can be described as a computer network technology that physically separates the traditional switch architecture's control and data planes into two systems. The main network elements in SDN consist of the SDN controllers, SDN-compliant switches, and their links [1] and these elements are often represented as a graph $G = (V, E, S)$, where V represents the set of switches, E the set of physical links, and S the set of controllers [2]. The separation simplifies the network administrators' day-to-day tasks of managing their networks as these SDN-compliant devices can now be viewed as a whole and not individually, using SDN controllers. In addition, SDN enables devices from different vendors to interoperate. Furthermore, these simplified devices require less processing power and are therefore less expensive to purchase whilst providing simple data forwarding functions [2]. However, the new switch-to-controller and inter-controller communication introduce additional latencies and network traffic [3], thus demanding urgent attention as this affects the overall network performance.

The SDN architecture comprises three layers: the application layer, the control layer, and the infrastructure layer. Figure 1 describes an SDN architecture.

Application Layer. The application layer consists of SDN software. The software provides programmable algorithms and protocols for the controllers to manage the network [2]. In addition, the application layer enables features such as load balancing, security monitoring, and access control to be implemented, thus eliminating the need for middleboxes such as load balancers [4].

Control Layer. With a global view of the network topology, the control layer's primary responsibility is to determine the network paths or flows and distribute the flow tables throughout the network to maintain synchronisation and prevent loops. The control layer consists of one or more SDN controllers and network services. A controller communicates with the software in the application layer via the Northbound API and switches in the infrastructure layer via the Southbound API. A famous example of the Southbound API control protocol is OpenFlow. A third interface is the East-West API, which is for the inter-controller communication within the control layer [4].

Infrastructure Layer. The infrastructure layer consists of SDN-compliant network elements such as switches or any packet-relaying node. These simplified switches have at least three components: secure channel, control protocol, and flow table [5]. A switch connects to a controller via the secure channel, communicates with the controller using the control protocol for configuration information, and processes flow based on its flow table—switches forward traffic based on primitive instructions given by their associated controller. Furthermore, the flow table consists of an entry identifier, statistics, and action fields to which a switch refers when determining whether a packet is to be forwarded or dropped [4].

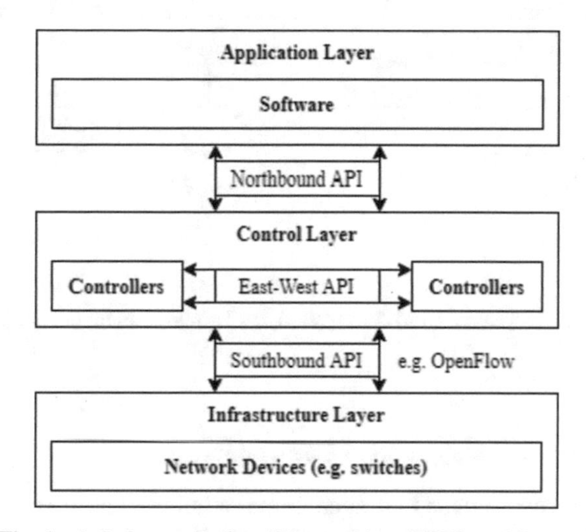

Fig. 1. A Software-Defined Networking (SDN) architecture.

1.2 Distributed Controller Architecture

Large-sized SDN-based networks rely on having distributed controllers. Thus the network has to have more than one controller in its control plane interacting with each other via the East-West API. There are two types of distributed controller architecture: the logically centralised but physically distributed and the fully distributed [6].

Horizontal (Flat) Design. In a logically centralised but physically distributed controller design, all the controllers are in the same level or *flat*, and all are logically designated as root controllers. Figure 2 describes an example of the horizontal (flat) design. Every controller is responsible for its local network topology, but because it is also a root controller, it must also maintain a global view of the network topology [6]. Hence, all changes happening in other local network topologies are communicated to all controllers, thus introducing unnecessary load to the controllers with every synchronisation.

Hierarchical Design. In a fully distributed design, the controllers consist of local controllers and a root controller. Figure 2 describes an example of the hierarchical design. The local controller maintains a local view of the network topology, whereas the root controller maintains the global view and is kept updated on any changes in the local topologies by the local controllers. Furthermore, any interdomain interaction between local controllers must go through the root controller [5]. Thus, only the root controller bears the majority of the synchronisation load.

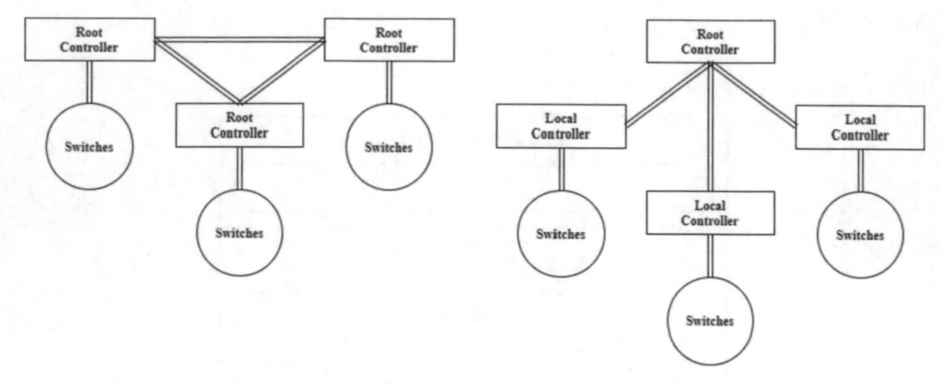

Fig. 2. A horizontal (flat) design (left) and a hierarchical design (right).

1.3 The Capacitated/Uncapacitated Controller

A controller's load corresponds to the maximum number of requests it can manage per second [7, 8]. Thus, the capacitated controller would imply the controller's capacity is considered, whereas, with an uncapacitated controller, the controller's capacity is negligible [7]. For example, Wang et al. formulated a problem based on controller capacity and proposed a solution to dynamically map switches to controllers according to variations in the network [8]. However, not all proposed solutions to the controller load imbalance consider the controller's capacity. Most literature that does consider controller capacity, however, views the controller as a single unit with fixed capacity instead of a virtualised instance or controller module that's dynamically configurable [9].

This paper reviews the most recent literature on the Controller Placement Problem (CPP) for Software-Defined-Wide Area Networks (SD-WAN) while highlighting the importance latency plays in it. The rest of this paper is organised as follows: Sect. 2 discusses the background and recent CPP literature and Sect. 3 concludes the paper.

2 Related Works

As the capacity of an SDN controller limits its capability to process its switches' requests, risks such as network bottlenecks and a Single Point of Failure (SPOF) are very likely to occur in a single controller setup. Therefore, the multi-controller solution can mitigate these risks to provide failover and load balancing capabilities. A decade ago, Heller et al. [10] introduced this NP-hard dilemma as the Controller Placement Problem (CPP), which focuses on discovering the SDN controllers' optimal number and placement in the SDN-based network topology. They analysed the average- and worst-case propagation switch-to-controller propagation latencies and concluded that a single controller is sufficient for most medium-sized networks. To this day, their initial study still prompts other researchers to investigate the topic further from various angles, mainly focusing on large-sized networks that would require multiple controllers.

Furthermore, determining controller placements in large-sized networks like the WAN is more significant due to its varying topologies and large non-negligible propagation latencies [11, 12]. Therefore, a near-optimal number of controllers is required to process the connected switches' load sufficiently and minimise costs, such as those that may incur from the unnecessary purchase of additional controllers, thus remaining within the approved budget. Subsequently, a near-optimal placement of controllers too is required to minimise switch-to-controller or inter-controller propagation latency. Most literature leverages the in-band control plane strategy [9], whereby both the control and data planes share the same links [13] instead of the out-of-band strategy. Minimising latency is a fundamental objective in any network as it affects its performance [1].

The following Sect. 2.1 reviews recent multi-latency-oriented controller placement in CPP literature.

2.1 Multi-latency Objectives

In recent CPP literature, Zhang et al. [12] investigated the propagation latency tradeoffs achievable with the switch-to-controller (southbound interface) and inter-controller (east-west interface) interactions. For example, evenly distributing the controllers reduced the switch-to-controller propagation latency but increased the inter-controller propagation latency. On the other hand, placing the controllers close to one another reduced the inter-controller propagation latency but increased the switch-to-controller propagation latency. Thus they viewed a controller's perceived reactivity time as being influenced by both and derived two operative models, namely the single and multiple data-ownerships models with similarities to the horizontal and hierarchical distributed controller designs.

Wang et al. [11] state that end-to-end switch-to-controller latency consists of three parts, namely packet transmission latency, packet propagation latency and switch processing latency. However, processing latency is negligible in large-sized networks [9], whereas transmission latency pertains to the data packets and port rates thus is usually a fixed value [2]. Their clustering-based network partitioning algorithm is a variant of the K-means that aims to shorten the worst-case end-to-end switch-to-controller and controller queuing latencies, calculating the shortest path using Dijkstra with Haversine distance, unlike the Euclidean distance typically used in K-means. However, it can be assumed that queuing latency is negligible in unobstructed networks [2].

Schütz et al. [14] proposed a heuristic mathematical approach to minimise the number of controllers and determine controller placement and switch assignments. In addition, they aimed to satisfy the capacity, load balancing, and propagation latency constraints. Particularly in switch assignments, they focused on minimising inter-switch distances to achieve acceptable switch-to-controller and inter-controller latencies. Torkamani-Azar et al. [15] had also considered heterogenous capacitated controllers to find the lowest switch-to-controller propagation latency that satisfies the controller's capacity and with ports in a meta-heuristic approach. They used the Knapsack 0–1 problem to calculate the controller's different processing rates and costs and investigated the local optima of meta-heuristic and cluster-based solutions by focusing on minimising intra-cluster versus inter-cluster link propagation delays. In comparison, Singh et al. [16] proposed another meta-heuristic approach to controller placement which focuses on propagation latency while considering the capacitated controllers and dynamic load of switches. In addition, they aimed to minimise the total average latency, and their results showed that optimisation-based solutions perform better than cluster-based solutions.

Another proposed solution that considered the dynamic load incurred from the number of switches associated with the controller and the frequency of these switches encountering new flows was proposed by Ul Huque et al. [17] who aimed to minimise switch-to-controller propagation latency. Liao et al. [18] and Jalili et al. [19] proposed variants of the Non-dominated Sorting Genetic Algorithm – II, a heuristic population-based algorithm to solve the multi-objective problem; in addition, both authors investigated how to minimise average switch-to-controller and inter-controller latencies with worst-case controller load imbalance, with the former incorporating PSO mutation and the latter a multi-start procedure.

In Virtualised SDN, switch-to-controller Packet_In messages pass through a hypervisor, thus introducing additional switch-to-hypervisor and hypervisor-to-controller propagation latencies. Therefore, Killi et al. [20] proposed a solution to optimise average- and worst-case propagation latencies while considering the optimal placement for both the hypervisors and controllers. They then referenced maximum latency as the switch-to-hypervisor-to-controller propagation latency, thus also aiming to optimise the maximum average and average maximum propagation latencies. Thus optimising controller placement would require balancing the different latencies to best suit an organisation's network. Finally, Hans et al. [21] proposed a swarm intelligence-based approach for controller placement in SD-IoT networks. They focused on minimising inter-controller propagation latency due to significant packet propagation latency and irregular placements of controllers in the topology.

However, all the above multi-latency solutions ignored the probabilities of link or controller failures. Thus the following subsection reviews CPP literature that combines multi-latency with other functional objectives while considering the link and controller failures.

2.2 Multi-latency with Other Functional Objectives

When a controller fails, its associated switches must be reassigned to another controller. However, the reassignment may cause a sharp increase in worst-case propagation latency [22]. Petale et al. [23] proposed a solution using decision making under uncertainty and aimed to minimise switch-to-controller and inter-controller latencies to achieve minimum latencies during controller failures. They also highlighted inter-switch latency as part of the overall network latency, which none of the other papers reviewed here have done. A disadvantage of heuristic algorithms is the local optima [15]. Thus Liao et al. [24] proposed a switch density-based clustering algorithm to partition the network according to the subnetwork's controller capacity. Furthermore, they state that the inter-controller propagation latency affects the performance of end-to-end propagation latency between different switches controlled by different controllers. Thus, controllers must be deployed close to other subnetworks. They had considered link failures but not controller failures. Killi et al. [22] had proposed a mathematical model for capacitated controller placement that minimises the worst-case propagation latencies with and without failures by assigning more than one controller to every switch while considering multiple constraints. However, according to [23], decision making under uncertainty yields better results when compared to mathematical methods.

Fan et al. [25] proposed a meta-heuristic approach for multi-objective controller placement. They considered at most one link failure and had focused on minimising propagation latency on both primary and backup switch-to-controller links. However, they ignored the controller and multiple link failures. In contrast, Kazemian et al. [26] had considered multiple switch-to-controller link failures, thus proposing a meta-heuristic based solution to minimise inter-controller and switch-to-controller propagation latencies by maximising multiple switch-to-controller connectivity paths. They state that network connectivity can be increased by maximising the average switch-to-controller disjoint paths. Similar to authors in [18] and [19], Hu et al. [13] had developed a variant of the NSGA-II, but they had considered multiple link failures during problem formulation. They aimed to minimise the number of controllers and worst-case propagation latency. However, controller failure was ignored.

Tanha et al. [7] state that a switch needs to be associated with more than one controller to achieve resilient controller placement. Switch-to-controller static assignments can further improve energy consumption and post-failure reassignment propagation latencies compared to dynamic assignments. Thus their solution required every switch to be associated with a primary master controller and a backup slave controller while satisfying the maximum allowable propagation switch-to-controller and inter-controller latencies during synchronisation. However, they did not consider multiple links failure. In contrast, Sahoo et al. [27] had proposed having primary and backup switch-to-controller links to achieve resiliency against single link failures while minimising propagation delay. Their work aims to minimise inter-controller and switch-to-controller propagation latencies while maximising multi-path connectivity. The flow conservation law had been applied to both primary and backup paths and was used to determine the number of switch-to-controller disjoint paths. However, they did not consider controller failure.

Huang et al. [28] state response time comprises the switch, controller, and scheduler's processing latencies, propagation latency, and transmission latency, although the transmission, switch and scheduler processing latencies are negligible. They highlighted the importance of controller scheduling, thus proposing a gradient descent-based solution to tackle both controller placement and scheduling. However, the scheduler introduced must be installed locally on switches and easily implemented as a Virtual Network Functions (VNF) component, thus requiring the SDN to be executed on a Network Functions Virtualisation (NFV) infrastructure. In an attempt to mitigate controller failure caused by security attacks, Samir et al. [29] proposed to change the controller's location virtually and dynamically to confuse attackers. They considered the latency metrics in their controller placement and shifting solutions. However, they split the network while having three potential substitute locations in every subnetwork, thus inevitably increasing deployment cost and energy consumption.

Table 1 describes the various combination of latencies in CPP literature.

Table 1. Latency combinations in CPP literature

Year	Solution	Focus	Method
2017	[12]	Propagation latencies' tradeoffs' impact on controller reactivity time perceived by switches	EVO-PLACE
2018	[11]	Propagation and queuing latencies' impact on overall network latency	CNPA
2020	[14]	Propagation latencies' impact on controllers' reaction to network events	Mathematical formalisation
2020	[15]	Propagation latencies with capacitated controllers	GSO with Knapsack 0–1
2020	[16]	Propagation latencies with capacitated controllers and dynamic load	Varna-based optimisation
2017	[17]	Propagation latencies with dynamic flow management	LiDy+
2021	[18]	Propagation latencies with load imbalance	MOGA with variant PSO
2017	[19]	Propagation latencies with memory	MHNSGA-II
2018	[20]	Propagation latencies with a hypervisor	JHCP with ILP
2022	[21]	Propagation latencies with adaptive fuzzy controllers	ESFO
2020	[23]	Propagation latencies with multiple link failures	Decision under uncertainty
2017	[24]	Propagation latencies with fault tolerance	DBCP
2016	[22]	Propagation latencies with controller failure	Mathematical model
2020	[25]	Propagation latencies with a single link failure	RALO
2021	[26]	Propagation latencies with multiple disjoint paths	Antlion optimisation
2021	[13]	Propagation latencies with multiple link failures	NSGA-II with HCPA
2018	[7]	Propagation latencies and capacitated controllers' impact on resiliency	Clique-based Graph Theory

(*continued*)

Table 1. (*continued*)

Year	Solution	Focus	Method
2018	[27]	Propagation latencies with multi-path connectivity	PSO with FFA
2020	[28]	Propagation and processing latencies with capacitated controllers and VNF scheduling component	CGA-CC with GD-based scheduling
2021	[29]	Propagation latencies with controller security	MTD with PAFR mechanism

3 Conclusion

To summarise, CPP is a fundamental component of the design phase of any large-sized SDN-based network as it ideally determines the requirements for (i) the number of controllers, (ii) their placement in the network, and (iii) the network's switch-controller/inter-controller mappings, whereby latency is known to play the utmost important role. However, only focusing on a solution based on multi-latency alone is insufficient and should be complemented with other functional objectives to achieve a well-rounded outcome that can be applied in real-life scenarios, even though combining these various latencies and functional objectives may prove conflicting. Therefore, it ultimately depends on what an organisation is willing to compromise to achieve the desired goal for their network.

References

1. Wang, G., Zhao, Y., Huang, J., Wang, W.: The controller placement problem in software defined networking: a survey. IEEE Network **31**, 21–27 (2017). https://doi.org/10.1109/MNET.2017.1600182
2. Lu, J., Zhang, Z., Hu, T., et al.: A survey of controller placement problem in software-defined networking. IEEE Access **7**, 24290–24307 (2019). https://doi.org/10.1109/ACCESS.2019.2893283
3. Alsaeedi, M., Mohamad, M.M., Al-Roubaiey, A.A.: Toward adaptive and scalable openflow-SDN flow control: a survey. IEEE Access **7**, 107346–107379 (2019). https://doi.org/10.1109/ACCESS.2019.2932422
4. Killi, B.P.R., Rao, S.V.: Controller placement in software defined networks: a comprehensive survey. Comput. Netw. **163**, 106883 (2019). https://doi.org/10.1016/j.comnet.2019.106883
5. Zhang, Y., Cui, L., Wang, W., Zhang, Y.: A survey on software defined networking with multiple controllers. J. Netw. Comput. Appl. **103**, 101–118 (2018)
6. Shirmarz, A., Ghaffari, A.: Taxonomy of controller placement problem (CPP) optimization in Software Defined Network (SDN): a survey. J. Ambient. Intell. Humaniz. Comput. **12**(12), 10473–10498 (2021). https://doi.org/10.1007/s12652-020-02754-w
7. Tanha, M., Sajjadi, D., Ruby, R., Pan, J.: Capacity-aware and delay-guaranteed resilient controller placement for software-defined WANs. IEEE Trans. Netw. Serv. Manage. **15**, 991–1005 (2018). https://doi.org/10.1109/TNSM.2018.2829661

8. Wang, T., Liu, F., Xu, H.: An efficient online algorithm for dynamic SDN controller assignment in data center networks. IEEE/ACM Trans. Netw. **25**, 2788–2801 (2017). https://doi.org/10.1109/TNET.2017.2711641
9. Das, T., Sridharan, V., Gurusamy, M.: A survey on controller placement in SDN. IEEE Commun. Surv. Tutorials **22**, 472–503 (2020)
10. Heller, B., Sherwood, R., Mckeown, N.: The controller placement problem. Comput. Commun. Rev. **42**(4), 473–478 (2012)
11. Wang, G., Zhao, Y., Huang, J., Wu, Y: An effective approach to controller placement in software defined wide area networks. In: IEEE Transactions on Network and Service Management. Institute of Electrical and Electronics Engineers Inc., pp. 344–355 (2018)
12. Zhang, T., Giaccone, P., Bianco, A., de Domenico, S.: The role of the inter-controller consensus in the placement of distributed SDN controllers. Comput. Commun. **113**, 1–13 (2017). https://doi.org/10.1016/j.comcom.2017.09.007
13. Hu, T., Ren, Q., Yi, P., et al.: An efficient approach to robust controller placement for link failures in Software-Defined Networks. Futur. Gener. Comput. Syst. **124**, 187–205 (2021). https://doi.org/10.1016/j.future.2021.05.022
14. Schütz, G., Martins, J.A.: A comprehensive approach for optimizing controller placement in Software-Defined Networks. Comput. Commun. **159**, 198–205 (2020). https://doi.org/10.1016/j.comcom.2020.05.008
15. Torkamani-Azar, S., Jahanshahi, M.: A new GSO based method for SDN controller placement. Comput. Commun. **163**, 91–108 (2020). https://doi.org/10.1016/j.comcom.2020.09.004
16. Singh, A.K., Maurya, S., Srivastava, S.: Varna-based optimization: a novel method for capacitated controller placement problem in SDN. Front. Comp. Sci. **14**(3), 1–26 (2019). https://doi.org/10.1007/s11704-018-7277-8
17. Ul Huque, M.T.I., Si, W., Jourjon, G., Gramoli, V.: Large-scale dynamic controller placement. IEEE Trans. Netw. Serv. Manage. **14**, 63–76 (2017). https://doi.org/10.1109/TNSM.2017.2651107
18. Liao, L., Leung, V.C.M., Li, Z., Chao, H.C.: Genetic algorithms with variant particle swarm optimization based mutation for generic controller placement in software-defined networks. Symmetry **13**, 1133 (2021). https://doi.org/10.3390/sym13071133
19. Jalili, A., Keshtgari, M., Akbari, R.: Optimal controller placement in large scale software defined networks based on modified NSGA-II. Appl. Intell. **48**(9), 2809–2823 (2017). https://doi.org/10.1007/s10489-017-1119-5
20. Killi, B.P.R., Rao, S.V.: On placement of hypervisors and controllers in virtualized Software Defined Network. IEEE Trans. Netw. Serv. Manage. **15**, 840–853 (2018). https://doi.org/10.1109/TNSM.2018.2823341
21. Hans, S., Ghosh, S., Kataria, A., et al.: Controller placement in software defined internet of things using optimization algorithm. Comput. Mater. Continua **70**, 5073–5089 (2022). https://doi.org/10.32604/cmc.2022.019971
22. Killi, B.P.R., Rao, S.V.: Optimal model for failure foresight capacitated controller placement in Software-Defined Networks. IEEE Commun. Lett. **20**, 1108–1111 (2016). https://doi.org/10.1109/LCOMM.2016.2550026
23. Petale, S., Thangaraj, J.: Failure-based controller placement in Software Defined Networks. IEEE Trans. Netw. Serv. Manage. **17**, 503–516 (2020). https://doi.org/10.1109/TNSM.2019.2949256
24. Liao, J., Sun, H., Wang, J., et al.: Density cluster based approach for controller placement problem in large-scale software defined networkings. Comput. Netw. **112**, 24–35 (2017). https://doi.org/10.1016/j.comnet.2016.10.014
25. Fan, Y., Wang, L., Yuan, X.: Controller placements for latency minimization of both primary and backup paths in SDNs. Comput. Commun. **163**, 35–50 (2020). https://doi.org/10.1016/j.comcom.2020.09.001

26. Kazemian, M.M., Mirabi, M.: Controller placement in software defined networks using multi-objective antlion algorithm. J. Supercomput (2021). https://doi.org/10.1007/s11227-021-04109-4
27. Sahoo, K.S., Puthal, D., Obaidat, M.S., et al.: On the placement of controllers in software-Defined-WAN using meta-heuristic approach. J. Syst. Softw. **145**, 180–194 (2018). https://doi.org/10.1016/j.jss.2018.05.032
28. Huang, V., Chen, G., Zhang, P., et al.: A scalable approach to SDN control plane management: high utilization comes with low latency. IEEE Trans. Netw. Serv. Manage. **17**, 682–695 (2020). https://doi.org/10.1109/TNSM.2020.2973222
29. Samir, M., Azab, M., Samir, E.: SD-CPC: SDN controller placement camouflage based on stochastic game for moving-target defense. Comput. Commun. **168**, 75–92 (2021). https://doi.org/10.1016/j.comcom.2020.11.019

Factors Influencing the Security of Internet of Things Systems

Fayez Hussain Alqahtani(✉)

King Saud University, Riyadh, Saudi Arabia
fhalqahtani@ksu.edu.sa

Abstract. The Internet of Things (IoT) is an IT-based innovation that could be implemented in various domains, such as manufacturing, logistics and healthcare. Things or objects in a particular domain can be tagged, sensed, and controlled over the Internet with technologies in object identification, wireless networks, sensors, and embedded systems. It is widely acknowledged that IoT systems are potential targets for malicious attacks, spread and actuated from the Internet to the physical world. Hence, IoT security is of utmost importance. This paper is part of a wider research project and aims to explore the factors responsible for security challenges that exist in IoT systems. A qualitative investigation was conducted by interviewing twenty IoT industry experts. The findings show that there are seven factors responsible for security challenges facing IoT systems, including a lack of IoT standards, heterogeneity, vulnerability, resource constraints, trust, pervasiveness, and manufacturing.

Keywords: Internet of Things · IoT security · Information security management

1 Introduction

The term Internet of Things (IoT) was first proposed by Ashton in [1] and Brock in [2] at the Auto-ID centre of the Massachusetts Institute of Technology (MIT). Auto-ID refers to identification technologies such as error reduction, improvement of efficiency, and automation used in several applications. Things can be tagged, sensed, and controlled over the Internet via wireless networks, sensors, embedded systems, and nanotechnologies. The IoT consists of a set of technologies to support communication and interaction among a broad range of networked devices and appliances [3]. Several applications for entertainment, manufacturing, administration, healthcare, logistics, etc. based on IoT enterprise systems have already been developed [4].

The key factor behind the changes in almost all business processes is IT-based innovation [5]. IT is not only an innovative factor, but also acts as an opportunity to manage innovative processes by acting as an enabler of innovation adoption. The use of IoT technologies in business processes is a recent innovative trend that acts as an extension to firms' IT-based systems. Commentators in [6] defined the IoT as 'the worldwide network of interconnected objects uniquely addressable based on standard communication protocols' (p. 1647).

F. Saeed et al. (Eds.): IRICT 2021, LNDECT 127, pp. 446–457, 2022.
https://doi.org/10.1007/978-3-030-98741-1_37

However, the practical realization of IoT subsystems depends on certain factors, such as cost, power, energy, and lifetime [7]. In addition, there is a wide consensus that the most challenging requirement is security [8]. It is a well-known fact that the potential for malicious attacks is greatly spread and actuated from the Internet to the physical world, and this highlights the importance of IoT security [9]. Securing information carried by wireless links in the IoT network is of utmost importance [10].

The identification of relevant factors and how they influence the security of IoT systems is critical. Therefore, the objectives of the current study are to 1) identify the relevant factors responsible for IoT security challenges, and 2) explore how these factors influence the security of IoT systems. Moreover, previous literature, such as [11–14], and [15], has discussed several security challenges faced by IoT systems. However, little attention has been paid in the literature to qualitatively investigating the factors that influence IoT security.

The current study extends previous studies and identifies the core factors responsible for security challenges encountered by present-day IoT systems based on empirical investigation with a number of industry practitioners. The snowball sampling method was used to recruit twenty IoT experts for individual interviews to enrich the understanding of how relevant factors could influence the security of IoT systems. This research is significant because it illustrates how the security of IoT systems can be threatened. Hence, the practice of IoT security can take the identified factors and their associated insights into consideration when implementing IoT systems.

The remainder of this paper is organised as follows. The Sect. 2 of this paper presents important concepts related to IoT and the challenges of implementing IoT systems, as discussed in the literature about IoT security. The Sect. 3 of this paper provides an illustration of the research approach followed in this study. Next, the Sect. 4 reveals the outcomes of this research. The Sect. 5 discusses the outcomes of this research, and finally, the paper is concluded.

2 Literature Review

IoT refers to a wide variety of Internet-connected devices, such as smart bulbs, smart locks, IP cameras, thermostats, electronic appliances, alarm clocks, and vending machines. In IoT networks, the number of devices and objects is linked with the Internet [15]. Such links with the Internet enable remote access and control of IoT devices and objects with minimal human involvement. Reference [16] provides a three-layer IoT framework and architecture consisting of perception, network, and application layers, as presented in Fig. 1. A detailed overview of the network architecture of cloud-based IoT has been presented by [17]. However, a number of issues result from linking different IoT systems with each other via the internet.

Generally, IoT systems do not focus on security being front-and-centre, leading to a scenario in which private information is disclosed to the public [18]. As mentioned in [19], along with unprecedented convenience, accessibility, and efficiency, IoT has caused acute security and privacy threats in recent years.

Several research projects have been conducted investigating a number of security challenges in the arena of IoT systems. The researchers in [11] analysed the existing

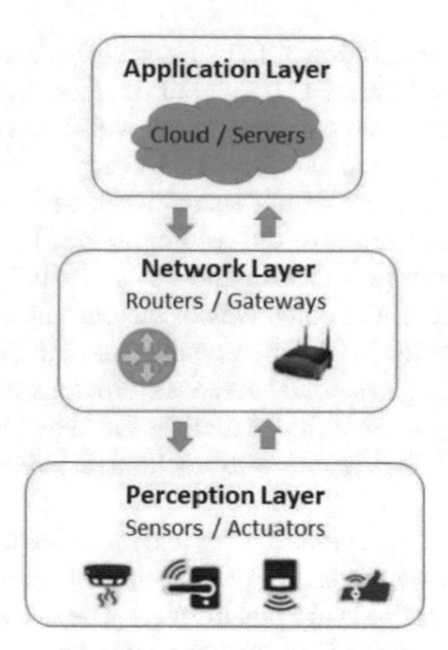

Fig. 1. Three-layer IoT architecture

protocols and mechanisms to secure communication in IoT networks, along with open security challenges. Kesavan and Prabhu [20] revealed in their findings that the level of service quality and the security of IoT systems and components are cornerstones in implementing this kind of network. Furthermore, security and privacy issues IoT systems have often attracted the interest of industry practitioners and those in academia, who have investigated IoT systems from multiple perspectives [21]. As noted in [22], issues such as the wide geographic spread of IoT devices and their limited power capacity and internet connectivity make IoT systems vulnerable to cyber security attacks.

Researchers in [23] investigated the challenges encountered when implementing security measures on the devices and components of IoT systems, which include limited resources such as the computation capabilities of IoT devices. Furthermore, this research identifies the resulting IoT security threats. These researchers [24] proposed a security framework model for authorising access to the IoT system. Several researchers have raised concerns about the generation of huge volumes of data and the processing capabilities of IoT systems. In [19], researchers divulged that due to the unique characteristics of resource constraints, self-organization, and short-range communication in IoT, it always resorts to the cloud for outsourced storage and computation. This has brought about a series of new, challenging security and privacy threats. Oracevic, Dilek, and Ozdemir [25] mentioned that the enormous number of connected devices in an IoT system are potentially vulnerable. This might generate a scenario in which highly significant risks emerge around issues of security, privacy, and governance, calling into question the future of IoT.

Clearly, from a review of the previews studies, IoT security receives researchers' attention. However, there is a need to further investigate this phenomenon for two reasons. First, the reviewed studies researched IoT conceptually, but lacked empirical support. Second, the literature has paid little attention to qualitatively investigating the factors that influence IoT security. Therefore, this research qualitatively explores insights into the factors that influence the security of IoT systems by interviewing IoT practitioners.

3 Methods

This study is based on the explorative acquisition and analysis of data. As stated in [26], a qualitative approach is better for explorative research. The present study aims to explore the factors responsible for IoT security challenges. This explorative study seeks to provide in-depth explanations for the responsible factors from an IoT practitioners' perspective. Recker [27] mentions that the study of the use of IT 'is multi-faceted and comprehensive, yielding insights from a variety of perspectives and lenses'. The qualitative research approach is the most suitable method for social science research when many uncontrollable variables are involved [28]. In our case, investigating IoT security based on practitioners from the industry is an appropriate situation for utilising the qualitative research approach. It was assumed that the industry experts might provide the best insight into the theme of this research. Thus, based on the findings in [29], the qualitative approach was selected due to its suitability for the explorative nature of the current study. Figure 2 presents the design of this study.

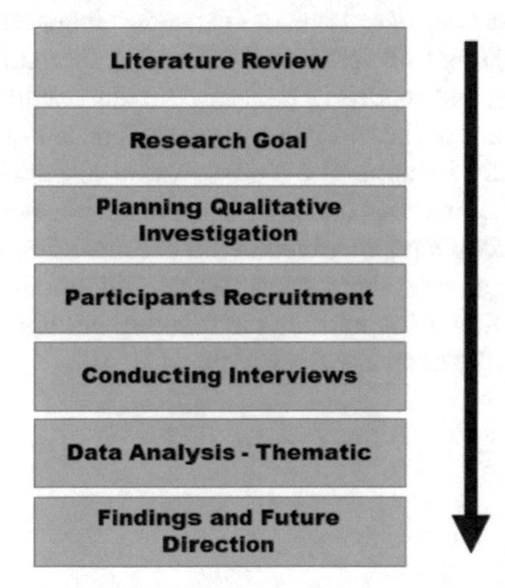
Literature Review
Research Goal
Planning Qualitative Investigation
Participants Recruitment
Conducting Interviews
Data Analysis - Thematic
Findings and Future Direction

Fig. 2. Research design of the current study

3.1 Data Collection

This study utilised semi-structured interviews conducted on focused samples (IoT industry experts) as they are capable of providing a deep illustration of the research issue under investigation. The interviews were performed using a number of predefined questions related to the issues in implementing IoT systems and how they can lead to the security challenges. The sole purpose of these interviews was to gather an in-depth and contextual understanding of the subject under investigation.

The snowball sampling method was used in this study. This method provides selective feedback wherein the researcher requests that every participant in the study suggests relevant persons to participate in the next interview [30]. The following assessment criteria were pre-set for the nominated participants: first, participants should be working or have worked in an organization regardless of the size or industry of these organizations. However, these organizations should have already started or completed building IoT systems. Second, participants have been actively involved in IoT implementation in their respective organizations.

The sample size in this study consisted of twenty selectively chosen participants. Out of these, ten participants were aged from twenty-five to twenty-nine; six were aged from thirty to thirty-nine, and the remaining four were aged from forty to forty-nine. The selected participants in this study are IoT cloud engineers, systems engineers, software developers, and IT security personnel. Due to the nature of qualitative research and its focus on meaning, the sample size of this study is adequate.

3.2 Data Analysis

Several qualitative data analysis techniques, such as content analysis, discourse analysis, grounded theory, and thematic analysis are used for exploratory studies [31]. Of these, thematic analysis is considered one of the predominant techniques for qualitative data analysis [32]. According to Braun and Clarke [31], thematic analysis is 'a method for identifying, analysing and reporting patterns (themes) within data'. Holloway and Todres [33] describes it as a foundational analysis method for qualitative data. The thematic analysis method can be applied across several epistemological and theoretical approaches, and that is the reason it better suits the objectives of this study.

Generally, there are six phases involved in the process of conducting thematic analysis: familiarising with gathered data, generating initial codes, searching for themes, reviewing the themes, defining and naming the themes, and finally producing the report [31]. The Table 1 below illustrates the data analysis steps.

Table 1. Thematic data analysis steps

Steps	Description
Familiarising with gathered data	This step involves transcribing the interview data, and reading the manuscript multiple times
Generate initial codes	This step involves generating initial codes/labels and grouping interviews data under each code
Search for themes	This step involves grouping initial codes/labels into potential themes
Review the themes	This step involves reviewing the initial themes with their associated interview data
Define and name the themes	This step involves refining themes, as well as developing theme definitions
Produce the report	This step involves writing up the finding by employing themes, discussion and extracted evidence from the interview data

After the interviews were conducted, they were transcribed with the help of a credible professional transcriber. Moreover, all the interviews' transcripts were reviewed and checked against the interviews' audio recordings. Data analysis of the interviews was conducted using the thematic analysis technique [31]. This analysis technique facilitates identifying important themes within the data. The research deductively analysed the data, searching for relevant insight into the predefined factors. Additionally, inductive examination of the data was used in this thematic analysis to identify emergent insights.

4 Findings

This study explores the causes or factors responsible for different security challenges that exist in current IoT systems. These factors are a lack of IoT standards, heterogeneity, vulnerability, resource constraints, trust, pervasiveness, and manufacturing (see Fig. 3).

4.1 Lack of IoT Standards

The worldwide development of IoT devices and applications does not have commonly recognised standards. This leads to the perception that the interoperability among those devices is difficult. As noted by one of the participants, there may be '*...mismatch among software in IoT systems, for example, with regard to authentication methods' (ex. 5)*. This complicates privacy and authentication in IoT systems. The participants in the current study divulged that the absence of common standards creates a vacuum in the establishment of proper security mechanisms, as noted: *'The absence of agreed upon standards lead to security concerns in this heterogeneous system' (ex. 18).*

Furthermore, according to one participant, *'it is very difficult for manufacturers in the area of IoT to design IoT devices while there is lack of secure IoT solutions' (ex. 2).*

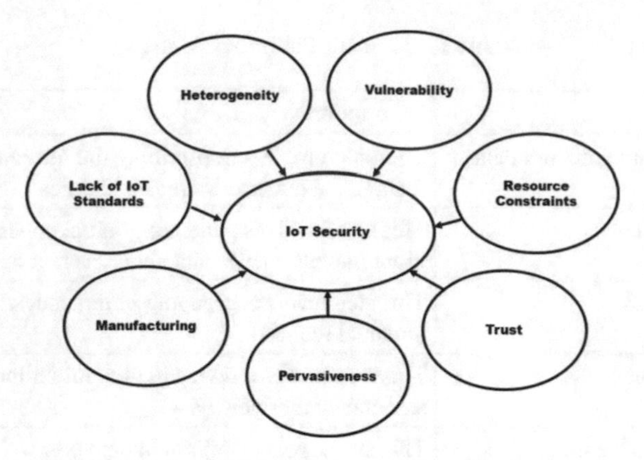

Fig. 3. Factors influencing the security of IoT systems

There is an understanding that the lack of standards is the reason for poor interaction among the devices; as mentioned: *'those common standards are essentials to illustrate the different methods of connecting different IoT devices and components with the IoT systems' (ex. 4).*

4.2 Heterogeneity

The heterogeneous devices being used in IoT systems are exponentially increasing. Different manufacturers utilise *'various models or frameworks for networking and various security mechanisms for security' (ex. 1).* Few participants are of the opinion that heterogeneity among IoT devices might be a hindrance to mutual interaction, and *'this is because deferent IoT devices vary regarding their security requirements' (ex. 9).*

Several participants believe that heterogeneity may limit security capabilities. Since different manufacturers set their own standards for various devices, some may stress enhancing security features, while others might be of the opinion to keep the things simple and easy going, bypassing the required security standards. As expressed by one of the participants, *'…it is very difficult to decide which security measure is most effective to be used because of the heterogeneity nature of the Internet of Things' (ex. 7).*

4.3 Vulnerability

It has been observed that thc fast growth of IoT devices and services has led to the deployment of many vulnerable and insecure nodes. One of the participants was of the opinion that: *'…networked system accessibility is a significant vulnerability' (ex. 17).* Others feel that attacks can be *'…conducted remotely due to the accessibility of IoT systems via the Internet' (ex. 9).*

Hardware vulnerability is another aspect of concern. Some of the participants pointed out that *'malicious people can physically access Internet of Things's devices and components of the IoT system as these component are widely spread outside buildings, neighbourhoods, or cities' (ex. 11).* The open environment can be cities, hospitals, farms, and universities, where hardware components and interfaces are running and are subject to attack. Therefore, it has been verified that vulnerability can be a cause of people losing faith in the confidentiality of this kind of system.

4.4 Resource Constraints

The small size of IoT system components, such as sensors, determines the limited resources of those components, such as memory and processing. Additionally, there is *'a networking constraint of IoT devices as these devices use low-power radio' (ex. 13).* All these constraints contribute to the challenge of implementing a strong algorithm to secure IoT devices.

Resource-constrained IoT devices are vulnerable to attack because *'...devices like IoT are with humble abilities regarding storage and processing' (ex. 15),* as well as *'the intention of IoT manufacturers in not to make devices with very effective measures in security' (ex. 4).* For example, encryption and decryption are resource-intensive tasks. As mentioned by one participant, *'the process of encryption and decryption requires huge computational capacity in terms of processing and storage*' (ex. 16).

4.5 Trust

The IoT mainly focuses on the machine-to-machine (M2M) mode of communication. For these communicating nodes, authentication is very important, as the intruders may take advantage of trust among IoT devices and infiltrate IoT systems via a forged node. This may create a security threat, as there are no authentication mechanisms for a massive number of IoT devices, which creates a security hole that needs to be filled. As mentioned by one participant, *'while two or more nodes communicate with each other, first those nodes should prevent themselves from being attacked by other nodes and this can be done if each one authenticates the others' (ex 16).*

It is noted that an important challenge related to trust is protecting users' private information, *'which importantly refers to preventing information discloser' (ex. 17).* As observed, there are hardly any security mechanisms during data communication in IoT systems due to trust among the devices. This may be a threat to the users' private information, as *'...the confidentiality of the data could be compromised due to the presence of a counterfeit node' (ex 12).*

4.6 Pervasiveness

Pervasiveness or ubiquitous computing is a useful concept and computing capability that *'support deceives and objects to connect and form a network of intelligent devices to collect and manipulate data on the go' (ex. 5).* The pervasive IoT environment leads to the emergence of several security challenges due to constrained resources, such as limited memory and processing capabilities, topology change, and latency in IoT devices. These constraints may be due to *'...the behaviour of the network, the features of an individual node, and constraints at the application level' (ex.13).* Most of these constraints are application dependent and are common in pervasive applications.

It has been observed that *'for such a ubiquitous environment to be useful and relevant, it should allow access, transmitting, and manipulating personal data of the users' (ex. 9)*. This is not a desired situation because the privacy and security of the system's users is at risk. Additionally, in a pervasive IoT ecosystem, there is a possibility that the *'...number of transmissions and receptions (communication) also increases' (ex. 15)*. This creates a situation in which demand becomes higher than available connectivity. This slows down the system, restricting its availability.

4.7 Manufacturing

Companies in the device manufacturing sector of IoT have increased their production manifold because of the wide acceptance of IoT applications around the world. Many of these companies try to embed security features during manufacturing. However, it is found that *'...this causes an increase of the cost and then the return of investment would be difficult to reach' (ex. 6)*. Contrary to this, a group of manufacturers produce cheaper IoT devices that are not equipped with security features and hence might be susceptible to security breaches. It is witnessed that this generates questions about the integrity of the system.

It is noted that with the increase of IoT, for example, in smart buildings, there is a dramatic increase in security issues harming smart home applications of IoT systems. This type of security threat is subject to end user awareness and compliance with security best practices, as noted: *'as users vary regarding their tending to regularly update their firmware' (ex. 19)*. This, at the end, leads to breaking down the level of security for these devices and presents an authentication challenge.

5 Discussion

The results of this study reveal that a lack of standards is a crucial factor in the weakness of an IoT system. The study further reveals that there is a greater chance of a forged node intrusion or authentication issues due to the existence of varying standards. Heterogeneity is yet another factor identified in this research. Due to the varying capabilities of the IoT devices developed by several manufacturers, a resistance to mutual interaction among the devices emerged. This study also found that network and hardware vulnerabilities have a negative impact on the confidentiality and availability of IoT systems. This might be the cause of security threats to IoT systems, such as disabling network availability and accessing users' personal information.

The focus of developing the IoT is to use devices that have the minimum power consumption and memory capacity. These resource constraints hinder the use of strong encryption algorithms and weaken the authentication process of the IoT system. Trust was also found to have a significant effect on the security of IoT systems. Trust is a highly complex factor gained by ensuring user safety and system security. Furthermore, pervasive computing has been found to be a core for several security challenges in IoT. The results of this research reveal that pervasiveness of the system can be the cause of threats to confidentiality and availability of the system. Users' privacy is at risk, as the pervasive environment autonomously deals with users' personal data.

Manufacturing of IoT devices in the absence of common standards was found to have a negative impact on the security of IoT systems. The findings also reveal that the manufacturers concentrate on cost-effective solutions that might lead to challenges in the authentication process.

6 Conclusions

The findings presented in this paper show that there are seven factors responsible for security challenges facing IoT systems, including a lack of IoT standards, heterogeneity, vulnerability, resource constraints, trust, pervasiveness and manufacturing. These findings add significantly to the existing literature, in which little empirical work has been done to explore the factors influencing IoT system security. Furthermore, this paper illustrates how the identified factors threaten IoT security. Hence, the practice of IoT security can take the identified factors and their associated insights into consideration when implementing IoT systems.

Like all research, this paper has limited scope, as it sheds light on the factors responsible for the security challenges in IoT systems. The aim of this paper was to explore the important factors that should be considered to enhance IoT security. These findings represent the context of the participants who were involved in the qualitative investigation. However, these findings might be applicable to other similar settings. Therefore, the next phase of the researcher's larger project is to build on the findings of this paper to generalise its findings. More specifically, a quantitative measure will be developed based on the seven factors of IoT security identified in this paper. The quantitative measure will help in collecting large quantitative data from representative samples to generalise the findings.

References

1. Ashton, K.: That "internet of things" thing. RFID J. **22**, 97–114 (2009)
2. Brock, D.L.: The Electronic Product Code™ (EPC™) as a Meta Code. Massachusetts Institute of Technology, USA (2003)
3. Yadav, K., Alharbi, A., Jain, A., Ramadan, R.A.: An IoT based secure patient health monitoring system. CMC-Comput. Mater. Continua **70**, 3637–3652 (2022)
4. Ancarani, A., Di Mauro, C., Legenvre, H., Cardella, M.S.: Internet of things adoption: a typology of projects. Int. J. Oper. Prod. Manag. **40**, 849–872 (2020)
5. Janiesch, C., et al.: The internet of things meets business process management: a manifesto. IEEE Syst. Man Cybern. Mag. **6**, 34–44 (2020)
6. Gubbi, J., Buyya, R., Marusic, S., Palaniswami, M.: Internet of things (IoT): a vision, architectural elements, and future directions. Futur. Gener. Comput. Syst. **29**, 1645–1660 (2013)
7. Rahmani, A.-M., et al.: Smart e-health gateway: bringing intelligence to internet-of-things based ubiquitous healthcare systems. In: 12th Annual IEEE Consumer Communications and Networking Conference (CCNC). IEEE, NV, USA (2015)
8. Samuel, R., Connolly, D.: Internet of things-based health monitoring and management domain-specific architecture pattern. Issues Inf. Syst. **16**, 58–63 (2015)
9. Agrawal, S., Vieira, D.: A survey on internet of things. Abakós, Belo Horizonte **1**, 78–95 (2013)

10. Alandjani, G.: Features and potential security challenges for IoT enabled devices in smart city environment. Int. J. Adv. Comput. Sci. Appl. **9**(8), 231–238 (2018)
11. Dihulia, S., Farooqui, T.: A literature survey on IoT security challenges. Int. J. Comput. Appl. **169**(4), 975–8887 (2017)
12. Rao, T., Ul Haq, E.: Security challenges facing IoT layers and its protective measures. Int. J. Comput. Appl. **179**(27), 31–35 (2018)
13. Lin, H., Bergmann, N.: IoT privacy and security challenges for smart home environments. Information **7**(3), 44 (2016). https://doi.org/10.3390/info7030044
14. Omitola, T., Wills, G.: Towards mapping the security challenges of the internet of things (IoT) supply chain. Procedia Comput. Sci. **126**, 441–450 (2018)
15. Pathak, P., Vyas, N., Joshi, S.: Security challenges for communications on IOT & big data. Int. J. Adv. Res. Comput. Sci. **8**(3), 431–437 (2017)
16. Mahmoud, R., Yousuf, T., Aloul, F., Zualkernan, I.: Internet of things (IoT) security: current status, challenges and prospective measures. In: 2015 10th International Conference for Internet Technology and Secured Transactions (ICITST), pp. 336–341 (2015)
17. Zhou, J., Cao, Z., Dong, X., Vasilakos, A.: Security and privacy for cloud-based IoT: challenges, countermeasures, and future directions. IEEE Commun. Mag. **55**(1), 26–33 (2017)
18. Liu, X., Zhao, M., Li, S., Zhang, F., Trappe, W.: A security framework for the internet of things in the future internet architecture. Future Internet **9**(3), 1–28 (2017)
19. Zhou, W., Jia, Y., Peng, A., Zhang, Y., Liu, P.: The effect of IoT new features on security and privacy: new threats, existing solutions, and challenges yet to be solved. IEEE Internet Things J. **6**(2), 1606–1616 (2019)
20. Kesavan, M., Prabhu, J.: A survey, design and analysis of IoT security and QoS challenges. Int. J. Inf. Syst. Model. Des. **9**(3), 48–66 (2018)
21. Frustaci, M., Pace, P., Aloi, G.: Evaluating critical security issues of the IoT world: present and future challenges. IEEE Internet Things J. **5**(4), 2483–2495 (2018)
22. Somani, G., Gaur, M., Sanghi, D., Conti, M., Rajarajan, M.: Scale inside-out: rapid mitigation of cloud DDoS attacks. IEEE Trans. Dependable Secure Comput. **15**(6), 959–973 (2018)
23. Yang, Y., Wu, L., Yin, G., Li, L., Zhao, H.: A survey on security and privacy issues in internet-of-things. IEEE Internet Things J. **4**(5), 1250–1258 (2017)
24. Bouij-Pasquier, I., El Kalam, A., Ouahman, A., De Montfort, M.: A security frame-work for internet of things. International conference on cryptology and network security, pp. 19–31. Springer, Chem (2015). https://doi.org/10.1007/978-3-319-26823-1_2
25. Oracevic, A., Dilek, S., Ozdemir, S.: Security in internet of things: a survey. In: International Symposium on Networks, Computers and Communications (ISNCC), pp. 1–6. Marrakech (2017). https://doi.org/10.1109/ISNCC.2017.8072001
26. Remler, D., Ryzin, G.: Research Methods in Practice: Strategies for Description and Causation. SAGE, Thousand Oaks CA (2011)
27. Recker, J.: Scientific Research in Information Systems: A Beginner's Guide. Springer, Heidelberg, New York (2013)
28. Wu, P.: Opening the black boxes of tam: Towards a mixed methods approach. In: The International Conference on Information Systems, Phoenix, Arizona (2009)
29. Dudley, J.: Research Methods for Social Work: Being Producers and Consumers of Research, 2nd edn. Allyn & Bacon, Boston, MA (2010)
30. Fink, A.: How to Sample in Surveys, 2nd edn. Sage Publications, Thousand Oaks, CA (2003)
31. Braun, V., Clarke, V.: Using thematic analysis in psychology. Qual. Res. Psychol. **3**(2), 77–101 (2006)
32. Christofi, M., Nunes, J., Peng, G.: Identifying and improving deficient business processes to prepare SMEs for ERP implementation. In: UK Academy for Information Systems (UKAIS) 14th Annual Conference, St Anne's College, University of Oxford, UKAIS, pp. 1–17

33. Holloway, I., Todres, L.: The status of method: flexibility, consistency and coherence. Qual. Res. **3**(3), 345–357 (2003)

Cyber Security

Facilitate Security Event Monitoring and Logging of Operational Technology (OT) Legacy Systems

Kenny Awuson-David[1](✉), James Thompson[2,3], Kiran Tuner[1,3], and Tawfik Al-Hadhrami[3]

[1] The Office of Gas and Electricity Markets Ofgem London, London, United Kingdom
{kenny.awuson-david,kiran.tuner}@ofgem.gov.uk
[2] EDF Energy United Kingdoms, Nottingham, United Kingdom
james.thompson@edfenergy.com
[3] School of Science and Technology, Nottingham Trent University, Nottingham, United Kingdom
tawfik.al-hadhrami@ntu.ac.uk

Abstract. Traditional networks with event monitoring and logging capability have been successfully deployed and implemented for years. However, these solutions are not always suited to be deployed and configured within an industrial control system (ICS) due to the legacy challenges and nature of devices running on this ecosystem. It is essential to understand what system, device and application to monitor, which logs to collect, where to collect them, how to acquire, secure, and preserve them as well as how best to use the collected logs. For example, users, assets, applications, and behaviours should be monitored and logged with an easy-to-read dashboard that adds context to the acquired logs. There has been a significant cyber threat to the ICS legacy system, such as malicious malware and advanced persistent threat (APT). In this paper, we propose a secure virtualised architecture based on the Purdue Enterprises Reference Architecture Model (PERA) for the ICS ecosystem that facilitates monitoring and logging of ICS legacy systems. The proposed architecture uses an enhanced open-source host-based intrusion detection system (HIDS) and network monitoring capability to maintain log integrity on transit and storage. The current Operational Technology (OT) monitoring and logging tools and software are ineffective in collecting and centralising OT legacy system logs. The novelty of the proposed virtualised architecture has an endpoint visibility feature and critical alert capabilities that detects an indication of compromise on the legacy and non-legacy systems in the ICS ecosystem.

Keywords: APT · Cyber attack · ICS · IDS · OT · PERA

1 Introduction

An industrial control system involves three major components namely the Supervisory Control And Data Acquisition (SCADA), Distributed Control Systems (DCS), and Programmable Logic Controller (PLC) [17, 18]. Securing the ICS system is vital as the

F. Saeed et al. (Eds.): IRICT 2021, LNDECT 127, pp. 461–472, 2022.
https://doi.org/10.1007/978-3-030-98741-1_38

SCADA and its legacy devices do not have the same functionality mechanisms as the traditional network [1, 19]. Furthermore, some of the OT core components are highly automated and require no human intervention. For instance, the Safety Instrumented System (SIS) reacts to a potentially unsafe system shutdown by restoring all functional processes to a safe state [1, 18]. Further investigation then revealed that it was a sophisticated malware designed to target the vulnerabilities of OT protocols [12–14]. Decades ago, OT networks were separate from traditional IT because they relied on different technologies and functionality, including different security mechanisms. OT security is highly safety-driven and needs constant availability of service [17, 18]. In contrast, traditional networks depend on the confidentiality, integrity and availability (CIA) and non-repudiation of data and applications associated with the network. The interconnection of these two different networks (OT and IT) have led to genuine concern about the ICS system's cyber resiliency, especially with the legacy challenges. In cyberspace, new malicious malware is created by cyber adversaries designed to invade system security mechanisms [15, 29, 31]. Research has revealed the sophistication of some of this malware. For instance, Stuxnet was designed with a zero-day payload in mind targeting an OT system and its components [28].

Cybersecurity experts are skilled to secure and maintain the CIA of a system by adopting cyber defence mechanisms learnt through practical experience. However, this notion is different in the OT environment as the system is designed with availability in mind. In addition, the convergence of OT and IT has also made the ICS ecosystem more complex to maintain security at every level of the Purdue architectural reference model. There is a need to make the ICS more resilient against cyber-attack using a security event monitoring and logging approach to react to any indication of an attack [17, 28]. There has been a significant shift within the ICS community to revaluate current ICS security measures through research and innovative ideas. Malicious malware such as ransomware has continued to pose a significant threat to ICS systems [2, 3]. In 2020 and 2021, ransomware attacks increased, targeting government institutions, universities, and national healthcare infrastructures, including the ICS system [4]. The threat of malicious malware targeting an industrial control system was of genuine concern when a cyber attack took down the Ukrainian power grid in 2015 [3, 4, 22]. The Ukrainian authorities initially suspected a simple virus attack facilitated through a phishing campaign. It is vital to have a real-time proactive logging and monitoring mechanism in the ICS system that enables incident response, forensics, and recovery [5, 28]. This paper introduces a virtualised architecture integrating Security Onion (SO), Wazuh, PfSense and Snort to facilitate security events logging and monitoring of ICS assets [33, 34, 36]. The virtualised ICS testbed is integrated with Siemens TIA Portal V16 running 1500 PLC. It also has an API interface of WinCC and S7 and Profinet protocol with a ladder logic program that mimics a hydro-power station. A single case study is used to evaluate the proactive logging and monitoring approach. A scenario is used to validate whether the acquired logs can highlight an indication of attack by alerting the ICS system security operator.

The next section of this paper will look at related works, the methodology, and a case study with the results of the proposed OT security event logging and monitoring virtualised architecture. Finally, the conclusion with direction for future work.

2 Related Works

The persistent cybersecurity threats to an industrial control system have prompted several academic studies to carry out research to understand the need for data flow integrity in the ICS ecosystem and to ensure operational safety at all times. This section introduces related works from ICS security logging and monitoring.

2.1 The Industrial Control System (ICS)

Research has demonstrated that Modbus lacks the most modern security features that could mitigate the ICS system malicious exploits [6, 17] proposed a high-level method where ICS text-based logs are viewed, with the data aggregated statistics using the Kibana dashboard. However, this paper could have been extended to enhance the Elastic Stack capability in real-time ICS monitoring and logging of all security events, including ICS application protocols [24, 35]. Additionally, [7] implemented a module for monitoring a Modbus TCP traffic to detect any anomaly behaviour in the industrial control system. This paper concept uses a multi-algorithm detection based on the EMERALD detection and correlation mechanisms. This paper could have considered monitoring other ICS protocols such as the Profinet, EtherNet/I.P. or Distributed Network Protocol (DNP3). [8] proposed a DNP3 analyser intrusion detection framework based on Bro. The DNP3 analysis is a scenarios based approach, which involves a formatted network packet. The concept of the DNP3 analyser is to detect any anomaly events associated with the DNP3 protocol. However, the limitation of the paper is that the DNP3 will not monitor Modbus and other vendors' protocols such as Profinet or BACnet. This paper [25] integrated an Elastic Stack approach where data is primarily observed as aggregated statistics and correlations in a SCADA environment.

3 Methodology

This paper adopted a virtual environment simulation methodology that validates a real-time simulation of an ICS environment [37]. It enables a virtual test environment for OT legacy system logging and monitoring that combines physical system components. The methodology was implemented in two phases. First, design and build an ICS architecture with legacy systems integration. Secondly, Kali Linux was used to generate security event network traffic. The logs were captured in real-time, and the server-generated incident alerts, as demonstrated in Fig. 4. The advantage of virtual simulation methodology is the ability to log and monitor legacy systems without impacting the operational environment of an ICS system.

3.1 The Integrated Architectural Tool

Security Onion was adopted and enhanced to suit our virtualised ICS logging and monitoring architecture and the traditional PERA. Security Onion is a free and open Linux distribution for threat hunting, enterprise security monitoring and log management. It includes a suite of well-known security applications such as TheHive, Playbook and

Sigma, Fleet, Osquery, CyberChef, Elasticsearch, Logstash, Kibana, Suricata, Zeek, Wazuh and supports many modules such as Sysmon.

Furthermore, the virtualised architecture environment logs are shipped from the OT devices, including SCADA and the engineering workstation, to the centralised Security Onion server for further analyses. The server will alert the system operator if there is any malicious traffic on the network. The enhanced Security Onion solution is suitable for endpoint visibility of the legacy devices, including network switches in the OT ecosystem. Another aspect to note is the capability of the solution to sniff all network traffic from our management LAN.

4 Security Logging and Monitoring in the ICS Ecosystem

This section describes how our architectural logging and monitoring testbed is designed and built to support and enhance the ICS infrastructure with security, uptime and resilience in mind. The paper looked at how possible it was to add endpoint visibility to the ICS system with the legacy system in mind. The paper examines security logging and monitoring in the ICS space and defines the three main methods of security monitoring and logging: passive, active, and threat hunting.

Passive Security Monitoring: There is a low risk in introducing passive monitoring to the OT environment as it doesn't disrupt the network, and the process makes this suitable for legacy networks that might be unstable if additional traffic is introduced. It provides extensive coverage of devices, and each switch configured includes a range of all devices connected to that switch. There is less security risk as all monitoring clients are separate from the ICS system, and there is no risk they could communicate to any node that is part of the ICS system.

Active Security Monitoring: This is accomplished by developing a software agent such as Wazuh to interrogate the host system and forward any anomaly behaviour with the host system to a centralised logging server. Agents provide much more detail about the computers. Current OT network monitoring and logging mechanisms detect only traffic activities on the network and do not know the state of each node. In our virtualised architecture solution, the agents can forward all logs, including monitoring security events and running processes, file operations, PLC, HMI's, USB etc. The novelty of the architecture is its active and passive monitoring and logging of security events of legacy and non-legacy systems within an ICS environment [1].

Threat Hunting: The threat hunting capability is still in its infancy in the ICS ecosystem. It is a process of actively interrogating all the security event evidence generated by the passive and active monitoring mechanism in the ICS environment. With a threat hunting capability, an incident responder could start investigating the generated suspicious flagged security events, alerts, software list, and captured network packets to prove or disprove if a security incident has occurred or not [27, 28].

4.1 Determine What to Monitor

There are hundreds of relevant event data generated by system devices within an ICS environment. With this high rate of events, there is a need to pinpoint what needs logging and monitoring on the different levels of the PERA. At the enterprise level, the following assets could be monitored and logged: applications, user information, databases server, Active Directory Domain Service (AD DS), client machines, firewall, wireless access points (AP) and the DMZ. However, it is a complex solution in deciding what to log in and monitor in the OT environment due to the critical nature of OT devices. OT assets such as the PLC, remote terminal units (RTUs), intelligent electronic devices (IEDs), human-machine interfaces (HMIs), and Historians servers should be monitored. The monitoring should also be extended to the OT protocols such as Modbus.

4.2 ICS Cybersecurity Challenges

Research has demonstrated the continued probing of the industrial control system by cybercriminals and nation-states whose mission is to disrupt and cause damage to their target both economically and socially. There is a need for ICS system security operators to be more effectively equipped with cybersecurity defence skills [20, 28, 32]. ICS asset owners could also consider taking further ICS cybersecurity training for their staff to improve their understanding of cyber threats and challenges. Figure 1 highlights a triangle approach that could be adopted in the ICS environment to ensure cyber resiliency. As shown in Fig. 1, if any of the three components, namely exploit, vulnerability and threat, are removed, ICS cyber resiliency will be achieved. This is like having the fire triangle components analogy for what a fire needs to burn: air, heat, and a fuel source must be present. However, remove any of the three components, and the fire will not start.

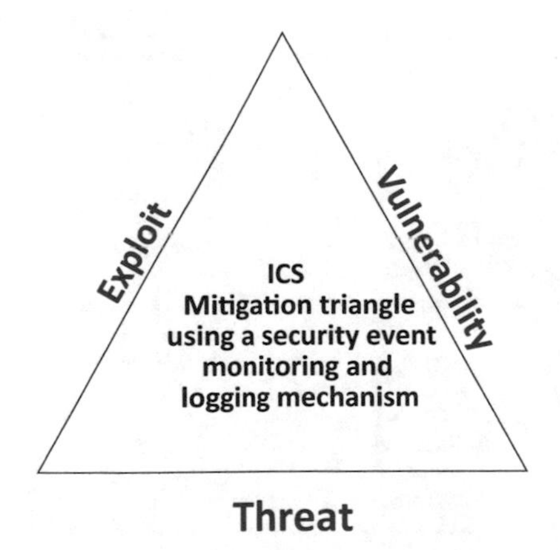

Fig. 1. Mitigation ICS triangle

There has been an increasing number of cyber-related attacks targeting the industrial control system (ICS) and the Operations Technology (OT), ranging from the Stuxnet attack in 2010 to the threats posed by the SolarWinds Orion/Sunburst breach and the persistent advance threat of ransomware attacks. As reported on 13 December 2020, the SolarWinds supply chain attack compromised about 300,000 organisations, of which 33,000 integrated the Orion platform, and 18,000 of their customers could have installed the malicious updates [21, 22]. Proactive security logging and monitoring mechanisms in the ICS ecosystem will strengthen the defence line of an ICS system by mitigating the challenges of endpoint visibility and enhanced forensic readiness [11].

5 ICS Logging and Monitoring Visualised Architecture

The virtualised ICS architectural testbed enables reliable testing of ICS logging and monitoring use cases. The virtual environment has its advantage. Firstly, it removes the concern of running logging and monitoring use cases on an operational ICS environment, given the legacy nature of the current ICS system. Secondly, the proposed ICS architecture is for a test environment rather than an operational one. However, as part of the research for this paper, the concept is now being deployed on ICS operational environment for a trial. Thirdly, the hardware components of the ICS virtualised environment are minimal and only requires a Windows 10 operating system with 32 GB of RAM and one terabyte hard disk space. Additionally, on the software side, a VMware workstation 16.

Pro was used to simulate the virtualised cloud environment highlighted in Fig. 2. At the same time, Siemens TIA Portal SIMATIC STEP 7 and WinCC V13 were integrated to mimic the ICS and SCADA environment. Furthermore, Kali Linux was used as an attacking node to represent an adversary [38]. Additionally, ICS reconnaissance experimental scenario was conducted using NMAP and Metasploit in a controlled environment.

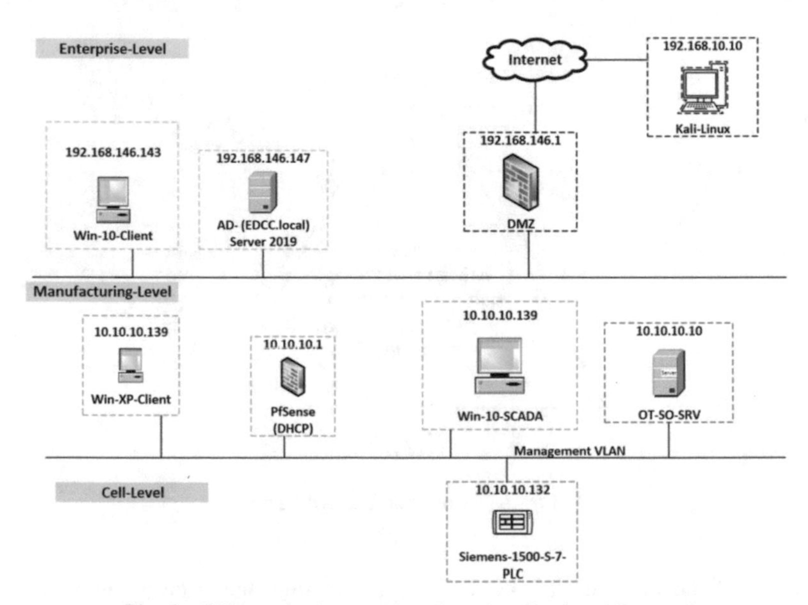

Fig. 2. ICS monitoring and logging visualised architectural

The Enterprise-level of the architecture has the Active Directory (AD) running on the Windows Server 2019 operating system. With an IP address of 192.168.146.147 and the domain name EDCC.local.

In addition, we deployed a Windows 10 client on the same Enterprise level with an IP address of 192.168.146.143. Furthermore, the LAN side of the pfSense firewall had an IP address of 10.10.10.1 The Manufacturing level has the engineering workstation with an IP address of 10.10.10.130 and the enhanced Security Onion centralised server with an IP address of 10.10.10.10. Another essential point of the proposed logging and monitoring architecture is the cell level where the Siemens TIA Portal SIMATIC STEP 7 with an IP address of 10.10.10.132 was integrated to simulate an OT environment. It is essential to point out that the proposed, designed ICS architecture is for a test environment rather than an operational one. However, as part of the research for this paper the concept is now being deployed on ICS operational environment for a trial.

6 Case Study Scenario

The case study scenario demonstrates how an insider threat compromised the SCADA system at the manufacturing level of the ICS and then went further to modify the users logging credentials and authorised access to the application and PLC database. Due to the sensitive nature of the experiment, the paper presents a result that highlights the importance of having security event logging and monitoring in the ICS environment. The paper demonstrated how a cyber-related incident was simulated to target OT devices through an insider with a basic knowledge of the network topology. The attack was captured, and an alert was flagged on the Kibana dashboard for the system administrator

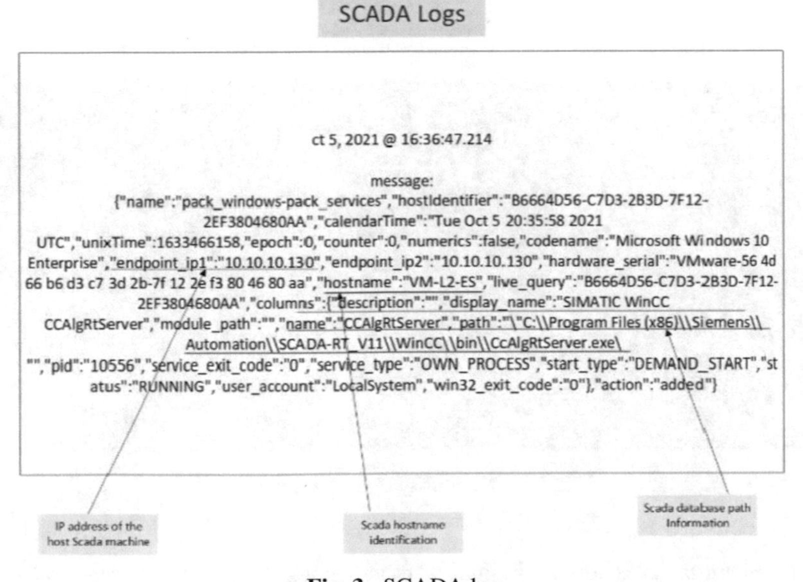

Fig. 3. SCADA log

to view. Figure 3 highlights how the security event logging and monitoring system captured SCADA activities with an accurate time stamp. Figure 4 captures all the legacy and non-legacy assets on the network, including the HMI and WinCC database entries in real-time. Furthermore, Fig. 5 captures the recognisance that the adversary initiated, and Kali Linux was highlighted as the host machine used for the NMAP active scan. Figure 6 and 7 present the security event logging and monitoring enhanced Security Onion server that uses low bandwidth resources from the network.

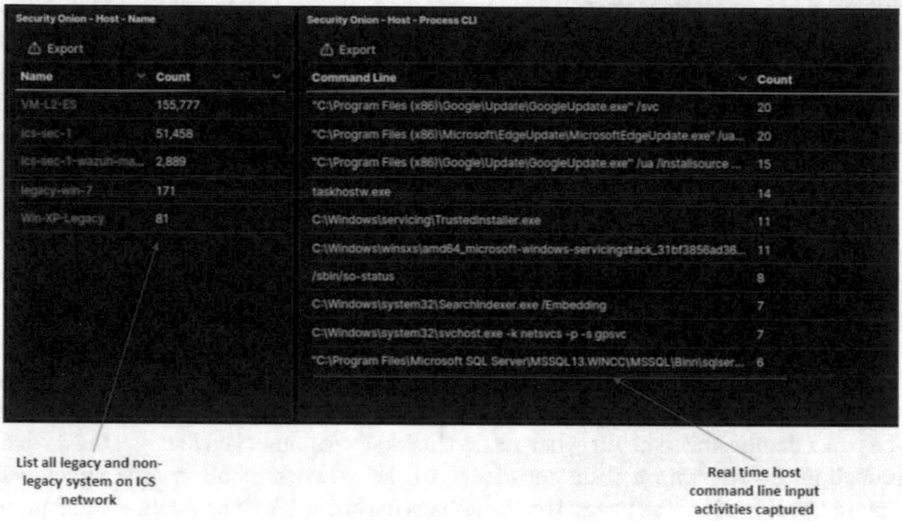

Fig. 4. Captured OT security events

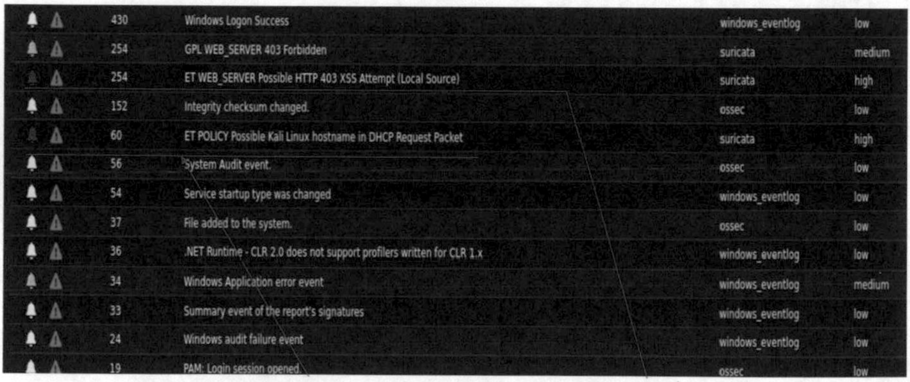

Fig. 5. ICS security event alert metrics

Figure 4 emphasises how the indication of attack was captured, then presents detailed alerting information of the attacker's intent including hostname as Kali Linux. The

Kibana dashboard's detailed information is crucial for ICS system operators and security administrators to activate mitigation mechanisms that could make it difficult for the attacker to succeed [30].

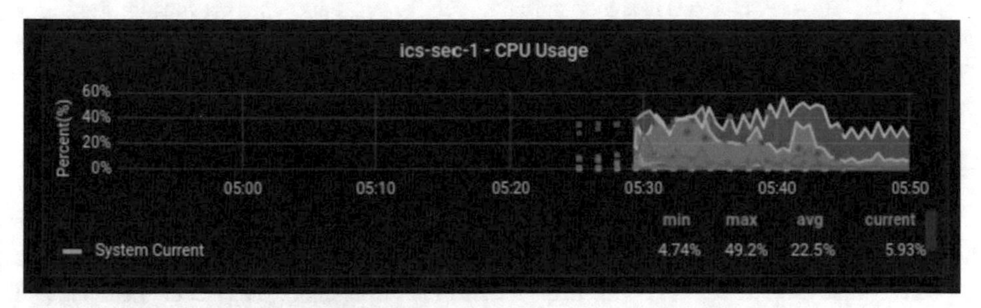

Fig. 6. ICS logging and monitoring server CPU usage

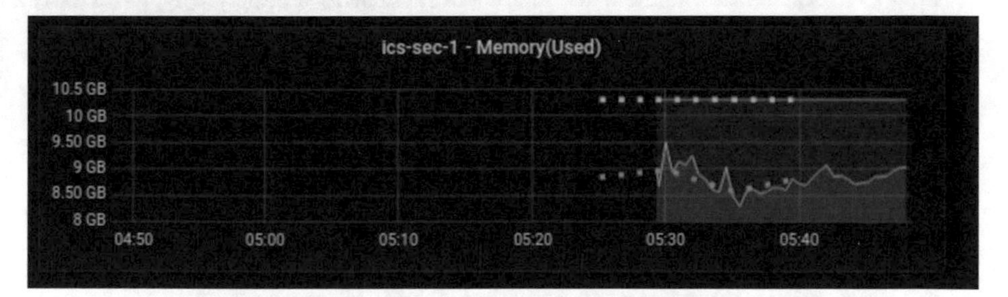

Fig. 7. ICS logging and monitoring server memory usage

7 Conclusion

This paper presents an industrial control system (ICS) virtualised architecture testbed that validates proactive security event logging and monitoring. Research has demonstrated that there is a need to solve ICS logging and monitoring challenges posed by the legacy nature of the system. Academic literature was reviewed for a solution that mitigates the complexity of endpoint visibility in the ICS ecosystem based on a centralised logging and monitoring mechanism. We selected Security Onion and Elastic Stack open-source tool to implement an ICS virtualised environment. An experimental scenario was conducted and evaluated. The results highlighted how the proposed solution enables proactive security monitoring and logging in the ICS ecosystem. The experiment demonstrated how the tools could be used to collect logs and analyse data of any type with high-performance metrics. The result of the experiment could facilitate incident response and a digital forensic readiness plan [30, 31]. The concept of this paper has been implemented into an operational environment. Furthermore, future research and development will focus on the integration of machine learning (ML) into the proposed architecture to add another layer of logging and monitoring in the ICS ecosystem [9, 10].

Acknowledgment. The bulk of the ICS monitoring and logging research work was funded by the UK Office of Gas and Electricity Markets (Ofgem) jointly with EDF Energy and Nottingham Trent University. We would like to thank all other parties who contributed to this paper. This paper is not intended as relevant guidance or as state of the art within the meaning of NIS Regulation 10 (3) and (4) [26]. Any reference to any organisation, service or product does not constitute or imply the endorsement, recommendation, or favouring by Ofgem or any of its employees or contractors acting on its behalf.

References

1. Look, B.G.: Handbook of SCADA/Control Systems Security. CRC Press, Boca Raton (2016)
2. Chen, Q., Bridges, R.A.: Automated behavioral analysis of malware: a case study of wannacry ransomware. In: 2017 16th IEEE International Conference on Machine Learning and Applications (ICMLA), pp. 454–460. IEEE (2017)
3. Zimba, A., Wang, Z., Chen, H.: Multi-stage crypto ransomware attacks: a new emerging cyber threat to critical infrastructure and industrial control systems. ICT Express **4**(1), 14–18 (2018)
4. Alladi, T., Chamola, V., Zeadally, S.: Industrial control systems: cyberattack trends and countermeasures. Comput. Commun. **155**, 1–8 (2020)
5. Khan, R., Maynard, P., McLaughlin, K., Laverty, D., Sezer, S.: Threat analysis of blackenergy malware for synchrophasor based real-time control and monitoring in smart grid. In: 4th International Symposium for ICS & SCADA Cyber Security Research 2016, vol. 4, pp. 53–63 (2016)
6. Hamilton, J., Schofield, B., Berges, M.G., Tournier, J.C.: SCADA Statistics monitoring using the elastic stack (Elasticsearch, Logstash, Kibana). In: International Conference on Accelerator and Large Experimental Physics Control Systems (2018)
7. Cheung, S., Dutertre, B., Fong, M., Lindqvist, U., Skinner, K., Valdes, A.: Using model-based intrusion detection for SCADA networks. In: Proceedings of the SCADA Security Scientific Symposium, vol. 46, pp. 1–12 (2007)
8. Lin, H., Slagell, A., Di Martino, C., Kalbarczyk, Z., Iyer, R.K.: Adapting bro into SCADA: building a specification-based intrusion detection system for the dnp3 protocol. In: Proceedings of the Eighth Annual Cyber Security and Information Intelligence Research Workshop, pp. 1–4 (2013)
9. Li, G., et al.: Detecting cyberattacks in industrial control systems using online learning algorithms. Neurocomputing **364**, 338–348 (2019)
10. Phillips, B., Gamess, E., Krishnaprasad, S.: An evaluation of machine learning-based anomaly detection in a SCADA system using the modbus protocol. In: Proceedings of the 2020 ACM Southeast Conference, pp. 188–196 (2020)
11. Cornelius, E., Fabro, M.: Recommended practice: creating cyber forensics plans for control systems (No. INL/EXT-08-14231). Idaho National Laboratory (INL) (2008)
12. Case, D.U.: Analysis of the Cyber Attack on the Ukrainian Power Grid. Electricity Information Sharing and Analysis Center (E-ISAC), p. 388 (2016)
13. Sullivan, J.E., Kamensky, D.: How cyber-attacks in Ukraine show the vulnerability of the US power grid. Electr. J. **30**(3), 30–35 (2017)
14. Sun, C.C., Hahn, A., Liu, C.C.: Cyber security of a power grid: state-of the-art. Int. J. Electr. Power Energy Syst. **99**, 45–56 (2018)
15. Ackerman, P.: Industrial Cybersecurity: Efficiently Secure Critical Infrastructure Systems. Packt Publishing Ltd, Birmingham (2017)
16. Stouffer, K., Falco, J., Scarfone, K.: Guide to industrial control systems (ICS) security. NIST Spec. Publ. **800**(82), 16 (2011)

17. Bodungen, C., Singer, B., Shbeeb, A., Wilhoit, K., Hilt, S.: Hacking Exposed Industrial Control Systems: ICS and SCADA Security Secrets & Solutions. McGraw Hill Professional, New York (2016)
18. Kim, H.: Security and vulnerability of SCADA systems over IP-based wireless sensor networks. Int. J. Distrib. Sens. Netw. **8**(11), 268478 (2012)
19. Stouffer, K.A., Falco, J.A., Scarfone, K.A.: Guide to industrial control systems (ICS) security: supervisory control and data acquisition (SCADA) systems, distributed control systems (DCS), and other control system configurations such as programmable logic controllers (PLC), pp. 800–882 (2011)
20. Auffret, J.P., et al.: Cybersecurity leadership: competencies, governance, and technologies for industrial control systems. J. Interconnection Netw. **17**(01), 1740001 (2017)
21. Quoted in Kari Paul et al.: 'SolarWinds Hack Was Work of "At Least 1,000 Engineers", Tech Executives Tell Senate', Guardian, 24 February 2021. https://www.theguardian.com/technology/2021/feb/23/solarwinds-hacksenate-hearing-microsoft
22. Willett, M.: Lessons of the SolarWinds Hack. Survival **63**(2), 7–26 (2021). https://doi.org/10.1080/00396338.2021.1906001
23. Knapp, E.D., Langill, J.T.: Industrial network security: securing critical infrastructure networks for smart grid, SCADA, and other Industrial control systems. In: Syngress (2014)
24. Chhajed, S.: Learning ELK Stack. Packt Publishing Ltd, Birmingham (2015)
25. UK statutory instruments 2018/506. https://www.legislation.gov.uk/uksi/2018/506/made
26. Coletta, A., Armando, A.: Security monitoring for industrial control systems. In: Security of Industrial Control Systems and Cyber Physical Systems, pp. 48–62. Springer, Cham (2015). https://doi.org/10.1007/978-3-319-40385-4_4
27. Knapp, E.D., Langill, J.: Industrial Network Security. Securing critical infrastructure networks for smart grid, SCADA, and other Industrial Control Systems. In: Syngress (2014)
28. Alsuhaym, F., Al-Hadhrami, T., Saeed, F., Awuson-David, K.: Toward home automation: an IoT based home automation system control and security. In: International Congress of Advanced Technology and Engineering (ICOTEN). IEEE (2021). https://doi.org/10.1109/ICOTEN52080.2021.9493464
29. Alanzi, A., Al-Hadhrami, T., Saeed, F., Awuson-David, K.: Wireless remote control-security system for entrances (WRC-SSE). In: International Congress of Advanced Technology and Engineering (ICOTEN). IEEE (2021). https://doi.org/10.1109/ICOTEN52080.2021.9493429
30. Awuson-David, K., Al-Hadhrami, T., Alazab, M., Shah, N., Shalaginov, A.: BCFL logging: an approach to acquire and preserve admissible digital forensics evidence in cloud ecosystem. Futur. Gener. Comput. Syst. **122**, 113 (2021)
31. Awuson-David, K., Al-Hadhrami, T., Funminiyi, O., Lotfi, A.: Using hyperledger fabric blockchain to maintain the integrity of digital evidence in a containerised cloud ecosystem. In: International Conference of Reliable Information and Communication Technology, pp. 839–848. Springer, Cham (2019). https://doi.org/10.1007/978-3-030-33582-3_79
32. Few, C., Thompson, J., Awuson-David, K., Al-Hadhrami, T.: A case study in the use of attack graphs for predicting the security of cyber-physical systems. In: 2021 International Congress of Advanced Technology and Engineering (ICOTEN), pp. 1–7. IEEE (2021)
33. Security Onion Homepage. https://securityonionsolutions.com/. Accessed 1 Nov 2021
34. Park, W., Ahn, S.: Performance comparison and detection analysis in snort and suricata environment. Wireless Pers. Commun. **94**(2), 241–252 (2016). https://doi.org/10.1007/s11277-016-3209-9
35. Hamilton, J., Schofield, B., Berges, M.G., Tournier, J.C.: SCADA Statistics monitoring using the elastic stack (Elasticsearch, Logstash, Kibana). In: International Conference on Accelerator and Large Experimental Physics Control Systems. Barcelona, Spain (2017)

36. Negoita, O., Carabas, M.: Enhanced security using elasticsearch and machine learning. In: Science and Information Conference, pp. 244–254. Springer, Cham (2020). https://doi.org/10.1007/978-3-030-52243-8_19
37. Abd-Alhamid, F., Kent, M., Bennett, C., Calautit, J., Wu, Y.: Developing an innovative method for visual perception evaluation in a physical-based virtual environment. Build. Environ. **162**, 106278 (2019)
38. Najera-Gutierrez, G., Ansari, J.A.: Web Penetration Testing with Kali Linux: Explore the Methods and Tools of Ethical Hacking with Kali Linux. Packt Publishing Ltd, Birmingham (2018)

Validating Mobile Forensic Metamodel Using Tracing Method

Abdulalem Ali[1] (✉), Shukor Abd Razak[1], Siti Hajar Othman[1], Rashiq Rafiq Marie[2], Arafat Al-Dhaqm[1], and Maged Nasser[1]

[1] School of Computing, Faculty of Engineering, Universiti Teknologi Malaysia, 81310 Johor Bahru, Johor, Malaysia
almaldolah2012@gmail.com

[2] Information System Department, College of Computer Science and Engineering, Taibah University, Medina, Kingdom of Saudi Arabia

Abstract. Mobile Forensic (MF) is a branch of digital forensic used to collect and analyze mobile device crimes. Several forensic models and frameworks have been proposed in the literature for the MF domain to identify, acquire, and investigate MF crimes. However, these models are redundant and developed for specific purposes. Therefore, the authors developed a metamodel to solve the redundancy and heterogeneity of the MF domain called Mobile Forensic Metamodel (MFM). However, the MFM has not been evaluated from the modeling perspective to evaluate the effectiveness of the MFM in terms of instantiation solution models for the MF domain. Thus, this paper aims to evaluate the effectiveness of the MFM using a tracing method. The tracing method is a common way of validating metamodels through reasonable reliability on the domain application of the metamodel to assess the logical consistency of metamodels against domain models. For this purpose, two real scenarios were selected to confirm the capabilities of developed MFM in instantiate solution models for problems in hands. From real scenarios, the developed MFM was found to be scalable, logical, complete, interoperable, coherent, and useful for the MFM domain.

Keywords: Mobile forensic · Metamodel · Tracing method

1 Introduction

Mobile devices such as smartphones have become one of the most popular technologies that exist today. The number of mobile phones subscriptions has increased to over 4.5 billion in 2017, and this number is growing exponentially [1, 2]. Advances in technologies related to smartphones lead to an increase in the functionality of mobile phones. Also, these devices are currently used for several activities in our daily lives. For instance, check e-mail, take photos, browse the Internet, business transactions, and location data, and do much more. In contrast, mobile phone crimes are rising, and cybercrime is now moving to mobile devices such as smartphones. For instance, committing fraud via e-mail, harassment through text messages, distribution of child pornography, terrorism, and selling drugs, etc. [3, 4].

F. Saeed et al. (Eds.): IRICT 2021, LNDECT 127, pp. 473–482, 2022.
https://doi.org/10.1007/978-3-030-98741-1_39

MF is a subfield of digital forensics concerning to the recovery of digital evidence from a mobile device under forensically sound conditions. Besides, MF is interconnected with various elements which involves people, authority, investigators team, resources, procedures, processes, and policies. The diversity of mobile devices as well as the sophistication of the digital crimes one of the major challenges to forensics investigators [5]. The previous research works viewed mobile forensics in terms of data acquisition and problem-solving scenarios as a subset of computer forensics. However, they did not extend mobile forensics beyond the computer forensics paradigm, nor did they focus on modelling case domain information in investigations.

Additionally, previous MF domain research did not focus on modeling case domain information involved in investigations. Therefore, Ali et al. [2] developed a complete/common framework called Mobile Forensic Metamodel (MFM) to solve complexity, heterogeneity, ambiguity, interoperability in the MF domain. The developed MFM recognized, documented, collected, and matched various MF activities, tasks, concepts, and processes from multiple MF models into a developed metamodel that allowed practitioners to derive solution models easily. However, the developed MFM was not evaluated by tracing method to prove its efficiency in the MF domain. Thus, this paper aims to assess the capabilities of the MFM using the tracing technique. The tracing method is presented to evaluate the rational consistency of metamodels compared to domain models. This evaluation method is more active than other evaluation methods. For this aim, a real scenario was selected to evaluate the developed MFM from the modeling perspective to ensure its consistency along with the MF domain.

The rest of this paper is prepared into five sections: Sect. 2 introduces the related works in the MF domain. Section 3 offers the methodology, while Sect. 4 displays discussion and analysis. The conclusion of this study is introduced in Sect. 5.

2 Related Works

Several research have been conducted in the MF domain. However, the majority of them solely focused on understanding the MF professionals' perception regarding the lack of digital investigation processes that can be used to prepare forensic reports for court cases [6, 7] stated that digital evidence in mobile phones is easily tampering with overwritten or remote commands from the wireless network. The rapid change of mobile phones on the market caused a demand for forensic examination of the devices, which existing computer forensics techniques could not meet [8, 9]. In addition, Casey et al. [10] mentioned that mobile devices hold a large amount of digital evidence for digital investigation processes. In recent years, forensic investigation has relied heavily on evidence gathered from mobile devices. In reference to real scenarios, mobile phone evidence was cited in the prosecution of Ian Huntley, who murdered two young girls, as well as in the search for and arrest of suspects in the 2007 failed attempt of London car bombings.

Despite that, validated frameworks and methods for extracting data from mobile devices are practically non-existent [11]. Casey [6] constanted growth of mobile devices makes it difficult to design a single forensic tool or set of standards for the MF domain that is specific to a single platform. In addition, Lessard and Kessler [12] stated that one of the major challenges in the MF domain is the lack of hardware, software, and standardisation in mobile devices which makes the investigation procedure harder. With the advancement in technology these days, as well as the wide range of mobile devices and operating systems, make the development of common framework or standards model a difficult effort [13–17]. Additionally, Khelalfa [18] stated that the main problem with mobile devices is that there is currently no standard forensic model or process for forensic analysis of smartphones. Therefore, forensic investigators face difficult challenges in conducting the forensic investigation processes in digital crimes, particularly for mobile phones [19, 20].

3 Methodology

A method has been adapted by [20–22] to validate the developed MFM [2]. It contains of two main stages as shown in Fig. 1. To find the proper/appropriate validation technique, this study should answer these two questions:

1) what are the existing metamodel validation techniques?
2) what are the pros and cons of the current metamodel validation techniques?

3.1 Stage I: Select Validation Technique

As long as this step aims to select the proper metamodel validation technique to verify the completeness, logicalness, coherence, scalability, and usefulness of the developed MFM, a list of existing metamodel validation techniques, and the advantages and disadvantages of these techniques are highlighted in this stage. Metamodels need to be validated before being utilized as a representation of real application domains. The quality of a metamodel is measured in view of how the metamodel can satisfy requirements during its creation [23]. In order to fulfill the completeness and effectiveness of the developed MFM, several validation techniques were applied during the validation stage. When the metamodel was developed, the question of how the metamodel can be used for real-world problems was often asked. According to Al-Dhaqm et al. [21], the criteria to select the best type of validation technique can be determined according to metamodel type and the goal of its development (e.g., agent-based modeling, semantic and conceptual modeling, and mathematical and statistical modeling). For example, the Bootstrap Approach [24], Cross-validation [25], and Multistage Validation [23] are usually used for the validation of simulation metamodels. These approaches involve a few cycles of comparison and need a large sample size to achieve validity. Since the MF models used in the developed MFM are limited and the sample size is small, these validation approaches were not suitable. With a smaller sample size, comparison against other models [26], which does not require a large sample to achieve validity, was more suitable. This study also needed to evaluate the metamodel's completeness, logicalness, coherence, scalability, and usefulness. Thus, the Tracing Technique [27] was used to validate the capabilities of the MFM in terms of instantiation/derivation solution models from the MFM.

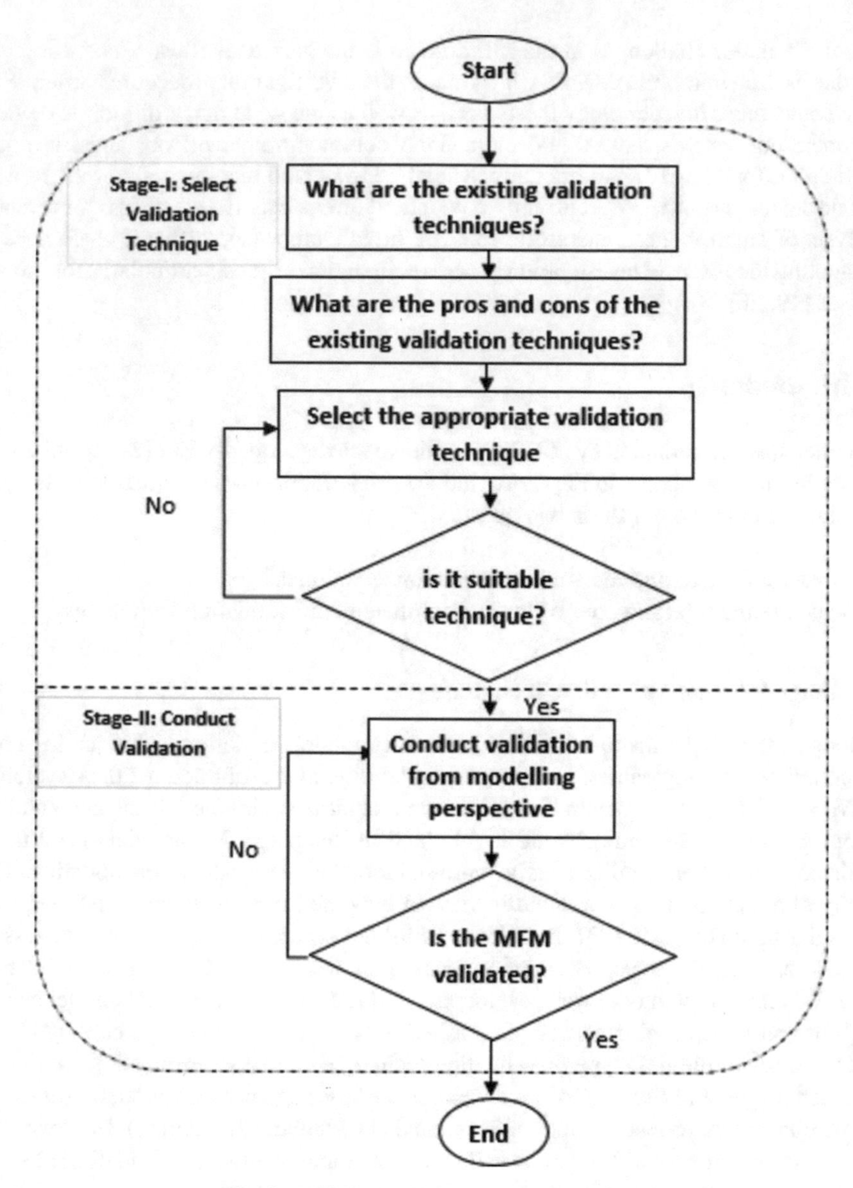

Fig. 1. Validate MFM using tracing method

Therefore, this paper validates the developed MFM using the tracing technique. The tracing approach generally leads to thinking about and capturing the hierarchical relations within a metamodel and ensuring that metamodel users can understand the relationships that exist within and across the metamodel [22]. The behaviors of different types of specific entities in the model are traced (followed) to determine if the logic of the model is correct and if the necessary accuracy is obtained. In this evaluation, the MFM is used to instantiate a specific mobile type. The behaviors of different kinds of particular entities in the model are traced (followed) to determine if the logic of the model is correct and if the necessary accuracy is obtained [20]. This tracing validation will determine an agreement between concepts in the metamodel and real MF scenarios.

3.2 Stage II: Conduct Validation

A real scenario was adapted to validate MFM from a modeling perspective [28], "*an employee at a large company has contacted HR regarding inappropriate messages and phone calls he has received from a co-worker. To confirm the unwanted behavior, management authorizes the analysis of the harasser's BlackBerry, which the company had issued for business purposes. Management does not want to alert the subject in question or other staff to the investigation. A note is sent to that group's manager explaining that their group is being targeted for BlackBerry firmware updates. A member of the desktop support staff is dispatched to each PC. The staff member asks each user to enter his/her PIN so that the device may be backed up. Support staff explains that a backup is needed just in case the firmware update does not go smoothly. All backups are copied to a network share, and the IPD file associated with the subject in question is taken for analysis.*"

Thus, to solve this scenario, an investigator needs to generate several M1-Models from M2-MFM using the UML stereotype <<>> [29].

Generate M1-Verfiication Model from M2-MFM: To verify/validate the incident in the scenario, author instantiated the M1-Verfication model from M2-MFM vertically to verify the incident. The M1-Vericication Model consists of eight (8) concepts as shown in the Fig. 2 <<Investigator>>, <<Identification>>, <<Crime>>, <<Mobile Device>>, <<Crime Scene>>, <<Authorization>>, <<Potential Evidence>>, and <<Recording>>. Therefore, the <<Investigator>> requires a <<Authorization>> to achieve the investigation, then, seizes the <<MobileDevice>> which has the <<Crime>> and conducts <<Verification>>. The <<Investigator>> will secure the <<Crime Scene>> and <<Recording>> crime events. The MFM has capabilities to instantiate the M1-Vrerfication model. Thus, concepts in the MFM covered most concepts in the scenario. For example, <<Crime>> concept in the MFM covers <<Inappropriate Messages>> in the scenario, and the <<MobileDevice>> in the MFM covers the <<BlackBerry>> concept in the scenario, and same thing for the <<Recording>> and <<Potential Evidence>>.

Generate M1- Acquisition Model from the MFM: According to the scenario, the investigator must acquire and preserve data from seized blackberry devices and other resources. Thus, the author nominates/selects appropriate concepts from the MFM to derive/instantiate a solution model, which is the M1-Acqussion model, as presented in Fig. 3. The instantiated model consists of ten (10) concepts: <<Investigator>>, <<Forensic Tools>>, <<Extraction>>, <<Acquired Data>>, <<Backup>>, <<MobileDevice>>,<<Imaging>>, <<Potential Evidence>>, <<Volatile Evidence>>, and <<Nonvolatile Evidence>>. The <<Investigator>>

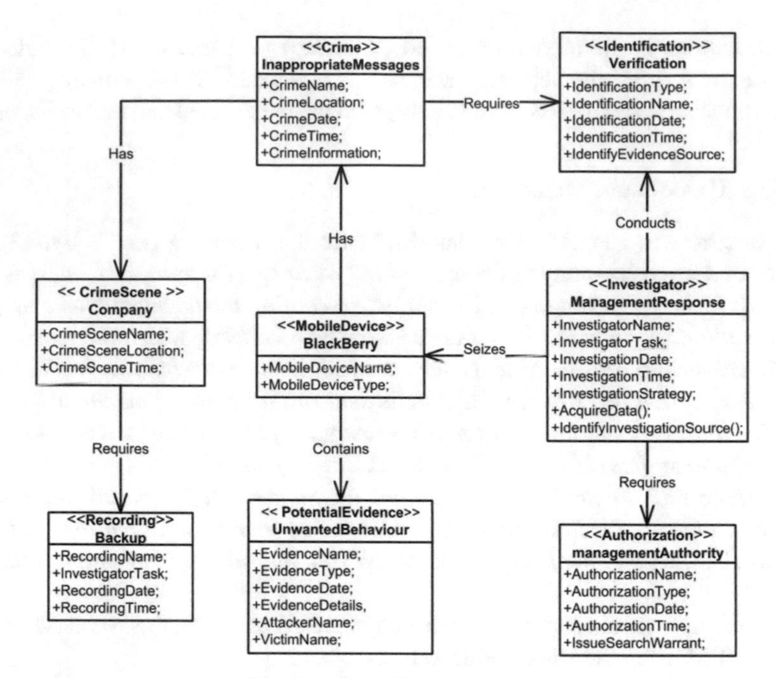

Fig. 2. M1-verification model

identified the <<MobileDevice>> which has the <<Potential Evidence>>, and conduct <<Imaging>> for whole mobile device. The <<Investigator>> will uses a special kind of <<Forensic Tools>> to conduct the <<Extraction>> from the mobile device. The purpose of this phase is to produce the <<Acquired Data>> from the mobile device and preserve it through <<Backup>>. Therefore, the MFM has successfully used to cover whole concepts to instantiate the M1-Acquisition model. The <<Acquired Data>> needs to move to the forensic lab for analysis purposes.

Generate M1-Examination and Analysis Model from the MFM: This model examines and analyzes the acquired data collected in the acquisition stage. To instantiate the M1-Examination and Analysis model from the MFM, the author selected appropriate concepts from the MFM that match/cover scenario concepts. Thus, the instantiated model consists of eight (8) concepts as shown in the Fig. 4: <<Forensic Specialist>>, <<Analysis Data>>, <<Evidence>>, <<Forensic Tools>>, <<Acquired Data>>, <<Examination Data>>, <<Reconstruction Events>>, and <<Examined Data>>. The first stage of this model is to verify the authentication of the acquired data. The investigator will check the integrity of the data via comparing collected data before hashing and after rehashing. Then, if the data is not original and has been tampered with, the investigator needs to go back and take another original copy of the collected data. The second stage is to reconstruct and analyze the acquired data and produces a list of evidence. Therefore, the MFM has been successfully used to instantiate the M1-Examination and Analysis Model. The whole concepts of the derived M1-Examination and Analysis Model match with MFM.

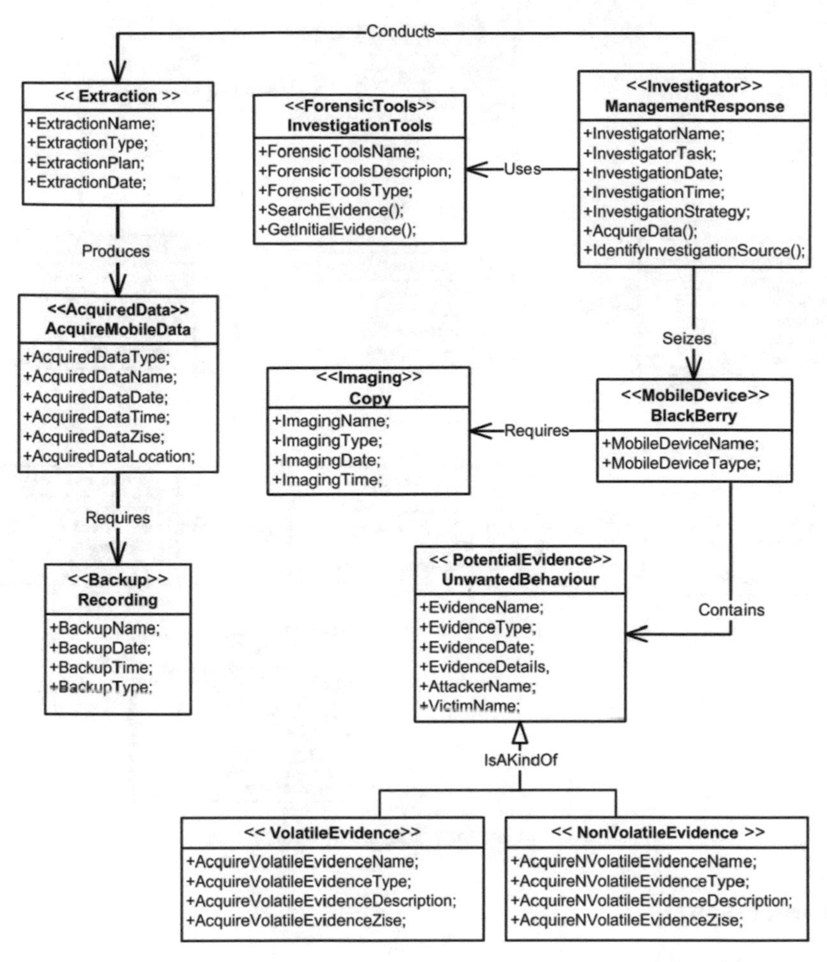

Fig. 3. M1-acquisition model

4 Discussion and Analysis

From the results, the MFM can instantiate different solution models to solve the problems at hand. Three user models (M1-user models) have been instantiated from the MFM to verify, acquire, preserve, examine and analyze mobile crime. Thus, the consistency/conformance between the MFM concepts and the real scenario concepts confirm that the MFM can cover different MF scenarios' concepts. For example, the <<Mobile>> concept in the MFM can instantiate/derive <<Blackberry Device>> in the real scenario, and the <<Potential Evidence>> in the MFM matching with <<UnwantedBehavior>>. Therefore, results in this study showed the MFM could derive different solution models from solving different problems.

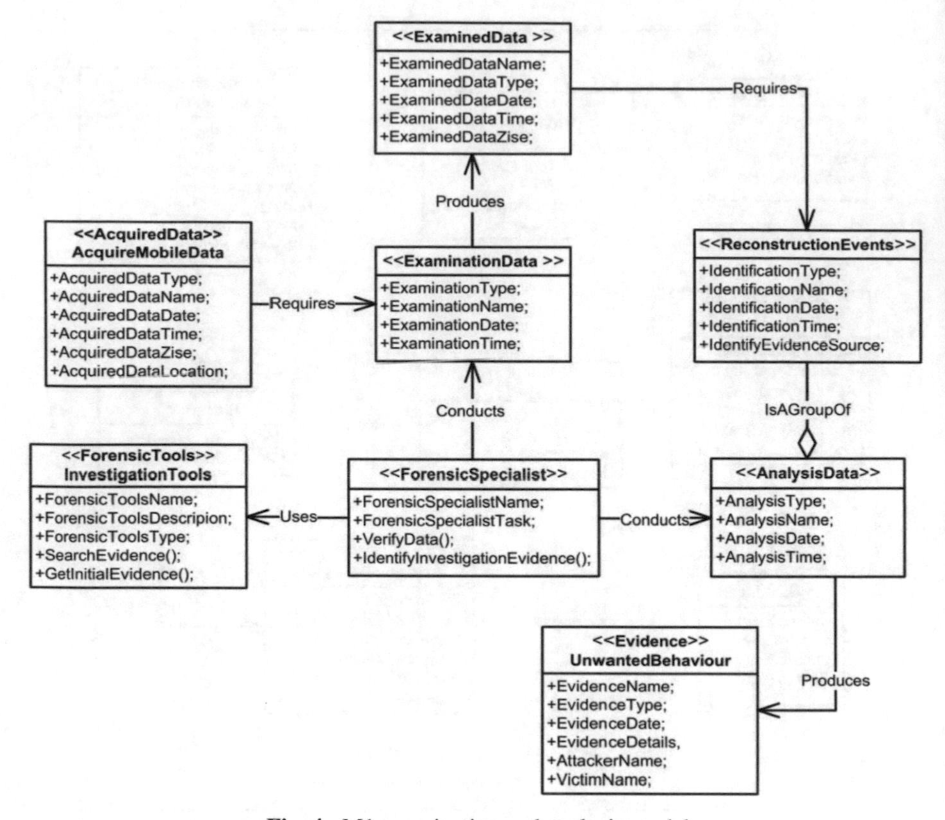

Fig. 4. M1-examination and analysis model

5 Conclusion

MF is a significant domain that is used to identify, acquire, preserve, reconstruct, analyze, and document MF crimes. Several models and frameworks have been proposed in the literature for the MF domain. These models are redundant and specific, which makes the MF domain complex and heterogenous among domain forensic practitioners. The MFM was developed to solve the heterogeneity and ambiguity of the MF domain. Therefore, this paper aimed to validate MFM from the forensic perspective to demonstrate the MFM's effectiveness in instantiating solution models for different specific problems. A scenario was selected for this purpose, and results showed the MFM could instantiate different solution models to solve the problem. The future work will include implementing the MFM in several real scenarios to ensure the applicability of the MFM on real mobile crimes.

References

1. Arts, I., Fischer, A., Duckett, D., van der Wal, R.: Information technology and the optimisation of experience–The role of mobile devices and social media in human-nature interactions. Geoforum **122**, 55–62 (2021)

2. Ali, A., Abd Razak, S., Othman, S.H., Mohammed, A., Saeed, F.: A metamodel for mobile forensics investigation domain. PloS one **12**(4), e0176223 (2017)
3. Al-Dhaqm, A., et al.: Digital forensics subdomains: the state of the art and future directions. IEEE Access **99**, 1 (2021)
4. Turnbull, B., Taylor, R., Blundell, B.: The anatomy of electronic evidence–Quantitative analysis of police e-crime data. In: 2009 International Conference on Availability, Reliability and Security. IEEE (2009)
5. Malware, S.: Security Threat Report 2014
6. Casey, E.: Digital Evidence and Computer Crime: Forensic Science, Computers, and the Internet. Academic press, New York (2011)
7. Al-Dhaqm, A., et al.: Categorization and organization of database forensic investigation processes. IEEE Access **8**, 112846–112858 (2020)
8. Al-Dhaqm, A., Ikuesan, R.A., Kebande, V.R., Razak, S., Ghabban, F.M.: Research challenges and opportunities in drone forensics models. Electronics **10**(13), 1519 (2021)
9. Saleh, M.A., Othman, S.H., Al-Dhaqm, A., Al-Khasawneh, M.A.: Common investigation process model for internet of things forensics. In: 2021 2nd International Conference on Smart Computing and Electronic Enterprise (ICSCEE). IEEE (2021)
10. Casey, E., Bann, M., Doyle, J.: Introduction to Windows Mobile Forensics. Elsevier, New York (2010)
11. Ahmed, R., Dharaskar, R.V.: Mobile forensics: an introduction from Indian law enforcement perspective. In: Prasad, S.K., Routray, S., Khurana, R., Sahni, Sartaj (eds.) ICISTM 2009. CCIS, vol. 31, pp. 173–184. Springer, Heidelberg (2009). https://doi.org/10.1007/978-3-642-00405-6_21
12. Lessard, J., Kessler, G.: Android forensics: simplifying cell phone examinations. Small Scale Digital Device Forensics J. **4**(1), 1 (2010)
13. Jansen, W., Ayers, R.: Guidelines on cell phone forensics. NIST Special Publication, pp. 800-101 (2007)
14. Al-Dhaqm, A., Razak, S., Othman, S.H., Ngadi, A., Ahmed, M.N., Ali Mohammed, A.: Development and validation of a Database Forensic Metamodel (DBFM). PloS one **12**(2), e0170793 (2017)
15. Ali, A., Razak, S.A., Othman, S.H., Mohammed, A.: Extraction of common concepts for the mobile forensics domain. In: Saeed, F., Gazem, N., Patnaik, S., Balaid, A.S.S., Mohammed, F. (eds.) Recent Trends in Information and Communication Technology, pp. 141–154. Springer International Publishing, Cham (2017). https://doi.org/10.1007/978-3-319-59427-9_16
16. Ali, A., Razak, S., Othman, S.H., Mohammed, A.: Towards adapting metamodeling approach for the mobile forensics investigation domain. In: International Conference on Innovation in Science and Technology (IICIST) (2015)
17. Al-Dhaqm, A., Razak, S., Othman, S.H.: Model derivation system to manage database forensic investigation domain knowledge. In: 2018 IEEE Conference on Application, Information and Network Security (AINS). IEEE (2018)
18. Khelalfa, H.M.: Forensics challenges for mobile phone security. In: Information Assurance and Security Technologies for Risk Assessment and Threat Management: Advances, pp. 72–133. IGI Global (2012)
19. Chang, W., Chung, P.: Knowledge management in cybercrime investigation – a case study of identifying cybercrime investigation knowledge in Taiwan. In: Chau, M., Hsinchun Chen, G., Wang, A., Wang, J.-H. (eds.) Intelligence and Security Informatics, pp. 8–17. Springer International Publishing, Cham (2014). https://doi.org/10.1007/978-3-319-06677-6_2
20. Ghabban, F.M., Alfadli, I.M., Ameerbakhsh, O., AbuAli, A.N., Al-Dhaqm, A., Al-Khasawneh, M.A.: Comparative analysis of network forensic tools and network forensics processes. In: 2021 2nd International Conference on Smart Computing and Electronic Enterprise (ICSCEE). IEEE (2021)

21. Al-Dhaqm, A., Razak, S., Ikuesan, R.A., Kebande, V.R., Hajar Othman, S.: Face validation of database forensic investigation metamodel. Infrastructures **6**(2), 13 (2021)
22. Ameerbakhsh, O., Ghabban, F.M., Alfadli, I.M., AbuAli, A.N., Al-Dhaqm, A., Al-Khasawneh, M.A.: Digital forensics domain and metamodeling development approaches. In: 2021 2nd International Conference on Smart Computing and Electronic Enterprise (ICSCEE). IEEE (2021)
23. Sargent, R.G.: Verification and validation of simulation models. J. Simul. **7**(1), 12–24 (2013)
24. Kleijnen, J.P., Deflandre, D.: Validation of regression metamodels in simulation: bootstrap approach. Eur. J. Oper. Res. **170**(1), 120–131 (2006)
25. Biles, W.E., Kleijnen, J.P., Van Beers, W.C., Van Nieuwenhuyse, I.: Kriging metamodeling in constrained simulation optimization: an explorative study. In: 2007 Winter Simulation Conference. IEEE (2007)
26. Sargent, R.G.: Verification and validation of simulation models. In: Proceedings of the 2010 winter simulation conference. IEEE (2010)
27. Kassab, M., Ormandjieva, O., Daneva, M.: A metamodel for tracing non-functional requirements. In: 2009 WRI World Congress on Computer Science and Information Engineering. IEEE (2009)
28. Do, Q., Martini, B., Choo, K.-K.R.: A forensically sound adversary model for mobile devices. PloS one **10**(9), e0138449 (2015)
29. Kuzniarz, L., Staron, M., Wohlin, C.: An empirical study on using stereotypes to improve understanding of UML models. In: Proceedings of 12th IEEE International Workshop on Program Comprehension, 2004. IEEE (2004)

Catching a Phish: Frontiers of Deep Learning-Based Anticipating Detection Engines

Hamzah Salah[1] and Hiba Zuhair[2](✉)

[1] Department of Networks Engineering, College of Information Engineering, Al-Nahrain University, Baghdad, Iraq
ha.salim94@gmail.com

[2] Department of Systems Engineering, College of Information Engineering, Al-Nahrain University, Baghdad, Iraq
hiba.zuhair.pcs2013@nahrainuniv.edu.iq

Abstract. In recent years, cyber-security gains high attention in the light of ethical hacking and social engineering attacks like phishing that riskily overshadow the development of social networking, e commerce, and information technology. Thus, mitigation of such risks via AI techniques represents the prime research direction in academia and industry. Amongst, are the detection engines integrating diverse deep learning algorithms to anticipate changeable phishing features over time into the classification models. However, extracting the mutual features and predicting the future changes in phishing attacks still need more concrete characterization and accurate classification with fewer faults in the online engine. Upon these needs, this paper aims to present future-oriented standpoints for long-term, hybrid, cognitive, and effective phishing detection about the existing deep learning-based classification models by appraising the prior research and compiling their outstanding problems. This aim is achieved through a comparative and critical review of the prior research and then discuss the possible solutions for future phishing detection approaches.

Keywords: Social engineering · Phishing attacks · Phishing detection · Deep learning-based models

1 Introduction

Recently and particularly in the COVID-19 pandemic, people's lives have become more reliant on cyberspace and web apps. By Global Digital Population Report, active web users have reached 4.66 billion (which accounts for 59.5% of the global population) via learning and education, healthcare, work meeting, business and social communicating that have switched from offline to online mode during the COVID-19 pandemic [1]. As such, lots of sensitive data have been exchanged and stored via cloud computing that has provided good chances to hackers for illegal impersonating and intruding on users' information systems by utilizing social engineering deceptions [1]. For more gains, hackers have never ended up bypassing the artificial intelligence secure mechanisms of the communicated information systems among organizations. Phishing has

F. Saeed et al. (Eds.): IRICT 2021, LNDECT 127, pp. 483–497, 2022.
https://doi.org/10.1007/978-3-030-98741-1_40

been utilized as the most perspective social engineering deception to closely resemble an organization's legitimate website, send mass notifications to users, redirect victimized users to a fake website, steal users' profiles, hack their exchanged data online, and intrude on the communicated information systems [1]. Furthermore, phishing attacks have evolved to successfully espionage many e-governments and e-commerce services for illegal monetary gains [2, 3].

To tackle these challenges, phishing detection has been acknowledged at a high level across diverse techniques such as list-based, heuristic-based, and visual similarity-based [2, 3]. However, the list-based detection techniques have needed updates regularly, the heuristic-based techniques have lacked the characterization of mutually relevant phishing features, and the visual similarity-based techniques have falsely resembled animated components and embedded objects in a phishing website [2, 3]. That, in turn, has fallen short at mitigating the dramatic evolution of phishing patterns and their over-time changeable features [2, 3]. Lately, AI has spotted the light to elaborate more effective techniques using machine and deep learning algorithms that are specially designed for phishing detection where the accuracy is extremely important [2, 3].

Machine learning-based detection, in their single and/or ensemble framework; has been constructed as features-based classifiers to identify phishing patterns from a batch of phishing and legitimate patterns [2, 3]. Yet, they have diverged in their classification accuracy on an escalating web stream (i.e. flow of phish/suspicious/legitimate website patterns) due to their diverse specifics, decision boundaries, and the set of features that they have deployed [2, 3]. Also, hackers have used to evolve zero-hour and different patterns carrying out phishing in advanced ways which have implied out-of-time and overlooked classification by the machine learning-based detection engines [2, 3].

As time progresses, evolved phishing patterns become an emerging problem that threatens information systems on mobiles and IoT domains by exploiting technical vulnerabilities and users' unawareness [2, 3]. That poses real growing threats not only to cyber-security but also to the global IT industries [2, 3]. Thus, researchers in academia and industry motive to develop pro-active phishing detection engines by leveraging deep learning algorithms [2, 3]. Unlike former detection engines, deep learning-based detection engines characterize mutually relevant features of phishing patterns without human tuning by self-learning and multi-classifying the unlabeled web stream in unsupervised, supervised, and hybrid models [2, 3]. However, some difficulties are encountered in applying deep learning due to phishing unpredictable activities over seconds not only hours which requires finding the line-level annotations of insider phishing activities and a stable model of truly legitimate patterns by training web stream continuously in an online fashion.

In this light, this paper addresses three main tracks: revisiting the existing deep learning-based phishing detection engines with the detail of their various phishing datasets for a better understanding of their frontiers and looking out the evolutionary solution scope for future phishing detection. To do so, the rest of this paper is organized into five sections as follows: zero-hour phishing detection; conceptual background of deep learning; phishing detection and the related works; critical issues and future solutions; then drawing our conclusions.

2 Zero-Hour Phishing Detection

Hackers have insisted on unlawfully accessing data and system files and then stealing the users' profiles for illegal monetary gains. Hence, they have targeted financial organizations, e-government services, IT industries, critical infrastructures, small-scale and large-scale enterprises. To do so, they have used sophisticatedly skilled and well-determined mechanisms to evolve their variable phishing patterns every hour (i.e., zero-hour patterns) and deliver them to the connected information systems via technical vulnerabilities in software or hardware of mobile and IoT devices. Also, they have leveraged various features to make their zero-hour phishing patterns persistent and to evade the existing detection engines for months and even years. Most features of zero-hour phishing patterns comprise misleading links, spoofed contents, and socially engineering deceptions that mimic victims to catch the bait and submit their confidential data via

Table 1. Evolutionary phishing detection engines [1, 4–6].

Detection engine	Mechanism
White and/or Black List	Whitelists sort a collection of authorized URLs that browsers can visit, and blacklists include phishing URLs to prevent browsers from downloading their web pages. When the browser downloads the related websites that are and/or are not banned, a significant number of true positives resulted. Otherwise, High false outputs resulted if the regular basis of these lists is not updated
Heuristics	Extract phishing common features (static traits) from sample phishing webpages and use them to qualify each visited webpage to detect any phishing activity. However, they produce a lower detection rate and false positives if they are not assisted by black or whitelist
Visual layout similarity	Usually, phishing patterns seem to look like legitimate websites for users' suspecting. Thus, successful detection can be achieved by comparing layouts of phishing replicas to legitimate websites and calculating the ratio of similarity. However, this requires a long execution time to process images, texts, and other visual contents. Dynamic contents like animations might be overlooked due to minimal resembling and then resulting in high false-negative rates
Machine learning	Machine learning classifiers are feature-based classifiers that predict the status of a visiting website (phishing or legitimate) by learning a set of extracted features on training and testing a set of samples. However, classifying new patterns of phishing websites might produce divergent accuracies due to the needs of actively learning of the features-based classifier on new samples
Deep learning	Beyond machine learning classifiers, the deep learning classifiers identify new phishing patterns proactively by automated extraction and analysis of unknown and relevant features and learning them actively

online transactions and web browsing. For that reason, most phishing detection engines strategies have developed features-based classification mechanisms. Such mechanisms are dependent on either checking up block lists of phishing URLs features, or phishing intrusion footprints (i.e., heuristics), or phishing replicas of the truly visual layouts of legitimate websites or characterizing phishing patterns actively and proactively throughout a trained set of features and machine learning deep learning classifiers, as presented in Table 1.

3 Conceptual Background of Deep Learning

As presented in Table 2 and shown in Fig. 1, deep learning is a machine learning approach that uses numerous layers of neural networks to show complicated ideas and relationships [7]. Deep learning is a branch of machine learning that uses artificial neural networks (ANN) to obtain results. A deep neural network is built up of layers that make up deep learning (DNN). Image classification, text mining, video recommendation, spam detection, and multimedia idea retrieval are just a few of the applications that use it. Deep learning approaches that have been recently created have demonstrated exceptional performance in a variety of applications, including natural language processing (NLP),

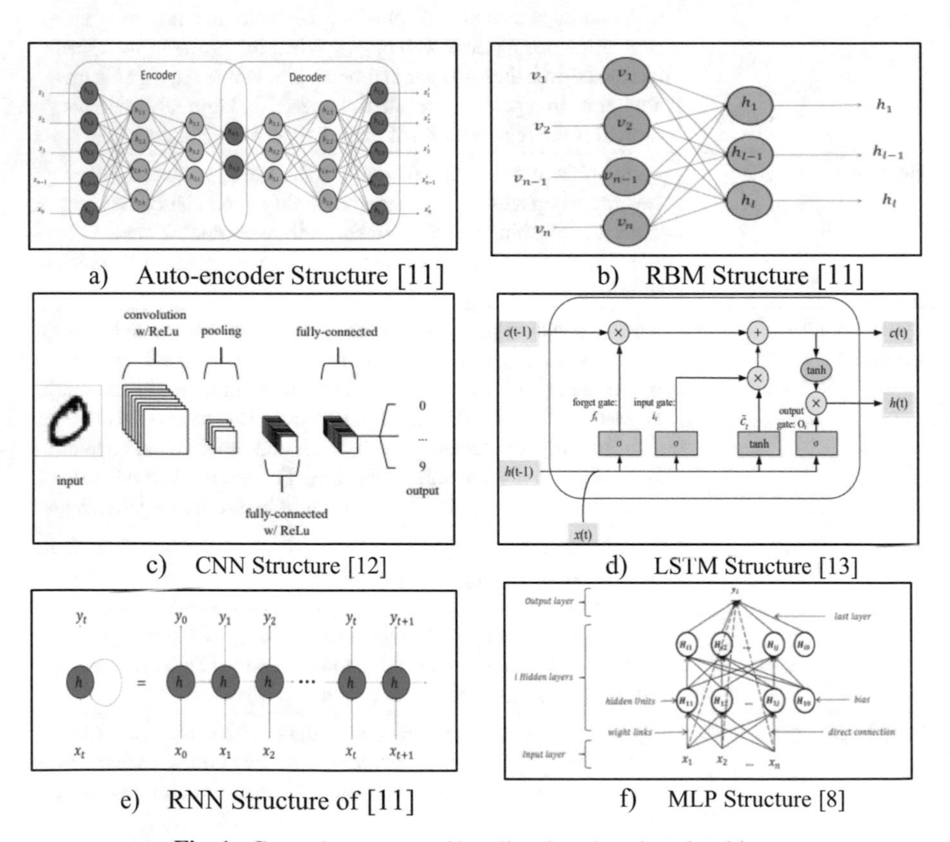

a) Auto-encoder Structure [11]
b) RBM Structure [11]
c) CNN Structure [12]
d) LSTM Structure [13]
e) RNN Structure of [11]
f) MLP Structure [8]

Fig. 1. General structures of baseline deep learning algorithms

Table 2. Baseline deep learning algorithms [8]

Method	Input data	Learning type	Characteristics
Deep Auto-encoders (AE)	Various	Unsupervised (generative)	• AE can operate with data instances that are unlabeled • The Output is a reconstructed version of the input data, and it is helpful for extracting features and reducing dimensionality
Convolutional Neural Network (CNN)	2-D (video, image, etc.)	Supervised (discriminative)	• Internal memory is used to process sequential data • Visual tasks need a large amount of training data (images and videos)
Multi-Layer Perceptron Neural Network (MLP)	Various	Supervised (discriminative)	• Learning that is adaptable, Non-linearity and MLP has a high fault tolerance
Recurrent Neural Network (RNN)	Sequence data, time-series	Supervised (discriminative)	• NTMA (Network Traffic Monitoring and Analysis) application scenarios with time-sensitive data are suitable • Use internal memory for processing sequential data
Restricted Boltzmann Machines (RBM)	Feature vectors	Unsupervised (generative)	• RBM can be trained single layer at a time • RBM does not have an intra-layer
Long Short-Term Memory (LSTM)	Sequence data, long time dependent data, time-series	Supervised (discriminative)	• Better performance than its predecessors in applications with lengthy time lag input data. And it can operate with labeled and unlabeled datasets

visual data analysis, and machine learning. DL is a subfield of machine learning in which Deep Neural Networks (DNN) used to identify data representation at each layer [8].

The term "deep" in the definition of "DL" relates to the concept of consecutive layers of representations. Furthermore, the depth of the model refers to the number of layers used to model the data [8]. There are three types of deep learning architectures: generative (unsupervised), discriminative (supervised), and hybrid architectures [9]:

- Generative Architecture (Unsupervised): It can learn from unlabeled raw data to achieve its goals. For data that does not provide the expected result, we might use the term "unsupervised."
- Discriminative Architectures (supervised): Typically used to find patterns in labeled data for prediction jobs [10]. In this learning type, a subset of training datasets is required, which includes both the input and intended outcomes. The training set has an impact on the classification of new data.
- Hybrid Architectures: This architecture combines both supervised and unsupervised models. This employs generative features at first and discriminative features later to recognize data.

Most deep learning-based detection engines have used different collections of data pieces that the computer may consider as a single entity for phishing prediction, but the acquired data must be understood and dealt with by the machines. Table 3 describes the utilized datasets along with their data sources and size. To testify and qualify the deep learning-based detection engines against zero-hour phishing patterns on scalable datasets, various evaluation criteria are used, and they are characterized as presented in Table 4.

Table 3. Summary of the utilized datasets in phishing detection

Dataset name	Size of dataset	Merits
Alexa database[14]	1M URLs	Top 1M site, Legitimate URLs
Common-Crawl [15]	940M URLs	2800M phishing URLs, Legitimate URLs
Mendeley [16]	88,647 instances, 111 features for full variant	Frequently published dataset
Phish-Tank [17]	6.8M URL's	Daily updated, Phishing URLs
Open-Fish [18]	4,253 URLs	Daily updated, Phishing URLs
UCI Machine learning repository [19]	11,055 URLs 30 features	Gathered from 2456 unique websites
Ebbu2017 [20]	73,575 URLs	Both phishing and legitimate URLs
Kaggle [21]	11,000 URL'S	Consists of many datasets
Best Websites [22]	5000 URLs	There is information about the website available

Table 4. Summary of evaluation criteria

Criterion	Description	Formula
Accuracy	It is the proportion of correctly identified samples to the total number of samples is that known as the right classification rate. When the dataset is well-balanced, it is a good metric	$Accuracy = (TP + TN)/(TP + TN + FN + FP)$
Precision	It defined as the percentage of legitimately positive samples to the anticipated legitimately positive samples	$P = TP/(TP + FP)$
Recall	It defined as the percentage of genuine positive samples among all positive samples	$R = TP/(TP + FN)$
F-measure	It is the harmonic average of accuracy and recall	$F = (2 * P * R)/(P + R)$

4 Frontiers of Deep Learning-Based Phishing Detection

Upon the revision of related works in phishing detection, this section demonstrates the main contribution of this paper by highlighting the frontiers of various deep learning-based phishing detection engines in terms of datasets sources, datasets size, extracted features, specifications, and their performance outcomes, as presented in Appendix Table A1. Then, justifying "why the revisited deep learning-based detection engines are still sub-optimum to classify zero-hour phishing patterns?".

To compile this questionable issue, their lacks and performance outcomes were synthesized and categorized as follows:

- Features. Each baseline deep learning algorithm emulated a feature-based classifier that projected the extracted features onto feature vectors. Then, it mapped these vectors back into the original extracted feature space to compare them versus the unexpected patterns. Unexpected patterns might be valid legitimate websites, valid phishing websites, and suspicious websites (neither phishing nor legitimate). Hence, not all features (as their types and their values) were part of classification boundaries and they were outliers in their mutual information, relevance, and redundancy across the feature space. That yielded a proportional feature-based classifier to the error of its reconstruction.
- Dataset. The web stream (collection of phishing and/or legitimate samples) might be anonymized eventually before being publicly simulated in the data repositories. Such anonymization obscured the potentially relevant features in these samples. Precisely, either the categorical features were absent in the open release datasets, or their values were missing.
- Tuning parameters. Developing and hybridizing multiple baselines deep learning algorithms in the detection engine needed to tune their functions/layers/layer dimension

on the same batch of data and batch size throughout a hyper-parameter search. Otherwise, the cost of missed detections would be substantially larger than the cost of mistaken detections.

To produce a superior performance on a vast web stream involving more sophisticated patterns and overtime changeable patterns of phishing, the aforementioned issues can be leveraged to improve deep learning in the phishing detection domain by the following disregarded facets:

- Eliminating the feature engineering mechanism that extracts a space of static phishing features by dramatically narrowing it into a vector of dynamic features which constitutes the insider activity of phishing patterns.
- Qualifying the best and richest cluster of phishing anticipating features amongst the literarily adopted deep learning algorithms for addressing their all-inclusive characterization and efficacious classification of zero-hour phishing patterns. That, in turn, could provide progressive configuration to deep learning algorithms and then would boost up the performance of detection engines towards maximal phishing detection rates in the near future as well as minimal processing and storage footprints on online mode.
- Applying deep learning-based detection engines on bigger web streams which may include more static and dynamic anomalies of phishing. Chronological aggregation of web streams will reveal less biased learning and the detection will be cost-sensitive against implicit and explicit class balance problems.
- Dual categorization of phishing patterns onto their granularities as well as their release time. Time of evolution will be a potential feature to characterize phishing patterns besides the prior examined features for minimal missing detections of different phishing patterns might be launch within a single hour.

5 Conclusions

The revision of existing deep learning-based phishing detection engines in this paper affirmed that they were computationally efficient but partially effective against zero-hour phishing patterns. This was due to their limitations in leveraging feature engineer-ing, dynamic features, big web stream, and functional parameters tuning. As stated in this paper, building proactive deep learning-based detection depends on dynamic fea-tures, datasets, and tuning parameters. Therefore, the paper restated the causality be-tween the observed limitations and the boost-up outlooks in phishing detection to pro-mote the detection of zero-hour phishing patterns on the evolving web stream. Such enhancement would maximize the detection accuracy and minimize the missing detections as well as reduce the computational cost. Overall, comparative, and critical review along with the underlined perspectives will serve as a navigating taxonomy to the re-searchers for their future work and extend the research facets.

Appendix

Table A1. Comparative performance outcomes of the revisited related works

<table>
<tr><th>Related Work</th><th>Deep Learning Algorithm</th><th>Description</th><th>Dataset (s)</th><th colspan="3">Performance Outcomes</th></tr>
<tr><td>Pavan Kumar et al. [23]</td><td>CNN</td><td>It is improved with Swarm Intelligence Binary Bat Algorithm to learn URL features</td><td>KAGGLE</td><td colspan="3">Accuracy: 94.8%
0.2% False detections</td></tr>
<tr><td>Xiao et al. [27, 28]</td><td>CNN</td><td>It is a multi-headed and self-attentional algorithm assisted by the Generative Adversarial Network (GAN) and URL features</td><td>Five thousand legitimate Websites, Phish Tank</td><td colspan="3">Accuracy: 97.20%
Detection Time: 174 as
Recall = 95.60%
Precision = 98.76%
F1 = 97.15%</td></tr>
<tr><td>Jiang et al. [25]</td><td>CNN</td><td>Classifies URL at character-level by the features of URL length, URL separators, number of dots, and other categorical and lexical features</td><td>Google, DMOZ Phish Tank, Virus Total</td><td colspan="3">Miss Rates: 4/1000 URLs</td></tr>
<tr><td rowspan="5">Ozcan et al. [26]</td><td rowspan="5">DNN + LSTM, DNN + Bi-LSTM</td><td rowspan="5">It is important for NLP features and character embedding features classification</td><td rowspan="3">Ebbu2017</td><td></td><td>Accuracy</td><td>F1</td></tr>
<tr><td>DNN + LSTM</td><td>98.62%</td><td>98.64%</td></tr>
<tr><td>DNN + BILSTM</td><td>98.79%</td><td>98.8%</td></tr>
<tr><td rowspan="2">Phish Tank</td><td>DNN + LSTM</td><td>98.98%</td><td>99.1%</td></tr>
<tr><td>DNN + BILSTM</td><td>99.21%</td><td>99.41%</td></tr>
</table>

(continued)

Table A1. (*continued*)

Related Work	Deep Learning Algorithm	Description	Dataset (s)	Performance Outcomes
Somesha et al. [1]	DNN + CNN + LSTM	It uses information gain (IG) for features ranking and optimizing a set of URL obfuscation features, hyperlink-based features, and third party-based features	Phish Tank, Alexa	Accuracy varied from: 99.57%, to 99.43%
Liang et al. [27]	DBN	Borderline Smote-based classification across a set of URL features, Page contents, and Images	Phish Tank	Recall: 90.7% Precision: 96.5%
Huang et al. [28]	CNN + RNN	It segments specific Viterbi and URL features for phishing classification	Phish Tank, Alexa, Open-Fish	Accuracy: 97.905% FPR = 0.020% Precision: 98.958%
Yang et al. [29]	CNN + LSTM	Integrating soft-max and dropout mechanisms for overfitting solution with Logistic Regression and XGBoost to classify URL features, and static contents of webpage code	Phish Tank, Dmoz	Recall = 98.57% Precision = 99.41% F1 = 99.9%
Yerima and Alzaylaee [30]	CNN 1D	Classifying URL features syntax	UCI Machine learning repository	Accuracy = 97.3% Recall = 98.2% Precision = 97% F1 = 97.6%
Su [31]	LSTM	Classifying URL features syntax	Phish Tank	Accuracy: 99.14% Recall: 98.91% Precision: 98.74% FNR: 02.12%
Yazhmozhi et al. [32]	LSTM + CNN	Classifying URL features syntax	Phish Tank	Precision: 97% Accuracy: 96%

(*continued*)

Table A1. (*continued*)

Related Work	Deep Learning Algorithm	Description	Dataset (s)	Performance Outcomes
Singh et al. [33]	CNN	Classifies embedding objects and URL features throughout two layers	https://github.com/ebbubekirbbr/pdd/tree/master/input	Accuracy: 98.0%
Rasymas and Dovydaitis [34]	CNN	Classifies URL features at multiple layers	Phish Tank	Accuracy: 94.4%
Wei et al., [35]	CNN	Classifies URL features at multiple layers	Phish Tank, Alexa, Common-Crawl	Accuracy: 99.98%
Zhang et al. [36]	AE and CNN	Classifies 30 features of URLs, webpage source code in a multi-modal classification	Phish Tank, UCI Machine learning repository	Accuracy: 97.68%
Lakshmi et al. [37]	DNN	Uses batch normalization of 30 hyperlinking features of phishing websites	UCI Machine learning repository	Not presented
Al-Ahmadi & Alharbi [38]	CNN	Recognizes URL and visual content as screenshots in a two-layered classification model	2000 webpage screenshots and URLs	Accuracy: 99.67% Precision: 99.43% F1 score: 99.28% Recall: 99.47%
Ali & Ahmed [39]	DNN	Utilizes a graphical feature and features ranking mechanisms to classify long URL, Server Form Handler (SFH), Having the IP Address, Request URL, URL of Anchor, Age of Domain, Website Traffic, Pop-Up window, HTTPS, and SSL,	UCI Machine learning repository	Not presented

(*continued*)

Table A1. (*continued*)

Related Work	Deep Learning Algorithm	Description	Dataset (s)	Performance Outcomes
Yao et al. [40]	R-CNN	It improved for Feature Pyramid Network (FPN) and Logo Recognition	FlickrLogos-32	Precision: 98.9% F1 score: 94.6% Recall: 90.6%
			FlickrLogos-32plus	Precision: 98.6% F1 score: 94.2% Recall: 90.1%
Xiao et al. [24]	CNN + LSTM	It classifies URL and website content features like images and frame elements	Common-Crawl, Phish Tank, 10,000 webpage screenshots	Precision: 93.3% F-measure: 94.2% Recall: 93.27% Accuracy: 93.28%
Chen et al. [41]	LSTM	It classifies features of domain names, subdomain length, URL length, prefixes and suffixes Length ratio, punctuation counts, TLDs, IP address, Port Number, and URL Entropy	Yahoo Directory, Phish Tank	Precision: 98.74% Recall: 98.91% Accuracy: 93.28%
Opara et al. [42]	CNN	It characterizes syntax and word embedding content of HTML code including tables, text, images, hyperlinks, and lists	Common-Crawl, Phish Tank, Alexa	Accuracy: 93%
Hema et al. [42]	DNN	DNN classifies 30 URL features	UCI Machine learning repository	Accuracy: 94.3%
Feng et al. [43]	Stacked Auto-encoder (SAE)	Soft-maxing source codes of HTML, URL, and the third-party services	Phish Tank, Alexa	Not clearly presented

References

1. Somesha, M., Pais, A.R., Rao, R.S., Rathour, V.S.: Efficient deep learning techniques for the detection of phishing websites. Sādhanā **45**(1), 1–18 (2020). https://doi.org/10.1007/s12046-020-01392-4
2. Zuhair, H., Selamat, A.: Phish webpage classification using hybrid algorithm of machine learning and statistical induction ratios. Int. J. Data Min. Model. Manag. **12**(3), 255–276 (2020)
3. Zuhair, H., Selamat, A.: Phishing classification models: issues and perspectives. Int. J. Digit. Enterpr. Technol. **1**(3), 219–240 (2019). https://doi.org/10.1504/ijdet.2019.10019065
4. Tang, L., Mahmoud, Q.H.: A Survey of machine learning-based solutions for phishing website detection. Mach. Learn. Knowl. Extr. **3**, 672–694 (2021). https://doi.org/10.3390/make30 30034
5. Routhu Srinivasa Rao, A.R.P.: Detection of phishing websites using an efficient feature-based machine learning framework. Neural Comput. Appl. **31**(8), 3851–3873 (2018)
6. Bai, W.: Phishing website detection based on machine learning algorithm. In: Proceedings - 2020 International Conference Computing Data Science CDS 2020, pp. 293–298 (2020). https://doi.org/10.1109/CDS49703.2020.00064
7. Josh Patterson, A.G.: Deep Learning. O'Reilly Media, Inc. (2017)
8. Abbasi, M., Shahraki, A., Taherkordi, A.: Deep learning for network traffic monitoring and analysis (NTMA): a survey. Comput. Commun. **170**, 19–41 (2021). https://doi.org/10.1016/j.comcom.2021.01.021
9. Mosca, P., Zhang, Y., Xiao, Z., Y.W.: Cloud security: services, risks, and a case study on amazon cloud services. Int'l J. Commun. Netw. Syst. Sci. **7**(12), 529 (2014)
10. Aldweesh, A., Derhab, A., Emam, A.Z.: Deep learning approaches for anomaly-based intrusion detection systems: a survey, taxonomy, and open issues. Knowledge-Based Syst. **189**, 105124 (2020). https://doi.org/10.1016/j.knosys.2019.105124.
11. Berman, D.S., Buczak, A.L., Chavis, J.S., Corbett, C.L.: A survey of deep learning methods for cyber security. Inf. **10**(4), 122 (2019). https://doi.org/10.3390/info10040122
12. O'Shea, K., Nash, R.: An Introduction to Convolutional Neural Networks. (2015)
13. Yuan, X., Li, L., Wang, Y.: Nonlinear dynamic soft sensor modeling with supervised long short-term memory network. IEEE Trans. Ind. Inform. **16**, 3168–3176 (2020). https://doi.org/10.1109/TII.2019.2902129
14. ALEXA Homepage. https://www.alexa.com/topsites. Accessed 21 Oct 2021
15. Commoncrawl Homepage. http://index.commoncrawl.org/. Accessed 21 Oct 2021
16. Vrbančič, G.: Phishing Websites Dataset. https://doi.org/10.17632/72ptz43s9v.1. Accessed 13 Nov 2021
17. Phish Tank Homepage. https://www.phishtank.com/. Accessed 21 Oct 2021
18. Openphish Homepage. https://openphish.com/. Accessed 21 Oct 2021
19. UCI Machine learning repository. https://archive.ics.uci.edu/ml/datasets/phishing+websites. Accessed 21 Oct 2021
20. Github Homepage. https://github.com/ebubekirbbr/pdd/tree/master/input. Accessed 21 Oct 2021
21. Kaggle Homepage. https://www.kaggle.com/datasets. Accessed 21 Oct 2021
22. 5000best Homepage. http://5000best.com/websites/. Accessed 21 Oct 2021
23. Pavan Kumar, P., Jaya, T., Rajendran, V.: SI-BBA – a novel phishing website detection based on Swarm intelligence with deep learning. Mater. Today Proc. (2021). https://doi.org/10.1016/j.matpr.2021.07.178
24. Xiao, X., et al.: Phishing websites detection via CNN and multi-head self-attention on imbalanced datasets. Comput. Secur. **108**, 102372 (2021). https://doi.org/10.1016/j.cose.2021.102372.

25. Jiang, J., et al.: A deep learning based online malicious URL and DNS detection scheme. In: Lin, X., Ghorbani, A., Ren, K., Zhu, S., Zhang, A. (eds.) SecureComm 2017. LNICSSITE, vol. 238, pp. 438–448. Springer, Cham (2018). https://doi.org/10.1007/978-3-319-78813-5_22
26. Ozcan, A., Catal, C., Donmez, E., Senturk, B.: A hybrid DNN–LSTM model for detecting phishing URLs. Neural Comput. Appl. 0123456789 (2021). https://doi.org/10.1007/s00521-021-06401-z.
27. Wang, G., Atiquzzaman, M., Yan, Z., Choo, K.-K. (eds.): SpaCCS 2017. LNCS, vol. 10658. Springer, Cham (2017). https://doi.org/10.1007/978-3-319-72395-2
28. Huang, Y., Yang, Q., Qin, J., Wen, W.: Phishing URL detection via CNN and attention-based hierarchical RNN. In: Proceedings - 2019 18th IEEE International Conference Trust Security Private Computing Communication IEEE International Confrence Big Data Science Engineering Trust 2019. 112–119 (2019). https://doi.org/10.1109/TrustCom/BigDataSE.2019.00024
29. Yang, P., Zhao, G., Zeng, P.: Phishing website detection based on multidimensional features driven by deep learning. IEEE Access. **7**, 15196–15209 (2019). https://doi.org/10.1109/ACCESS.2019.2892066
30. Yerima, S.Y., Alzaylaee, M.K.: High accuracy phishing detection based on convolutional neural networks. In: ICCAIS 2020 - 3rd International Conference Computing Application Information Security, pp. 19–21 (2020). https://doi.org/10.1109/ICCAIS48893.2020.9096869
31. Su, Y.: Research on website phishing detection based on LSTM RNN. In: Proceedings 2020 IEEE 4th Information Technology Networking, Electronic Automation Control Conference ITNEC 2020, pp. 284–288 (2020). https://doi.org/10.1109/ITNEC48623.2020.9084799
32. Yazhmozhi, V.M., Janet, B., Reddy, S.: Anti-phishing system using LSTM and CNN. In: 2020 IEEE International Conference for Innovation in Technology INOCON 2020, pp. 1–5 (2020). https://doi.org/10.1109/INOCON50539.2020.9298298
33. Singh, S., Singh, M.P., Pandey, R.: Phishing detection from URLs using deep learning approach. In: Proceedings of 2020 International Conference on Computing, Communication and Security ICCCS 2020, pp. 16–19 (2020). https://doi.org/10.1109/ICCCS49678.2020.9277459
34. Rasymas, T., Dovydaitis, L.: Detection of phishing URLs by using deep learning approach and multiple features combinations. Balt. J. Mod. Comput. **8**, 471–483 (2020). https://doi.org/10.22364/BJMC.2020.8.3.06
35. Wei, W., Ke, Q., Nowak, J., Korytkowski, M., Scherer, R., Woźniak, M.: Accurate and fast URL phishing detector: a convolutional neural network approach. Comput. Netw. **178** (2020). https://doi.org/10.1016/j.comnet.2020.107275
36. Zhang, X., Shi, D., Zhang, H., Liu, W., Li, R.: Efficient detection of phishing attacks with hybrid neural networks. In: International Conference on Communication Technology Proceedings, ICCT. 2019-October, pp. 844–848 (2019). https://doi.org/10.1109/ICCT.2018.8600018
37. Lakshmi, L., Reddy, M.P., Santhaiah, C., Reddy, U.J.: Smart phishing detection in web pages using supervised deep learning classification and optimization technique ADAM. Wirel. Pers. Commun. **118**(4), 3549–3564 (2021). https://doi.org/10.1007/s11277-021-08196-7
38. Al-Ahmadi, S., Alharbi, Y.: A deep learning technique for web phishing detection combined Url features and visual similarity. Int. J. Comput. Networks Commun. **12**, 41–54 (2020). https://doi.org/10.5121/ijcnc.2020.12503
39. Ali, W., Ahmed, A.A.: Hybrid intelligent phishing website prediction using deep neural networks with genetic algorithm-based feature selection and weighting. IET Inf. Secur. **13**, 659–669 (2019). https://doi.org/10.1049/iet-ifs.2019.0006

40. Yao, W., Ding, Y., Li, X.: Deep learning for phishing detection. In: Proceedings - 16th IEEE International Symposium Parallel Distribution Processing with Application 17th IEEE International Conference Ubiquitous Computing Communication 8th IEEE International Conference Big Data Cloud Computing, vol. 11t, pp. 645–650 (2019). https://doi.org/10.1109/BDCloud.2018.00099
41. Chen, W., Zhang, W., Su, Y.: Phishing detection research based on LSTM recurrent neural network. In: Zhou, Q., Gan, Y., Jing, W., Song, X., Wang, Y., Lu, Z. (eds.) ICPCSEE 2018. CCIS, vol. 901, pp. 638–645. Springer, Singapore (2018). https://doi.org/10.1007/978-981-13-2203-7_52
42. Opara, C., Wei, B., Chen, Y.: HTMLPhish: enabling phishing web page detection by applying deep learning techniques on HTML analysis. In: Proceedings of International Joint Conference Neural Networks, pp. 1–8 (2020). https://doi.org/10.1109/IJCNN48605.2020.9207707
43. Hema, R., Ramya, V., Sahithya, K., Sekharan, R.: Detecting of phishing websites using deep learning. J. Crit. Rev. **7**, 3606–3613 (2020)
44. Feng, J., Zou, L., Nan, T.: A phishing webpage detection method based on stacked autoencoder and correlation coefficients. J. Comput. Inf. Technol. **27**, 41–54 (2019). https://doi.org/10.20532/cit.2019.1004702

Applying an Enhanced Elliptic Curve Integrated Encryption Scheme ECIES to Enhance Smart Energy IoT Platform Security Based on Constrained Protocol

Ayoub Ech-Chkaf[1](✉), Salma Ait Oussous[1], Abdelhadi El Allali[1], Siham Beloualid[1], Taoufiq El Harrouti[2], Sanaa El Aidi[1], Abderrahim Bajit[1], Habiba Chaoui[1], and Ahmed Tamtoui[3]

[1] Laboratory of Advanced Systems Engineering (ISA), National School of Applied Sciences, Ibn Tofail University, Kenitra, Morocco
{ayoub.ech-chkaf,salma.aitoussous,siham.beloualid,sanaa.elaidi, habiba.chaoui}@uit.ac.ma, aelallali@gmail.com, abderrahim.bajit@gmail.com

[2] Department of Computer Science, Logistics and Mathematics (ILM) Engineering Science Laboratory National School of Applied Sciences, Ibn Tofail University, Kenitra, Morocco
taoufiq.elharrouti@uit.ac.ma

[3] Laboratory of Advanced Systems National Institute of Posts and Telecommunications, SC Department, Mohammed V University, Rabat, Morocco
tamtaoui@inpt.ac.ma

Abstract. The smart city is a new urban development idea whose purpose is to improve people's quality of life while also protecting the environment by utilizing new technologies that rely on an ecosystem of objects and services to make cities more adaptable and efficient. And the Internet of Things (IoT) is at the heart of practically all smart city gadgets and solutions. Data cannot be collected and presented in the different ways required by the city without it. It allows smart city sensors to regulate lighting, water and waste management, sound and air quality sensors, parking management, etc. Real-time data from buildings, streets, and infrastructure can now be actionable and valuable to all parties involved due to the IoT. In our work, we developed an intelligent and secure IoT Smart energy platform to monitor and control energy use in various parts of a smart city, utilizing the CoAP communication protocol to transport data from smart meters to a web server. We also used different topologies such as STAR, TREE, MESH, and CLUSTER to optimize the performance of our platform in terms of execution time and memory consumption, and we evaluated the impact of the ECIES security protocol compared to other security protocols such as AES-SHA256, RSA, and EEECC.

Keywords: IoT Smart energy platform · CoAP IoT protocol · STAR · TREE · MESH · CLUSTER topologies · AES-SHA256 · RSA-SHA256 · EEECC · ECIES security protocols

F. Saeed et al. (Eds.): IRICT 2021, LNDECT 127, pp. 498–511, 2022.
https://doi.org/10.1007/978-3-030-98741-1_41

1 Introduction

Smart city initiatives around the world are being enabled by new IoT applications. It enables remote monitoring, management, and control of devices, as well as the extraction of fresh insights and actionable data from huge quantities of real-time data. A high degree of information technology integration and a broad application of information resources are two of the most important characteristics of a smart city. Moreover, smart technology, smart industry, smart services, smart management, and smart grid are all vital components of urban growth for a smart city [1]. IoT has an important role which is presented in sensor's installation, then connect them to the internet via a protocol for transmitting data and enabling the communication, to generate a huge amount of data to be collected, transferred and examined to distribute results, and to obtain for example intelligent recognition, monitoring, and managing the energy production and consumption in a changing area. With the help of IoT, Smart cities must have three characteristics: they must be instrumented, networked, and smart. Then, at this advanced degree of IoT development, Smart City can be constructed by combining all of these intelligent components. The rapid expansion of it and IoT applications has created science and engineering issues that necessitate creative research from academia and business, particularly for the development of efficient, flexible, and dependable Smart Cities based on IoT [2]. A smart grid component is a modern electrical grid that employs analog or digital data and communication technology to make the most efficient use of widely available energy resources [3]. Renewable energy is an important topic in the study because of its wide availability, usability, and environmental responsibility, and the use of the smart grid in renewable energy expands its potential. This combination helps in the proper use of renewable sources, which is a big issue [4].

The present work attempts to develop an IoT smart energy platform to monitor and control the energy consumption of any area in a city while using the sustainability factor as a goal to ensure a green living lifestyle using the CoAP protocol, which is a customized web transfer protocol designed for IoT devices with limited resources, and it's made for M2M applications like smart energy [5, 6]. Then, we studied the impact of the ECIES security algorithm in our platform, by applying a set of topologies STAR, TREE, MESH, and CLUSTER to choose the appropriate topology for each zone in terms of memory consumption and execution time. Star topology is composed of a single network coordinator and one or more terminal devices that only interact with the coordinator, and it establishes centralized management for network operations and makes it simple to add a new node [7]. A Tree is based on a child-parent relationship, where the coordinator is connected to routers that can also be connected to others or leaf nodes [8]. Mesh is different, it has no hierarchical relationship, the communication is more flexible, and it is characterized by its increased reliability as more alternate pathways become accessible [9]. The Cluster is the most complex since it is a combination of the other topologies, then it can handle a large volume of traffic. In addition, it also has a hierarchy of child parents like a tree [10].

2 Smart Grid IoT Platform and Aims

The objective of our work is to develop an intelligent and secure smart grid IoT platform for a smart city in real-time, which is used to collect, analyze and control the energy consumption in each area in the smart city such as tourist area, industrial area, commercial area, etc.

As shown in Fig. 1, we used IoT smart meter nodes for each zone to measure the amount of energy consumed over a specified period, and then, we send data to the CoAP server via routers. The CoAP server sends the data to the webserver for modeling and analysis. This analysis provides an overview of our city's energy consumption and allows us to discover which areas are consuming more energy and the reason, to improve the consumption in the different areas of the city, as well as to choose the topology that suits it.

To accomplish this task, we employed four distinct topologies, in which the IoT smart meter nodes are connected directly to the coordinator, or each End device is connected to the coordinator via routers that operate as an intermediary. And to guarantee the security of the data that circulates, we have added the ECIES security layer.

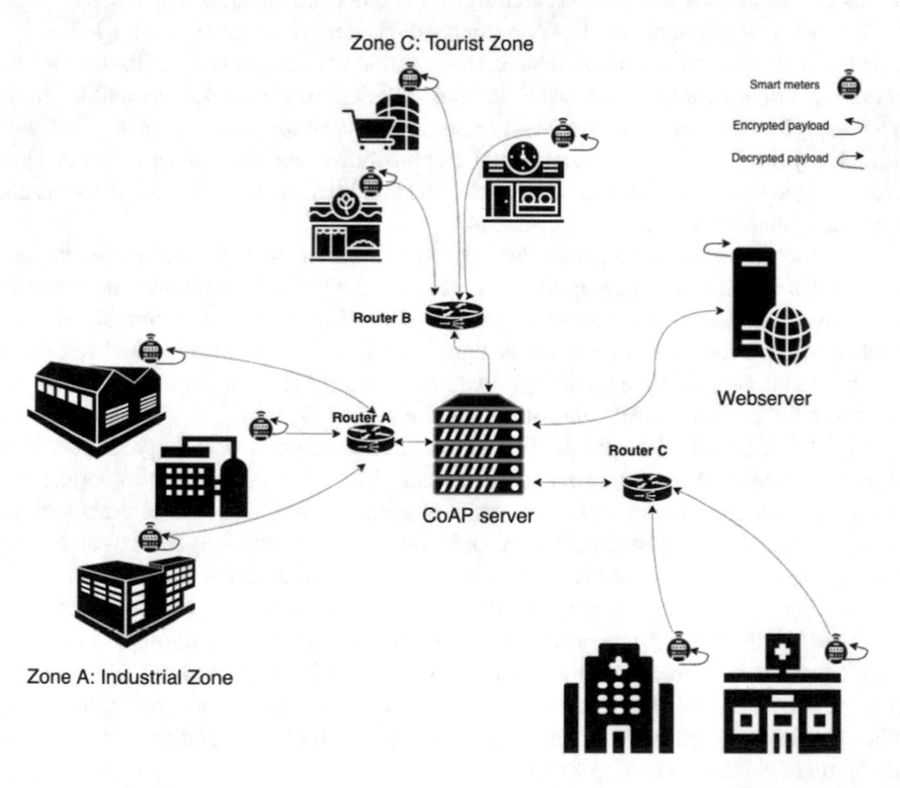

Fig. 1. IoT smart grid platform architecture based on CoAP protocol.

3 Methodology

To model and improve effective energy management by adopting environmental resources to control and power modern life devices in smart cities and contribute to better air quality and lower environmental nuisance, we used an IoT platform model interested in handling resource analysis and optimization needs by collecting stable and accurate information. And to avoid any kind of data loss, this data must be secured.

Data security has become an important topic. The majority of the data we use is insecure. As a result, we must search for solutions to secure them. And cryptography is one of several methods for securing information [11].

Elliptic Curve Cryptography (ECC) is a type of cryptography that can be used to encrypt data, create digital signatures, and manage key exchanges. ECC cryptography is considered the most suitable current successor to the Cryptosystem since it employs shorter keys and signatures for the same degree of security as RSA and allows for extremely quick key generation, key agreement, and signatures [12].

Moreover, it offers a range of approaches that rely on the mathematics of elliptic curves over finite fields, including ECC encryption algorithms and hybrid encryption schemes such as the ECIES Elliptic Curve Integrated Encryption Scheme, integrated and EEECC Energy-efficient Elliptic Curve cryptography, to ensure that authentication and key distribution issues are solved [13].

The present algorithms are known as hybrid cryptosystems since they combine symmetric and asymmetric techniques. The ECIES is the most well of the hybrid cryptosystems based on ECC, it may be found in various cryptographic standards as a result [14]. It is a public key encryption system that is based on the ElGamal encryption algorithm and is developed for Elliptic curve groups. It is ANSI X9.63 and ISO/IEC 15946-3 standardized, as well as IEEE P1363a. In addition, adaptively selected plaintext and chosen-ciphertext attacks are protected by this method. It combines encryption, key exchange, and digital signature capabilities. Because it is a hybrid scheme that uses a public key system to transmit a session key for use by a symmetric cryptosystem, it is dubbed Integrated Encryption Scheme [15].

The ECIES standard mixes ECC-based asymmetric cryptography with symmetric ciphers to offer data encryption and decryption using an EC private key and an EC public key. It employs ECC cryptography (public key cryptosystem) in conjunction with a key-derivation function, symmetric encryption, and the MAC algorithm. For decryption, the ECIES produces the original plaintext message by combining the output of the encryption with the recipient's private key [16].

Finally, our work is based on this security algorithm to ensure authentication, confidentiality, and availability of data in good condition.

4 Related Works

The authors provide secure and lightweight authentication algorithms for IoT devices based on this notion [16]. The devices in the perception layer are mutually authenticated with the system's gateway, in a centralized network paradigm. A mutual authentication approach that employs symmetric key negotiation with Elliptic Curve Diffie-Hellman

(ECDH) in the registration part of the protocol to preserve device credentials while minimizing device calculation costs. After the authentication, the sensor devices and the gateway form a key agreement based on symmetric-key cryptography. Furthermore, in the registration step of the preceding protocol, the Elliptic Curve Integrated Encryption Scheme (ECIES) approach is employed to avoid the risk of a man-in-the-middle attack (MITM). The protocols are subjected to an informal security verification, which shows that they are resistant to perception layer assaults. After the protocol has been simulated in the Cooja simulator under the Contiki OS environment, the performance of the protocol has been evaluated using metrics such as execution time, communication cost, and calculation cost. Furthermore, as compared to existing protocols, the suggested system is lightweight since it has a cheap calculation cost and a faster execution time.

Second, the authors give a survey of ECC in the context of lightweight cryptography in their article [17]. The goal of this work is to establish the parameters that make an ECC-based system lightweight and useful in limited situations. The key factors examined in ECC designs for lightweight realizations are systematically reviewed in representative works. As a result, this work establishes the concept and specifications for elliptic curve lightweight cryptography for the first time.

Based on those works, and from the previous work [18], which we created a smart grid platform for a smart city that aims to monitor and analyze energy consumption, using smart meter IoT nodes for each area. First, from the comparison performed on the data sent by the IoT nodes in terms of execution time and memory occupancy using the CoAP and MQTT protocols, we concluded that the CoAP protocol is better than the other one because it uses a small packet size, it consumes less memory and it takes less time to execute.

Then, we studied the impact of the topologies in terms of execution time and memory consumption, with and without security. The test is done on the following security protocols RSA-SHA256 and ECC, and we focused our study on the impact of the ECC to compare it with RSA. From this study, we found that ECC is better than RSA since it offers high data security, as well as it is fast, efficient, and consumes little memory thanks to its small size keys. The present work is a continuity of the previous work, we aim to achieve the same objectives as the previous, but this time we will focus our study on the impact of another security algorithm that ECC uses which is ECIES that must be compared with AES-SHA256 and EEECC to choose the best one using multi topologies.

5 The Proposed Approach

Our approach is focused on developing an IoT smart grid platform for a smart city, which collects, analyzes, and manages energy usage in each zone. To fix that, we employed IoT smart meters to quantify the quantity of energy spent in each zone; using the CoAP protocol. Moreover, it is based on different parts, where each zone uses one or more topologies. The use of these topologies is based on several criteria like surface, smart meter's number, and the distance between smart meters, routers, and coordinators. For securing our data circulates between them, we added the ECIES algorithm.

We choose to work with the CoAP protocol because it is asynchronous takes little time to execute and consumes less memory compared to MQTT according to these works [19, 20]. However, ECC is considered the most modern and secure protocol, it is a combination of the EEECC algorithm and the ECIES algorithm. And since it generates keys and computes message signatures faster than the RSA algorithm, additionally, it is capable to provide the same level of security as RSA.

We decided to study the impact of the ECIES algorithm to approve that it is the best in terms of memory consumption and execution time, by doing tests. Then we compared it with AES-SHA256 which is a security protocol faster in processing with high performance, low resource and memory requirements, as well as the possibility of encrypting and decrypting a large amount of data quickly compared to RSA [21], because it uses symmetric encryption with a smaller key size in which the sender and receiver of a communication share a single common key to encrypt and transmit the information.

6 Discussion and Results

To achieve the goal of our work, we made many tests for studying the performance of our platform in terms of execution time and memory consumption using different topologies Start, Tree, Mesh, and Cluster, with and without security layers.

In this section, we will discuss the results obtained to choose the best security layer. So, we focused to work with four versions of security: secured with RSA-SHA256, AES-SHA256, EEECC, and ECIES, using the CoAP protocol.

Firstly, Fig. 2 shows the results of all versions of the security layer mentioned before in terms of execution time by each type of topology. According to these results, we observed that the ECIES algorithm takes little time to execute which is the opposite of EEECC and RSA-SHA256. For AES-SHA256, we can say that it is almost the same as ECIES.

Secondly, Fig. 3 shows the results of all versions of the security layer in terms of memory consumption by topologies. From these results, we found that RSA- SHA256 consumes a lot of memory compared to ECIES. Moreover, ECIES consumes also more memory compared to EEECC and AES-SHA256.

Thirdly, Fig. 4 shows the average execution time and the average memory consumption for each topology by different versions of security. From these tests, we found that EEECC takes a lot of time to execute compared to the others, and ECIES is the least time-consuming. However, for the average memory consumption by topology and security layer, we found that RSA consumes more, then ECIES, AES-SHA256, and EEECC is the less consuming.

Additionally, Table 1 shows the average execution time according to the type of topology and security version, where we found that ECIES takes less time, On the other hand, RSA-SHA256 and EEECC take more time to execute.

However, Table 2 represents the average memory consumption by topology and security, we found that RSA-SHA256 consumes a lot of memory than the others. Fourthly, Table 3 represents the gain of execution time by topology and security layer, and Table 4 shows the memory consumption gain by topology and security layer, we found that ECIES saves time compared to RSA-SHA256, AES-SHA256, and EEECC, on the other hand at the level of memory consumption, we found that ECIES saves memory compared to RSA-SHA256 but it causes a loss of memory compared to AES-SHA256.

From all these results, we can deduce that ECIES is the suitable security algorithm for our platform. Since RSA-SHA256 takes time to execute and consumes a lot of memory, it causes us a great loss. Moreover, ECIES takes more time compared to RSA-SHA256, which also causes a loss, even if it consumes less memory. As for AES-SHA256, since it is symmetric, it can cause problems in managing several keys when we have a lot of

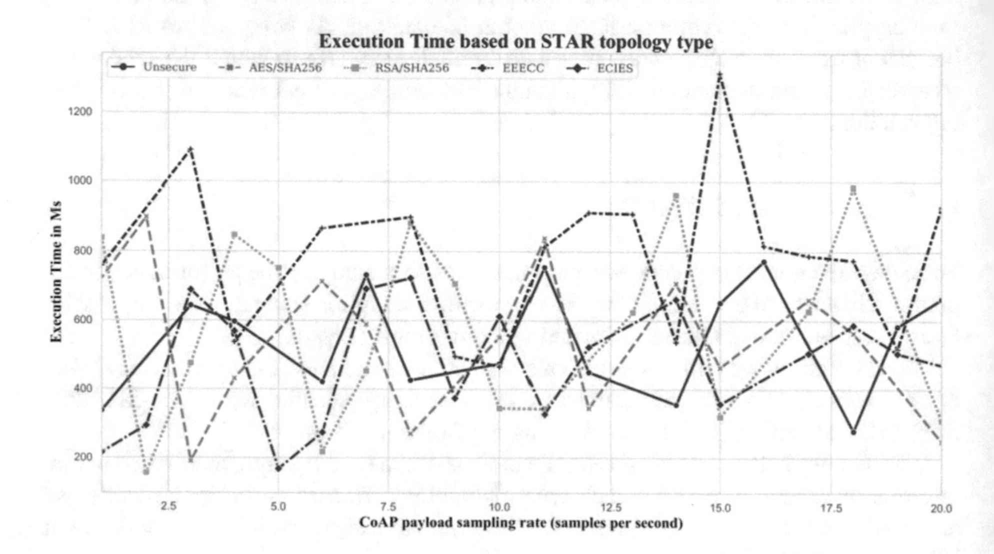

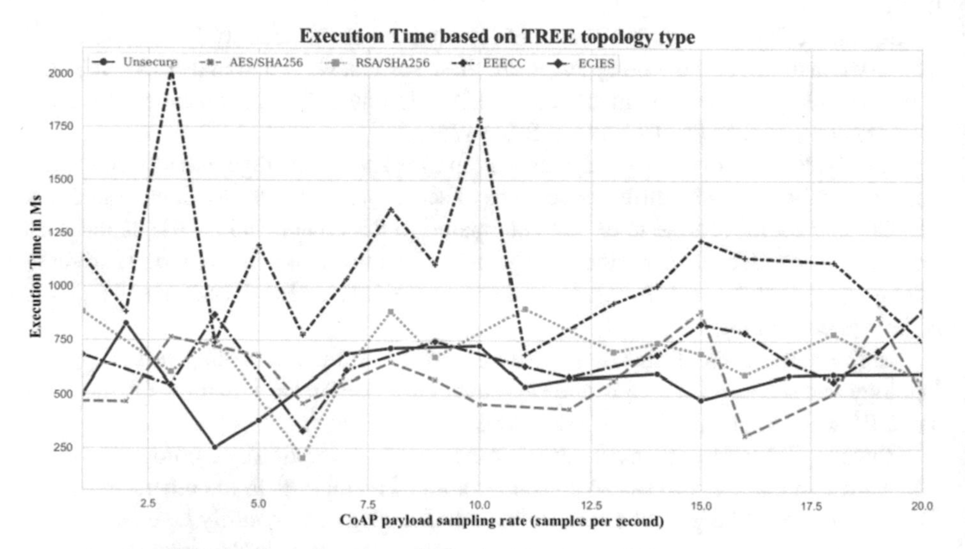

Fig. 2. Execution time with and without security by topologies.

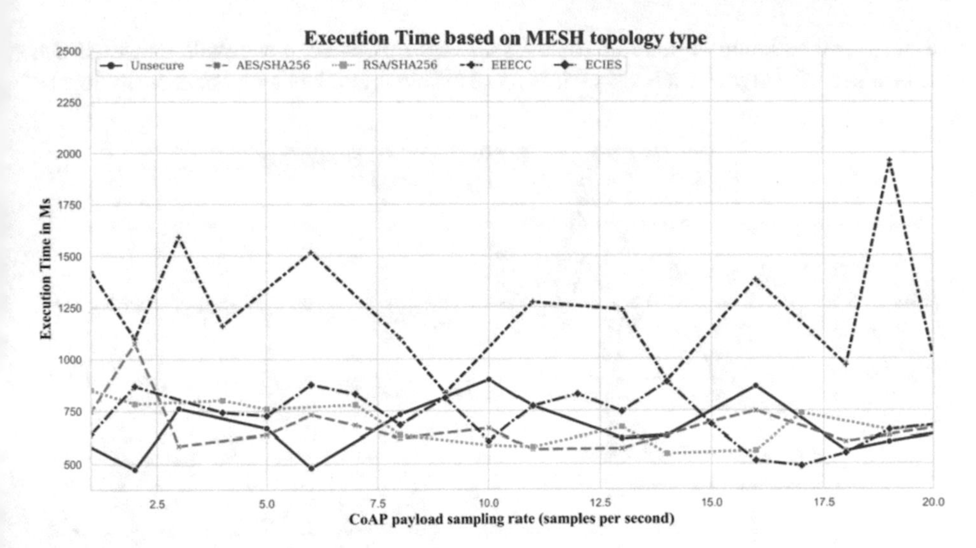

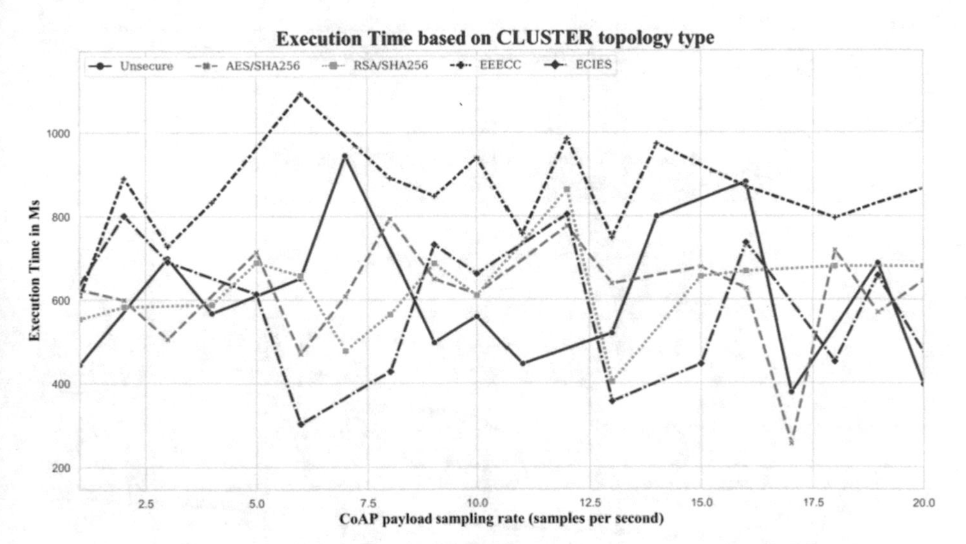

Fig. 2. continued

keys, as well as being vulnerable to attacks. From this, we can conclude that ECIES is the best security algorithm because it is more efficient and has a higher security level.

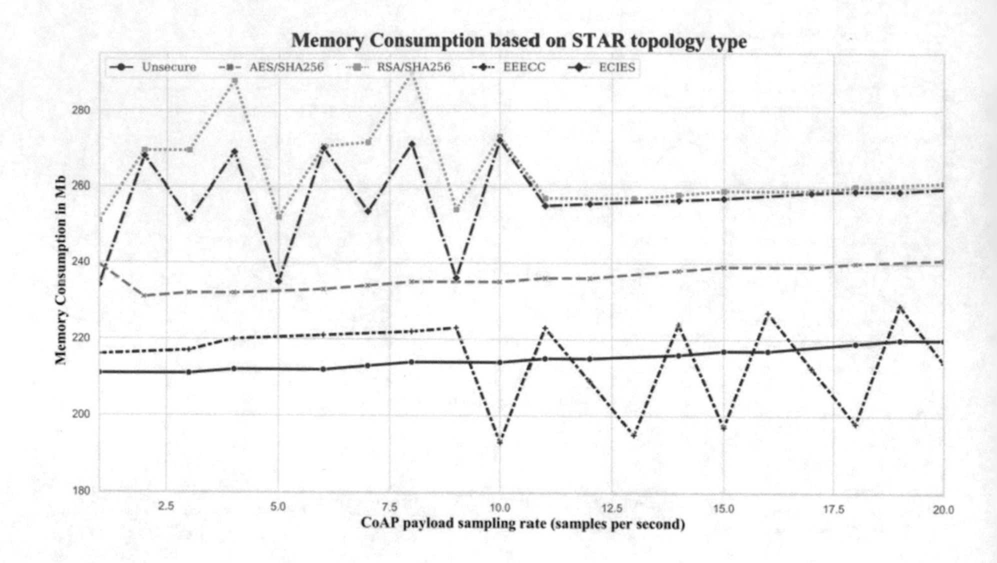

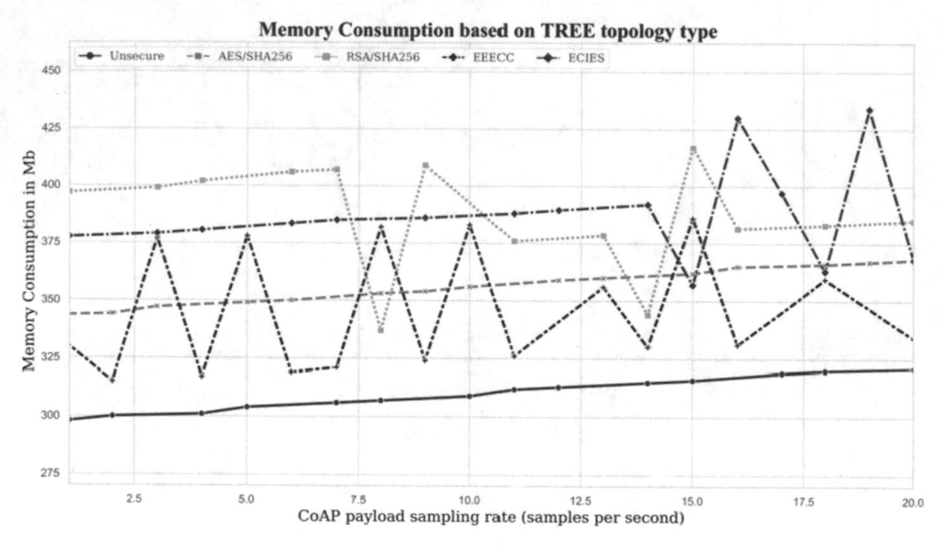

Fig. 3. Memory consumption with and without security by topologies.

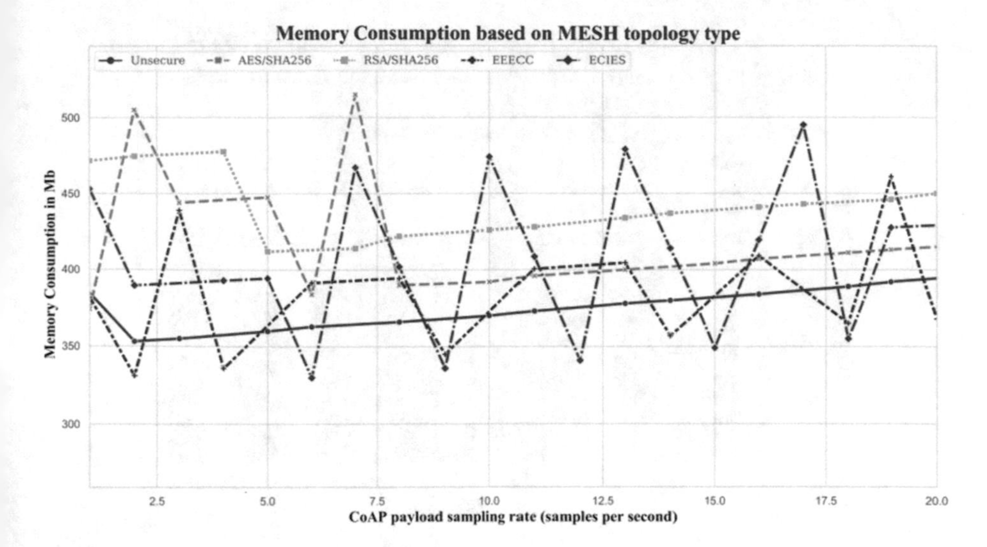

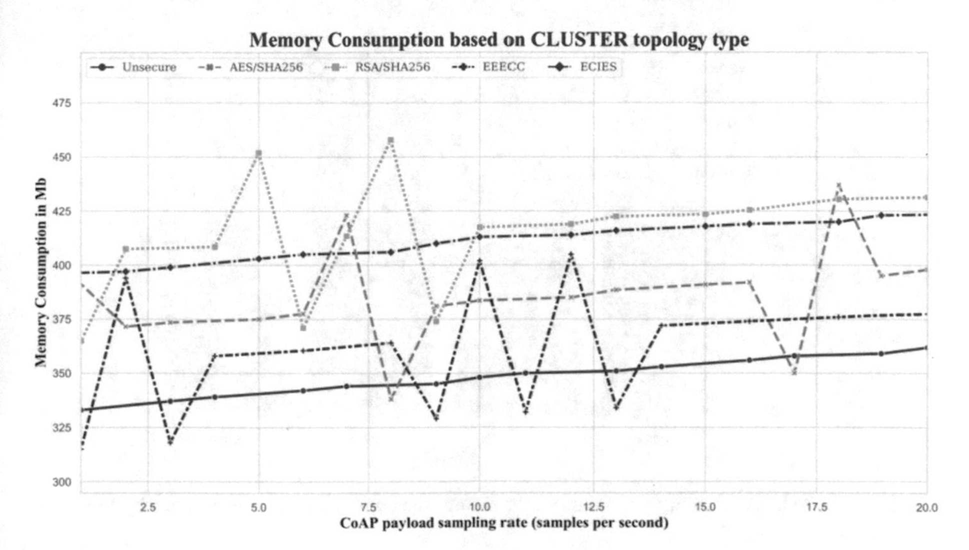

Fig. 3. continued

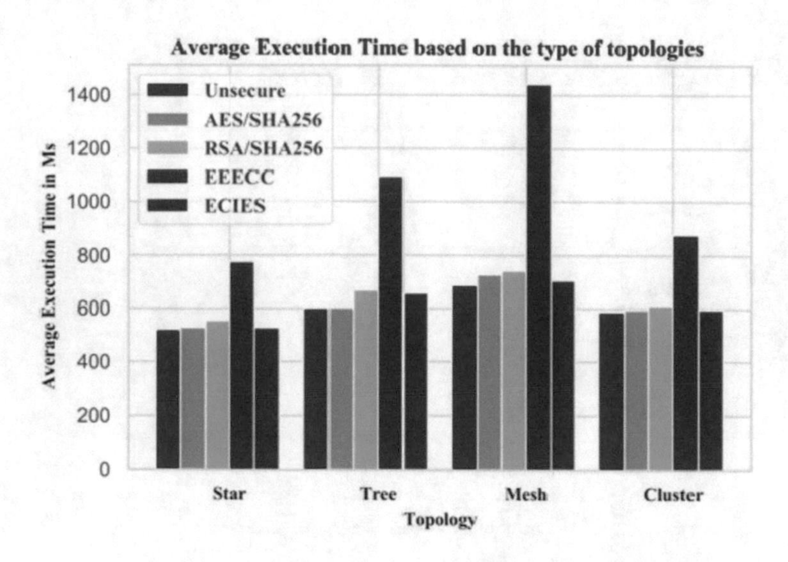

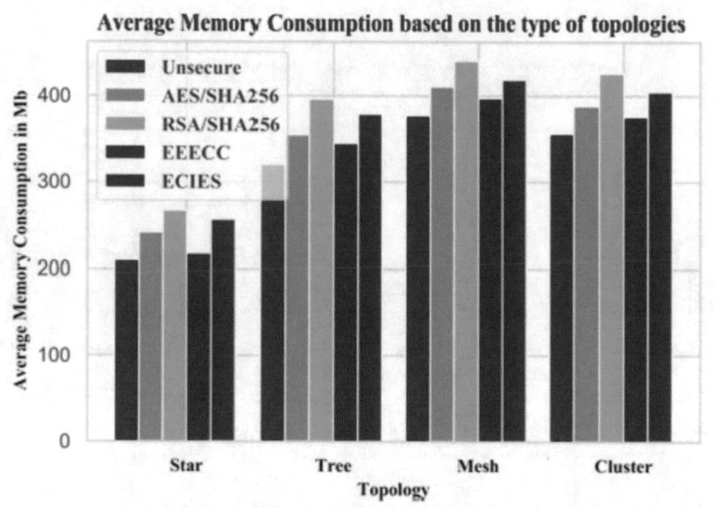

Fig. 4. Average Execution time and memory consumption with and without security by topology.

Table 1. Average time execution for the IoT smart grid platform.

		Star	Tree	Mesh	Cluster
Time (MS)	RSA	554.21	665.47	740.56	611.85
	AES	528.15	601.41	726.13	596.1
	EEECC	774.86	1095.34	1441.93	704.45
	ECIES	527.77	655.83	704.45	597.28
	Unsecured	520.58	600.35	685.68	588.04

Table 2. Average memory consumption for the IoT smart grid platform.

		Star	Tree	Mesh	Cluster
Memory	RSA	266.65	395.98	440.31	426.03
	AES	241.28	354.33	410.58	388.43
	EEECC	216.98	344.5	397.28	375.91
	ECIES	256.28	378.93	418.85	404.81
	Unsecured	209.28	320.26	377.08	355.81

Table 3. The gain of the execution time of ECIES compared to AES, RSA, and EEECC by topology.

	Time ECIES % RSA	Time ECIES % AES
Star	4.77%	0.07%
Tree	1.44%	–9.04%
Mesh	4.87%	2.98%
Cluster	2.38%	–0.19%

Table 4. The gain of memory consumption of ECIES compared to AES, RSA and EEECC by topology.

	Memory ECIES % RSA	Memory ECIES % AES
Star	3.88%	– 6,24%
Tree	4.30%	– 6.94%
Mesh	4.87%	– 2.01%
Cluster	4.98%	– 4.21%

7 Conclusion and Perspectives

In this work, we created a smart grid platform for a smart city that aims to monitor and analyze energy consumption, using smart meter nodes for each zone. This work is done with the CoAP protocol to study the impact of topologies and different types of security on the functioning of our platform because the goal was to apply an enhanced Elliptic Curve Integrated Encryption Scheme ECIES to enhance Smart Energy in IoT Platform. So, the results show that ECIES is the most suitable.

In the next work, we will improve this platform by working on the optimization of the costs of transmission of electrical energy, in order to propose a model that reduces costs and greenhouse gas emissions. And we will apply the Zigbee protocol to compare it with CoAP, as well as we will integrate the Blockchain.

References

1. Serban, A.C., Lytras, M.D.: Artificial intelligence for smart renewable energy sector in Europe smart energy infrastructures for next generation smart cities. IEEE Access **8**, 77364–77377 (2020). https://doi.org/10.1109/AC-CESS.2020.2990123
2. Mohammed, T.-H.: Smart city and IoT. Futur. Gener. Comput. Syst. **76**, 159–162 (2017). https://doi.org/10.1016/j.future.2017.03.034
3. Vineetha, C.P., Babu, C.A.: Smart grid challenges, issues and solutions. In: 2014 International Conference on Intelligent Green Building and Smart Grid (IGBSG), pp. 1–4 (2014). https://doi.org/10.1109/IGBSG.2014.6835208
4. Sharma, H., Kaur, G.: Optimization and simulation of smart grid distributed generation: a case study of university campus. In: 2016 IEEE Smart Energy Grid Engineering (SEGE), pp. 153–157 (2016). https://doi.org/10.1109/SEGE.2016.7589517
5. Bellavista, P., Zanni, A.: Towards better scalability for IoT-cloud interactions via combined exploitation of MQTT and CoAP. In: 2016 IEEE 2nd International Forum on Research and Technologies for Society and Industry Leveraging a better tomorrow (RTSI), pp. 1–6 (2016). https://doi.org/10.1109/RTSI.2016.7740614
6. Kayal, P., Perros, H.: A comparison of IoT application layer protocols through a smart parking implementation. In: 2017 20th Conference on Innovations in Clouds, Internet and Networks (ICIN), Paris, pp. 331–336 (2017). https://doi.org/10.1109/ICIN.2017.7899436
7. Pramono, S., Putri, A.O., Warsito, E., Basuki, S.B.: Comparative analysis of star topology and multihop topology outdoor propagation based on Quality of Service (QoS) of wireless sensor network (WSN). In: 2017 IEEE International Conference on Communication, Networks, and Satellite (Comnetsat), pp. 152–157 (2017). https://doi.org/10.1109/COMNETSAT.2017.8263591
8. Celtek, S.A., Durdu, A., Kurnaz, E.: Design and simulation of the hierarchical tree topology based wireless drone networks. In: 2018 International Conference on Artificial Intelligence and Data Processing (IDAP), pp. 1–5 (2018). https://doi.org/10.1109/IDAP.2018.8620755
9. Yu, L., Kin-Fai, T., Xiangdong, Q., Ying, L., Xuyang, D.: Wireless Mesh Networks in IoT networks. In: 2017 International Workshop on Electromagnetics: Applications and Student Innovation Competition, pp. 183–185 (2017). https://doi.org/10.1109/iWEM.2017.7968828
10. Ouadou, M., Zytoune, O., Aboutajdine, D., ElHillali, Y., Menhaj-Rivenq, A.: Improved Cluster-tree topology adapted for indoor environment in Zigbee Sensor Network. Procedia Comput. Sci. **94**, 272–279 (2016). https://doi.org/10.1016/j.procs.2016.08.041
11. Di Matteo, S., Baldanzi, L., Crocetti, L., Nannipieri, P., Fanucci, L., Saponara, S.: Secure elliptic curve crypto-processor for real-time IoT applications. Energies **14**(15), 4676 (2021). https://doi.org/10.3390/en14154676
12. Sadkhan, S.B.: Elliptic curve cryptography- status, challenges, and future trends. In: 2021 7th International Engineering Conference "Research & Innovation amid Global Pandemic" (IEC), pp. 167–171 (2021). https://doi.org/10.1109/IEC52205.2021.9476090
13. Salim, A., Abbas, A., Abdul, B.M.: Data security for cloud computing based on elliptic curve integrated encryption scheme (ECIES) and modified identity-based cryptography (MIBC). In: International Journal of Applied Information Systems (IJAIS) – ISSN: 2249-0868 Foundation of Computer Science FCS, New York, USA, vol. 10, no.6 (Mar 2016). www.ijais.org
14. Vinchoo, M.M., Kadam, S.S., Shaikh, I.A., Vora, D., Nayak, D.: Grey Immune: Security in hybrid cloud. In: 2017 International Conference on Intelligent Sustainable Systems (ICISS), pp. 492–495 (2017). https://doi.org/10.1109/ISS1.2017.8389460

15. Milen, S., Marina, S.: Practical book cryptography for developers. https://cryptobook.nakov.com/
16. Oh, J., Yu, S., Lee, J., Son, S., Kim, M., Park, Y.: A secure and lightweight authentication protocol for IoT-based smart homes. Sensors **21**, 1488 (2021). https://doi.org/10.3390/s21041488
17. Lara-Nino, C.A., Diaz-Perez, A., Morales-Sandoval, M.: Elliptic curve lightweight cryptography: a survey. IEEE Access **6**, 72514–72550 (2018). https://doi.org/10.1109/ACCESS.2018.2881444
18. Rao, V., Prema, K.V.: Lightweight authentication and data encryption scheme for IoT applications. In: 2020 IEEE International Conference on Distributed Computing, VLSI, Electrical Circuits and Robotics (DISCOVER), pp. 12–17 (2020). https://doi.org/10.1109/DISCOVER50404.2020.9278048
19. Yachou, M., et al.: Applying lightweight elliptic curve cryptography ECC to smart energy IOT platforms based on the CoAP protocol. In: The International Conference on Information, Communication & Cybersecurity (ICI2C 21). https://doi.org/10.1007/978-3-030-91738-8_20
20. ElAidi, S., Bajit, A., Barodi, A., Chaoui, H., Tamtaoui, A.: An optimized security vehicular Internet of Things-IoT-application layer protocols MQTT and COAP based on cryptographic elliptic-curve. In: 2020 IEEE 2nd International Conference on Electronics, Control, Optimization and Computer Science, ICECOCS 2020, pp. 9314579 (2020)
21. El Aidi, S., Bajit, A., Barodi, A., Chaoui, H., Tamtaoui, A.: An advanced encryption cryptographically-based securing applicative protocols MQTT and CoAP to optimize medical-IOT supervising platforms. Lect. Notes Data Eng. Commun. Technol. **72**, 111–121 (2021)

Applying Lightweight Elliptic Curve Cryptography ECC and Advanced IoT Network Topologies to Optimize COVID-19 Sanitary Passport Platforms Based on Constrained Application Protocol

Fatima Zahra Hamza[1](✉), Sanaa El Aidi[1], Abdelhadi El Allali[1], Siham Beloualid[1], Abderrahim Bajit[1], and Ahmed Tamtaoui[2]

[1] Laboratory of Advanced Systems Engineering (ISA), National School of Applied Sciences, Ibn Tofail University, Kenitra, Morocco
{fatimazahra.hamza,sanaa.elaidi,siham.beloualid, abderrahim.bajit}@uit.ac.ma, aelallali@gmail.com

[2] National Institute of Posts and Telecommunications (INPT-Rabat), SC Department, Mohamed V University, Rabat, Morocco
tamtaoui@inpt.ac.ma

Abstract. Being in a period of covid-19 urges us to develop platforms that help in minimizing the spread of the virus. Thus, this paper proposes a Medical IoT platform that is created to control citizens' access to public areas. Our platform focuses on three scenarios on which a citizen is admitted to: being vaccinated which means that the person holds a vaccine pass that contains a unique QR code, possessing a PCR test which means that the person holds a unique barcode, and having an RFID tag which contains a unique identifier. All scenarios start with the same test which allows us to detect the presence of a citizen using a PIR IoT Client node, and end with one last test which is the face recognition to verify the present citizen is indeed who he/she claims to be. Only if one of the scenarios is valid can the citizen be allowed to access the public space. To ensure communication between the IoT nodes we developed our platform based on the Constrained Application Protocol CoAP. As for the security of the payloads, we have implemented RSA, AES, and ECC encryption algorithms to protect the integrity of the data and prevent any attacks. We also based our platform on 4 types of network topologies namely star, tree, mesh, and cluster. The use of different topologies and different encryption methods will allow us to eventually choose which one best matches the platform's requirements, and that is in terms of execution time and memory occupation.

Keywords: CoAP Protocol · Star · Tree · Cluster · Mesh · AES · RSA · ECC · Vaccine pass · PCR · QR · Barcode · RFID · IoT · COVID-19

F. Saeed et al. (Eds.): IRICT 2021, LNDECT 127, pp. 512–523, 2022.
https://doi.org/10.1007/978-3-030-98741-1_42

1 Introduction

The Internet of things is the most emerging technology that is growing exponentially, providing new opportunities in the technology arena. It can be defined as devices or 'things' interconnecting to achieve a network through which data is created, transmitted, received, and can yield analytical insight [1].

IoT has enabled the healthcare system to improve its supervision quality with real-time information in addition to strengthening the healthcare services provided to the patient, this makes IoT receive huge attention in the healthcare domain, where IoT's use is necessary and plays an important role to predict, prevent and control emerging infectious diseases such as COVD-19 [2, 4]. The worldwide is now aware of this innovative technology and its significant applications since it provides practical and cost-effective solutions to face the problems that came with this pandemic [2, 3].

Most of the countries in the world have imposed travel restrictions, containment measures, and social distancing, so it is obligatory to respect the sanitary rules to reopen the public spaces. In this scope, this paper proposes an IoT platform that supervises and controls the citizens' access to public areas, by either granting them access or denying them access. The decision is made through the results of several tests that are divided into three scenarios, and thanks to the use of four types of IoT devices which are: PIR node, RFID tag, temperature sensor, and a camera node.

To elaborate, the first scenario of our platform concerns the people who are vaccinated so they hold a vaccine pass with a unique QR code, the second scenario is for the citizens who hold a PCR test which also contains a unique barcode, and the last scenario is for the citizens who are not vaccinated and don't have a PCR test but they possess a unique RFID tag. So, to grant access to a person, he/she must have a vaccine pass, a PCR test, or an RFID tag, in addition to passing some tests such as face recognition, else their access is unauthorized. These scenarios are discussed and elaborated more in the next section.

In this platform, we have used face recognition as a final test in each scenario. Face recognition is an important element in our platform since it provides another layer of access security and allows us to identify the detected citizen through analyzing the facial structure and comparing it to the information in the database [5].

The platform relies on the Constrained Application protocol CoAP as a communication protocol that connects the nodes and is developed based on different types of topologies namely star, tree, mesh, and cluster. AES, RSA, and ECC cryptography algorithms were also used to encrypt the payloads shared through the network by the IoT nodes. This will eventually allow us to deduct results about each network topology and encryption method to finally adopt which ones will suit best the requirements of the platform, in terms of efficiency, time consumption, memory occupation, and power consumption. Figure 1. Shows the Medical IoT Architecture.

2 Related Works

Various researchers have addressed smart solutions for combatting covid-19 pandemic. Researchers in [21] have proposed a medical supervising platform that serves to detect a citizen with PIR Node, measure the body temperature through a temperature sensor, and then verify the identity through the combination of an RFID and facial recognition test

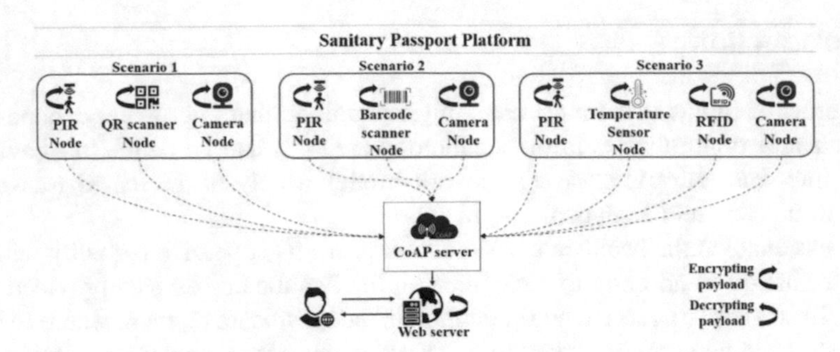

Fig. 1. Medical IoT architecture

to allow the citizen to access the public area. However, nowadays vaccines have been developed, a huge number of PCR tests is made on a daily basis, which will guide us to the questionable issue of if those tests are sufficient to allow access to a public space.

As for cybersecurity, researchers in [13] say that to elevate the security level of RSA, the necessary key size must be increased exponentially. And since IoT devices only have access to limited resource, it is not convenient to use RSA as a cryptography algorithm for these resource-constrained environments. And so, the researchers propose that ECC, even with a small key size, can provide the same level of security as RSA.

In this paper, we develop an optimized IoT platform that controls citizens' access to public areas, in addition to evaluating the performance of each cryptosystem, communication protocol, and wireless network topology implemented, when combined with each other.

3 Functional Medical IoT Scenarios

This paper proposes a Medical IoT platform that is developed to supervise and control citizens' access to public areas, and it focuses on three scenarios: being vaccinated, possessing a PCR test, and having an RFID tag (Fig. 2). All scenarios start with the same test which allows us to detect the presence of a citizen using a PIR IoT Client node, then it moves to the other tests of each scenario. For the first scenario, the vaccination of the person is checked thanks to his/her vaccine pass, from which we scan the QR code that contains a unique identifier to see its validity. If the citizen does not have a vaccine pass, we move to the second scenario and scan the barcode in the presented PCR test which also contains a unique identifier as well as an indication of its date, since we need it to verify that the PCR test did not exceed 48 h. The third scenario is where the citizen does not possess a vaccine pass nor a PCR test, so we check his body temperature as well as his RFID's unique identifier to see if they're valid. All of these three scenarios end with one last test which is the face recognition to verify that the present citizen is indeed who he/she claims to be. Only if one of the scenarios is valid can the citizen be allowed to access the public space.

4 The Proposed Approach

The development of this IoT intelligent medical platform is to control citizens' access to public space. As we mentioned before, we have implemented three scenarios in the platform: the first one for those who are vaccinated, the second one for those who have a PCR test, and the last one for those with an RFID tag. As explained before, if all of the scenarios do not apply to the person, or if one of the tests is not correct, the access will not be granted to the person.

This work consists of implementing different approaches in the platform's functioning, by encrypting the communication protocol's payloads with various encryption algorithms which are RSA, AES, and ECC, in addition to developing the platform according to different network topologies. In the end, this will allow us to carry out comparative results of each approach, and adopt the one that is most suitable and effective for our platform.

The application layer protocol plays a significant part in the IoT framework as it enables the communication between things, devices, or objects with the application interfaces [6]. The constrained Application Protocol CoAP is a simple and lightweight protocol that is used in networks with limited resource. It is a specialized web transfer protocol for constrained devices and constrained networks [7], even though its characteristics and operations are similar to those of a Hypertext Transfer Protocol (HTTP). Also, CoAP supports the usage of DTLS which adds more security guarantees [8].

Cryptography is the process of secret writing, which allows converting plain text into a non-readable format. It consists of two types: symmetric-key/private-key cryptography and asymmetric-key/public-key cryptography [12]. In asymmetric key cryptography, a key pair is generated; a public and a private key, which is why it is also called Public Key cryptography. The public key is used for encryption, while only the corresponding private key is used for decryption [9]. RSA is a well-known public-key cryptography algorithm that is the most widely used. It is incredibly onerous to crack since the algorithm is based on the fact that it is of great difficulty to factorize large integers into prime factors. However, the RSA algorithm has been considered too resource-consuming for constrained devices, where storage, memory, and speed are limited [10, 11]. Another known Public Key cryptography algorithm is the Elliptic Curve Cryptography (ECC), which's security is based on the elliptic curve discrete logarithm problem [12]. Being able to provide the same level of security as RSA with reduced key size makes ECC the best alternative choice. In other words, the use of smaller key sizes by the Elliptic Curve means it has a compact key size which is the main advantage of ECC [13, 14].

Concerning the other cryptography type, symmetric-key cryptography uses only one key to encrypt and decrypt, hence, the name of private-key cryptography. So, the sender encrypts the plain text with the private key and the receiver applies the same key to decrypt the message. Two types of cipher are used in Symmetric Key Cryptography, and they are stream cipher and block cipher. Advanced Encryption Standard (AES) is one of the most common symmetric block cipher algorithms. It encrypts the information by breaking it down into fixed-sized blocks and encrypting data in each block with a powerful and complex structure [15].

When it comes to network topologies, it is mandatory to understand the method within which the nodes communicate with each other, and how they are arranged. A star network consists of one central hub to which all other nodes in the network are linked. This means that each end node has only one path to transmit the data, which is through the central node, and that's what allows it to act as a coordinator for the network [16,

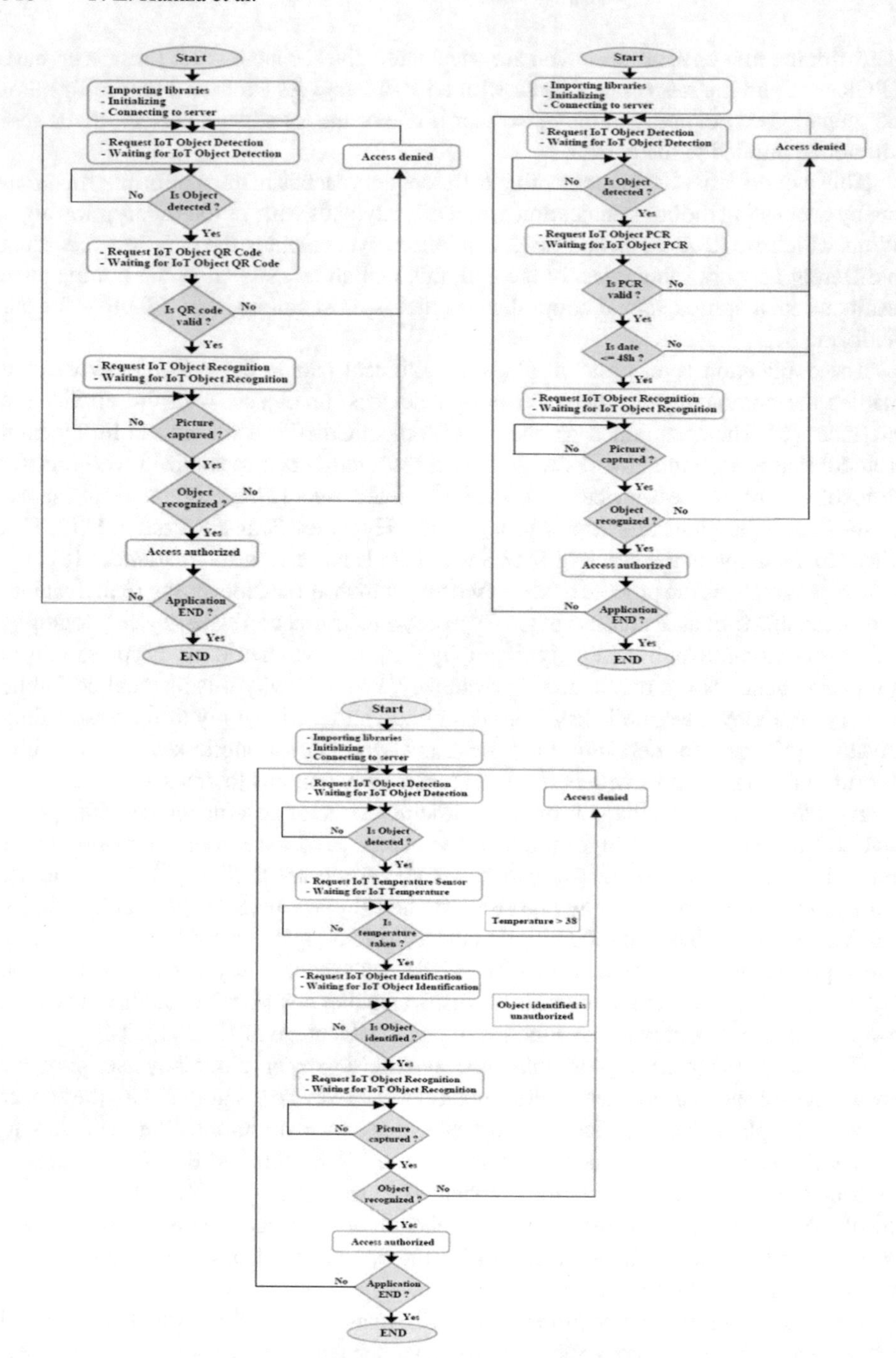

Fig. 2. Functional algorithm

17]. The elements of the star, as well as bus topology, are incorporated in a tree topology. A tree topology is structured just like a tree: all nodes are connected in a way that looks like branches of a tree, so we have parent nodes and child nodes. This makes it flexible since we can add one or more nodes without affecting other nodes [18]. As for mesh topology, it is characterized by its higher fault tolerance and robustness to the fall of one or more nodes, and this is because each node is allowed to communicate with several other nodes, thanks to the paths created within the network, unlike star. This allows the message to multi-hop until it reaches the assigned gateway [19, 20]. The advantages of this topology, as well as star topology, are combined in another topology called cluster, where the nodes of a star are clustered around routers that communicate with each other and the gateway in a mesh [19, 20], or where the nodes of a cluster are connected in a way that forms another type of topology. This makes cluster very useful when wanting to apply different topologies in different parts of the network.

5 Discussion and Results

This paper aims to minimize the spread of covid-19 by developing an IoT platform that controls citizens' access to public areas. We have applied the AES, RSA, and ECC encryption methods on our platform, as well as developed it according to different topologies in order to analyze the impact of each one on the platform, in addition to implementing the right communication protocol, keeping in mind that it is a high constraint resource environment, thus it is important to preserve the power of the IoT nodes, and to shrink their memory occupation and execution time. This is why we have made a comparative study between the topologies, the encryption methods, and communication protocols to finally see what matches best our platform.

CoAP protocol has a small fixed-length binary header compared to MQTT which's packet is loaded, and, MQTT has slower transmission cycles which make CoAP more practical for use in constrained resource environments, which was also concluded in the results published in the ICI2C conference (Fig. 3). We can see that MQTT consumes more time and occupies more memory, resulting in using more energy to work properly. As for security, CoAP is built over UDP and not on TCP like MQTT.

Securing the payloads with different encryption methods enables us to compare them in terms of efficiency, robustness, and resource consumption to eventually adopt the right encryption algorithm for our platform. Figure 4 shows the time consumption and memory occupation of each encryption method applied to a CoAP's payload. Using two large keys to encrypt and decrypt makes the RSA algorithm hard to crack and allows it to offer great security of the data. However, it makes it very expensive when it comes to resource constrained environments, and having limited resource consumption of IoT devices eliminates the use of RSA in our platform. As for AES, it is a symmetric algorithm that consumes much less resource than RSA, thanks to its use of only one shared key, does not require a lot of energy, and is fast in processing. This is clearer in Table 1 which shows the big consumption difference between RSA and AES (as well as ECC), in terms of average memory occupation and average time consumption, wherein each scenario, and in each topology applied, RSA always has higher memory and time consumption than AES (and ECC). What we need now is a cryptography algorithm that matches the security level of RSA, but has low resource consumption to -if not the same as- AES. This is what we notice when implementing the ECC algorithm to our platform. Using a key pair to encrypt and decrypt allows it to offer better security than AES, a very high-security level as RSA, but less resource consumption than AES if not the same. Table 2 shows the percentage of time and memory we gain by implementing it in our platform with the different topologies and scenarios, and from which we can say that ECC adopts the advantages of RSA by using a key pair which makes it strong against attacks, and the advantages of AES by having light resource requirements, in addition to having its own benefits such as allowing faster keys generation thanks to the reduced key size [13, 14], which also leads to less processing power and faster response time, as seen in the results.

We must take into consideration some attributes to choose a wireless network, for example, latency, fault resiliency, scalability. From the results of Fig. 5, we can notice that star has the lower memory and time consumption, followed by cluster, tree, and then mesh being last since it has the higher numbers. This makes the performance of star predictable and fast, also the data travels only through one hop to reach its destination. Star is also reliable thanks to the ease of detecting faults in devices since each one uses its own link. However, more energy must be spent to deliver messages when the communication link between the coordinator and the end node is long. Adding to that, star's range is limited to the transmission range of a single device, and, if the coordinator failed, all the nodes attached are interrupted. A tree topology incorporates the elements of both bus topology and star topology. Between any two connected nodes, there is an existence of only one connection. This topology is known for its flexibility and easy expansion without any issue since it follows a hierarchy pattern. Also, the removal of an end node will not affect the performance of the network. Nonetheless, the uses of tree topology are limited due to its difficult installation process and cost, also its maintenance and configuration because of its large size. If the backbone connection, on which the entire network depends, fails, the point where the failure occurs will decide the level of loss. In other words, the nodes related to the branch damaged will face problems functioning, while others that are not associated with it will continue to work. Mesh topology is a growing network topology commonly found in IoT deployments, since it can withstand high traffic, there is always an alternative path if a node failed so the transfer of the data will not be affected. However, there is a high latency in mesh networks due to multiple hops to transmit data from an end node to the gateway, and that is clear in the results (Fig. 5) since mesh has the higher consumption amongst the other topologies. Cluster tree network combines the advantages of star and mesh networks: the low latency and low power consumption of star, plus extended range and fault tolerance of mesh. We can see that it comes right after star for the low resource consumption. This topology is perfect for a platform where we want to apply different topologies in different parts of the network in the form of clusters. In addition, that even when applying ECC with cluster, the resource consumption is still low. So, to sum up our discussion, we will opt for CoAP as a communication protocol, ECC as a cryptography method, and cluster as a wireless sensor network.

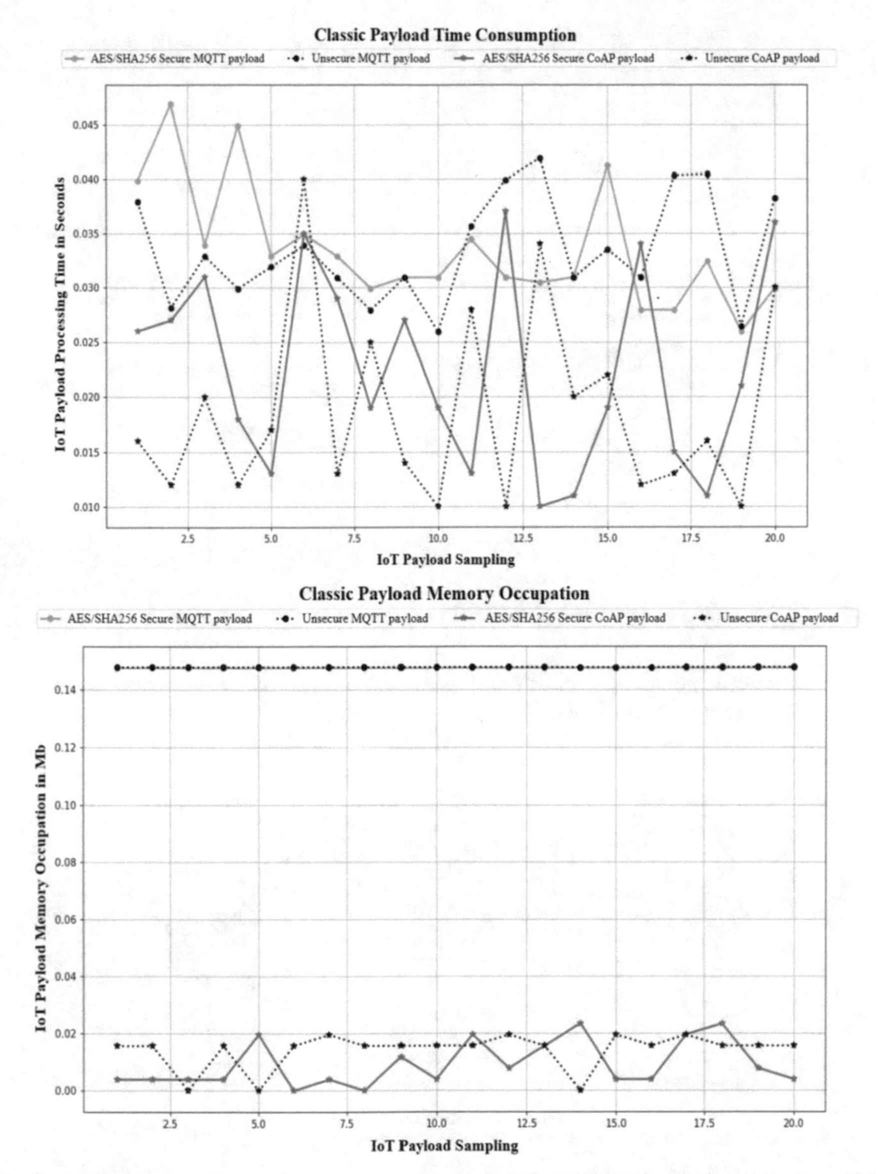

Fig. 3. Time consumption and memory occupation of CoAP/MQTT classic payload combined with AES/SHA256.

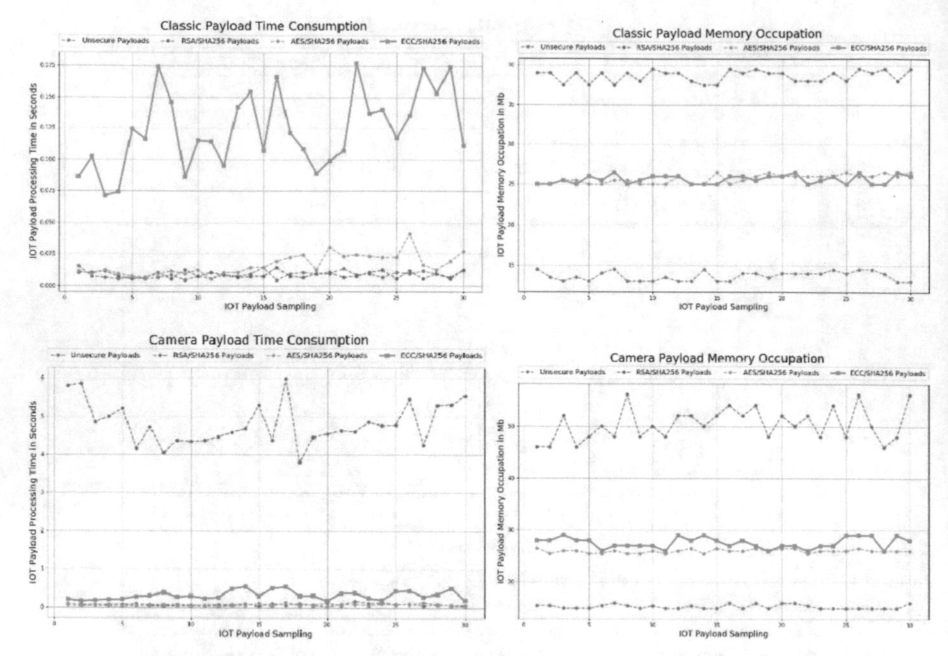

Fig. 4. Time consumption and memory occupation of a CoAP camera payload and Classic Payload secured with RSA, AES, and ECC.

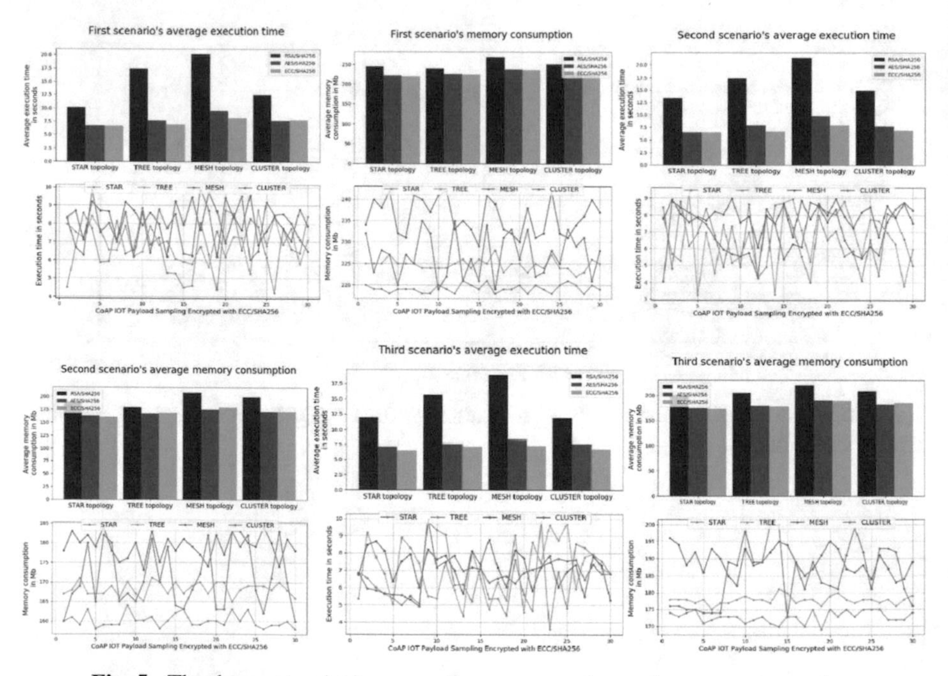

Fig. 5. The three scenarios' average time consumption and memory occupation.

Table 1. Average time consumption (s) and memory occupation (Mb) of the three scenarios.

		Star	Tree	Mesh	Cluster
Scenario 1 Time (s)	RSA	10.13	17.46	20.12	12.47
	AES	6.71	7.72	9.56	7.70
	ECC	6.69	6.96	8.19	7.78
Scenario 2 Time (s)	RSA	13.38	17.46	21.38	14.91
	AES	6.42	7.92	9.76	7.71
	ECC	6.48	6.60	7.95	6.91
Scenario 3 Time (s)	RSA	11.93	15.72	18.95	11.89
	AES	7.07	7.52	8.51	7.61
	ECC	6.54	7.05	7.22	6.80
Scenario 1 RAM (Mb)	RSA	244.6	249.4	268.0	251.0
	AES	222.3	225.6	237.4	230.2
	ECC	219.2	224.7	235.8	226.9
Scenario 2 RAM (Mb)	RSA	189.3	179.5	207.5	199.5
	AES	162.9	167.3	175.1	171.1
	ECC	160.0	168.2	179.2	171.1
Scenario 3 RAM (Mb)	RSA	200.7	204.8	219.0	208.7
	AES	173.9	179.4	190.0	181.9
	ECC	172.8	177.8	189.2	185.1

Table 2. Scenarios' gain percentage of ECC compared to RSA and AES in terms of time consumption and memory occupation.

		Star	Tree	Mesh	Cluster
Scenario 1 (time)	ECC%RSA	33.9%	60.1%	59.2%	37.6%
	ECC%AES	0.3%	9.8%	14.3%	–1.0%
Scenario 2 (time)	ECC%RSA	51.5%	62.1%	62.8%	53.6%
	ECC%AES	–0.9%	16.6%	18.5%	10.3%
Scenario 3 (time)	ECC%RSA	45.1%	55.1%	61.8%	42.8%
	ECC%AES	7.5%	6.2%	15.1%	10.6%
Scenario 1 (ram)	ECC%RSA	10.3%	9.9%	12.0%	9.6%
	ECC%AES	1.4%	0.4%	0.6%	1.4%
Scenario 2 (ram)	ECC%RSA	15.4%	6.2%	13.6%	14.2%
	ECC%AES	1.7%	–0.5%	–2.3%	0.0%
Scenario 3 (ram)	ECC%RSA	13.9%	13.1%	13.6%	11.3%
	ECC%AES	0.6%	0.9%	0.4%	–1.7%

6 Conclusion and Perspectives

This work enabled us to create a sanitary passport platform that serves to control the access of vaccinated as well as non-vaccinated citizens to minimize the spread of the Covid-19 virus. The platform was built and based on different approaches from which we were able to carry out and deduct comparative results, that helped us, in the end, to extract the approach that fits best the requirements of the platform, when it comes to the communication protocol, cryptography algorithm, and network topology.

Eventually, and after studying the results, CoAP was chosen combined with ECC cryptography algorithm to ensure light and secure communication, in addition to adopting Cluster topology to ensure the reliability and efficiency of the platform.

For future works, we will propose a blockchain architecture that will give data more security, we will also implement other communication protocols such as Zigbee and 6LowPan, and deploy other security methods like ECIES.

References

1. Nord, J.H., Koohang, A., Paliszkiewicz, J.: The Internet of Things: review and theoretical framework. Expert Syst. Appl. **133**, 97–108 (2019)
2. Singh, R.P., Javaid, M., Haleem, A., Suman, R.: Internet of things (IoT) applications to fight against COVID-19 pandemic. Diab. Metab. Syndr. Clin. Res. Rev. **14**(4), 521–524 (2020)
3. Rahman, M.S., Peeri, N.C., Shrestha, N., Zaki, R., Haque, U., Hamid, S.H.A.: Defending against the Novel Coronavirus (COVID-19) outbreak: How can the Internet of Things (IoT) help to save the world? Health Policy Technol. **9**(2), 136–138 (2020). https://doi.org/10.1016/j.hlpt.2020.04.005
4. Nasajpour, M., Pouriyeh, S., Parizi, R.M., Dorodchi, M., Valero, M., Arabnia, H.R.: Internet of Things for current COVID-19 and future pandemics: an exploratory study. J. Healthcare Inf. Res. **4**(4), 325–364 (2020). https://doi.org/10.1007/s41666-020-00080-6
5. Masud, M.: Deep learning-based intelligent face recognition in IoT-cloud environment. Comput. Commun. **152**, 215–222 (2020)
6. Gupta, P., Indhra Om Prabha M.: A survey of application layer protocols for Internet of Things. In: 2021 International Conference on Communication information and Computing Technology (ICCICT), pp. 1–6 (2021). https://doi.org/10.1109/ICCICT50803.2021.9510140
7. Suwannapong, C., Khunboa, C.: Congestion control in CoAP observe group communication. Sensors **19**, 3433 (2019). https://doi.org/10.3390/s19153433
8. Nebbione, G., Calzarossa, M.C.: Security of IoT application layer protocols: challenges and findings. Future Internet **12**, 55 (2020). https://doi.org/10.3390/fi12030055
9. Dhakar, R.S., Gupta, A.K., Sharma, P.: Modified RSA Encryption Algorithm (MREA). In: 2012 Second International Conference on Advanced Computing & Communication Technologies, pp. 426–4292012https://doi.org/10.1109/ACCT.2012.74
10. Lihua, G., Kaide, Q., Chengzhi, D., Nanrun, Z.: An optical image compression and encryption scheme based on compressive sensing and RSA algorithm. Opt. Lasers Eng. **121**, 169–180 (2019)
11. Kothmayr, T., Schmitt, C., Hu, W., Brünig, M., Carle, G.: DTLS based security and two-way authentication for the Internet of Things. Ad Hoc Netw. **11**(8), 2710–2723 (2013)
12. Mahto, D., Yadav, D.K.: RSA and ECC: a comparative analysis. Int. J. Appl. Eng. Res. **12**(19), 9053–9061 (2017)

13. Shaikh, J.R., Nenova, M., Iliev, G., Valkova-Jarvis, Z.: Analysis of standard elliptic curves for the implementation of elliptic curve cryptography in resource-constrained E-commerce applications. In: 2017 IEEE International Conference on Microwaves, Antennas, Communications and Electronic Systems (COMCAS), pp. 1–4 (2017). https://doi.org/10.1109/COMCAS.2017.8244805
14. Albalas, F., Alsoud, M., Almomani, A., Almomani, O.: Security-aware CoAP application layer protocol for the Internet of Things using elliptic-curve cryptography. Int. Arab J. Inf. Technol. **5**(3A), Special Issue (2018)
15. Abdullah, A.: Advanced encryption standard (AES) algorithm to encrypt and decrypt data. In: Cryptography and Network Security (2017)
16. Network topology guide for the internet of things. https://www.rcrwireless.com/20161017/big-data-analytics/network-topology-guide-tag31-tag99. Accessed 04 Oct 2021
17. Topologies driving IoT networking standards. http://radar.oreilly.com/2014/04/3-topologies-driving-iot-networking-standards.html. Accessed 04 Oct 2021
18. Tree Topology Advantages and Disadvantages. https://www.aplustopper.com/tree-topology-advantages-and-disadvantages/. Accessed 04 Oct 2021
19. Wireless Topologies. https://www.emerson.com/documents/automation/training-wireless-topologies-en-41144.pdf. Accessed 04 Oct 2021
20. Bilbao, J., Bravo, E., Varela, C., et al.: Developing the IoT through wireless communication networks: analysis of topologies. Int. J. Biosen. Bioelectron. **3**(4), 327–331 (2017)
21. El Aidi, S., Bajit, A., Barodi, A., Chaoui, H., Tamtaoui, A.: An advanced encryption cryptographically-based securing applicative protocols MQTT and CoAP to optimize medical-IOT supervising platforms. In: Saeed, F., Mohammed, F., Al-Nahari, A. (eds.) IRICT 2020. LNDECT, vol. 72, pp. 111–121. Springer, Cham (2021). https://doi.org/10.1007/978-3-030-70713-2_12

Challenges on Digital Cyber-Security and Network Forensics: A Survey

Omar Ismael Al-Sanjary[1(✉)], Ahmed Abdullah Ahmed[2], M. N. Mohammed[3], and Kevin Loo Teow Aik[1]

[1] Faculty of Information Sciences and Engineering, Management and Science University, 40100 Shah Alam, Malaysia
omar_ismael@msu.edu.my
[2] Faculty of Engineering and Computer Science, Qaiwan International University (QIU), Slemani Heights, Sulaymaniyah, Iraq
[3] Mechanical Engineering Department, College of Engineering, Gulf University, Sanad, Kingdom of Bahrain

Abstract. There are minimal studies have attempted to shed light on the reality of the challenges and as such, the present paper brings forth studies identifying, quantifying, and prioritizing the challenges to motivate future authors to focus on the issues affecting the domain. Accordingly, a survey was conducted among researchers and practitioners (at the level of law enforcement and organizations) in order to investigate actual challenges and differentiate them from perceived challenges for the purpose of providing insight into the effects upon digital forensic domain in the near future. The study provided and collated a compact survey of the top significant challenges highlighted in the design/development of modern digital forensics tools. The study contributes to the identification of the important, mid- and long-term opportunities and issues that need to be taken into account by the security experts and network forensics in the field investigations fields.

Keywords: Cybersecurity · Cyberattack · DDOS · Network threats · Cybercrime

1 Introduction

Internet has a key role in the network information technology realm, with security of information being the top challenge presently considering the amount of activities done using digital information [1]. In relation to this, cybersecurity combines processes and the protection of secrecy, integrity, practices, technologies design and computer network availability from attacks, damages or access from unauthorized individuals [2, 3]. According to Cybersecurity Ventures, global cybercrime costs is looking at 15% growth every year for the next five years, which will reach to U.S.$10.5 trillion by 2025, a $4 trillion increase from 2020 [4]. Aligned with this is the increased cyberattacks – which on the basis of the Symantec survey involving 20,000 individuals throughout 24 nations, 69% had experienced cyber-attacks in their lifetimes. The survey also found that every second, 14 adults experience cyber-attacks, equating to over one million attacks daily

F. Saeed et al. (Eds.): IRICT 2021, LNDECT 127, pp. 524–537, 2022.
https://doi.org/10.1007/978-3-030-98741-1_43

[5]. The costs incurred for tackling cybercrime covers data damage and destruction, stolen money, lows productivity, intellectual property theft, personal and financial data theft, embezzlement, fraud, fraud, post-attack disruption to the normal business activities, forensic investigation, hacked data/system restoration and deletion, and harm to the reputation. (See Fig. 1.) depicts the costs predicted throughout the period.

On the other hand, cyber criminals need only to incur a few costs relating to obtaining a computer and Internet connection, and are unhindered by geography and distance, difficult to identify and prosecute because of the Internet's anonymous nature. Considering the easy and feasibility that involves in attacking information technology systems, it is predicted that cyber-attacks will continue to grow in number and sophistication. Therefore, this paper conducts an assessment of the cyber security field through a thorough review of literature dedicated to current and less traditional aspects in the field. The study primarily aims to determine significant focus areas in the current academic cyber security research. Given the level of human ability, this part of the study is not intended to develop a detailed information and ontology of cyber security, however inferences are drawn from the findings to determine and highlight current trends, and for the reviewed papers are grouped into general fields [6].

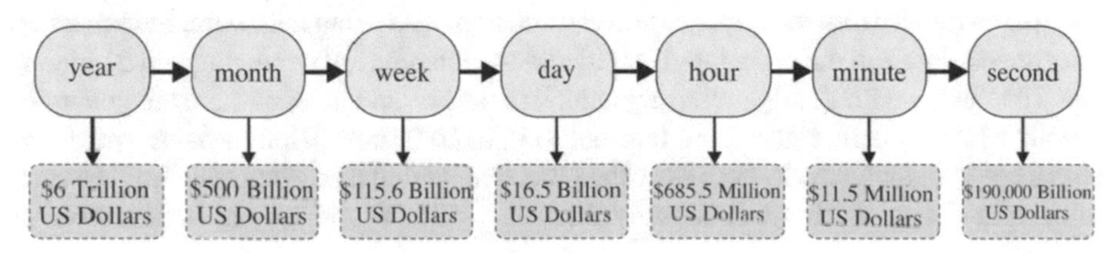

Fig. 1. Global cybersecurity attack cost

The paper furnishes speculative observations as to the directions that future authors can follow, which include; privacy concerns to protect increasing personal information volumes that are entered into the Internet, requirement to have a current secure Internet from scratch while considering the subjected growth and patterns of use, which differs from the scenario of today's internet, and a trustworthy system with a distinct fundamental architecture from its inception in order to address the constantly changing malware. Along with the above are the need to identify and keep track of the attacks source through the development of global scale identity management system and trace-back methods, and also a clear stress on usable security to provide security controls to individuals for their comprehension and control [7, 83]. The survey's objective is to establish and prioritize the major future challenges that digital forensics face with a clear perspective of the various forensic practitioners and forensic researchers' points of view. It is assumed that various researchers' motivations, which focus on longer-term may be distinct from practitioners, who focus on near-term as this may affect the major challenge.

2 Digital Cyber-Security and Network Forensics Methods

In this background, digital forensics also referred to as computer forensics is about using scientific methods to preserve, gather, validate, identify, analyze, interpret, document and present digital evidence obtained from digital sources in order to bring about the development of criminal events. Throughout its history, since its inception, computers have become the target of viruses/worms attacks, and this has urged businesses to consider this security risk. Nevertheless, the present methods used for deploying attacks and penetrating networks are quite covert in a sense that they remain undetected until the attack happens [5, 8].

In addition, literature contains studies that touch upon areas of broad fields that have not been explicitly outlined – for instance, some authors craft ontologies concerning cyber security using manual and automated methods [10–12], Efforts along this line often use fewer inputs, initiating with fundamental phrase of cyber security and conducting automated searches for papers containing the same, and hence, such studies may fall short of covering the complete cyber security scope [9, 84].

It is surprisingly clear that the information security terminology is often aligned with that of national security discourses – in that both are concerned with threats, vulnerabilities, agents, and the like but each of the terms have distinct meanings that should be used with caution. In relation to this, threats can be categorized into various failures, accidents and attacks, with failures being potentially damaging occurrences stemming from the system deficiencies/external element that the system is dependent on. Failures may also originate from the errors in software design, degrading hardware, human errors or corrupted data. On the other hand, accidents cover a range of occurring and damaging events that happen randomly including natural disasters, and most of them are generated external of the system, rather than internal to it, as in failures. Both passive and active attacks could damage the system as is the objective behind a human rival. Attacks form the primary focus of the cyber-security discourse [13, 14] and they are categorized as follows:

i. **Passive attack** – this type of attack takes the form of listening to system passwords, releasing message content, analysing traffic and capturing data.
ii. **Active attack** – in active attack, various activities are adopted including attempts to log into accounts, wire taps, service denial, masquerading, and modifying messages.

Notably, it may be useful for future research to identify with the above for further opportunities, however it is not suggested that any terms in this level be employed as paper keywords. On the whole, the optimal range contains candidate standard terms, while the minimum range contains candidate terms. In the latter range, searching using terms are not covered in the former range and as such, this should be carried out through the combination of many terms in order to obtain accurate results. In the present study, the rejection and suggestion of standard terms involved the consideration of optimal range of cybersecurity terms and cyberattack terms total hits, and this is used when assessing the meeting of required term guidelines (refer to Table 1). The use of suboptimal terms and phrases may be an invaluable research progression aspect in order to make sure that the publications are acceptable.

In the present work, digital cybersecurity and cyberattacks are referred to as using scientifically obtained and proven methods and techniques to identify, preserve, reconstruct, and present digital evidence of the attack/incident obtained from the digital devices. This definition covers digital evidence recovered from the computer as well as digital evidence recovered from the device that are not computers, and from digital activity that falls under an attack or incident [87].

3 Digital Cyber-Security Model

In a security model, significant security aspects and their connections to system behavior are described, with the primary objective of providing the required understanding level of implementation success of major security requirements [73, 82]. In this regard, the security policy has a key role in the determination of the security model contents and as such, good security model development calls for a clear, well-rounded security policy. As for a formal model, development should place reliance on suitable mathematical equations of description and form analysis. Evaluation and usage success should be followed by the model's explanation of security-relevant aspects of the functionality of the system and later on, in the maintenance stage, it should lay down the guidance of undergoing security-relevant changes when needed. Moreover, individual security control and security vulnerability requires one or more key concepts. The fundamental Cyber-Security Model components are; Information Security Properties and Information States and Security Measures [74, 75] (refer to Fig. 2). Every organization and management should consider information security properties as a top priority in a business plan. Such properties entail the protection of organizational data and optimal information systems. Information security assists in the prevention of breaches in confidential assets, data losses, erroneous deletion of data, and inaccurate production of data [73, 76]. The Central Intelligence Agency (CIA) represents the four basic supports of information security as confidentiality, integrity, availability and non-repudiation. In sum, confidentiality involves limitation of data access, integrity ensures accurate data, and availability ensures access to data of those who are authorized and in need This triad is used as the basis for robust information security policies development.

Table 1. Keywords extracted from related methods and additional cybersecurity terms and cyberattack terms

Cybersecurity	Cybersecurity	Cyberattacks	Cyberattacks
CISO [15]	Honey pots [45]	Hacker attack [33]	Zeus Gameover attack [72]
Cloud computing [16]	wireless security [42]	Cracker attack [33]	Carberp attack [85]
Computer abuse [17]	Blockchain technology [46]	Spamming attack [33]	Torpig attack [15]
Critical infrastructure [18]	Digital Watermarking [47]	Ransomware attack [33]	Secure Sockets Layer SSL [28]

(continued)

Table 1. (*continued*)

Cybersecurity	Cybersecurity	Cyberattacks	Cyberattacks
Cryptanalysis [19]	IoT security [48]	Spoofing attack [33]	Router attack [33]
Cryptography [19]	Social protection application [38]	Active attack [14]	Cryptowall attack [71]
Cryptology [19]	Digital Forensics [40]	Denial-of-service (DoS) attack [63]	Emotet attack [19]
Crypto-assets [20]	Privacy settings [49]	Distributed Denial-of-service (DDoS) attack [63]	Cryptojacking attack [28]
Cryptocurrencies [17]	cyber-physical security [22]	Phishing attack [64]	Virtual private network [11]
Cybercrime [20]	Cybersquatting [50]	IP attack [37]	Shellshock attack [22]
Cyberlaw [20]	CyberSlam [23]	Drive-by attack [18]	Browser attack [13]
Cyberoperation [21]	Computer Intrusions [31]	Password attack [37]	Brute force attack [14]
Cyberphysical [22]	Cyber sextortion [51]	SQL injection attack [68]	Internal attack [15]
Cyberthreat [23]	Cyber Criminology [52]	Cross-site scripting (XSS) [68]	External attack [16]
Cyberwar [24]	Cyber Deterrence [53]	Eavesdropping attack [37]	Man-in-the-middle attack [17]
Antivirus programs [25]	Cybernetics [54]	Malware attack [64]	Social engineering attacks [10]
Antispyware software [25]	Cyber Extortion [55]	Trojan Horses [37]	Adversarial attacks [11]
Monitored internet access [26]	Cyber Vandalism [79]	Birthday attack [27]	Panic attacks [12]
Cloud security [27]	Cyberterrorism [56]	Botnets attack [31]	Server attack [14]
Cryptojacking [28]	Cybertherapy [57]	Access control attack [26]	DNS attack [33]
Cyberbullying [29]	Cyberharassment [58]	Asset attack [17]	Address Resolution Protocol (ARP) attacks [37]
Cyberspace [29]	Cybergeddon [56]	Data Structure attack [17]	Smurf attack [37]
Digital Signature [30]	Hacktivism [56]	Unstructured attack [66]	Hijacking [33]
Demilitarized Zone (DMZ) [31]	Cyber physical systems [18]	Passive attack [14]	BlackHole attack [46]

(*continued*)

Table 1. (*continued*)

Cybersecurity	Cybersecurity	Cyberattacks	Cyberattacks
Steganography [32]	Cybercriminal [20]	Risk Management [39]	Wormhole attacks [67]
Firewall [31]	Rogue security software [37]	URL attack [37]	Sybil attack [69]
Internet service provider (ISP) [31]	Cryptovirology [59]	Water Hole Attack [33]	Sinkhole attack [70]
Intrusion detection system (IDS) [31]	Cloud computing security [16]	Zero-Day Exploits [67]	jamming attack [71]
Intrusion prevention system (IPS) [31]	Mobile cloud security [38]	Viruses/Worms attack [37]	Wrapping Attack [17]
Incident Response (IR) [33]	Automotive security [91]	Vulnerability [42]	Online Auction Fraud [37]
Security information and event management (SIEM) [34]	Cyber information warfare [25]	Spyware [37]	Non-Delivery Merchandise fraud [37]
Cyberconflict [35]	CyberStrike [60]	Backdoor attack [19]	Fake Escrow Services [9]
Cyberdomain [36]	CyberGames [61]	Email attacks [19]	Slowloris attacks [72]
Countermeasures [37]	Cyberethics [62]	Teardrop attacks [12]	Session Downgrade Attacks [21]
Cyber Stalking [37]	Cyber forensics [40]	SYN Flood attack [13]	Data scraping attack [22]
Network Security [37]	Cybergeography [19]	Buffer Overflow attack [54]	Byzantine Attacks [23]
Application Security [38]	Cybergogy [59]	Credit/Debit Card Fraud [28]	Fabrication Attacks [24]
Mobile Security [38]	Cyberweapon [24]	Identity Theft [42]	Honeypot attack [45]
Security Assessments [39]		Investment Fraud [17]	User Emulation attack [26]
Anti-forensics [40]		Freight Forwarding/ Reshipping scheme [17]	Shellcode attack [28]
Computer Forensics [40]		Ponzi and Pyramid Schemes [66]	Fork bombs [23]
Darknet [41]		File Inclusion attacks [15]	Fraudulent dialers [24]
Hybrids Security [42]		Malicious attack [16]	Logic bombs [25]
CryptoLocker [43]		Adware attack [17]	Evil Maid attack [29]
Dedicated Internet Access (DIA) [31]		Crimeware attack [24]	Image tampering [65]

(*continued*)

Table 1. (*continued*)

Cybersecurity	Cybersecurity	Cyberattacks	Cyberattacks
CAPTCHA Security [44]		Mobile Malware attack [64]	Video tampering [65]
Threat Detection [42]		Rootkit attack [20]	Data tampering attacks [65]
System Security [42]		Bot attack [21]	Code injection [28]
Prevention System [31]		SpyEye attack [12]	

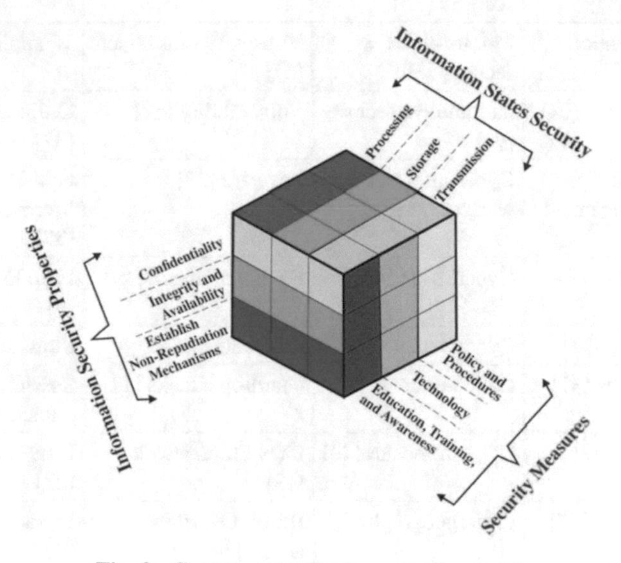

Fig. 2. Components of cyber-security model

4 Cybercrime Investigation Process

Extensive and expansive processes of cybercrime investigations are a must for the standardization of terminology, requirements definition and enabling new techniques development and investigation tools [65, 77]. Cybercrime scene investigation involves an activity within which judicial entity observes and inspects the crime scene based on law to comprehend the case circumstances and to gather required evidence. In addition, an effective cybercrime investigation process is crucial in providing an abstract reference framework, which is not dependent on specific technological/organizational context, based on which techniques and technologies for supporting the investigators work can be discussed. It can also function as a basis for common terminology for expertise sharing. The investigation process is useful in developing and applying methodologies to new emerging technologies as they become the topic behind the investigations. In the same way, a relevant model can be useful in identifying opportunities for development and use of technology so that work of investigators are enabled and the requirements for investigative tools are captured and analyzed - this is particularly true for advanced automated analytical tools. Presently, processes that are directed specifically to cybercrime investigations are still lacking, with the proposed models focusing only towards a part of the investigative process (gathering, analyzing and presenting evidence), while overlooking other important aspects.

Literature evidences several investigation processes, which are briefly described in this section. The models are limited to the investigations of the crime scene and the evidence is not as extensive in their encapsulation compared to the proposed models. To begin with, [78, 79] brought forward a process consisting of four stages, namely recognition, preservation, classification and reconstruction. This process mimics with that presented by [104, 108] in the initial and final stage, and it focuses on a systematic and methodical investigation technique of any digital crime case. However, the process is limited to digital forensic process and does not cover data acquisition (preparation and presentation). Added to the above, digital forensic research workshop (DFRWS) [65, 81] developed and proposed a model with the steps involving, identification, preservation, collection, examination, analysis, presentation and decision [78, 107]. The model can be considered as a comprehensive one as it has a tendency to include stages that were not included by prior models (e.g., presentation stage).

The previous section elaborated on the processes utilized and now the question arises as to how to develop and update digital forensic investigation process. The present process failed to focus on the entire cybercrime investigation aspects, but rather emphasized on the digital evidence processing [78, 80]. The design of the existing models failed to indicate the information process flow and address issues like chain of custody or chain of identity. In fact, in most of the presented investigation processes, the latest gap exists in tackling fragile evidence and data acquisition process [78]. Lack of stages addressing such aspect could mean an unstable cybercrime investigation. The new steps of cybercrime investigation proposed are displayed in the following Fig. 3. In the figure, the cybercrime investigation process begins with the identification phase which assumes the recognition and determination of the incident type – this step is crucial as all the remaining steps hinges on it. This is followed by the preparation step, where tools, techniques, search warrants, monitoring authorization and management support are prepared. The approach strategy is then introduced in a step that maximizes the evidence collection while at the same time mitigating the impact on the victim through approaches/procedures formulation [85, 86]. The next phase involves preserving the acquired data by isolating and securing them to maintain their authenticity. The entire digital evidence is also duplicated and the physical scene recorded on the basis of standardized procedures under the collection step. The examination step involves in-depth systematic analysis of evidence that links to the case and this is followed by the analysis phase which determines the probative value of the examined evidence. Presentation phase summarizes the develop process, while returning evidence step culminates the investigation process by returning physical and digital evidence to their owner.

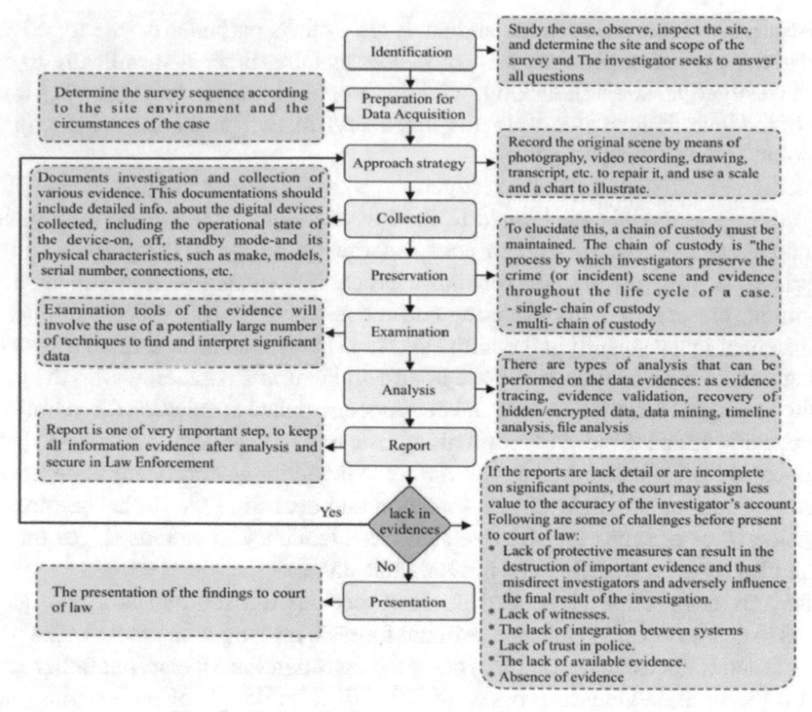

Fig. 3. Steps of cybercrime investigation process

5 Conclusion

Throughout the past decade and a half, attack of digital cybersecurity and network forensics has been rampant. Because the Internet has become the chosen medium of communication for billions of web users through which they can share their interests, photos, videos and engage with their friends without geographic and economic barriers. Using such services however could leave users vulnerable to serious cyber security risks and this paper provided a state-of-the-art study of various privacy/security issues in digital cyber-security. The paper provided a summary of the recent attack statistics and security reports documented by security organizations and cyber security and cyber-attacks blogs. The paper also addressed the security state of cyber-security by presenting three malicious code attacks categories, namely vulnerabilities, threat and risk management. Based on the presentation, a new analysis of cybercrime investigation process is proposed to assist relevant research respond to developments in technology and investigations.

References

1. Jang-Jaccard, J., Nepal, S.: A survey of emerging threats in cybersecurity. J. Comput. Syst. Sci. **80**(5), 973–993 (2014)
2. Li, L., He, W., Xu, L., Ash, I., Anwar, M., Yuan, X.: Investigating the impact of cybersecurity policy awareness on employees' cybersecurity behavior. Int. J. Inf. Manage. **45**, 13–24 (2019)

3. Kshetri, N.: Blockchain's roles in strengthening cybersecurity and protecting privacy. Telecommun. Policy **41**(10), 1027–1038 (2017)
4. Internet Security Threats Report. Cybercrime Magazine. https://cybersecurityventures.com/cybercrime-damage-costs-10-trillion-by-2025/. Accessed 13 Nov 2020
5. https://pcmag.com/article2/0.2817.2392570.00.asp. Accessed June 2013
6. Ishak, Z., Rajendran, N., Al-Sanjary, O.I., Razali, N.A.M.: Secure biometric lock system for files and applications: a review. In: 2020 16th IEEE International Colloquium on Signal Processing & Its Applications (CSPA), pp. 23–28. IEEE , February 2020
7. Mohammed, T.L., Ahmed, A.A., Al-Sanjary, O.I.: KRDOH: kurdish offline handwritten text database. In: 2019 IEEE 7th Conference on Systems, Process and Control (ICSPC), pp. 86–89. IEEE (2019)
8. Al-Sanjary, O.I., Ibrahim, O.A., Sathasivem, K.: A new approach to optimum steganographic algorithm for secure image. In: 2020 IEEE International Conference on Automatic Control and Intelligent Systems (I2CACIS), pp. 97–102. IEEE, June 2020
9. Al-Sanjary, O.I., Ahmed, A.A., Zangana, H.M., Ali, M., Aldulaimi, S., Alkawaz, M.: An investigation of the characteristics and performance of hybrid routing protocol in (MANET). Int. J. Eng. Technol. **7**(4.22), 49–54 (2018)
10. Iannacone, M., et al.: Developing an ontology for cyber security knowledge graphs. In: Proceedings of the 10th Annual Cyber and Information Security Research Conference, pp. 1–4, April 2015
11. Takahashi, T., Kadobayashi, Y.: Reference ontology for cybersecurity operational information. Comput. J. **58**(10), 2297–2312 (2015)
12. Khairkar, A.D., Kshirsagar, D.D., Kumar, S.: Ontology for detection of web attacks. In: 2013 International Conference on Communication Systems and Network Technologies, pp. 612–615. IEEE, April 2013
13. Ahmed, A.A., Hasan, H.R., Hameed, F.A., Al-Sanjary, O.I.: Writer identification on multi-script handwritten using optimum features. Kurdistan J. Appl. Res. **2**(3), 178–185 (2017)
14. Nasr, M., Shokri, R., Houmansadr, A.: Comprehensive privacy analysis of deep learning: passive and active white-box inference attacks against centralized and federated learning. In: 2019 IEEE symposium on security and privacy (SP), pp. 739–753. IEEE, May 2019
15. Tari Schreider, S.S.C.P., CISM, C., CISO, I.: Building Effective Cybersecurity Programs: A Security Manager's Handbook. Rothstein Publishing (2017)
16. Zissis, D., Lekkas, D.: Addressing cloud computing security issues. Futur. Gener. Comput. Syst. **28**(3), 583–592 (2012)
17. Corbet, S., Meegan, A., Larkin, C., Lucey, B., Yarovaya, L.: Exploring the dynamic relationships between cryptocurrencies and other financial assets. Econ. Lett. **165**, 28–33 (2018)
18. Yusta, J.M., Correa, G.J., Lacal-Arántegui, R.: Methodologies and applications for critical infrastructure protection: state-of-the-art. Energy Policy **39**(10), 6100–6119 (2011)
19. Stinson, D.R., Paterson, M.: Cryptography: Theory and Practice. CRC Press (2018)
20. Butkovic, A., Mrdovic, S., Uludag, S., Tanovic, A.: Geographic profiling for serial cybercrime investigation. Digit. Investig. **28**, 176–182 (2019)
21. Kim, Y.G.: Deception tree model for cyber operation. In: 2019 International Conference on Platform Technology and Service (PlatCon), pp. 1–4. IEEE , January 2019
22. Alguliyev, R., Imamverdiyev, Y., Sukhostat, L.: Cyber-physical systems and their security issues. Comput. Ind. **100**, 212–223 (2018)
23. Mavroeidis, V., Bromander, S.: Cyber threat intelligence model: an evaluation of taxonomies, sharing standards, and ontologies within cyber threat intelligence. In: 2017 European Intelligence and Security Informatics Conference (EISIC), pp. 91–98. IEEE (2017)
24. Kaiser, R.: The birth of cyberwar. Polit. Geogr. **46**, 11–20 (2015)

25. Shukla, J.B., Singh, G., Shukla, P., Tripathi, A.: Modeling and analysis of the effects of antivirus software on an infected computer network. Appl. Math. Comput. **227**, 11–18 (2014)
26. Tynes, B., Reynolds, L., Greenfield, P.M.:Adolescence, race, and ethnicity on the Internet: a comparison of discourse in monitored vs. unmonitored chat rooms. J. Appl. Dev. Psychol. **25**(6), 667–684 (2004)
27. Kandukuri, B.R., Rakshit, A.: Cloud security issues. In: 2009 IEEE International Conference on Services Computing, pp. 517–520 (2009)
28. Eskandari, S., Leoutsarakos, A., Mursch, T., Clark, J.: A first look at browser-based cryptojacking. In: 2018 IEEE European Symposium on Security and Privacy Workshops (EuroS&PW), pp. 58–66 (2018)
29. Slonje, R., Smith, P.K., Frisén, A.: The nature of cyberbullying, and strategies for prevention. Comput. Hum. Behav. **29**(1), 26–32 (2013)
30. Harn, L.: Group-oriented (t, n) threshold digital signature scheme and digital multisignature. IEEE Proc. Comput. Digit. Tech. **141**(5), 307–313 (1994)
31. Chowdhary, A., Dixit, V.H., Tiwari, N., Kyung, S., Huang, D., Ahn, G.J.: Science DMZ: SDN based secured cloud testbed. In: 2017 IEEE Conference on Network Function Virtualization and Software Defined Networks (NFV-SDN), pp. 1–2. IEEE, November 2017
32. Cheddad, A., Condell, J., Curran, K., Mc Kevitt, P.: Digital image steganography: survey and analysis of current methods. Signal Process. **90**(3), 727–752 (2010)
33. Schneier, B.: The future of incident response. IEEE Secur. Priv. **12**(5), 96 (2014)
34. Miller, D.R., Harris, S., Harper, A., VanDyke, S., Blask, C.: Security Information and Event Management (SIEM) Implementation. McGraw Hill Professional (2010)
35. Karatzogianni, A.: The Politics of Cyberconflict. Routledge (2006)
36. Hoffman, R.R., Lee, J.D., Woods, D.D., Shadbolt, N., Miller, J., Bradshaw, J.M.: The dynamics of trust in cyberdomains. IEEE Intell. Syst. **24**(6), 5–11 (2009)
37. Hazelwood, S.D., Koon-Magnin, S.: Cyber stalking and cyber harassment legislation in the United States: a qualitative analysis. Int. J. Cyber Criminol. **7**(2), 155–168 (2013)
38. Li, Q., Clark, G.: Mobile security: a look ahead. IEEE Secur. Priv. **11**(1), 78–81 (2013)
39. Kirschen, D.S., Jayaweera, D.: Comparison of risk-based and deterministic security assessments. IET Gener. Transm. Distrib. **1**(4), 527–533 (2007)
40. Stamm, M.C., Liu, K.R.: Anti-forensics of digital image compression. IEEE Trans. Inf. Forensics Secur. **6**(3), 1050–1065 (2011)
41. Biddle, P., England, P., Peinado, M., Willman, B.: The darknet and the future of content protection. In: Feigenbaum, J. (eds) Digital Rights Management. DRM 2002. Lecture Notes in Computer Science, vol. 2696, pp. 155–176 Springer, Berlin, Heidelberg (2002). https://doi.org/10.1007/978-3-540-44993-5_10
42. Stamm, M.C., Lin, W.S., Liu, K.R.: Forensics vs. anti-forensics: a decision and game theoretic framework. In: 2012 IEEE International Conference on Acoustics, Speech and Signal Processing (ICASSP), pp. 1749–1752. IEEE, March 2012
43. Liao, K., Zh, Z., Do, A., Ahn, G.J.: Behind closed doors: measurement and analysis of CryptoLocker ransoms in Bitcoin. In: 2016 APWG Symposium on Electronic Crime Research (eCrime) p. 113 (2016)
44. von Ahn, L., Blum, M., Hopper, N.J., Langford, J.: CAPTCHA: using hard AI problems for security. In: Biham, E. (eds) Advances in Cryptology — EUROCRYPT 2003. EUROCRYPT 2003. Lecture Notes in Computer Science, vol. 2656, pp. 294–311. Springer, Berlin, Heidelberg. https://doi.org/10.1007/3-540-39200-9_18
45. Dagon, D. et al.: HoneyStat: local worm detection using honeypots. In: Jonsson, E., Valdes, A., Almgren, M. (eds.) Recent Advances in Intrusion Detection. RAID 2004. Lecture Notes in Computer Science, vol. 3224. Springer, Berlin, Heidelberg, pp. 39–58 (2004). https://doi.org/10.1007/978-3-540-30143-1_3

46. Mohanta, B.K., Jena, D., Panda, S.S., Sobhanayak, S.: Blockchain technology: a survey on applications and security privacy challenges. Internet Things **8**, 100107 (2019)
47. Cox, I.J., Miller, M.L., Bloom, J.A., Honsinger, C.: Digital Watermarking, vol. 53. Morgan Kaufmann, San Francisco (2002)
48. Xiao, L., Wan, X., Lu, X., Zhang, Y., Wu, D.: IoT security techniques based on machine learning: How do IoT devices use AI to enhance security? IEEE Sign. Process. Mag. **35**(5), 41–49 (2018)
49. Ghazinour, K., Matwin, S., Sokolova, M.: YOURPRIVACYPROTECTOR, A recommender system for privacy settings in social networks (2016). arXiv preprint arXiv:1602.01937
50. Mercer, J.D.: Cybersquatting: Blackmail on the information superhighway. BUJ Sci. Tech. L. **6**, 290 (2000)
51. Clark, J.F.: Growing threat: Sextortion. US Att'ys Bull **64**, 41 (2016)
52. Jaishankar, K.: Cyber criminology as an academic discipline: history, contribution and impact. Int. J. Cyber Criminol. **12**(1), 1–8 (2018)
53. Crosston, M.D.: World gone cyber MAD: how mutually assured debilitation is the best hope for cyber deterrence. Strat. Stud. Q. **5**(1), 100–116 (2011)
54. Krippendorff, K.: The cybernetics of design and the design of cybernetics. In: Fischer, T., Herr, C. (eds.) Design Cybernetics. Design Research Foundations. Springer, Cham. pp. 119–136 (2019). https://doi.org/10.1007/978-3-030-18557-2_6
55. Ibarra, J., Jahankhani, H., Kendzierskyj, S.: Cyber-physical attacks and the value of healthcare data: facing an era of cyber extortion and organised crime. In: Jahankhani, H., Kendzierskyj, S., Jamal, A., Epiphaniou, G., Al-Khateeb, H. (eds.) Blockchain and Clinical Trial. Advanced Sciences and Technologies for Security Applications, pp. 115–137. Springer, Cham. https://doi.org/10.1007/978-3-030-11289-9_5
56. Denning, D.E.: Activism, hacktivism, and cyberterrorism: the Internet as a tool for influencing foreign policy. Netw. Netwars Future Terror Crime Milit. **239**, 288 (2001)
57. Spagnolli, A., Bracken, C.C., Orso, V.: The role played by the concept of presence in validating the efficacy of a cybertherapy treatment: a literature review. Virt. Real. **18**(1), 13–36 (2014)
58. Van Laer, T.: The means to justify the end: combating cyber harassment in social media. J. Bus. Ethics **123**(1), 85–98 (2014)
59. Young, A.L., Yung, M.: Cryptovirology: the birth, neglect, and explosion of ransomware. Commun. ACM **60**(7), 24–26 (2017)
60. Vandaele, K., van der Velden, S., Dribbusch, H., Lyddon, D., Vandaele, K.: From the Seventies Strike Wave to the First Cyber-Strike in the Twenty-First Century, pp. 196–205. Aksant, Amsterdam (2007)
61. Wimmer, J.: Digital game culture(s) as prototype(s) of mediatization and commercialization of society: the world cyber games 2008 in cologne as an example. In: Fromme, J., Unger, A. (eds.) Computer Games and New Media Cultures. Springer, Dordrecht, pp. 525–540 (2012) . https://doi.org/10.1007/978-94-007-2777-9_33
62. Pusey, P., Sadera, W.A.: Cyberethics, cybersafety, and cybersecurity: preservice teacher knowledge, preparedness, and the need for teacher education to make a difference. J. Digit. Learn. Teach. Educ. **28**(2), 82–85 (2011)
63. Kandula, S., Katabi, D., Jacob, M., Berger, A.: Botz-4-sale: Surviving organized DDoS attacks that mimic flash crowds. In: Proceedings of the 2nd conference on Symposium on Networked Systems Design & Implementation-Volume 2, pp. 287–300 (2005)
64. Leukfeldt, E.R., Kleemans, E.R., Stol, W.P.: Cybercriminal networks, social ties and online forums: social ties versus digital ties within phishing and malware networks. Br. J. Criminol. **57**(3), 704–722 (2017)
65. Al-Sanjary, O.I., Ahmed, A.A., Sulong, G.: Development of a video tampering dataset for forensic investigation. Forensic Sci. Int. **266**, 565–572 (2016)

66. Suo, H., Liu, Z., Wan, J., Zhou, K.: Security and privacy in mobile cloud computing. In: 2013 9th International Wireless Communications and Mobile Computing Conference (IWCMC), pp. 655–659. IEEE (2013)
67. Sun, X., Dai, J., Liu, P., Singhal, A., Yen, J.: Using Bayesian networks for probabilistic identification of zero-day attack paths. IEEE Trans. Inf. Forensics Secur. **13**(10), 2506–2521 (2018)
68. Lee, I., Jeong, S., Yeo, S., Moon, J.: A novel method for SQL injection attack detection based on removing SQL query attribute values. Math. Comput. Model. **55**(1–2), 58–68 (2012)
69. Abbas, S., Merabti, M., Llewellyn-Jones, D., Kifayat, K.: Lightweight sybil attack detection in manets. IEEE Syst. J. **7**(2), 236–248 (2012)
70. Salehi, S.A., Razzaque, M.A., Naraei, P., Farrokhtala, A.: Detection of sinkhole attack in wireless sensor networks. In: 2013 IEEE international conference on space science and communication (IconSpace) , pp. 361–365. IEEE, July 2013
71. Shi, Y., Sagduyu, Y.E., Erpek, T., Davaslioglu, K., Lu, Z., Li, J.H.: Adversarial deep learning for cognitive radio security: jamming attack and defense strategies. In: 2018 IEEE international conference on communications workshops (ICC Workshops), pp. 1–6. IEEE (2018)
72. Shorey, T., Subbaiah, D., Goyal, A., Sakxena, A., Mishra, A.K.: Performance comparison and analysis of slowloris, goldeneye and xerxes ddos attack tools. In: 2018 International Conference on Advances in Computing, Communications and Informatics (ICACCI), pp. 318–322. IEEE (2018)
73. Peltier, T.R.: Implementing an information security awareness program. Inf. Secur. J. A Glob. Perspect. **14**(2), 37–49 (2005)
74. Kao, D.-Y.: Cybercrime investigation countermeasure using created-accessed-modified model in cloud computing environments. J. Supercomput. **72**(1), 141–160 (2015). https://doi.org/10.1007/s11227-015-1516-7
75. Al-Sanjary, O.I., Ghazali, N., Ahmed, A.A., Sulong, G.: Semi-automatic methods in video forgery detection based on multi-view dimension. In: Saeed, F., Gazem, N., Patnaik, S., Saed Balaid, A.S., Mohammed, F. (eds.) IRICT 2017. LNDECT, vol. 5, pp. 378–388. Springer, Cham (2018). https://doi.org/10.1007/978-3-319-59427-9_41
76. Ahmed, A.A., Al-Sanjary, O.I., Kaeswaren, S.: Reserve parking and authentication of guest using QR Code. In: 2020 IEEE International Conference on Automatic Control and Intelligent Systems (I2CACIS), pp. 103–106. IEEE (2020)
77. Casey, E.: Handbook of Digital Forensics and Investigation. Academic Press (2009)
78. Ciardhuáin, S.Ó.: An extended model of cybercrime investigations. Int. J. Digit. Evid. **3**(1), 1–22 (2004)
79. Abushahma, R.I.H., Ali, M.A., Al-Sanjary, O.I., Tahir, N.M.: Region-based convolutional neural network as object detection in images. In: 2019 IEEE 7th Conference on Systems, Process and Control (ICSPC), pp. 264–268. IEEE (2019)
80. Reust, J., Friedburg, S.: DFRWS 2005 Workshop Report. http://www.dfrws.org/2005/download/2005final.Pdf (2006)
81. Al-Sanjary, O.I., et al.: Deleting object in video copy-move forgery detection based on optical flow concept. In: 2018 IEEE Conference on Systems, Process and Control (ICSPC), pp. 33–38. IEEE (2018)
82. Al-Sanjary, O.I., Sulong, G.: Detection of video forgery: a review of literature. J. Theor. Appl. Inf. Technol. **74**(2) (2015)
83. Al-Sanjary, O.I., Ahmed, A.A., Jaharadak, A.A.B., Ali, M.A., Zangana, H.M.: Detection clone an object movement using an optical flow approach. In: 2018 IEEE Symposium on Computer Applications & Industrial Electronics (ISCAIE), pp. 388–394. IEEE (2018)

84. Alkawaz, M.H., Steven, S.J., Hajamydeen, A.I.: Detecting phishing website using machine learning. In: 2020 16th IEEE International Colloquium on Signal Processing & Its Applications (CSPA), pp. 111–114 (2020)
85. Che Hamid, H.E., et al.: Disaster management support model for Malaysia. In: Badioze Zaman, H., et al. (eds) Advances in Visual Informatics. IVIC 2019. LNCS, vol. 11870, pp. 570–581. Springer, Cham (2019). https://doi.org/10.1007/978-3-030-34032-2_50
86. Hajamydeen, A.I., Udzir, N.I.: A detailed description on unsupervised heterogeneous anomaly based intrusion detection framework. Scalable Comput. Pract. Exper. **20**(1), 113–160 (2019)
87. Aidee, N.A.N., Johar, M.G.M., Alkawaz, M.H., Hajamydeen, A.I., Al-Tamimi, M.S.H.: Vulnerability assessment on ethereum based smart contract applications. In: 2021 IEEE International Conference on Automatic Control & Intelligent Systems (I2CACIS), pp. 13–18 (2021)

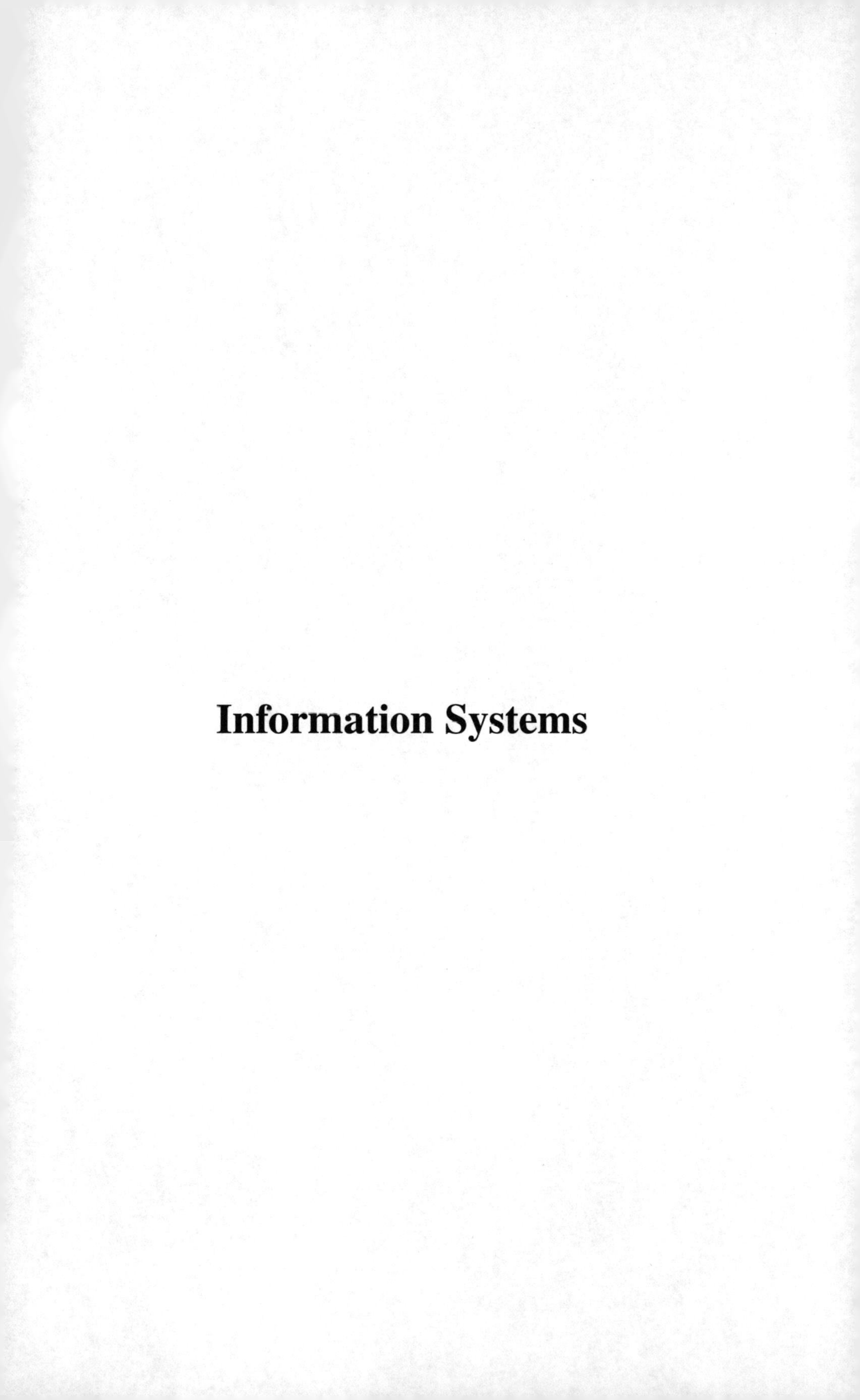

Information Systems

A Model of Trusted Factors of Video Word of Mouth (vWOM) in Social Commerce

Humaira Hairudin and Halina Mohamed Dahlan(✉)

Information System Department, Azman Hashim International Business School (AHIBS), Universiti Teknologi Malaysia (UTM) Skudai Johor, Skudai Johor, Malaysia
humairahairudin@graduate.utm.my, halina@utm.my

Abstract. In this digital era, many people often searching information before make purchase decision. The vWOM might be considered as resources for customer to searching beneficial information that can increase customer trust to purchase online. However, there is still less study conducted about what is significant attributes of vWOM that make them effective in influence purchase intention. This study identified trusted factors of vWOM that can influence purchase intention and also identified a suitable theory for develop a model of trusted factors of vWOM. Therefore, this study identify Rhetoric theory is suitable theory and developed a conceptual model of trusted factors of vWOM in social commerce which consists of seven factors which is informative, credible, perceived transparency, perceived benefit, perceived emotion, expertise and attractiveness. All the factors identified are categorized under definition of each Rhetoric theory's elements.

Keywords: Video word of mouth · Purchase intention · vWOM

1 Introduction

With the emergence of internet, product review using video format is considered as a new and developing trend. Video word of mouth or shortly called as vWOM is defined as a product review using video format that provide individual faces and vivid demonstrations [1]. The vWOM is created by the reviewer to convey their real experience and provides helpful information which can help customers to find trusted product information through online platform [2]. The vWOM also defined as audiovisual content that display characteristics of product to introduce the product to customer, which can convey the product information to help customer purchase decision making [3]. Therefore, the vWOM is determined have powerful persuasive effects that can increase customers trust and influence their purchase intention [1].

During online shopping, customers often exposed to being inconveniently to physical touch of the products and feeling unsatisfactory to make high quality decision by plainly depending with product information provided by seller [4]. Hence, by using trusted vWOM, customer has ability to see the product in action, where customer cannot test the product as in physical store [5]. Moreover, it can help customers to understand the product affordances such as functionalities of different parts of the product. Customer

F. Saeed et al. (Eds.): IRICT 2021, LNDECT 127, pp. 541–550, 2022.
https://doi.org/10.1007/978-3-030-98741-1_44

also can watch the interaction between the reviewer and the product featured in the video that enhance customer understanding about the product affordances [7]. In social commerce, there many customers are rely on vWOM before make purchase decision. However, there is still less study conducted about what is significant attributes of vWOM that make them effective and help generate favorable perceptions among customers [6].

Apparently, vWOM has a much more powerful persuasive effective due to the multimedia presentation because it can show how the products work or not. However, how such vWOM can be trusted is still unknown [1]. Numerous studies have found that vWOM posted using online video sharing platform to share information with online customers [18, 9, 10, 13, 8], but to date lack of studies looking on the how communication is carried out through the video that can be trusted and can influence purchase intention. Besides, a number of authors have reported the characteristics of reviewer in the video [11, 12], however, far too little attention has been paid to video content that the reviewer can conveyed to the audiences to increase customer trust [13]. Therefore, this study will develop a conceptual model of trusted factors of vWOM in social commerce that can influence purchase intention and help customer to avoid wasteful purchase.

This paper is organized into five sections. The first section is about the introduction of vWOM and the research problem. The literature review is explained in Sect. 2, while Sect. 3 is about the research methodology applied in this study. Then, Sect. 4 explains about the findings and last but not least, Sect. 5 is about the conclusion of this study.

2 Literature Review

2.1 Video Word of Mouth (vWOM)

vWOM is video based on eWOM that refer to online product review video that created by individual and posted through social commerce platform. The vWOM is online product review using video based format, which is show the individual faces and provide product demonstrations to share information to the customers and lead to purchase intention [1]. vWOM is defined as the reviewer can convey a great deal of information to the customers using videos through language verbally and non-verbally [11]. The reviewer can convey the information by explain briefly about the characteristics of product to introduce them to the customer through vWOM that can ease customer purchase decision making [3].

By using YouTube as online video sharing platform for upload vWOM, it can enhance consumer's perception towards the value of products and it is easy to searching the information that matching with the customer's needs. This can strengthen customer's awareness about the products by include relevant information into the video created [25]. Besides, the reviewer also can upload vWOM through TikTok platform where it is more convenient to create and share vWOM packed with music and special effects that typically lasting between 15 s to a few minutes [26].

2.2 Research Related Video Word of Mouth (vWOM)

Many people use social media for entertainment platform but it is should be viewed as communicating platform as well. Previous scholar identified that video theme is important for creator to choose the suitable topics or specific information that can give benefits to the viewer [8]. Besides, the credible information is important in order to delivering factual description about products, attributes, and people that can increase customer trust [9]. The informative video content could provide specific information to customers which help in their purchase decision making [10]. Previous study explains that informativeness can be measured by which explanations or completeness of the information from reviewers that conveys to the customers can help them to searching credible product information through online platform [11].

Nowadays, communication is important to convey the information in the vWOM. Previous scholar also pointed out that in the vWOM normally have individual character being shown most in the video and playing the leading role. The good image and have professional background would encourage people more believe with the individual who communicate in the video [8]. The credible speaker should have high knowledge background to provide valid information and evidence to the audience [12, 13]. In addition, the speaker also tends to focus on what they can convey the information, so communication appears more reliable and professional [11]. Moreover, the reviewer that has attractiveness, skilled, abilities and expertise in certain field to be qualified to convey effective and valid information to the customers can influence purchase intention [14].

Another previous scholar discuss about emotion focused has either positive or negative emotion. Positive emotion is give good impressions of the product such as love, joy, and excitement. While negative emotion and expressing negative feelings are such as sadness, shame and anger [1, 9]. In addition, emotion that could be found in the vWOM is enjoyable, fun, and pleasing may attract them to watch the vWOM without feel boring [10, 11]. Perceived enjoyment is an active feeling which activity conducted is considered pleasurable that can contribute to customer behaviour [11]. The reviewer provides right expression to stir with the audience's emotion, which the expression look like a representation of customer feeling toward the product. A few cheerful and smiles expression also needed to applied in some humor messages to entertain the customer [12].

2.3 Rhetoric Theory

The rhetoric theory is based on Aristotle's persuasive communication method that consists of three effective elements of rhetoric which include Logos, Ethos, and Pathos, where it is expected to provide enrichment in communication theory. Logos refers to the validity of arguments, Ethos refers to speaker's credibility or characteristics, and Pathos refers to the ability of emotions [15]. Based on previous study, three effective elements of rhetoric which is consist of logos, pathos and ethos applied in order to examine how the vWOM help strengthen the connection between customers and the reviewer [16].

The logos is verbal messages that contain information such as evidence and arguments [12]. Moreover, Logos refer to the arguments in favor of strengthening of the connection or information presented by the speaker due to the exposure of social media marketing activities [16]. Logos used in this study refer to provide valid and accurate information in the video that might helpful and useful for customer. Meanwhile, the pathos appears in serious nonverbal messages to influence the emotions of the audience [12]. In other words, Pathos refer to the feelings evoked to the customers which expressed through the communication [16]. Phatos used in this study refers to how to deliver the communication with emotion in the vWOM. Besides, another element which is Ethos refers to the credibility of the sources or speaker [16]. Therefore, Ethos is use credible speaker that have high knowledge background to convey information to the audience [12]. Ethos used in this study refers to character of the reviewer in the vWOM.

3 Research Methodology

The methodology used in this paper consists of two phases which are:

Phase 1: Identification of trusted factors of vWOM that can influence purchase intention based on literature review. In finding the trusted factors, this study using database platform such as Google Scholar, Scopus, ScienceDirect, IEEE Xplore, and other institution available database access. The searching strategy for identify the factors is based on the keywords used which related to the domain of this study. The information will be taken from each article to derive the factors of vWOM. There are 371 selected studies from online database platform that relevant and related to this domain study. According to the selected studies, there are 30 factors of vWOM are identified. Next, all the identified vWOM factors will be analyzed based on weight of criteria and definition of trust. The weight of criteria of the vWOM factors are calculated which results only seven factors of vWOM achieved weight of criteria more than 0.5. Seven factors identified from previous literature review which is perceived emotion, informative, credible, perceived transparency, perceived benefit, expertise, and attractiveness.

Phase 2: The development model of trusted video word of mouth (vWOM) which consists of seven factors identified from previous literature review which is perceived emotion, informative, credible, perceived transparency, perceived benefit, expertise, and attractiveness. In addition, this study also identifies the relevant theory for adapt in the model development which is Rhetoric theory. Hence, this steps results the development model of trusted factors of vWOM that adapted Rhetoric theory. The Rhetoric theory identified is suitable to provide enrichment in communication theory. Moreover, Rhetoric refers to competency of individual to identify existing means to convince another individual [15].

4 Findings

4.1 Trusted Factors of Video Word of Mouth (vWOM)

Based on the literature review, the selected factors are analyzed based on definition of trust which is considered as trusted factors of vWOM that can influence purchase intention. The definition of trust explains that vWOM provided is able to act in the customer's interest which involves honest, competent, benevolent, and predictable [27]. Therefore, trust is important in the social media platform where the vWOM created and delivered must effectively provide trusted information, advice and service [28]. The trusted factors of vWOM identified are informative, credible, perceived transparency, perceived benefit, expertise, attractiveness, and perceived emotion.

Informative refer to the amount of information could provide to customers in the video which is beneficial in customer purchase decision making. The information provided must be a good source of product information to explain the useful of product reviewed in the video, which can lead to purchase intention. The informative factor considered as utmost priority in the vWOM when customers seeking for online product information [10]. In general, informative consists of product features, the use of product, price, and news for upcoming events that can give knowledge to the customer and can influence purchase intention. Moreover, the informative vWOM may maintain the interest of potential customer that seeking for information through vWOM before make purchase decision [17].

The video credibility is defined as the believability and trustworthiness based on customer perception towards the video. The video is perceived credible as provide credible information that may help to enhance customer trust toward the product effectiveness and this will leading to purchase intention about the product [10]. The video that provide credibility to the audiences is to enhance trust of customer toward the video content. Customer will put a trust on the video if the video is trustworthiness and useful in aided customer to make purchase decision [18].

The video review is considered as perceived benefit if it can confirm the customer the positive and negative things about the product before to purchase. The perceived benefit video can help customer to make a good purchase and can avoid the purchase risk [19]. If the reviewer provides information that has benefit through vWOM, it will help customer to think carefully to determine whether the purchase made will be worthy. The benefit of information is perceived by customer that may influence them toward perceptions of product value. Therefore, information that perceived benefit is depends on the reviewer experience for consuming the product either feel satisfied or unsatisfied [20].

Perceived transparency is described as an effort to provide clear and relevant information regarding products and business to the customers. For example, transparent communication about the product related cost and price is perceived higher level of information sensitivity. Hence, the practice of disclosing cost and product information can help build perception of customer towards the perceived product transparency and authenticity [21]. Besides, the vWOM should provide specific information such as features and functions of product in order to facilitate customer's understanding of a product. By provide product feature information, it can help customer to have better understanding and can determine whether the product features can satisfy their needs [22].

In the vWOM, emotions are one of the most influential factors during process of decision making. By showing positive emotions in the video, it has positive effect on customer satisfaction and may be influenced with the reviewer to purchase the product exposed in the vWOM. There are nine positive emotions can be identified in the vWOM such as joy, love, pride, hope, amusement, compassion, contentment and gratitude [20]. The emotion provided may convince customer to purchase the product if the emotion shown is satisfy the customer. It is because positive emotion expression in the vWOM can create the feeling among the audience to feel the same way as the reviewer. Moreover, it also can make the audience feel good and have positive mood to purchase [9].

Expertise can be described by how much a reviewer is capable of providing valid and credible information in the video. The individual who share informative sources and helpful information to the customers is believed as credible and reliable reviewer. It can be seen through the reviewer's words that show his/her competence, reliability, and good will [16]. Hence, the reviewer tend to be more professional in convey the relevant information, which make the customers respond more favorably towards the reviewer. The expertise of the reviewer perceived by the customers after watching vWOM will influence their attitude towards the product exposed in the vWOM [23].

Physical attractiveness is defined as an attractiveness and beautiful face which determine the first impression in a moment. Besides, the attractiveness of reviewer perceived by customers after watching vWOM will lead the customers to have positive attitude toward information sharing and product exposed through the vWOM [23]. Customers are more easily influenced by the physical attractiveness of the reviewer during review the product. It is because the attractiveness of the reviewer is considered as a strong factor in determining an ability of the reviewer to persuade customers to make purchase decision [24].

4.2 Trusted Video Word of Mouth (vWOM) Model

In order to understanding the trusted factors of vWOM in influencing purchase intention, this study needs to identify the suitable theory used for develop a model. This study identify the Rhetoric theory is suitable for model of trusted factors of vWOM. Rhetoric theory consist of Therefore, the figure below shows a model of trusted factors of vWOM (see Fig. 1).

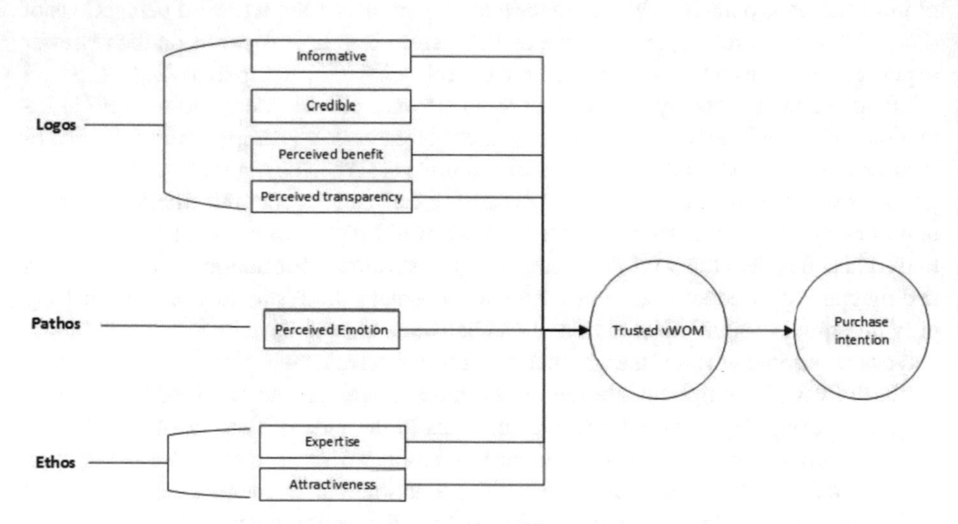

Fig. 1. Trusted vWOM model.

Based on the Fig. 1 above, the four factors identified which is informative, credible, perceived benefit and perceived transparency are categorized under logos. Logos used in this study refer to provide valid and accurate information in the video that might helpful and useful for customer [12]. Next, Phatos used in this study refers to how to deliver the communication about the vWOM [16]. Hence, Perceived emotion is categorized under

Phatos because the reviewer can show their emotion expression in the vWOM. Lastly, two factors identified which is expertise and attractiveness is categorized under ethos. Ethos used in this study refers to character of the reviewer in the video [15]. It is because expertise and attractiveness are related to character of the user who talking in the video. The operational definition of rhetoric elements and its factors is as in Table 1 below.

Table 1. Trusted factors and rhetoric elements

Trusted factors	Definition of trusted factors	Rhetoric elements	Definition of rhetoric elements
Informative	Completeness and sufficient of information or explanation from reviewer can be conveyed to the customers [10]	Logos	The arguments on the subject presented by the speaker [16]
Credible	The truthfulness and believability of the vWOM [12]		
Perceived benefit	Beneficial information which helpful for purchase decision [29]		
Perceived transparency	The information provided in the video need to be truthful and balance [11]		
Perceived emotion	The emotion expression presented in the video [8]	Pathos	Expressed emotions between the speaker and audiences [30]
Expertise	The reviewer that has background knowledge and expert in certain field to be qualified [31]	Ethos	The credibility of the speaker [16]
Attractiveness	The degree of attraction of the reviewer to the customers [31]		

5 Conclusion

In conclusion, this study identifies the trusted factors of vWOM based on literature review that can increase customer trust and influence purchase intention. Due to pandemic, customers often exposed to being inconveniently to physical touch of the products because customer cannot test the product as in physical store. Therefore, this study develops a model of trusted factors of vWOM that can help customer who seeking credible information about the product through online platform. Literature review is adapted in this study in order to identify the trusted factors of vWOM and suitable theory. The selected trusted factors of vWOM are calculated which is achieved weight of criteria and analyzed based on trust definition. Besides, Rhetoric theory is identified in this study as suitable theory for a model of trusted factors of vWOM because it is related with communication theory. The findings from this paper is development conceptual model of trusted factors of vWOM in social commerce which consists of informative, credible, perceived transparency, perceived benefit, perceived emotion, expertise, and attractiveness. In the future, this study can be extended in order to develop hypothesis and evaluate the model.

References

1. Bi, N.C., Zhang, R., Ha, L.: Does valence of product review matter?: the mediating role of self-effect and third-person effect in sharing youtube word-of-mouth (vWOM). J. Res. Interact. Mark. **13**(1), 79–95 (2019)
2. Diwanji, V.S., Cortese, J.: Contrasting user generated videos versus brand generated vide-os in ecommerce. J. Retail. Consum. Serv. **54**, 102024 (2020)
3. Orús, C., Gurrea, R., Flavián, C.: Facilitating imaginations through online product presentation videos: effects on imagery fluency, product attitude and purchase intention. Electron. Commer. Res. **17**(4), 661–700 (2016). https://doi.org/10.1007/s10660-016-9250-7
4. Lah, N.S.B.C., Hussin, A.R.B.C., Dahlan, H.B.M.: Information relevance factors of argument quality for e-commerce consumer review. Adv. Intell. Syst. Comput. **843**, 871–881 (2019)
5. Yu, Y.W., Natalia, Y.: The effect of user generated video reviews on consumer purchase intention. In: Proceedings - 7th International Conference on Innovative Mobile and Internet Services in Ubiquitous Computing, IMIS 2013, pp. 796–800 (2013)
6. Ghosh, T.: How to make effective product review videos: the influence of depth, frame, and disposition on consumers. J. Electron. Commer. Organ. **18**(4), 73–92 (2020). https://doi.org/10.4018/JECO.2020100104
7. Fang, K., et al.: Demo2Vec: reasoning object affordances from online videos. In: Proceedings of the IEEE Computer Society Conference on Computer Vision and Pattern Recognition, pp. 2139–2147. https://doi.org/10.1109/CVPR.2018.00228 (2018)
8. Zhu, C., Xu, X., Zhang, W., Chen, J., Evans, R.: How health communication via tik tok makes a difference: a content analysis of tik tok accounts run by Chinese provincial health committees. Int. J. Environ. Res. Public Health **17**(1), 1–13 (2020)
9. Tellis, G.J., MacInnis, D.J., Tirunillai, S., Zhang, Y.: What drives virality (sharing) of online digital content? the critical role of information, emotion, and brand prominence. J. Mark. **83**(4) pp. 1–20 (2019).
10. Bezbaruah, S., Trivedi, J.: Branded content: a bridge building gen Z's consumer-brand relationship. Vision **24**(3), 300–309 (2020)
11. Fitriani, W.R., Mulyono, A.B., Hidayanto, A.N., Munajat, Q.: Reviewer's communication style in YouTube product-review videos: does it affect channel loyalty?, Heliyon, **6**(9), e04880 (2020)

12. Sofian, F.A.: YouTubers creativity in creating public awareness of COVID-19 in Indonesia: a youtube content analysis. In: International Conference on Information Management and Technology (ICIMTech), (August), pp. 881–886 (2020)
13. Sokolova, K., Kefi, H.: Instagram and YouTube bloggers promote it, why should I buy? How credibility and parasocial interaction influence purchase intentions. J. Retail. Consum. Serv. 53, 101742 (2020)
14. Chen, J.-L., Dermawan, A.: The Influence of youtube beauty vloggers on Indonesian Consumers' purchase intention of local cosmetic products'. Int. J. Bus. Manag. **15**(5), 100 (2020)
15. Aristotle: On Rhetoric: A Theory of Civic Discourse. Edited by G. A. Kennedy and G. A. Kennedy. Oxford University Press (1991)
16. Panigyrakis, G., Panopoulos, A., Koronaki, E.: All we have is words: applying rhetoric to examine how social media marketing activities strengthen the connection between the brand and the self. Int. J. Advert. **39**(5), 699–718 (2020)
17. Kefi, H. and Maar, D.: The power of lurking: assessing the online experience of luxury brand fan page followers. J. Bus. Res. (2017), pp. 0–1 (2018) .https://doi.org/10.1016/j.jbusres.2018.08.012
18. Yang, K.C., Huang, C.H., Yang, C., Yang, S.Y.: Consumer attitudes toward online video advertisement: YouTube as a platform. Kybernetes **46**(5), 840–853 (2017)
19. Mumuni, A.G., Lancendorfer, K.M., O'Reilly, K.A., MacMillan, A.: Antecedents of consumers' reliance on online product reviews. J. Res. Interact. Mark. **13**(1), 26–46 (2019)
20. Bueno, S., Gallego, M.D.: eWOM in C2C platforms: combining IAM and customer satisfaction to examine the impact on purchase intention. J. Theor. Appl. Electron. Commer. Res. **16**(5), 1612–1630 (2021). https://doi.org/10.3390/jtaer16050091
21. Yang, J., Battocchio, A.F.: Effects of transparent brand communication on perceived brand authenticity and consumer responses. J. Prod. Brand Manag. (September) (2020). https://doi.org/10.1108/JPBM-03-2020-2803
22. Zhou, L., et al.: Perceived information transparency In B2C e-commerce: an empirical investigation. Inf. Manag. **55**(7), 912–927 (2018). https://doi.org/10.1016/j.im.2018.04.005
23. Choi, W., Lee, Y.: Effects of fashion vlogger attributes on product attitude and content sharing. Fashion Text. **6**(1), 1–18 (2019). https://doi.org/10.1186/s40691-018-0161-1
24. Benito, S.M., Illera, A.E., Fernández, E.O.: Youtube celebrity endorsement: audience evaluation of source attributes and response to sponsored content a case study of influencer verdeliss. Commun. Soc. **33**(3), 149–166 (2020). https://doi.org/10.15581/003.33.3.149-166
25. Yadav, M.S. et al.: Social commerce: a contingency framework for assessing marketing potential. J. Inter. Mark. **27**(4), 311–323 (2013). https://doi.org/10.1016/j.intmar.2013.09.001
26. Shao, T., Wang, R., Hao, J.X.: Visual destination images in user-generated short videos: an exploratory study on Douyin. In: 2019 16th International Conference on Service Systems and Service Management, ICSSSM 2019, (2), pp. 1–5 (2019). https://doi.org/10.1109/ICSSSM.2019.8887688
27. McKnight, D.H., Chervany, N.L.: What trust means in e-commerce customer relationships: an interdisciplinary conceptual typology. Int. J. Electron. Commer. **6**(2), 35–59 (2001). https://doi.org/10.1080/10864415.2001.11044235
28. Abdulgani, M.A., Suhaimi, M.A.: Exploring factors that influence Muslim intention to purchase online. In: 2014 the 5th International Conference on Information and Communication Technology for the Muslim World, ICT4M 2014, pp. 1–6 (2014). https://doi.org/10.1109/ICT4M.2014.7020637
29. Xu, P., Chen, L., Santhanam, R.: Will video be the next generation of e-commerce product reviews? Presentation format and the role of product type',. Decis. Supp. Syst. **73**, 85–96 (2015). https://doi.org/10.1016/j.dss.2015.03.001

30. Huber, A., Pable, J.: Aristotelian appeals and the role of candidate-generated videos in talent assessment. Int. J. Art Des. Educ. **38**(1), 90–109 (2019). https://doi.org/10.1111/jade.12176
31. Ananda, A. F. and Wandebori, H.: The impact of drugstore makeup product reviews by beauty vlogger on youtube towards purchase. In: International Conference on Ethics of Business, Economics, and Social Science, vol. 3, no. 1, pp. 264–273 (2016)

Information Quality Requirements for a Nutrition App Based on Experts Interviews

Siti Asma Mohammed(✉), Mohamed Aden Ighe, and Azlin Nordin

Kulliyyah of Information and Communication Technology, IIUM, Selangor, Malaysia
siti_asma@iium.edu.my

Abstract. Many people nowadays are using nutrition and dietary apps to manage their health by monitoring their food and calorie intake. Online health information enables people to search for specific health-related information that may concern them in the comfort and privacy of their home. Thus, the quality of such information is crucial to ensure people are getting the right and reliable information. The objective of this paper is to present the information quality requirements for nutrition app by analysis of experts' interviews. The interview was conducted using semi structured interview with five nutritionists. The finding from the interviews show that a nutrition app should include a complete, reliable, accurate and updated information.

Keywords: Information quality · Nutrition app

1 Introduction

There is an increasing number of nutrition health applications which are reaching more and more people with a new kind of nutrition information [1, 2]. Many internet users are seeking for information on diet, nutrition, vitamins or nutritional supplements [3]. Consequently, credibility and reliability of the massive information produced in nutrition app has become the major concern to the healthcare providers [1]. Due to outdated references or sources from the food composition database, several applications have failed to offer exact, dependable and consistent information about specific foods to their users [4, 5] and lack of quality-control procedures [6]. Nutritionists and system developers should collaborate early on in the development process to implement the information quality criteria [6, 7] in order to avoid rework and poor information in nutrition apps. Most research on nutrition apps information are focusing on the user's behavior change and influence of the use of nutrition information to healthy eating [1, 5]. However, research on the kind of quality information that are required in order to have a quality by design nutrition app is still limited. As a result, this paper goal is to suggest the dimensions of information quality for nutrition apps. The significance of this research is that users with inadequate internet skills and lower computer literacy might unknowingly access inaccurate information that is potentially dangerous to their health. Searching online nutrition or dietary information are becoming a trend as many people are trying to manage their own nutrition intakes nowadays and willing to change their lifestyle [1].

F. Saeed et al. (Eds.): IRICT 2021, LNDECT 127, pp. 551–558, 2022.
https://doi.org/10.1007/978-3-030-98741-1_45

2 Information Quality for Online Health Information

Information quality is known as fitness for use, which means that the information must corresponds with user tasks according to the context usage [8, 9]. The information should also have clear purpose and created under certain policies and procedures [10]. In terms of online health information, Health on the Net (HON) is a quality instrument that certifies medical and health websites, which provides high quality and transparent health information [11, 12]. Table 1 explains the HON principles [13].

Table 1. The HON principles and their definition. (Source [13])

Principle	Definition
Authoritative	Medical and health information provided are only given by medically trained and qualified professionals
Complementarity	The information is meant for supplementary rather than replace the user-physician interactions
Privacy	Information of the users are kept confidential
Attribution	The information is supported by clear references to source data and the most recent date of updated information is clearly mentioned
Justifiability	Any claims about the efficacy of a treatment, a product or a service must be backed up by scientific proof
Authorship transparency	Contact information should be available for users who require additional information or assistance from the site or app
Financial disclosure	Identities of the funder for the site or app should be acknowledged
Advertising policy	Advertising policy should be displayed

Nevertheless, poor information quality can still be found in some nutrition apps. Several existing studies that evaluated nutrition apps highlighted the common issues found often related to accuracy, completeness, timeliness and reliability of the information, in which this research has chosen to investigate further. For example, [14] and [15] found that the information on food composition in some free nutrition apps are inaccurate. Poor information was found in five apps, where the information from food database are not relevant and are not based on reliable sources [5, 14]. As for [16], they found that some food database information are not updated regularly.

3 Methodology

This research uses qualitative method to get in-depth understanding of nutrition information and the quality requirements from nutrition experts by applying Goal-Questions-Metric (GQM) approach to design a semi structured interview questions. GQM is a suitable approach to design an interview protocol for a specific measurement setting [17].

3.1 The Objective of the Interview

The main objective of the interview is to investigate the perception of the experts on the important information requirements for a nutrition application based on the chosen information quality dimensions. Table 2 presents the interview protocol based on GQM approach, including the aim of the interview, the questions to investigate and the metrics to support the purpose of each inquiry.

Table 2. The interview protocol based on GQM approach.

Goal: To investigate the information quality requirements for nutrition apps	
Question	Metric
Q1: Tell me what kind of information should be included in the nutrition app?	M1: Personal opinion on including the actual use of information the nutrition app
Q2: Who are responsible for providing the information?	M2: Personal opinion on the information ownership or authorship - relating to reliability dimension
Q3: How do you make sure the information in a nutrition app always available to the users?	M3: Personal opinion on the information completeness in the nutrition app - relating to completeness and accuracy dimension
Q4: What are the information that needs to be updated from time to time?	M4: Personal opinion on updated information that should be in the app - relating to timeliness dimension

3.2 Selection of Experts

The experts from this interview were 5 nutritionists. The selection criteria includes within 5 years of experience in the nutrition field, has practicing or non-practicing background with formal education background in nutrition. Purposive sampling was used because it is the most effective method when one needs to study a certain domain with knowledgeable experts [18]. Table 3 explains the background of nutritionists based on years of experience and relevance.

3.3 Data Collection and Analysis

All conversations during the interview were audio recorded. The duration for each interview lasted between 45 min to 1 h. Every recorded interview was transcribed carefully into text document for analysis. Thematic analysis was used to analyze the collected data for interpretation.

4 Results

The result from thematic analysis are divided into three. First, the stakeholders and their roles, which indicate to reliability or authorship of the information. Second is types

Table 3. Background of nutritionists.

Nutritionist	Relevance	Years of experience
N1	Nutritional science officer	5+
N2	Nutritional science officer	5+
N3	Lecturer and researcher for nutrition and diets	5+
N4	Lecturer and researcher for nutrition and diets	15+
N5	Researcher and developer for nutrition apps	9+

of information required for a nutrition app to ensure the accuracy, completeness and timeliness of the information, and third is the overall information quality requirements for a nutrition app.

4.1 Stakeholders and Roles

According to the nutritionist experts, there are three types of stakeholders for a nutrition app. First stakeholder is the nutritionist. The nutritionist is the person who provides the app with food, nutrition and weight management information. Nutritionist is responsible of ensuring that the information offered in the nutrition app is of high quality. The information provided should come from valid sources such as the World Health Organization (WHO) and Malaysia Food Composition Database (MyFCD). MyFCD includes all the food composition targeting for Malaysia local population. The second stakeholder is the app developer. According to all the experts, the app developer is responsible to ensure that all the provided information coming from the nutritionists should be translated into the app accurately and completely, while the app end-user is the third stakeholder that will provide information relating to his or her nutrition intake, weights, calories, physical activities and diets including feedback in the app. Nutritionist 1 and 2 explained that end-users are also responsible for the accurate and complete information of their own personal data and the information on their food intake, which they provide through the app in order to manage their weight. Other than that, users also can provide comments and feedback in the app if they find any inaccurate and incomplete information from the app. This will help the nutritionist to always improve the quality of the app information.

4.2 Types of Information

The major functions that should be included in a nutrition app, according to all the nutritionist experts, are the Body Mass Index (BMI) calculator, food calorie dictionary, meal diary, weight record and the user's calorie intake. All experts believe that the information should include a variety of local and popular food lists,as well as a BMI classification and calculation based on Asian or International standards. Expert 1 said the current MyFCD that is being used currently in Malaysia is dated back in 1997. He agrees that the food database needs to be updated as there are many food recipes are being invented in the market and restaurant, especially on hipster food as the people nowadays call.

4.3 Information Quality Requirements

All the experts agree that accuracy, completeness, timeliness and reliability are among the important dimensions that indicate the quality of information in nutrition app. Table 4 depicts the definition of each dimension with regard to the information that should be in a nutrition app. These four dimensions are also among the existing issues that contribute to the poor information quality as found in the literature.

Table 4. Information quality requirements for nutrition app.

Dimension	Description
Reliability	• Reliability of nutrition and dietary guidelines for the local population. For example, MyFCD • Reliability of the food database, food diary, its servings and nutrition facts • Reliability of the references and sources originality • Reliability of authority to the nutrition app. For example, Ministry of Health
Accuracy	• Accuracy of the nutrition information • Accuracy of the provided information coming from valid references or sources • Accuracy of the BMI, ideal weight range index and calorie intake calculations • Accuracy of the user feedback in the app
Completeness	• Complete records of food composition data and nutrition facts provided in the app • Complete records of food servings, calorie intakes, weight by the app user for BMI calculation • Complete information on frequently asked questions (FAQs) in the app for the users
Timeliness	• Update frequency of the nutrition information • Timeliness of the information provided • Timeliness for the food composition database and its nutrition facts • Timeliness of users provided information and feedbacks

In terms of authorship and reputation, all experts agree that the information in nutrition app must be trustworthy and reliable. As Nutritionist 4 mentioned "*..user will trust the information as long as the nutritionist able to give the correct information and can validate that the information comes from reliable reference..*". Nutritionist 3 also agreed that reliability is an important criterion for a nutrition app as according to him, "*..the issues that we have found with many app, less than 50% of the apps, the data and information they have are not really reliable..*"

As for accuracy, the information is considered true and free from errors with respect to valid and reliable sources. Nutritionist 3 mentioned "*Accuracy of the content must go into proper procedure…we have to go into validation with nutritionist expert as well as the users…*".

The completeness of the input records by the nutritionists and the app users in the nutrition app are perceived importance as Nutritionist 4 mentioned "*..the information* *from the app should cater on user needs including food portions and calorie intake that can manage the eating habit of the user*". On the other hand, Nutritionist 3 said completeness of information also include the frequent question and answer feature so that expert can always add new information in order to make it complete and available to the users. "*..there should be something like Q&A in which user can ask whatever information that are not there (in the app)..*" as mentioned by Nutritionist 3.

In term of timeliness, the nutrition app's information must constantly be up to date for the users and must be based on the most recent evidence. Nutritionist 3 mentioned that even the data used by Malaysia nutritionists is from MyFCD, which is last updated in 1997, the information are still valid. It is the responsibility of the nutritionist to make sure the information is always recent and to answer the user feedback and queries with the latest information.

5 Discussion

This research is conducted to investigate the information quality requirements for a nutrition app. Identifying the quality requirement at the early stages of development is crucial to ensure high quality information in the app. This research found that inaccurate and untrustworthy content such as unavailable references and authorship can make the user misunderstand [19] as well as complicating their decision making options to manage their health [20]. Other than that, the findings shows that information quality can be achieved when all the stakeholders - nutritionist, app developer and app end-user are aware of their responsibility in providing the correct and complete input into the app. Information quality is important and need to be defined in the early phase of system/app development to avoid rework. The app has to be designed in such a way it fits the usage of various stakeholders, otherwise becomes useless or lack of use.

6 Conclusion

This research presents the information quality requirements by analysis of experts' opinions on the meaning of reliability, accuracy, completeness and timeliness for developing a nutrition app. Lack of study has been focusing on identifying the quality requirements at the beginning of system or app development, which becomes the motivation for conducting this research. The overall results show that in order to determine the quality requirements, stakeholders and their roles will also determine the quality of the information. All the experts agree that reliability, accuracy, timeliness and completeness are important in order to have quality information in nutrition app. Our future research is to develop a nutrition app that is based on the information quality requirements from this study.

Acknowledgments. We would like to express gratitude to the Ministry of Higher Education Malaysia to fund this project under Fundamental Research Grant Scheme (FRGS19–075-0683) and to our university, International Islamic University Malaysia (IIUM) for the invaluable support.

References

1. Zarnowiecki, D., et al.: A systematic evaluation of digital nutrition promotion websites and apps for supporting parents to influence children's nutrition. Int. J. Behav. Nutr. Phys. Activ. **17**(1), 1-19 (2020)
2. Adamski, M., Truby, H., M Klassen, K., Cowan, S., Gibson, S.: Using the internet: Nutrition information-seeking behaviours of lay people enrolled in a massive online nutrition course. Nutrients. **12**(3), 750 (2020)
3. Ahmad, N., Rahman, A.B., Jasman, N., Zaman Salleh, K., Harun, S.,N.F., Krishnan, M.: Usage of internet for health information seeking among elderly in Malaysia. EPRA Int. J. Multidiscipl. Res. (IJMR) **6**(5), 187–193 (2020)
4. Tosi, M., et al.: Accuracy of applications to monitor food intake: Evaluation by comparison with 3-d food diary. Nutrition. **84**, 111018 (2021)
5. Ferrara, G., Kim, J., Lin, S., Hua, J., Seto, E.: A focused review of smartphone diet-tracking apps: usability, functionality, coherence with behavior change theory, and comparative validity of nutrient intake and energy estimates. JMIR mHealth uHealth. **7**(5), e9232 (2019)
6. Holzmann, S.L., Proll, K., Hauner, H., Holzapfel, C.: Nutrition apps: Quality and limitations. an explorative investigation on the basis of selected apps. Ernaehrungs Umsch. **64**, 80–9 (2017)
7. Gabrielli, S., et al.: Design of a mobile app for nutrition education (TreC-LifeStyle) and formative evaluation with families of overweight children. JMIR mHealth uHealth **5**(4), e7080 (2017)
8. Wang, R.Y., Strong, D.M.: Beyond accuracy: What data quality means to data consumers. J. Manag. Inf. Syst. **12**(4), 5–33 (1996)
9. English, L.P.: Information Quality Applied: Best Practices for Improving Business Information, Processes and Systems. Wiley Publishing (2009)
10. Liaw, S.T., et al.: Quality assessment of real-world data repositories across the data life cycle: a literature review. J. Am. Med. Inform. Assoc. **28**(7), 1591–1599 (2021)
11. Boyer, C., et al.: Health on the net's 20 years of transparent and reliable health information. In: Exploring Complexity in Health: An Interdisciplinary Systems Approach, pp. 700–704. IOS Press (2016)
12. Daraz, L., et al.: Can patients trust online health information? a meta-narrative systematic review addressing the quality of health information on the internet. J. Gen. Intern. Med. **34**(9), 1884–1891 (2019)
13. Health on the Net foundation, HONcode, Health on the Net Foundation. http://www.hon.ch/HONcode. Accessed 28 Sept 2021
14. Braz, V.N., de Moraes Lopes, M.H.: Evaluation of mobile applications related to nutrition. Public Health Nutr. **22**(7), 1209–1214 (2019)
15. DiFilippo, K.N., Huang, W.H., Chapman-Novakofski, K.M.: Mobile apps for the dietary approaches to stop hypertension (DASH): app quality evaluation. J. Nutr. Educ. Behav. **50**(6), 620–625 (2018)
16. Schumer, H., Amadi, C., Joshi, A.: Evaluating the dietary and nutritional apps in the google play store. Healthc. Inform. Res. **24**(1), 38–45 (2018)
17. Ya'u, B.I., Nordin, A., Salleh, N.: Analysis of expert's opinion on requirements patterns for software product families framework using GQM method. In: Alfred, R., Lim, Y., Haviluddin, H., On, C.K. (eds.) Computational Science and Technology. LNEE, vol. 603, pp. 135–144. Springer, Singapore (2020). https://doi.org/10.1007/978-981-15-0058-9_14
18. Patton, M.Q.: Qualitative Research & Evaluation Methods: Integrating Theory and Practice. Sage Publications (2014)

19. Wong, D.K., Cheung, M.K.: Online health information seeking and ehealth literacy among patients attending a primary care clinic in Hong Kong: a cross-sectional survey. J. Med. Internet Res. **21**(3), e10831 (2019)
20. Xiao, Y., et al.: Challenges in data quality: the influence of data quality assessments on data availability and completeness in a voluntary medical male circumcision programme in Zimbabwe. BMJ open. **7**(1), e013562 (2017)

Design of Test Data Generation Method for Dynamic- Functional Testing in Automatic Programming Assessment Using Flower Pollination Algorithm

Nurhidayah Mokhtar[1](✉), Rohaida Romli[1], Rusnida Romli[2], Alawiyah Abd Wahab[1], and Nooraini Yusoff[3]

[1] School of Computing, Universiti Utara Malaysia, Kedah, Malaysia
kroerysher2@gmail.com, {aida,alawiyah}@uum.edu.my
[2] Faculty of Electronic Engineering Technology, Universiti Malaysia Perlis (UniMAP), Perlis, Malaysia
rusnida@unimap.edu.my
[3] Institute For Artificial Intelligence and Big Data (AIBIG), Universiti Malaysia Kelantan (UMK), Kota Bharu, Kelantan, Malaysia
nooraini.y@umk.edu.my

Abstract. Automatic Programming Assessment (APA) is one of the vital methods that has been applied around Computer Science education in realizing automated marking and grading on students' programming exercises or assignments. APA is fundamentally relying upon a test data generation process to perform a dynamic testing. Recently in Software Testing (ST) research, it has been proven that the adoption of any Meta-Heuristic Search Techniques (MHSTs) is able to improve the efficiency of generating adequate and optimal test data. Unfortunately, current studies on APA have not yet usefully incorporated the techniques to include a better quality program testing coverage by considering the optimal size of generated test data. Thus, our study propose a method of generating and locating an adequate test data with optimal in size by adapting a MHST to satisfy the dynamic-functional testing in APA (or is called DyFunFPA-TDG method). In this paper, we merely focus on revealing the design of the method with a sample of the generated test cases to be used in APA. This method able to assist educators of elementary programming courses to provide the means of deriving and generating adequate test data with optimal in size regardless of having the expertise in specific knowledge of test cases design.

Keywords: Automatic programming assessment · Test data generation · Dynamic testing · Flower pollination algorithm

1 Introduction

Practically, learning programming has become a common challenge among students of Computing related disciplines particularly when they are at the basic level of programming efficiency. As acquiring certain extend of programming skills towards the end of

F. Saeed et al. (Eds.): IRICT 2021, LNDECT 127, pp. 559–570, 2022.
https://doi.org/10.1007/978-3-030-98741-1_46

learning process is vital, hence the students need to be provided with lots of programming exercises and assignments to allow them getting familiar and consistently practice the programming concepts and principles accordingly. Programming skills are usually evaluated by practical programming tasks which are typically either based on homework assignments or laboratory hands-on [1]. Unfortunately, this circumstance causes burdensome to the educators when dealing with programming exercises' assessment and evaluation manually. Also, manual way of assessing these exercises through hardcopies and softcopies has been deemed as costly, inflexible and time-consuming [2]. Thus, Automatic Programming Assessment (or APA) has been identified as a method to overcome this challenge so as to improve the accuracy, consistency, and efficiency of assessing the programming assignments [3]. There have been several APA tools were developed such as Assyst [4], BOSS [5], TRAKLA2 [6], CourseMaster [7], SAC [8] and Bottlenose [9] to realize APA and particularly in assisting educators.

The fundamental concept of programming assessments is related to Software Testing (ST) [4, 10]. Static analysis and dynamic testing have been acknowledged as the main testing techniques or strategies that are typically implemented in ST. The dynamic testing needs a tested program to be executed against a set of inputs or test data. Test data generation is one of the processes of identifying a set of test data which satisfies a given testing criterion [11]. Process of preparing high quality test data manually is commonly known as a hard, time consuming, and impractical task in practice [12]. Thus, as resolving these difficulties, Automated Test Data Generation (ATDG) has become desirable and vital among researchers for decades [13].

Nowadays, Meta-Heuristic Search Techniques (or MHSTs) have been demonstrated to be the significant techniques to resolve ATDG issues [14]. The techniques able to explore the search area efficiently and find the best solution for any particular problem [14]. One of the new optimization algorithms for solving global problem optimization is the Flower Pollination Algorithm (FPA) [16]. Due to the reduced parameter required to solve the tuning parameter problem, FPA is easy to implement compared to other algorithms [15]. Thus far, studies as proposed by [16] have proven FPA can be successfully applied in supporting efficient ATDG in ST field. There is a significant gap in the use of ATDG and MHST in APA, especially for functional testing. Thus far, merely a study conducted by [17] attempted to integrate ATDG and MHST in APA (see Sect. 2). Therefore, our study proposes a method for generating test data to produce and locate a suitable collection of test data with an optimum size that satisfies the dynamic-functional testing in APA that is called DyFunFPA-TDG method. In this paper, the focus is on the design of test cases for the method with a relevant sample of programming exercises.

The content of the remaining sections is organized as follows: Sect. 2 provides a brief discussion on some related works. Section 3 details out the design of DyFunFPA-TDG method. Section 4 briefly depicts the realization of the DyFunFPA-TDG method as a test cases design based on a sample of programming exercise, and finally, Sect. 5 concludes the paper.

2 Related Work

In a software development cycle (in terms of time and cost), Software Testing (ST) is vital and considered as an expensive phase. Practically, in this phase, the process of generation of test data is commonly known as one of the main issues. Test data generation is one of the processes of identifying a set of test data which satisfies a given testing criterion [11]. Also, it is one of the difficult tasks in ST and can be very burdensome and effortful process [18]. Thus, as an alternative, Automated Test Data Generation (ATDG) has become crucial and attentive among researchers for decades [13].

To date, in current literatures, a lot of studies proposed approaches for automating the process of test data generation [13] to furnish the better means of generating adequate test data. Also, in ST field, Meta-Heuristic Search Techniques (MHST) have been empirically proven as the technique that able to derive and generate adequate and optimal test data. Among the most common MHSTs used in test data generations include Simulated Annealing (SA), Gradient Descent, Taboo Search (TS), Ant Colony Optimization (ACO) and Evolutionary Algorithms such as Genetic Algorithm (GA) [19]. The techniques were broadly applied to resolve the test data generation problems due to the fact that the techniques can be formulated as an optimization [20]. Latest study by Nasser et al. [21] found out that Flower pollination algorithm (FPA) has promising result to be implemented in ATDG.

The integration of MHST into APA only began in 2014 [17] and the focused merely on structural testing. In this study, a Particle Swarm Optimization (PSO) algorithm was utilized to automatically generate test cases and then being applied for Online Programming Assessment or Judge (UOJ) system. The focus is not concerned with ATDG but more on test cases generation only. Based on this finding, it can be deduced that utilizing MHST to support testing in APA is still at its early stages, and to the very best of our knowledge, none of the studies attempted to utilize the technique as to support more efficient ATDG in APA. Realizing the benefits of FPA and supported by a signification impact of utilizing MHST in ATDG, hence, there is massive room of research to show up to look upon resolving the existing gaps of ATDG in APA.

3 Methodology

This study was carried out by following the research procedures as shown in Table 1.

Table 1. Research procedures

Phase	Activity	Method
Theoretical study	• Study related terminology and concepts involved in the research • Searching for related issues • Investigation of earlier works related to APA, ATDG, an integration of APA and ATDG, MHSTs utilization on ATDG and ATDG in APA • Explore possible solution by utilizing Flower Pollination Algorithm (FPA) in supporting ATDG in APA	• Literature survey
Construction of the DyFunFPA-TDG method	• Construct criteria of test data and test set schema • Mapping and integrating FPA and the identified test data and test set schema • Design DyFunFPA-TDG method	• Positive and negative testing criteria for functional testing + FPA • Algorithm of DyFunFPA-TDG method
Test data generator Implementation and Testing	• Develop a test data generator (a prototype) to realize DyFunFPA-TDG method • Testing the prototype	• Prototyping • Unit testing (Black-box testing)
Evaluation and conclusion	• Evaluating the prototype • Analysis of results and discussion	• Controlled experiment [one group pre-test and post-test design] – completeness of test data adequacy

4 Design of DyFunFPA-TDG Method

This study is an extension of the study proposed by Romli [13]. FPA has been utilized to select the optimal number of test cases and test data that are adequate for executing functional testing in APA. The following sub-sections details out the design of DyFunFPA-TDG method.

4.1 Criteria of Deriving Test Set

A test set (that is test cases with test data) are derived by integrating the specification-derived test and boundary value analysis techniques, as proposed by Romli [13]. Based on the study, test case design depends on integration of test specification and boundary value analysis techniques with the combination of positive and negative test criteria. Table 2 shows the means of deriving test data as proposed by Romli [13]. Meanwhile,

Fig. 1 shows the criteria of input conditions (or input space) that has been embedded in DyFunFPA-TDG method.

As shown in Table 3, each input condition is given certain weightage so that it will be used as an additional criterion in choosing pollens with best fitness in FPA. The higher the weight value indicating that the more critical is the test case and test data to be selected as among the most optimal test set by FPA.

Table 2. The division of input conditions with their respective category of data type value and type of data [13].

Type of variable	Category of data type value	Input conditions
Numeric (integer, float, double, short, long, byte)	Global (all numeric values $\mathbb{R}$, $\mathbb{Z}$)	V_b
		$V_{ulb\text{-}left}$
		$V_{ulb\text{-}right}$
		IL
	Positive ($\mathbb{R}^+$, $\mathbb{Z}^+$)	V_b
		V_{ulb}
		IV_{ulb}
		IL
	Negative ($\mathbb{R}^-$, $\mathbb{Z}^-$)	V_b
		V_{ulb}
		IV_{ulb}
		IL
	Range ($\mathbb{R}$, $\mathbb{Z}$)	$V_{b\text{-}Range1}$
		$V_{b\text{-}Range2}$
		V_{ulb}
		$IV_{ulb\text{-}Range1}$
		$IV_{ulb\text{-}Range2}$
		IL
	Specific ($\mathbb{R}$, $\mathbb{Z}$)	V_b
		$IV_{ulb\text{-}left}$
		$IV_{ulb\text{-}right}$
		IL
Character	Global (any characters)	V_b
	Specific	V_b
		IV_b
String	Global (any strings)	V_b
	Specific	V_b
		IV_b
Boolean	Global (true or false)	V_b
		IL
	Specific	V_b
		IV_b
		IL

4.2 Flower Pollination Algorithm

Yang [22] proposed the Flower Pollination Algorithm (FPA) as a new heuristic algorithm in 2012. The FPA can solve multi-objective optimization, high-dimensional function

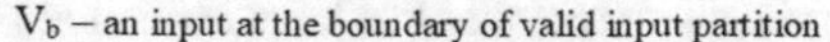
V_b – an input at the boundary of valid input partition
$V_{b\text{-}Range1}$ – an input at the boundary-Range 1 of valid input partition
$V_{b\text{-}Range2}$ – an input at the boundary-Range 2 of valid input partition
V_{ulb} – an input between the upper and lower boundaries of valid input partition
IV_b – an input at the boundary of invalid input partition
IV_{ulb} – an input between the upper and lower boundaries of invalid input partition
$IV_{ulb\text{-}left}$ – an input between the upper and lower boundaries-left of valid input partition
$IV_{ulb\text{-}right}$ – an input between the upper and lower boundaries-right of valid input partition
$IV_{b\text{-}Range1}$ – an input at the boundary-Range 1 of invalid input partition
$IV_{b\text{-}Range2}$ – an input at the boundary-Range 2 of invalid input partition
IL – an illegal input at an error prone point

Fig. 1. Criteria of input conditions [13]

Table 3. The division of input conditions with their respective weight values.

Input Condition	Weight value
Valid input conditions - V (V_b, V_{ulb}, $V_{ulb\text{-}left}$, $V_{ulb\text{-}right}$, $V_{b\text{-}Range1}$, $V_{b\text{-}Range2}$)	5
Invalid input conditions - IV (IV_b, IV_{ulb}, $IV_{ulb\text{-}Range1}$, $IV_{ulb\text{-}Range2}$, $IV_{ulb\text{-}left}$, $IV_{ulb\text{-}right}$)	4
Illegal input conditions - L	1

optimization, and engineering optimization thanks to its good searching capability, fewer parameters, and simple structure [23]. Even though the pollination algorithm was only proposed for a brief period, it quickly became a common research subject. Figure 2 shows the original version of FPA. In this study, the existing FPA has been modified by adding additional process of selecting best fitness. Best fitness has been chosen based on the weightage criteria as depicted in Table 2. Thus, the optimal number of adequate test set can be chosen from the test set that are initially derived based on the test set and weighted scoring criteria as shown in Fig. 1 and Table 3.

4.3 Flower Pollination Algorithm (FPA) in DyFunFPA-TDG

Figure 2 depicts the flow of the original FPA procedure. Meanwhile, Fig. 3 depicts the modified FPA used in the DyFunFPA-TDG technique. The original FPA has been modified in certain ways. The first change is made during the initialization of a population, where a weightage scoring criterion is assigned to each pollen. The second change occurs in the second step, when the best pair of pollens is added to a collection of test cases (TC). The third modification occurs during the computation of the objective function of a new solution, which occurs after local or global pollination is completed. Weightage is added to the evaluation throughout this procedure, which acts as a new criterion for picking the pollen with the best fitness. The last modification is the inspection of each pollen to determine the score of each input condition. The greater the weight value, the more important it is for the test case and test data to be selected as part of FPA's most optimal test set.

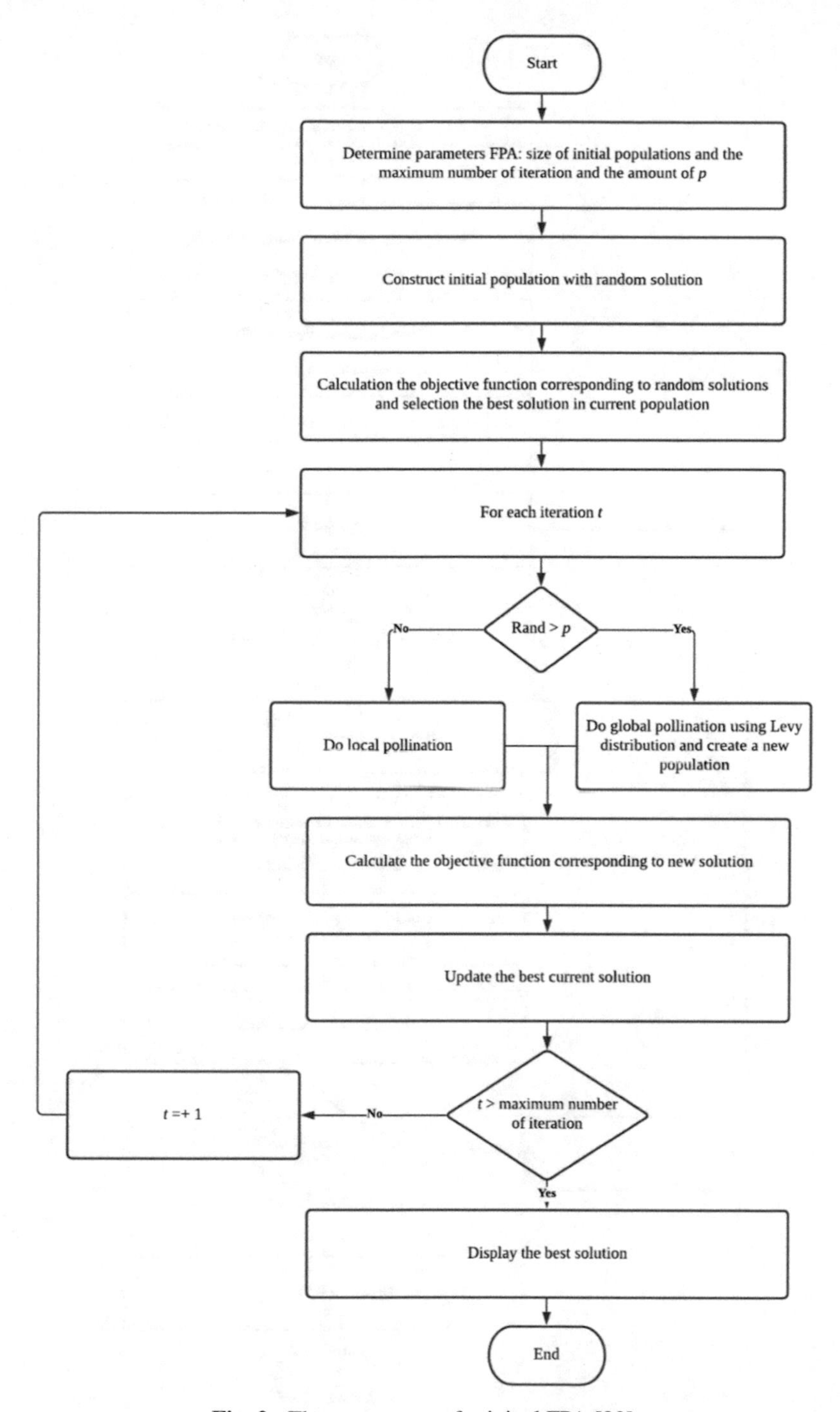

Fig. 2. Flow processes of original FPA [23]

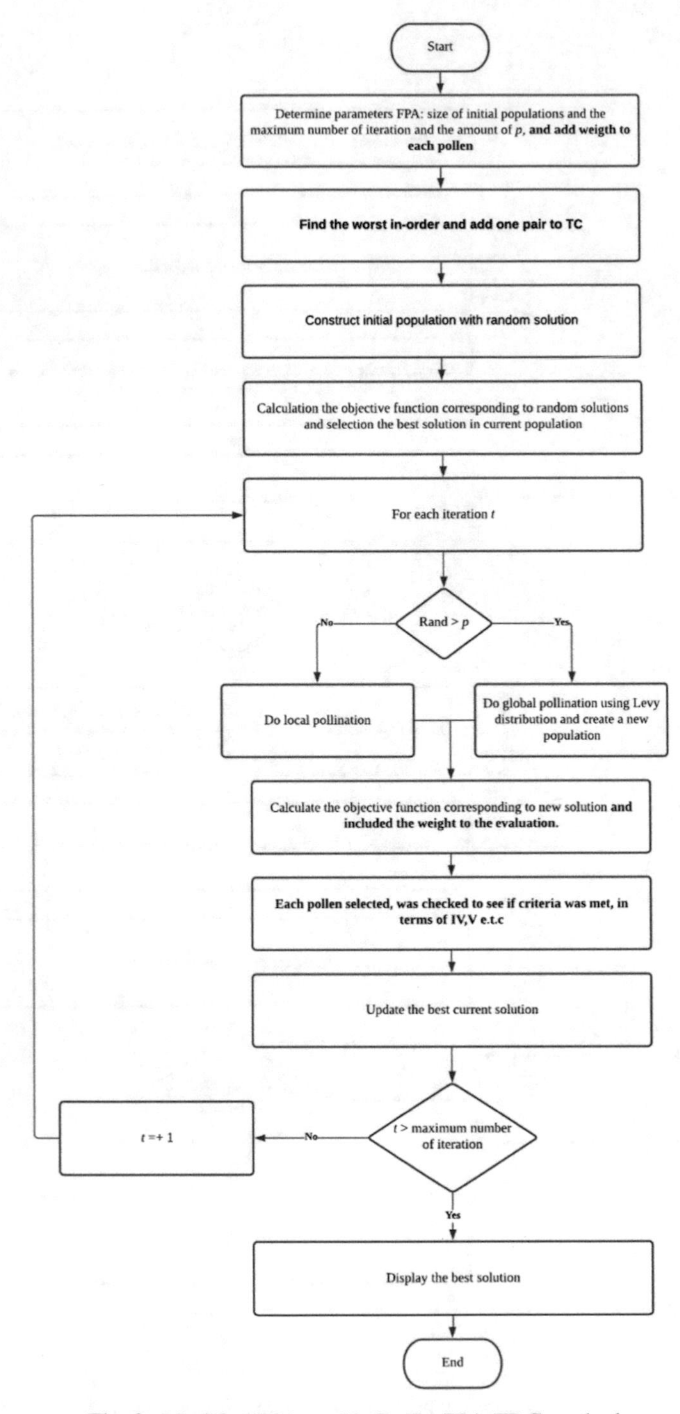

Fig. 3. Modified FPA used in DyFunFPA-TDG method

5 DyFunFPA-TDG Method by Example

In this paper, we include one example of programming exercise to illustrate and provide a clearer understanding of how DyFunFPA-TDG method is mapped to APA. The programming exercise is categorized as Numeric Global (refer Table 1) with three input variables and having a selection control structure. Figure 4 depicts the example of programming exercise with its specifications. The generated test set with test data for the given sample programming exercise is tabulated in Table 4.

Question: Write a program called MinMax3 that prompts user for three integers, num1, num2 and num3. The program shall read the inputs and will find the minimum and maximum of the three integers. Print the result.

Functional Specification:

Input – Three (3) integer numbers: num1, num2 and num3

Output – The min number is: 2 (evaluate three number using if..else if)

The max number is: 5 (evaluate three number using if..else if)

Functional process:

if the inputs are integer numbers, then the min and max are also integer numbers.

format of program input and output are as follows:

Input:

2

3

5

Output:

The min number is: 2

The max number is: 5

Fig. 4. Sample programming exercise and its specifications for numeric global-three input variables–selection

Initially, as the programming exercise consists of three input variables (*num1*, *num2*, and *num3*), then the total number of test cases produced is sixty-four (64). This result is based on as proposed by Romli [13]. For the Numeric Global category with three input variables, in involves four input conditions which are *Vb*, *Vulb-left*, *Vulb-right* and *IL* (see Table 1). The DyFunFPA-TDG method reduces the amount of test cases initially created by Romli [13]. Table 4 shows the generated schema of test set as produced by DyFunFPA-TDG method. The produced test set is reduced by around 56.25% as compared to test set generated by the previous method. The DyFunFPA-TDG method trains all the test cases and picks the best optimal test data, resulting 28 test cases. As mentioned in Table 3, each input condition is assigned with certain weightage value as an extra criterion in choosing the pollen with best fitness in FPA. The higher the weight value indicates the more critical is the test data. Most critical test data will be having higher tendency to be selected as the most optimal test set by DyFunFPA-TDG. Thus, unfit test data will be omitted from the test set selection.

Table 4. Generated schema of test set by DyFunFPA-TDG for the sample programming exercise in Fig. 4.

Test Case (TC)	Input			Output	Test Case Description
	num1	num2	num3		
TC1	5	8	9	The min number is: 5 The max number is: 9	Vb of num1, num2 and height
TC2	2	3	-11110	The min number is: -11115 The max number is: 3	Vb of num1 and num2 Vulb-left of num3
TC3	8	7	12021	The min number is: 7 The max number is: 12021	Vb of num1 and num2 Vulb-right of height
TC4	6	-11111	6	The min number is: 6 The max number is: -11111	Vb of num1, Vulb-left of num2 and Vb of height
TC5	8	-12000	-12222	The min number is= -12000 The max number is= 8	Vb of num1, Vulb-left of num2 and Vulb-left of height
TC6	1	-15000	11002	The min number is= -15000 The max number is= 11002	Vb of num1, Vulb-left of num2 and Vulb-right of height
TC7	3	11100	5	The min number is= 3 The max number is= 11100	Vb of num1, Vulb-right of num2 and Vb of height
TC8	2	12222	-11111	The min number is= -11111 The max number is= 12222	Vb of num1, Vulb-right of num2 and Vulb-left of height
TC9	9	13333	11111	The min number is= 9 The max number is= 13333	Vb of num1, Vulb-right of num2 and height
TC10	-11111	2	2	The min number is= -11111 The max number is= 2	Vulb-left of num1, Vb of num2 and height
TC11	-12222	3	-10001	The min number is= -12222 The max number is= 3	Vulb-left of num1, Vb of num2 and Vulb-left of height
TC12	-13000	4	10001	The min number is= -13000 The max number is= 4	Vulb-left of num1, Vb of num2 and Vulb-right of height
TC13	-11000	-10000	3	The min number is= -11000 The max number is= -10000	Vulb-left of num1 and num2, Vb of height
TC14	-10000	-10001	-10002	The min number is= -10001 The max number is= -10000	Vulb-left of num1,num2 and height
TC15	-17000	-10002	10002	The min number is= -17000 The max number is= -10002	Vulb-left of num1 and num2, Vulb-right of height
TC16	-13000	10001	4	The min number is= -13000 The max number is= 10001	Vulb-left of num1, Vulb-right of num2 and Vb of height
TC17	-11001	10002	-10002	The min number is= -11001 The max number is= 10002	Vulb-left of num1, Vulb-right of num2 and Vulb-left of height
TC18	-12002	10003	10001	The min number is= -12002 The max number is= 10003	Vulb-left of num1, Vulb-right of num2 and height
TC19	11111	5	6	The min number is= 5 The max number is= 11111	Vulb-right of num1, Vb of num2 and height
TC20	12222	6	-10004	The min number is= 6 The max number is= 12222	Vulb-right of num1, Vb of num2 and Vulb-left height
TC21	13000	7	10004	The min number is= 7 The max number is= 13000	Vulb-right of num1, Vb of num2 and Vulb-right height
TC22	11000	-10004	9	The min number is= -10004 The max number is= 11000	Vulb-right of num1, Vulb-left of num2 and Vb height
TC23	15000	-10005	-10000	The min number is= -10005 The max number is= 15000	Vulb-right of num1, Vulb-left of num2 and Vulb-left height
TC24	17000	-10006	10000	The min number is= -10006 The max number is= 17000	Vulb-right of num1, Vulb-left of num2 and Vulb-left height
TC25	13000	10005	8	The min number is= 10005 The max number is= 13000	Vulb-right of num1, Vulb-right of num2 and Vb height
TC26	10001	10006	-10001	The min number is= -10001 The max number is= 10006	Vulb-right of num1, Vulb-right of num2 and Vulb-left height
TC27	12002	10007	10001	The min number is= 10007 The max number is= 12002	Vulb-right of num1, Vulb-right of num2 and Vulb-right height
TC28	jsp	4	perl	Error	IL of num1,Vb of num2, IL of height

6 Conclusion

This paper has highlighted the design of our proposed work namely DyFunFPA-TDG method. The proposed method has improved the current work as proposed by Romli [13] on the part of selecting the optimal number of test set such that there is a certain extend of test set reduction from the initial generated test set. The proposed DyFunFPA-TDG method is able assist lecturers or educators of programming course to derive and generate adequate set of test data with optimal in its size and without the need to master on certain specific test cases design. Having this method as a part of APA tool will significantly reduce lecturers time and effort related to assessing students' programming exercises or assignments as well as providing students with timely feedbacks on their programming assignments.

Acknowledgement. This research was supported by Ministry of Higher Education (MoHE) of Malaysia through Fundamental Research Grant Scheme (FRGS/1/2017/ICT01/UUM/03/1).

References

1. Ala-Mutka, K.M.: A survey of automated assessment approaches for programming assignments. Comput. Sci. Educ. **15**(2), 83–102 (2005). https://doi.org/10.1080/08993400500150747
2. Yusof, N., Zin, N.A.M., Adnan, N.S.: Java programming assessment tool for assignment module in moodle e-learning system. Procedia - Soc. Behav. Sci. **56**, 767–773 (2012). https://doi.org/10.1016/j.sbspro.2012.09.714
3. Blumenstein, M., Green, S., Nguyen, A., Muthukkumarasamy, V.: GAME: a generic automated marking environment for programming assessment. Int. Conf. Inf. Technol. Coding Comput. ITCC **1**(May), 212–216 (2004). https://doi.org/10.1109/ITCC.2004.1286454
4. Jackson, D., Usher, M.: Grading student programs using ASSYST. ACM SIGCSE Bull. **29**(1), 335–339 (1997). https://doi.org/10.1145/268085.268210
5. Luck, M., Joy, M.: A secure on-line submission system. Softw. - Pract. Exp. **29**(8), 721–740 (1999)
6. Arivazhagan, S., Nidhyanandhan, S.S., Shebiah, R.N.: Texture categorization using statistical and spectral features. In: Proceedings of 2008 International Conference Computing Communication Networking, ICCCN 2008, vol. 3, no. 2, pp. 267–288 (2008). https://doi.org/10.1109/ICCCNET.2008.4787722
7. Motivation et al., Automated Assessment and Experiences of Teaching Programming COLIN A. HIGGINS, GEOFFREY GRAY, PAVLOS SYMEONIDIS, ATHANASIOS TSINTSIFAS The University of Nottingham, Nottingham, UK Thi, vol. 5, no. 3, pp. 1–21, (2005). https://doi.org/10.1145/1163405.1163410
8. Auffarth, B., Lopez-Sanchez, M., Campos i Miralles, J., Puig, A.: System for Automated Assistance in Correction of Programming Exercises (SAC), Congr. Univ. Teach. Innov., pp. 104–113 (2008)
9. Sherman, M., Bassil, S., Lipman, D., Tuck, N., Martin, F.: Impact of auto-grading on an introductory computing course. J. Comput. Sci. Coll. **28**(6), 69–75 (2013)
10. Rajamanickam, L., Saat, N.A.B.M., Daud, S.N.B.: Software testing: the generation tools. Int. J. Adv. Trends Comput. Sci. Eng. **8**(2), 231–234 (2019). https://doi.org/10.30534/ijatcse/2019/20822019

11. Korel, B.: Automated software test data generation. IEEE Trans. Softw. Eng. **16**(8), 870–879 (1990). https://doi.org/10.1109/32.57624
12. Monpratarnchai, S., Fujiwara, S., Katayama, A., Uehara, T.: Automated testing for java programs using JPF-based test case generation. ACM SIGSOFT Softw. Eng. Notes **39**(1), 1–5, (2014). https://doi.org/10.1145/2557833.2560575
13. Romli, R.: Test data generation framework for Automatic Programming Assessment, PHD Thesis (2014)
14. Bin, L.: Automatic test data generation tool based on genetic simulated annealing algorithm. In: 2007 International Conference on Computational Intelligence and Security Workshops (CISW 2007), pp. 183–186 (2007)
15. Mejia, J., Muñoz, M., Feliu, T.S.: Test cases minimization strategy based on flower pollination algorithm. RISTI - Rev. Iber. Sist. e Tecnol. Inf. **26**, ix–xiii (2018). https://doi.org/10.4304/risti.35.0
16. Nasser, A.B., Zamli, K.Z., Alsewari, A.A., Ahmed, B.S.: Hybrid flower pollination algorithm strategies for t-way test suite generation, pp. 1–24 (2018)
17. Foong, O., Tran, Q., Yong, S., Rais, H.: Swarm inspired test case generation for online C ++ programming assessment, pp. 2–6
18. Tahbildar, H., Kalita, B.: Automated software test data generation: direction of research.pdf. Int. J. Comput. Sci. Eng. Surv. **2**(1), 99–120 (2011)
19. Romli, R., Sulaiman, S., Zamli, K.Z.: Test data generation framework for automatic programming assessment. In: 2014 8th Malaysian Software Engineering Conference MySEC 2014, vol. 110, no. 1, pp. 84–89 (2014). https://doi.org/10.1109/MySec.2014.6985993
20. Mcminn, P., Street, P., Holcombe, M.: Evolutionary testing using an extended chaining approach. Evol. Comput. **14**(1), 41–64 (2006)
21. Nasser, A.B., Sariera, Y.A., Alsewari, A.A., Zamli, K.Z.:Assessing optimization based strategies for t-way test suite generation : the case for flower-based strategy. In: 2015 IEEE international conference on control system, computing and engineering (ICCSCE), pp. 27–29, (2015)
22. Yang, X.S.: Metaheuristic algorithms for self-organizing systems: a tutorial. In: International Conference on Self-Adaptive and Self-Organizing Systems SASO, vol. 40, no. 3, pp. 249–250 (2012). https://doi.org/10.1109/SASO.2012.40
23. Yang, X.: Nature-Inspired Algorithms, pp. 297–323 (2018)

A Comparative Evaluation on Methods of Teaching Computer Programming

Asmalinda Adnan and Rohaida Romli(✉)

School of Computing, Universiti Utara Malaysia, Sintok, Kedah, Malaysia
aida@uum.edu.my

Abstract. Learning programming is typically regarded as a challenging task by both educators and learners. The face-to-face learning method alone is likely insufficient to promote effective teaching and learning solutions. Thus, having a suitable teaching method can be useful in various situations and encourages learners to actively and effectively participate in programming classes. Likewise, having appropriate formation of different programming learning methods and environments to influence learners' computational thinking is something significant. As such, this paper presents an analysis and comparison of the related works on any promising methods that are able promote a better and efficient way of learning programming. In the meantime, it suggests any possible direction for future work by conducting a comparative evaluation. As far as this study is concerned, several methods of teaching programming such as visualization, game-based, robotics, problem-solving, code tracing, simulation and pair programming have been analyzed and compared. Results of this study indicated that visualization and game-based method are the most effective formation methods. Using visualization and games-based methods in teaching programming can help to enhance learners' programming concepts in terms of enhancing the learners' cognitive ability to develop a mental model, increase their engagement and stimulate their abstract thinking in cognitive development.

Keywords: Teaching and learning programming · Visualization · Code tracing · Game-based · Robotic · Problem-based · Simulation and pair programming

1 Background

Programming concepts, syntax, and logic-building processes are commonly tough and difficult tasks for most novice learners to grasp. The key issue is to encourage learners to build meaningful programs in a short number of times by emphasizing computational thinking and problem-solving skills [1]. As compared to traditional lecture approaches, most learners prefer to be involved and to discover material through discovery, involvement, and fun [2].

Teaching programming is commonly known as a demanding task that has its own set of challenges [3]. In that sense, educators must master the subject of teaching, which is the process of converting knowledge into understandable knowledge for learners by

F. Saeed et al. (Eds.): IRICT 2021, LNDECT 127, pp. 571–582, 2022.
https://doi.org/10.1007/978-3-030-98741-1_47

using correct teaching methods. Meanwhile, teaching method is a systematic overall plan to deliver instruction that is influenced by the nature of the learners' language [4].

In the context of the programming subject teaching method, a study by Costelloe [5] has shown that the problem-solving teaching method is used as a teaching method for programming subjects. To ensure more effective teaching and programming learning to improve students' achievement and computational thinking levels, the problem-solving method should be accompanied by a suitable teaching method. These methods are visualization, game-based, robotic tool application, simulation, code-tracing, problem-solving and pair programming. Accordingly, the comparative evaluation in this paper aims to promote appropriate formation teaching methods with a successful implementation that can be applied in teaching and learning computer programming.

This paper focuses on a comparative evaluation that has been done to analyse and compare the existing teaching methods of computer programming course to address the mentioned issues and by then suggesting any possible effective teaching methods that are able to promote better programming teaching methods understanding. The content of this article is structured as follows: Sect. 2 briefly addresses some fundamental concepts of teaching programming methods with regard to visualization, game-based, code tracing, robotic, problem-based, simulation and pair programming; Sect. 3 provides a detailed discussion of the methodology used in this study; Sect. 4 reveals the analysis and results of the conducted comparative evaluation and Sect. 5 concludes this paper and provides suggestion for future research direction.

2 Methods of Teaching Programming and Its Fundamental Concepts

Previous researchers [6] have conducted studies to review programming teaching methods. However, in terms of comparative methods, there is a study by Kanika [7] covers five methods which are visual programming, game-based learning, pair and collaborative programming, robot programming, and assessment system, while the focus is only on the advantages and challenge parameters. Meanwhile, this paper extends the comparison in terms of the teaching programming methods based on the current literature review as well as the parameter of the evaluation. There are three additional methods presented in this paper which are simulation, code tracing, and problem-solving. The other three added parameters such as the teaching approach, the method applied as a digital application, and effectiveness have been reviewed to comprehend the existing study.

Recently, the theme of programming teaching has becomes an emphasis to researchers and educators because it is among the difficult subjects to teach in any computing discipline program [8]. In addition, the teaching method chosen to teach programming should be able to maintain learners' motivation and engagement [9]. These teaching methods will be discussed further in the subsequent sections.

2.1 Visualization

Yehezkel [10] asserted that visuals have the potential to enhance the cognitive ability to develop a mental model if exploited effectively in a conducive learning environment. The use of visual software aims to facilitate the process of demonstration of basic concepts to facilitate learners to generate ideas and make hypotheses in teaching that are not feasible by traditional methods [11]. This method helps these learners to strengthen computational thinking [12], and problem-solving skills [13], make things easy to correct errors [14], stimulate learners engagement with illustrations [15], reduce the involvement of technical skills [16], is user-friendly and accessible at all times using mobile devices [17], bridge the learner's grade gap [18], support distance learning [19], be able to demonstrate real situations [20] and they are mostly syntactic-error free [21]. A study [22] stated that the main platforms of visual tools are web and mobile devices.

2.2 Game-Based Learning

Game-Based Learning (GBL) in education is known as one of the branches of Serious Game (SG) [23]. SG is a video (visual) game in which the main purpose is not for entertainment but is used to convey teaching objectives in line with the curriculum guidelines [24]. In addition, the basic principles of gamification design include: the principle of learners engagement; the principle of freedom of choice; the principle of freedom to fail, and the need to provide quick feedback [25]. SG is generally able to increase learners' engagement [26], stimulate their abstract thinking in cognitive development, turn and develop their high-level thinking skills [27]. Although this method has shown a positive effect on educational institutions, SG is still not widely used in the classroom [28]. This is due to the lack of involvement of educators and field experts to prove the benefits of its use and necessity in the development of SG applications [29].

2.3 Robotics

In terms of a robotic method, it allows learners to write programs to control robots in performing simple tasks in real-time and be able to promote active learning as well as opening some space for constructive learning [30]. In particular, this method empowers collaborative work, increase motivation and promote cognitive development by supporting the learners' knowledge construction. However, its application in the classroom is not an easy task and must be accompanied by appropriate methods for effective learning [31]. Among the concepts of programming applied using this robot are the sequential execution of statements, conditional statements, iterative statements [32], and algorithms [33].

2.4 Problem-Solving

Boud and Feletti [34] defined problem-solving-based teaching as; "A way of constructing and teaching courses using problems as the stimulus and focus for learners activity". The statement is also supported by Hsu, Chang, and Hung [35] who stressed that problem-solving learning supports learners in building new knowledge through problem-solving concepts. In this method, learners gain experience with mind creation, speaking, writing, and learning independently, expressing their ideas by creating simulation models [36] and learning collaboratively [37]. Problem-solving learning is not only used to solve problems but also to enhance learners' understanding of new knowledge through appropriate questions [38].

2.5 Simulation

Simulation is the use of visual technology that can facilitate learners to learn the learning content that is abstract and very difficult to understand [39]. It is also suitable for use in experimental learning and discovery methods [40]. There are various educational benefits of using simulation in engineering and computing [41], interactively [42]. This learning has successfully demonstrated a strong relationship between the dimensions of behavior, emotional cognitive, learners engagement, and help in shaping learning experiences that span various areas of teaching [43]. Yet, researchers have suggested the prospect of a simpler intuitive control design for ease of operating mobile devices without the need for high technical knowledge. However, aspects that focus on individual relationships (user-study) such as the implications of the role of instructors and the role of learners' peers are still poorly studied.

2.6 Code Tracing

Code tracing and code writing are two processes to trace values in memory alignment for all variables to understand the programme manually and to compare the actual results of the programme [44]. Nelson [18] stated that mastering programming code detection is to understand the set of all mappings among syntax, semantics and code compilation. Once students develop a semantic reading understanding, they can trace the code, determine situations and ascertain the output in the middle and at the end. This is in line with the teaching theory to build on programming skills highlighted by [45]. The theory outlines code tracing as an important skill in programming that needs to be mastered in addition to writing the right syntax and applying it to solve problems. Pinter [46] said students would not be able to write code if they did not learn to trace code first. This is because students who are skilled in code tracing skills will have more potential to write code correctly.

2.7 Pair Programming

The programming teaching and learning in pair programming/peer programming/peer sharing or "*pairgogy*" encompasses a variety of learning modes supported by digital resources. The statement was supported by [47] who stated that pair-based techniques include face-to-face mode in computer labs and online. Pair programming is also defined as a programming activity in which two individuals sit side-by-side, sharing one keyboard and a monitor [48]. There are two roles in pair programming, namely driver and browser. The driver focuses on encoding while the browser actively observes the work and proposes an appropriate code to the driver [49]. However, this role may change while programming is carried out [50].

3 Methodology

In this paper, a comparative evaluation has been adopted as a method to guide the process of analysis and comparison to be done. The comparison is made for the purpose to comprehend the different teaching programming methods when implemented in teaching programming sessions. This comparative evaluation can be considered as a well-analyzed picture to illustrate distinct programming teaching methods. The method used in this study was introduced by Vartiainen [51] to explain the comparative evaluation study. The following illustrates detailed explanations of each phase of the method.

3.1 A Theoretical Study

A theoretical study consists of the concepts of visualization, game-based, robotics, problem-solving, code tracing, simulation and pair programming together with their definition and existing theories that are used for a particular study [52]. Through the theoretical study of the existing work, it helps to identify various teaching programming methods that are used to teach programming as well as the advantages, disadvantages, and effectiveness of review methods. The outcome of this theoretical study is the proposed teaching programming methods to support teaching programming.

3.2 Comparative Evaluation

The comparative evaluation phase comprises of four main activities as follows:

i. Selection of the object evaluation - The object evaluation identified is the teaching methods used to teach programming. In this practice, the comparative evaluation process has been focusing on the implementation of the teaching method on teaching computer programming.
ii. Determine the level of comparison - The level of comparison involved the parameters for comparison inclusive of teaching approach that has been supported, applied as a digital application, effectiveness of the method as well as the advantages and disadvantages of the considered methods. The evaluation is based on these parameter points.
iii. Conceptual Comprehension - In this phase, the concepts used in analysis and comparison are determined by the fundamental concepts of each method of teaching programming. The definition of the concept that applied in this study are utilized during evaluation and when comparing the result of the analysis.
iv. Analysis of the findings of an evaluation - In this phase, the analysis and findings are discussed in identifying any effective method (s) and then providing suggestions on the possible direction of future work. On the other hand, the findings make it possible to interpret the operative teaching methods throughout the concepts, definitions, and theories.

3.3 Conclusion and Suggestion

This phase is in concern with reporting the findings obtained from the conducted comparative evaluation in consequence to suggest any applicable teaching programming methods that have promising insights to support teaching computer programming. Hence, by completing this phase, the aim of this study has been achieved.

4 Analysis and Result of Comparative Evaluation

This section discusses the analysis and result of comparative evaluation based on reviewed teaching programming methods. There are seven (7) types of programming teaching methods that have been identified. Table 1 below illustrates a list of comparative analysis of the teaching programming methods.

Table 1. Comparative analysis of programming teaching methods.

Teaching programming methods	Parameters					
	Teaching approach	Applied as a digital application	Effectiveness	Advantages	Disadvantages	Source
Visualization	Collaborative, active	Yes	90% of learners were satisfied with animation, and 83% did better programming than expected using animation [53]	Strengthens computational thinking and problem-solving skills; stimulates engagement; reduces technical skill; mostly free of syntax error; supports distance learning	Provides poor debugging skills	[2]
Game-based	Collaborative, active learning	Yes	Impact of pass rate between 59.27% to 80.64% and 86% learners preferred games over traditional classes [53]	Supports the cognitive engagement and active learners' involvement	Not widely used in the classroom due to the lack of involvement of educators and field experts	[55]
Robotics	Collaborative, active learning	Yes	Physical robots and robot simulators contribute to learners interest and participation in lessons [56]	Empowers collaborative work, increases motivation; promotes cognitive development	Specialized learning environment settings - requires special technical skills and expensive equipment and continuous power supply	[57]

(*continued*)

Table 1. (*continued*)

Teaching programming methods	Parameters					
	Teaching approach	Applied as a digital application	Effectiveness	Advantages	Disadvantages	Source
Problem-solving	Collaborative, active learning, scaffold	Yes	Increases learners' self-efficacy in group learning [58]	Supports learners to build new knowledge; enhances critical thinking, analysis, synthesis and creative thinking	High-level cognitive skills give the impact of heavy cognitive load	[17]
Simulation	Collaborative, active learning,	Yes	78.6% effectiveness of course content and 76.84% of course outcomes effectively [59]	Suitable for experimental learning and discovery methods;	Hard to construct a suitable design	[60],
Pair Programming	Collaborative, active learning,	Yes	Students are more likely to complete courses and have higher passing rates [61]	Capable of influencing students' ability to learn a programming language	Limitation of physical encounters for sharing the use of tools and for collaboration	[62]
Code tracing	Active learning	Yes	69% of students were able to speed up their understanding of tracking algorithms [63]	Skilled students of code tracing skills will have more potential to write code correctly	Students need to practise over and over again	[21]

Based on previous studies, the discussion of the strengths and weaknesses that are illustrated in Table 1 is to determine among the most effective method(s) that can be applied by educators of programming courses in improving their teaching method. Visualization, game-based, robotics, problem solving, code tracing and simulation are the teaching methods that can be applied to produce digital-based applications like web-based systems or mobile apps. The digital learning environment allows full support to contribute to the effectiveness of learning and teaching thus increasing student motivation. The digital application (online tool and mobile application) helps the students understand, learn, revise, and practise coding, at their pace and convenience. However, game-based and robotics techniques require learning environment settings that are not often designed for curriculum alignment. Likewise, robotics needs specialized learning environment settings to implement robotics technology in the classroom. Thus, it requires special technical skills, expensive equipment, and a continuous power supply. Nevertheless, visualization helps in establishing the user interface but the design needs to focus on the concept of syntax and semantic.

In programming subject, [64] mentioned about the ability to solve a problem as the main factor of programming success which involves cognitive function but it is built based on behaviour. Furthermore, activities in pair programming also use cooperative techniques such as brainstorming in problem-solving. Nevertheless, the disadvantage of pair programming is the limitation of physical encounters for sharing the use of tools and for collaboration [65]. Although this technique shapes active learning, increases confidence and builds interest in solving problems, there is still less research on asynchronous online learning pair programming [66]. In addition, code tracing focuses on performance and optimizes the process of coding.

Visualization, game-based, code tracing and simulation are programming teaching methods that support collaborative and active learning approaches and have also commonly applied as digital applications. In comparison to other methods, the visualization method is able to increase learners' computational thinking, stimulate engagement, higher rate of learner's satisfaction (90%), and also enhances active and collaborative learning in their learning session. Meanwhile, game-based learning promotes cognitive engagement and participation among learners and has become the most learners' preferred method with 86% score. Contrarily, the simulation showed the difference between the effectiveness of course content (78.6%) and course outcomes (76.84%). Therefore, this method is recommended for educators to use in their learning sessions because of its effectiveness as well as its ability to develop students' computational thinking.

5 Conclusion

In this paper, a comparative evaluation was conducted to identify among the effective teaching programming methods that can be applied by existing educators or instructors. An improvement to the comparative evaluation from the aspect of parameter is shown in Table 1. In the comparative evaluation, there are five comparison parameters recognized that include teaching approach; has been applied as a digital application or not, effectiveness, advantages, and disadvantages of the teaching programming methods. Isiaq and Jamil [43] stated that values of teaching and learning activities are reliant on a meaningful learning environment and learners' engagement.

Based on the conducted comparative evaluation, it can be concluded that visualization and game-based teaching methods are among the promising solutions to support teaching and learning programming courses. The reason is that, game-based teaching has a significant impact to encourage critical thinking [67]; helps in problem-solving; increases student engagement and motivation [68] and offers a comfortable environment to learn and collaborate with others. However, this method requires a specific focus on the design requirements that underlie the curriculum requirements.

On the contrary, visualization provides a simplified learning process by visualizing complex topics in a simpler form, helps to store longer information, and assists students to understand a program flow better. In this regard, it would be essential in future work to explore any teaching programming approaches and techniques that have been applied as digital applications as this will be able to resolve any issues related to remote and online learning particularly during the Covid-19 pandemic.

References

1. Wing, J.M. Computational thinking. Commun. ACM **49**(3), 33–35 (2006)
2. Rahman, M.M., Paudel, R.: Visual programming and interactive learning based dynamic instructional approaches to teach an introductory programming course. In: IEEE Frontiers in Education Conference (FIE), pp. 1–6 (2019)
3. Koulouri, T., Lauria, S., Macredie, R.D.: Teaching introductory programming: a quantitative evaluation of different approaches. ACM Trans. Comput. Educ. **14**(4), 1–28 (2014)
4. Anthony, E.M.: Approach, Methods and Technique (1965)
5. Costelloe, E.: Teaching Programming the State of the Art, Institute of Technology Tallaght (2004)
6. Vihavainen, A., Airaksinen, J., Watson, C.: A systematic review of approaches for teaching introductory programming and their influence on success. In: 10th Annual International Conference on International Computing Education Research, pp. 19–26 (2014)
7. Kanika, Chakraverty, S., Chakraborty, P.: Tools and techniques for teaching computer programming: a review. J. Educ. Technol. Syst. **49**(2), 170–198 (2020)
8. Apiola, M., Tedre, M.: New perspectives on the pedagogy of programming in a developing country context. Comput. Sci. Educ. **22**(3), 285–313 (2012)
9. Attard, L., Busuttil, L.: Teacher perspectives on introducing programming constructs through coding mobile-based games to secondary school students. Inform. Educ. **19**(4), 543–568 (2020)
10. Yehezkel, C.: A taxonomy of computer architecture visualizations. In: Proceedings Annual SIGCSE Conference Innovation Technology Computer Science Education, pp. 101–105 (2002)
11. Hrabovskyi, Y., Brynza, N., Vilkhivska, O.: Development of information visualization methods for use in multimedia applications. Phys. Eng. **1**, 3–17 (2020)
12. Kyfonidis, C., Moumoutzis, N., Christodoulakis, S.: Block-C: a block-based programming teaching tool to facilitate introductory C programming courses. In: IEEE Global Engineering Education Conference, EDUCON (2017)
13. Hooshyar, D., Ahmad, R.B., Yousefi, M., Fathi, M., Horng, S.J., Lim, H.: SITS: A solution-based intelligent tutoring system for students' acquisition of problem-solving skills in computer programming. Innov. Educ. Teach. Int. **55**(3), 325–335 (2018)
14. Jawad, H.M.: Gamifying the code genie programming tool. In: IEEE International Conference on Electro Information Technology, pp. 555–559 (2019)
15. Kölling, M.: The greenfoot programming environment. ACM Trans. Comput. Educ. **10**(4), 1–21 (2010)
16. Lin, S., Kafura, D., Tech, V.: PDL : scaffolding problem solving in programming courses. In: 26th ACM Conference on Innovation and Technology in Computer Science Education V. 1 (ITiCSE 2021), June 26-July 1, 2021, Virtual Event, Germany (vol. 1, Issue 1). Association for Computing Machinery (2021)
17. Mathew, R., Malik, S.I., Tawafak, R.M.: Teaching problem solving skills using an educational game in a computer programming course. Inform. Educ. **18**(2), 359—373 (2019)
18. Nelson, G.L., Xie, B., Ko, A.J.: Comprehension first: evaluating a novel pedagogy and tutoring system for program tracing in CS1 (2017)

19. Selwyn-smith, B., Anslow, C., Homer, M., Wallace, J.R.: Co-located Collaborative Block-Based Programming, pp. 107–116 (2019)
20. Suh, S., Lee, M., Xia, G., Law, E.: Coding Strip: a pedagogical tool for teaching and learning programming concepts through comics. In: Proceedings of IEEE Symposium on Visual Languages and Human-Centric Computing, VL/HCC, 2020-Augus(c) (2020)
21. Vasilopoulos, I.V., van Schaik, P.: Design, development, and evaluation of an educational visual tool for Greek novice programmers. J. Educ. Comput. Res. **57**(5), 1227–1259 (2019)
22. Kuhail, M.A., Farooq, S., Hammad, R., Bahja, M.: Characterizing visual programming approaches for end-user developers: a systematic review. IEEE Access **9**, 14181–14202 (2021)
23. Anastasiadis, T., Lampropoulos, G., Siakas, K.: Digital game-based learning and serious games in education. Int. J. Adv. Sci. Res. Eng. **4**(12), 139–144 (2018). https://doi.org/10.31695/ijasre.2018.33016
24. Perrotta, C., Featherstone, G., Aston, H., Houghton, E.: Game-based learning: Latest evidence and future directions (2013)
25. Dicheva, D., Dichev, C., Agre, G., Angelova, G.: Gamification in education: a systematic mapping study. Educ. Technol. Soc. **18**(3), 75–88 (2015)
26. De Freitas, S.: Are games effective learning tools? a review of educational games. J. Educ. Technol. Soc. **21**(2), 74–84 (2018)
27. Abbasi, S., Kazi, H., Khowaja, K.: A systematic review of learning object oriented programming through serious games and programming approaches. In: 4th IEEE International Conference on Engineering Technologies and Applied Sciences (2018). https://doi.org/10.1109/ICETAS.2017.8277894
28. Almeida, F., Simoes, J.: The role of serious games, gamification and industry 4.0 tools in the education 4.0 paradigm. Contemp. Educ. Technol. **10**(2), 120–136 (2019)
29. Manuel, P.C.V., José, P.C.I., Manuel, F.M., Iván, M.O., Baltasar, F.M.: Simplifying the creation of adventure serious games with educational-oriented features. Educ. Technol. Soc. **22**(3), 32–46 (2019)
30. Linder, S.P., Nestrick, B.E., Mulders, S., Lavelle, C.L.: Facilitating active learning with inexpensive mobile robots. J. Comput. Sci. Coll. **16**(4), 21–33 (2001)
31. Aparicio, J.T., Pereira, S., Aparicio, M., Costa, C.J.: Learning programming using educational robotics. In: IEEE 14th Iberian Conference on Information Systems and Technologies (CISTI), pp. 1–6 (2019)
32. Feijóo García, P.G., De la Rosa, F.: RoBlock - web app for programming learning. Int. J. Emerg. Technol. Learn. **11**(12), 45–53 (2016)
33. Fagin, B., Merkle, L.: Measuring the effectiveness of robots in teaching computer science. SIGCSE Bull. **35**(1), 307–311 (2003)
34. Boud, D., Feletti, G.: The Challenge of Problem-Based Learning, 2nd edn. Biddle Ltd, Guilfford and King's Lynn, London (1991)
35. Hsu, T.C., Chang, S.C., Hung, Y.T.: How to learn and how to teach computational thinking: Suggestions based on a review of the literature. Comput. Educ. **126**, 296–310 (2018)
36. Janpla, S., Piriyasurawong, P.: The development of problem-based learning and concept mapping using a block-based programming model to enhance the programming competency of undergraduate students in computer science. TEM J. **7**(4), 708–716 (2018)
37. Chang, C.-S., Chung, C.-H., Chang, J.A.: Influence of problem-based learning games on effective computer programming learning in higher education. Educ. Tech. Res. Dev. **68**(5), 2615–2634 (2020). https://doi.org/10.1007/s11423-020-09784-3
38. Wood, F.D.: ABC of Learning and Teaching in Medicine. Occup. Med. (Chic. Ill) **61**(6), 446 (2003)

39. Mohd Syahrizad, E., Ahmad Zamzuri, M.: a. Penggunaan simulasi packet tracer dalam meningkatkan pemahaman pelajar terhadap konsep abstrak dalam matapelajaran rangkaian komputer: Suatu tinjauan awal. In: Proceedings of International Conference Integration Knowledge (ICIK 2012), pp. 69–77 (2012)
40. De Jong, T., Van Joolingen, W.R.: Scientific discovery learning with computer simulations of conceptual domains, Rev. Educ. Res. **68**(2), 179–201 (1998)
41. Xie, C., Schimpf, C., Chao, J., Nourian, S., Massicotte, J.: Learning and teaching engineering design through modeling and simulation on a CAD platform. Comput. Appl. Eng. Educ. 26(4), 824–840 (2018)
42. Connolly, T.M., Stansfield, M.: From e-learning to games-based e-learning: using interactive technologies in teaching an IS course. Int. J. Inf. Technol. Manag. **6**(2–4), 188–208 (2007)
43. Isiaq, S.O., Jamil, M.G.: Enhancing student engagement through simulation in programming sessions. Int. J. Inf. Learn. Technol. (2018)
44. Schoeman, M., Gelderblom, H., Smith, E.: A tutorial to teach tracing to first-year programming students. Progressio **34**(3), 59–80 (2012)
45. Xie, B., et al.: A theory of instruction for introductory programming skills, Comput. Sci. Educ. 29(2–3), 205–253 (2019)
46. Pinter, R., Čisar, S.M., Kovari, A., Major, L., Čisar, P., Katona, J.: Case study: students' code-tracing skills and calibration of questions for computer adaptive tests. Appl. Sci. **10**(20), 1–21 (2020)
47. Sulaiman, S. Pairing-based approach to support understanding of object-oriented concepts and programming, Int. J. Adv. Sci. Eng. Inf. Technol. **10**(4) (2020)
48. Choi, K.S., Deek, F.P., Im, I.: Exploring the underlying aspects of pair programming: the impact of personality. Inf. Softw. Technol. **50**(11), 1114–1126 (2008)
49. Arisholm, E., Gallis, H., Dybå, T., Sjøberg, D.I.K.: Evaluating pair programming with respect to system complexity and programmer expertise. IEEE Trans. Softw. Eng. **33**(2), 65–86 (2007)
50. Nawahdah, M., Taji, D.: Work in progress: investigating the effects of pair-programming on students' behavior in an advanced computer programming course. In: Proceedings 2015 IEEE International Conference Teaching, Assessment Learning Engineering TALE 2015, December, pp. 157–160 (2016)
51. Vartiainen, P.: On the principles of comparative evaluation. Evaluation **8**(3), 359–371 (2002)
52. Sekaran, U.: Research and Markets: Research Methods for Business - A Skill Building Approach (2003)
53. Yulianto, B., Prabowo, H., Meyliana. Effective digital contents for computer programming learning: a systematic literature review. Adv. Sci. Lett. **23**(5), 4733–4737 (2017)
54. Faja, S.: Pair programming as a team based learning activity: a review of research. Issues Inf. Syst. **XII**(2), 207–216 (2011)
55. Fornós, S.: Game making as a learning strategy for chemical engineering. In: CHI PLAY 2020 –Extended Abstracts of the 2020 Annual Symposium on Computer-Human Interaction in Play, pp. 234–236 (2020). https://doi.org/10.1145/3383668.3419888
56. Kurniawan, O., Lee, N.T.S., Datta, S., Sockalingam, N., Leong, P.K.: Effectiveness of physical robot versus robot simulator in teaching introductory programming. In: Proceedings of 2018 IEEE International Conference Teaching, Assessment, Learning Engineering TALE 2018, pp. 486–493 (2019)
57. Rodríguez, C., Guzman, J.L., Berenguel, M., Dormido, S.: Teaching real-time programming using mobile robots. IFAC-PapersOnLine **49**(6), 10–15 (2016)
58. Wang, X.-M., Hwang, G.-J.: A problem posing-based practicing strategy for facilitating students' computer programming skills in the team-based learning mode. Educ. Tech. Res. Dev. **65**(6), 1655–1671 (2017). https://doi.org/10.1007/s11423-017-9551-0

59. Chandrasekaran, J., Anitha, D., Thiruchadai Pandeeswari, S.: Enhancing student learning and engagement in the course on computer networks, J. Eng. Educ. Transform. **34**, 454–463 (2021)
60. Mecca, G., Santoro, D., Sileno, N., Veltri, E.: Diogene-CT: tools and methodologies for teaching and learning coding. Int. J. Educ. Technol. High. Educ. **18**(1), 1–26 (2021). https://doi.org/10.1186/s41239-021-00246-1
61. Chigona W., Pollock, M.: Pair programming for information systems students new to programming: students' experiences and teachers' challenges. In: PICMET'08-2008 Portland International Conference on Management of Engineering \& Technology, pp. 1587–1594 (2008)
62. Asnawi, A.L., et al.: The needs of collaborative tool for practicing pair programming in educational setting. Int. J. Interact. Mob. Technol. (2019)
63. Bahig, H.M., Khedr, A.Y.: MonitTDPA: a tool for monitoring the tracing of dynamic programming algorithms. Comput. Appl. Eng. Educ. **25**(2), 179–187 (2017)
64. Mayer, R.E., Dyck, J.L., Vilberg, W.: Learning to program and learning to think: what's the connection?. Commun. ACM **29**(7), 605–610 (1986)
65. Hanks, B.: Empirical evaluation of distributed pair programming. Int. J. Hum. Comput. Stud. **66**(7), 530–544 (2008)
66. Zin, A.M., Idris, S., Subramaniam, N.K.: Improving learning of programming through E-learning by using asynchronous virtual pair programming. Turkish Online J. Dist. Educ. **7**(3), 162–173 (2006)
67. Cicchino, M.I.: Using game-based learning to foster critical thinking in student discourse, Interdiscip. J. Probl. Learn (2015)
68. Hussein, M.H., Ow, S.H., Cheong, L.S., Thong, M.K., Ale Ebrahim, N.: Effects of digital game-based learning on elementary science learning: a systematic review. IEEE Access **7**, 62465-62478 (2019)

Attitude Towards Intention to Use Mobile-Based Teaching Assessment Based on TAM and a Novel Extended TAM Model

Abdullahi Ahmed Abdirahman[1](✉), Marzanah A. Jabar[2], Abdirahman Osman Hashi[1], Mohamed Abdirahman Elmi[1], and Octavio Ernesto Romo Rodriguez[3]

[1] Faculty of Computing, SIMAD University, Mogadishu, Somalia
{aaayare,m.abdirahman}@simad.edu.so

[2] Department of Information System and Software Engineering, Faculty of Computer Science and Information Technology,, Universiti Putra Malaysia, Seri Kembangan, Malaysia
marzanah@upm.edu.my

[3] Department of Computer Science, Faculty of Informatics, Istanbul Teknik Üniversitesi, 34469 Maslak, İstanbul, Turkey

Abstract. In recent years the combination of a rapid development in mobile technology and the pandemic scenario in which currently the world is still in, have caused an increasing demand for online systems that can replace the traditional methods in a variety of areas. For instance, the rising usage of e-learning and e-health are evidence of this reality. Consequently, Mobile Based Teaching Assessment (MBTA) has become the ideal candidate to replace traditional classroom evaluation. The intention of end users to use MBTA as an alternative to traditional evaluation is the main indicator of its adoption in a regular basis. This study has two main goals, the first one is to use the Technology Acceptance Model (TAM) to evaluate how people's feelings towards the usage of MBTA, the second goal is to propose an extended TAM that incorporates intrinsic motivation to the traditionally extrinsic regular TAM. Partially least squares (PLS) were used in this study, and data was gathered from 75 students and academic support personnel using a simple sampling technique, as well as structural model to evaluate the proposed model. Based on the findings of this research, the attitude of individuals directly influences their desire to use MBTA. Along with that, individual's attitude is influenced by a variety of factors, this is more evident in the extended TAM proposed. Despite the indications achieved with TAM regarding the implementation of mobile-based teaching assessment in an academic context, the claimed user attitude explains 75% of the variance in user intention towards MBTA. The importance of the suggested paradigm, as well as the accuracy of the extended TAM proposed, is shown in the results of this work.

Keywords: Partial least squares · Technology acceptance model · Mobile assessment in mobile devices

F. Saeed et al. (Eds.): IRICT 2021, LNDECT 127, pp. 583–593, 2022.
https://doi.org/10.1007/978-3-030-98741-1_48

1 Introduction

With global acceptance of technologies for the improvement of learning activities, various portable personal computing, and communication devices (like Smartphone and tablets) made adoption of such technologies a reality. Also, the rapid growth of IT has led to new applications such as e-learning, e- health to replace traditional methods [1]. As a result, mobile-based teaching assessment (MBTA) has developed as a useful supplement to traditional classroom evaluation methods.

Among academics, mobile learning has become a frequent occurrence. Furthermore, it is becoming more widely accepted owing to its accessibility and the fact that it provides users with a variety of capabilities, such as 3G and 4G networks [2]. In accordance with this, O' Malley et al. [3] described m-learning as a kind of learning that allows students to study at any time and from any location while also allowing them to communicate through mobile devices. Mobile technologies support a variety of activities in the educational setting, including dynamic, location-aware, context-aware, collaborative, peer, and self-assessment practices [4]. However, contemporary educational evaluations are not intended to be completed on mobile terminals, but rather on a desktop computer. It demonstrates that students' ease in using the system at any time and from any location receives less attention. As a result, mobile devices should be used in classroom assessment to improve academic services [5].

More specifically, the wide array of a proliferation of technology applications in education environment necessitates a mobile-based teaching assessment. However, learners' recognition of mobile-based teaching assessment has been overlooked, and the effectiveness of the adoption of MBTA raises a question among academics, practitioners, and developers. To that end, special attention is given to the adoption of MBTA. Since the previous literature highlighted the suitability of assessing the computers [6–8]. While other literature stated that mobile learning is encouraged to be adopted in an academic environment [9, 10]. Therefore, from the viewpoint of the Technology-Acceptance-Model, this provides sufficient scope to examine the attitude toward the intention to utilize Mobile-Based Teaching Assessment. In fact, this research will be one of the first to predict the acceptability of Mobile-Based Teaching Assessment.

The paper is structured as follows: the background of Assessments by the mobile technology is presented in section two. Followed by and Technology Acceptance Model (TAM) in section three. Research model and formulation of hypotheses are reported in section four. A methodology is presented in section five. The data analysis is shown in section six. Section seven presents discussions and conclusion.

2 Background and Related Work

2.1 Assessments on the Basis of Mobile Technology

Technology innovation brought portable devices like tablets, notebooks, and Smartphones allowing academicians gain access to digital content in learning which leads to a new learning mode called mobile learning. In addition, technology innovation offered not only mobile learning but also enabled users to make communication, entertainment, and multiple purpose information processing tools. Therefore, the usage of mobile devices in higher education improved due to conjunctions with near universal 3G/4G wireless connectivity. In addition to that, mobile learning has features that include ubiquity, portability, low cost, mobility and flexibility engaging users to use the Mobile-learning [11]. On the other hand, mobile devices have a potential effect on improving the outcomes and motivations of the students besides the enhancement of their attitudes since mobile technology has already integrated into learning activities [12]. Consequently, the ubiquitous and mobility features at mobile devices plus the growth of technology enable to perform possible evaluations and create a new technique for the assessments, called Mobile-Based Testing (MBT).

Context-aware adaptation provides support to the educational activities in a mobile learning platform. Economides [13] demonstrates the essential features that affect the quality of using mobile learning devices. Adaptive mobile learning and mobile learner are two ideas in mobile technology, with adaptive mobile learning serving as an engine that personalizes educational activities in a given environment, and the mobile learner doing educational activities. Moreover, mobile devices make a possible extension of services due to their mobility. For instance, mobile learning plays a vital role in various education-related activities, namely performing formative assessment or self-assessment [14]. For that reason, mobile technology can be alternatively adoptable in teaching assessment. Therefore, the mobile devices become inevitable in the adoption of the implications in a real world, and that renders mainly teaching evaluation to benefit them.

2.2 Technology Acceptance Model

Due to technology applications proliferation in the academics, a new approach for mobile assessment was innovated to replace the existing traditional methods of evaluation such as paper-and-pencil based or web-based. The mobile devices can access the contents anytime and anywhere. Thus, it is imperative to explore student's acceptance of mobile-based teaching assessment adoption in academic institutions. Various studies were conducted about users' the acceptance to adopt the information system for their lives [15, 16]. For example, a study by Hussein [17] revealed that intention to use the e-learning depends on users' attitude which has a significant part for making the system well performed.

This paper puts forward the technology-acceptance-model (TAM) to explain the relationship between the variables of interest. Perceived ease of use (EoU), perceived usefulness (PU), and attitudes (ATT) are three variables in this theory that characterize and predict system adoption. They have different meanings, since perceived usefulness captures how much a user believes utilizing a specific technology would improve his or her work performance (PU). This factor determines the usefulness and efficacy of mobile teaching assessment in academics. The ease of understandability of such mobile teaching assessment is defined by its ease of use (EoU), which relates to the ease-of-use (EoU) of TAM, since ease-of-use refers to the extent/degree to which a person has strong views that he or she can utilize the system with ease [18]. Finally, the third component of the theory provides light on the users' attitudes that motivate them to utilize mobile-based instructional assessment. In an e-learning system, the attitude relates to the degree to which the user is interested in the MBTA. Furthermore, the voluntary adoption of MBTA in academics is motivated by a behavioral purpose that is affected by attitude. The user's desire to utilize the mobile to manage teaching-related evaluations is predicted by the general dimensions described above. As a result, the purpose of this study is to look at user acceptability of the MBTA's usage of TAM. It is critical to examine the underlying variables that drive MBTA, which are influenced by the user's behavioral goals and attitude toward technology adoption, either directly or indirectly. Given that TAM is the theory that may be used to verify the interrelationships between the variables in this research. To put it another way, acceptance of mobile learning has previously been used in TAM assessment with a variety of changes and extensions to incorporate a variety of external factors [10, 20]. However, the research on the acceptability of mobile-based instructional evaluation is still lacking. Moreover, the empirical existing literature about mobile based assessment by users shows contradictory results. Mobile users have positive attitude towards MBA according to Chen [21], while other show negative attitude towards MBA [22, 23]. Therefore, this study is first step forward by examining the users' (students and academic support) attitudes which lead to the behavioral intention which results in driving mobile-based teaching assessment.

2.3 Research Model and Hypothesis

The reliability of TAM has proven by an extensive number of research. Nonetheless, TAM has an emphasis on the notion of instrumentality, focusing mainly on functional and extrinsic motivations. Such a perception could be limited when dealing with situations out of an organizational environment, where the motivations behind the choices of individuals are not so obvious.

According to research in the field of Psychology and Psychoanalysis, motivations can be classified in two categories, extrinsic and intrinsic motivators. Extrinsic motivation is when an individual is motivated to do an activity to obtain a reward, the focus is on the outcome of the activity. Intrinsic motivation is naturally the opposite, when an individual chooses to do an activity because it is internally rewarding, the activity is satisfactory by itself, therefore the focus is on the activity and not the outcome of it.

Given that psychological principle, it has been proven that intrinsic motivation plays a key role in decision making of individuals, particularly among young people. Taking that into consideration, it becomes clear that TAM, as reliable as it might be in some cases, does not cover the whole spectrum of the motivations behind the decisions of people in this case, mainly because the environment is more varied and the individuals targeted are younger, thus with a higher tendency to base their decisions on intrinsic motivation.

That is the main reason why it was decided to extend the previously presented model, using a regular TAM model, and introduce an extended TAM model including intrinsic motivation. This motivation has been included in the form of two factors: System Quality Perception (SQP) and Enjoyment (E). The relation between these two new factors and the previous model is based on research in the fields of psychology, pedagogy and information systems, as well as data gathered in this research to prove the reliability of the proposed model.

Established on the factors mentioned, the extended model proposed is the following:

The first introduced factor is System Quality Perception (SQP). This involves aspects such as system quality, information quality and content quality, as well as the availability of the system as a whole. Instinctively, the quality of a system influences the Ease of Use

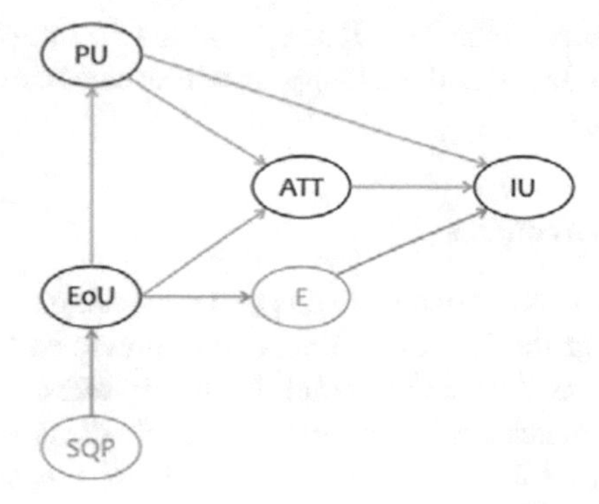

Fig. 1. Describes the proposed extended model to be adopted in this research

(EuO), since a good quality system consists of well documented and planned features that will allow users to navigate in the system and use its resources efficiently. With that said, quality can be interpreted in a variety of ways, objective and subjectively.

Given that the focus of this research is the intention of people to use mobile-based teaching assessment, and that the targeted demographic consists of mostly young people who tend to base their decisions on intrinsic motivation, the interpretation given to quality in this model has an additional aspect, which is the perception. Hence, System Quality Perception conveys the objective and subjective features of quality in a system, such as the actual usability and availability of the system, as well as the statics of the system, that influence enormously the perception of the end user regarding to the quality of the system.

The second new factor is Enjoyment (E). This is entirely an intrinsic motivation and as the name suggests it refers to the enjoyment while using the system. It is directly influenced by the Ease of Use of the system, naturally a user-friendly system increases the enjoyment of the end users, that is the reason why social media developers put so much effort in making their systems as intuitive as possible. If the user enjoys using their system, he will come back to use it again.

Continuing with those principles, Enjoyment is indirectly influenced by the System Quality Perception. Given that this factor consists subjective aspects like the appreciation of statics, it is clear that these also influence the overall enjoyment of the user while using the system. Regardless of that, these aspects are not directly influencing the Enjoyment factor due to the fact that subjective aspects like the statics of a system cannot make the end user enjoy using the system if the system is not functional itself. It is the combination of functional and static aspects that influences the enjoyment of the end user. Such a relationship is portrayed in the proposed model.

3 Proposed Methodology

3.1 Participants

Random sampling technique was conducted to select participants for the survey. A Total of 75 participants were collected from undergraduates, graduates studies, and academic support of Universiti Putra Malaysia (UPM). In which 50 out of 75 making (66.67%) were students and 25 (33.33%) academic support, while males constituted of 46 (61.33%) and 29 females (38.67%).

3.2 Procedure and Instrument

A quantitative approach was conducted in this paper by using a survey. A questionnaire was formulated based on the TAM constructs from previously validated instruments. The English language was designed to build the survey questionnaire. All items were graded on a 5-point Likert scale ranging from 1 (strongly disagree) to 5 (strongly agree) (strongly agree). Construct three items for Perccived Usefulness (PU) and three items for Perceived Ease of Use from [26]. We utilized six questions from [27] to evaluate Attitudes toward (ATT) and Intention to Use (IU) of Mobile-Based Teaching Assessment, and we upgraded the items slightly to reflect the current research environment (mobile-based teaching assessment). The item "In the future, I plan to utilize e-learning" was changed with "In the future, I want to use mobile devices for teaching evaluation. "In addition to that, to describe and explain the features of the Mobile-Based Teaching Assessment, we have given to the participants 10 min presentation before answering the questionnaire, and 15 min to complete the questionnaires. To validate and analyzing data for the variables that effect the implementation of teaching assessment through mobile technologies. Smart PLS Version 3.0 software was used to test the measurement and structural model of this analysis.

4 Data Analysis

We utilized Smart PLS Version 3.0 to offer the study model's convergent and discriminant validity in order to evaluate and verify its quality. As a result, to verify that the concept indicators are genuine, the convergent validity must be assessed. The model's validity must meet the following measurement requirements: (1) constructs with factor loadings higher than 0.700 are acceptable; (2) each variable's composite reliability must exceed 0.700; and (3) each construct's Average Variance Extracted (AVE) must likewise exceed 0.700.

The results in Table 1, indicates that all the measures for convergent validity passed and verified. In the factor loadings, the results of all variables are in between 0.755–0.942 that means they exceed 0.700. Also, the Average Variance Extracted (AVE) values indicate that they are in the range of 0.665 to 0.760 (AVE $>$ 0.5). In addition, the values of root squared of AVE as shown in Table 2 are greater than correlation of corresponding constructs. As a result, all AVE square root values are higher than the construct inter-correlation values. As a result, the suggested research model's convergent and discriminant validity are both confirmed.

We used PLS-Graph to complete the SEM by calculating the R-squared values and Path coefficients. We also tested whether hypotheses formulated are in line with the study expectations or not. Therefore, the results reveal that all hypotheses tested are in accordance with expected signs. These imply that relationships among variables are statistically significant and positive.

Table 1. Convergent validity of the model

Items	Factor loading (>0.7)	Cronbach's (>0.7)	Composite Reliability (>0.7)	Average Variance Extracted (>0.5)
EoU		0.746	0.856	0.665
EoU 1	0.799			
EoU 2	0.878			
EoU 3	0.764			
U		0.780	0.872	0.695
U1	0.755			
U2	0.878			
U3	0.863			
IU		0.841	0.904	0.760
BIU 1	0.816			
BIU 2	0.923			
BIU 3	0.873			
ATT		0.795	0.880	0.712
ATT 1	0.873			
ATT 2	0.942			
ATT 3	0.801			

EoU: Ease of Use, PU: Perceived Usefulness, IU: Intention to Use, ATT: Attitude.

Table 2. Discriminant Validity of the Model

Item	ATT	IU	EoU	PU
ATT	**0.844**			
IU	0.764	**0.872**		
EoU	0.641	0.603	**0.815**	
PU	0.832	0.867	0.622	**0.834**

Bold values: the square root of the average variance extracted (AVE) of each construct.

Table 3. Hypothesis testing results

H	Path	Path Coefficient	t statistics	Support
H1	EoU -> PU	0.622***	8.124	Supported
H2	EoU -> ATT	0.201***	2.071	Supported
H3	PU - > IU	0.554***	4.724	Supported
H4	PU -> ATT	0.707***	7.008	Supported
H5	ATT -> BIU	0.754***	5.781	Supported

*** $p < 0.1$, ** $p < 0.05$, *** $p < 0.01$**

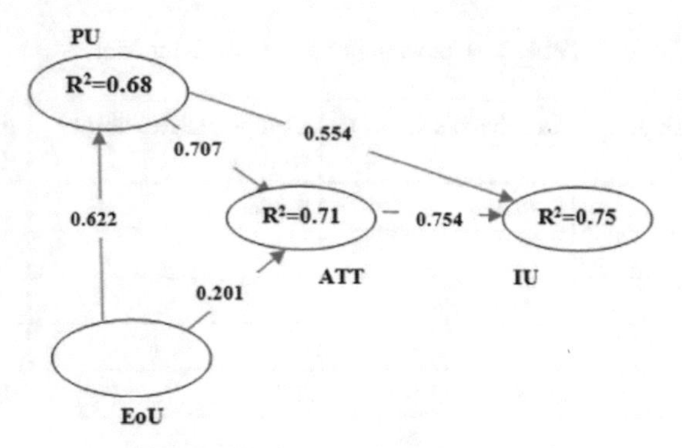

Fig. 2. The structural model results

Structural equation modeling was used to examine the newly added variables and their connections (Table 4). The calculation of the values produced findings that showed a good match of the structural model to the data for the specified research model [31].

It can be noticed that the values in the table are given within a range. The decision and direction of the result also confirms the validity of the proposed model.

Table 4. A summary of the results achieved is shown in the following table:

Relationship	Path	t-value	p-value	Direction	Support
SQP → PU	– 0.006	0.114	0.914	Neg	No
SQP → EoU	0.103	2.498	0.011	Pos	Yes
E → EoU	– 0.203	2.673	0.009	Neg	Yes
E → IU	0.133	2.112	0.035	Pos	Yes
EoU → PU	0.295	5.160	0.000	Pos	Yes
EoU → ATT	0.150	3.123	0.002	Pos	Yes
PU → ATT	0.522	9.697	0.000	Pos	Yes
EoU → IU	0.086	1.867	0.040	Pos	Yes
PU → IU	0.195	2.832	0.005	Pos	Yes
ATT → IU	0.341	5.132	0.000	Pos	Yes
IU → Actual Usage	0.192	3.486	0.001	Pos	Yes

Structural model results (significant at $p^{**} < = 0.01$, $p^{*} < 0.05$).

It is important to notice the accuracy of the proposed model in accordance to the results achieved in Table 4. For instance, in the proposed model System Quality Perception directly influences Ease of Use, in the previous table this hypothesis is confirmed since it shows a positive relationship between these two factors.

In a similar manner, in the proposed model a relationship between Ease of Use and Enjoyment was introduced, this relationship is also confirmed in the third row of the table, showing a negative relationship between Enjoyment and Ease of Use. The direction is also consistent with the proposed model since it was proposed that Ease of Use influences Enjoyment and not the other way around, which is proven right in the structural model results.

Additionally, the last introduced relationship in the proposed model is also present in the results achieved. The fourth row of the table shows a positive relationship between Enjoyment and Intention to Use, which is precisely what the proposed model describes.

5 Discussion

Using the Technology Acceptability Model, this research investigates the acceptability of mobile-based teaching assessment (TAM). This is the first study to use the Technology Acceptance Model to assess mobile-based teaching (TAM). It adds to the theoretical body of knowledge in the area of mobile apps. The mindset of the user, according to the idea, is the most important element that affects their desire to use the MBTA. User attitude has a favorable and substantial effect on their intention to use the MBTA, according to the findings, accounting for 75% of the variance in user intention to use the MBTA. The result is that the user's intention has an impact on whether or not mobile-based teaching assessment (MBTA) is utilized, since a positive attitude leads to a greater willingness to use mobile-based teaching assessment (MBTA).

Furthermore, these results corroborate both hypotheses, and previous research has shown that the user's attitude influences their intention to utilize an e-learning system [28, 29]. TAM has a strong predictive value in describing how academic arena could be adopted mobile-based-teaching-assessment (MBTA) in the, according to the data. The purpose of users of mobile-based teaching assessment (MBTA) changes with their attitudes, according to TAM. As a result, users' attitudes and other associated variables that may enhance or reduce user acceptance of online educational tools must be given top priority in the success of such a model in the educational environment. Since TAM included attitude as the most important main explanatory variable, the study recommends that variables that increase attitude be studied in the future.

Through the mediation of attitude, the ease of use has a substantial beneficial impact on the intention to use. Students and academic support staff develop a strong proclivity to utilize MBTA with ease as they get a better understanding of mobile apps in teaching assessments. The MBTA's perceived utility (PU) has a direct positive impact on the desire to use it. Students and support groups have a greater conviction in the use of mobile applications in teaching assessment as an alternate or complementary method to paper-based and computer-based assessment delivery modalities that may be used both within and outside of the school.

6 Conclusions

The implications of this study include motivation of both students and academic support groups to perform the teaching assessment for their convenience and encourage developer should design mobile applications that appeal needs of students and academic support groups on one side and education administration on the other. Implementation of teaching assessment based on mobile applications depends on the positive attitude of the administration.

Although the current research represents an early effort at developing MBTA acceptability, it does not imply that it is without limits. The present proposed model calls to be tested to other theories than TAM. It further needs to account for individual differences among users of mobile applications in teaching assessment. For future research, proposed model calls for applying in other settings as well as adding additional variables.

Acknowledgment. It is imperative to acknowledge the support given by SIMAD Research Center in order to make this research a success.In addition to that, the authors of this paper are honored to thank SIMAD University for making this research possible by granting the Research University Grant.

References

1. oAlsabawy, F., Younis, A., Aileen, C.S., Soar, J.: Determinants of perceived usef e- learning systems. Comput. Hum. Behav. **64**, 843- 858 (2016)
2. Cerratto-Pargman, T., Järvelä, S.M., Milrad, M.: Designing Nordic technology-enhanced learning. Internet High. Educ. **15**(4), 227–323 (2012)
3. O'Malley, C., et al.: Guidelines for learning/teaching/tutoring in a mobile environment (2005)
4. Berge, Z.L, Muilenburg, L.: Handbook of Mobile Learning, Routledge (2013)
5. Tulloch, M., et al.: Case studies to enhance online student evaluation: Charles Sturt University–Evaluation, analytics and systems integration (2015)
6. Terzis, V., Economides, A.A.: The acceptance and use of computer based assessment. Comput. Educ. **56**(4), 1032–1044 (2011)
7. Terzis, V., Moridis, C.N., Economides, A.A.: Continuance acceptance of computer based assessment through the integration of user's expectations and perceptions. Comput. Educ. **62**(50–6), 1 (2013)
8. Terzis, V., Moridis, C.N., Economides, A.A., Mendez, G.R.: Computer based assessment acceptance: A cross-cultural study in Greece and Mexico. J. Educ. Technol. Soc. **16**(3), 411 (2013)
9. Abu-Al-Aish, A., Love, S.: Factors influencing students' acceptance of m-learning: an investigation in higher education. Int. Rev. Res. Open Distrib. Learn. **14**(5), 82-107 (2013)
10. Park, S.Y., Nam, M.-W., Cha, S.-B.: University students' behavioral intention to use mobile learning: evaluating the technology acceptance model. Br. J. Edu. Technol. **43**(4), 592–605 (2012)
11. Cheung, W.S., Hew, K.F.: A review of research methodologies used in studies on mobile handheld devices in K-12 and higher education settings. Australas. J. Educ. Technol. **25**(2) (2009)
12. Hwang, G.-J., Chang, H.-F.: A formative assessment-based mobile learning approach to improving the learning attitudes and achievements of students. Comput. Educ. **56**(4), 1023–1031 (2011)
13. Economides, A.A.: Requirements of mobile learning applications. Int. J. Innov. Learn. **5**(5), 457–479 (2008)
14. Huang, Y.-M., Lin, Y.-T., Cheng, S.-C.: An adaptive testing system for supporting versatile educational assessment. Comput. Educ. **52**(1), 53–67 (2009)
15. Hsu, H.-H., Chang, Y.-Y.: Extended TAM model: impacts of convenience on acceptance and use of moodle. Online Submiss. **3**(4), 211–218 (2013)

16. King, W.R., He, J.: A meta-analysis of the technology acceptance model. Inf. Manag. **43**(6), 740–755 (2006)
17. Hussein, Z.: Leading to intention: the role of attitude in relation to technology acceptance model in e- learning. Procedia Comput. Sci. **105**, 159–164 (2017)
18. Davis, F.D., Bagozzi, R.P., Warshaw, P.R.: User acceptance of computer technology: a comparison of two theoretical models. Manage. Sci. **35**(8), 982–1003 (1989)
19. Saadé, R.G., Galloway, I.: Understanding intention to use multimedia information systems for learning. Inf. Sci. Int. J. Emerg. Transdiscipl. **2**, 287–296 (2005)
20. Liu, Y., Han, S., Li, H.: Understanding the factors driving m-learning adoption: a literature review. Campus-Wide Inf. Syst. **27**(4), 210–226 (2010)
21. Chen, C.-H.: The implementation and evaluation of a mobile self-and peer-assessment system. Comput. Educ. **55**(1), 229–236 (2010)
22. Huff, K.C.: The comparison of mobile devices to computers for web-based assessments. Comput. Hum. Behav. **49**, 208–212 (2015)
23. Wang, Y.-S., Wu, M.-C., Wang, H.-Y.: Investigating the determinants and age and gender differences in the acceptance of mobile learning. Br. J. Edu. Technol. **40**(1), 92–118 (2009)
24. Ju, T.L., Sriprapaipong, W., Minh, D.N.: On the success factors of mobile learning. In: Paper presented at 5th International Conference on ICT and Higher Education (2007)
25. Bangkok
26. Terzis, V., Moridis, C.N., Economides, A.A.: The effect of emotional feedback on behavioral intention to use computer based assessment. Comput. Educ. **59**(2), 710–721 (2012)
27. Venkatesh, V., Morris, M.G., Davis, G.B., Davis, F.D.: User acceptance of information technology: toward a unified view. MIS Q. **27**(3), 425e478 (2003)
28. Chang, H.H.: Task-technology fit and user acceptance of online auction. Int. J. Hum.-Comput. Stud. **68**(1e2), 69e89 (2010). http://dx.doi.org/https://doi.org/10.1016/j.ijhcs.2009. 09.010
29. Altawallbeh, M., Soon, F., Thiam, W., Alshourah, S.: Mediating role of attitude, subjective norm and perceived behavioural control in the relationships between their respective salient beliefs and behavioural intention to adopt elearning among instructors in jordanian universities. J. Educ. Pract. **6**(11), 152–159 (2015)
30. Sujeet, K.S., Jyoti, K.C.: (2013) 'Technology acceptance model for the use of learning through websites among students in Oman. Int. Arab J. E- Technol. **3**(1), 44–49 (2013)
31. Salloum, S.A.S.: Investigating students' acceptance of E-learning system in Higher Educational Environments in the UAE: Applying the Extended Technology Acceptance Model (TAM) (Doctoral dissertation, The British University in Dubai)sss (2018)

The Roles of Information Presentation on User Performance in Mobile Augmented Reality Application

Nur Intan Adhani Muhamad Nazri and Dayang Rohaya Awang Rambli(✉)

Universiti Teknologi PETRONAS, Perak, Malaysia
{nur_9113,dayangrohaya.ar}@utp.edu.my

Abstract. Mobile Augmented Reality (AR) has an interesting and interactive method of presenting information because it is the combination of real and virtual environments. Thus, a large amount of information is required and some of the necessary information is not fit to the screen due to the small screen display. Hence, lead to user dissatisfaction and not getting the right and accurate information. This study herein aims to examine the roles and optimal combination of information presentation to improve user performance in mobile AR applications. A possible combination of information modalities is created and a study was conducted by comparing two different conditions: 1) without sound and haptic feedback; 2) with sound and haptic feedback. Results showed the optimal combination of information modalities is with sound feedback and haptic feedback based on statistical analysis and user preferences. Moreover, the roles of information presentation indeed able to support visual information modality in the mobile AR application.

Keywords: Mobile augmented reality · Multimodal information presentation · User performance

1 Introduction

Augmented Reality (AR) technology has become an ideal platform due to the advancement of technology such as a high-quality camera, powerful microprocessor, tracking technology and others. Thus, provide an interactive technique to interact with the physical and virtual environment. Consequently, AR uncovers unique ways to present data and information. Though AR has been introduced more than a decade, these still a very important area of future research [1]. By embedding AR within applications, it can offer an interactive experience by providing creative details such as data and information through the use of augmentation added to it. Some features that make AR practical to use is, it makes users aware of their surrounds while interacting with virtual content in the mobile AR application [2]. This is different compared to users who may be texting or scrolling content on their mobile devices, which may narrow their eyes vision resulting in accidents while walking.

In spite of its ubiquity, it is found that when creating mobile AR application, designers, developers and researchers barely see from the user's point of view. This in the

F. Saeed et al. (Eds.): IRICT 2021, LNDECT 127, pp. 594–603, 2022.
https://doi.org/10.1007/978-3-030-98741-1_49

long run driven to the low commercialization of versatile AR applications within the market. This is because presenting meaningful information in effective ways is still an ongoing challenge due to the nature of AR technology, which involves a large amount of data and information required to be presented [3–5]. Therefore, due to the small screen display of a mobile device, some required and meaningful data, content and information are not fitted into it. Eventually, it will make user feel frustrated and disappointed. Moreover, it will lead to an error in getting the right and accurate information [6] due to the impact of ineffective information presentation. Hence, there is a need to mapping types of information to tasks in and understand the roles of information presentation, which will allow exploration of possible uses and benefits of various modalities that can eventually improve the user performance [7].

This paper addresses a question on what is the roles of information presentation and the optimal combination of output modalities in mobile AR application. Thus, the objectives of this study are to examine and identify the optimal combination and investigate the roles of information presentation in mobile AR application.

In the next section, related works of this study are highlighted. Followed by methods to conduct this study. Then, results and discussion are described in detail.

2 Related Work

2.1 Mobile Augmented Reality

Today, smartphones have become a popular mobile AR platform due to its sufficient processing powers which improve the AR functions [8–10] and widely used. This is because of it features that offers mobility, lightweight and small. To experience mobile AR, users do not have to carry a bulky hardware. With the widespread adoption of AR using smartphone, it encouraged users to look at the screen and interact with the AR content inside it.

In order to make mobile AR experience possible, as a start, it only takes processing power, camera, internet connection, a basic understanding of geometry and 3D graphics to deliver augmented reality experiences for users. The development of AR applications is very accessible and basic application are easy to get. This allows developers to reach the most users because people already own AR capable smartphones.

2.2 Information Presentation Theory

Information presentation is generally referring to a manner in which a system or interfaces present information to user [7]. In order to expand the knowledge of the users, the role of information presentation is to create a creative visual representation of data to be meaningful and can be easily understood.

The main role of information presentation is to offer a simple, yet concise and compact presentation content to support users in working and exploring the content of an application [12]. At the same time, the information needs to be accurate, meaningful and are able to be perceived by user. Furthermore, with respect to its projection on the eye level, there is a need to ensure the displayed information is well organized [11, 13] and provide interactive and intuitive user interface.

Below is some of the terms that were used interchangeably in many existing literatures related to information presentation: -

- Information presentation: common ways of presenting data. Example type of medias are icon, text, image, audio and video. It is generally used as a type of information presentation. The purpose and objective of information presentation are to increase users' knowledge, awareness and engagement by providing interactive media. [14–16].
- Information representation: The same information can have few alternative representations. For example, icon 'Printer' represents to print a document.

2.3 Information Presentation in Mobile AR

Compared to the traditional method, information presentation in mobile AR is far more challenging as it combines information from the real environment and information that needs to be augmented. Furthermore, to fit onto the screen of mobile devices, the relevant data and information need to be squeezed and become compact information [17].

Moreover, identifying the type and style of information of each presentation mode will eventually speak its purpose within the user interface (UI). According to Lombard & Ditton [18], there is always a relation between the form in which information is displayed with the content of the information and features exclusive to the user.

Therefore, information presentation in mobile AR has become a unique way to provide a form of interactive communication, engagement and provide a better mutual understanding between users as it is effective and memorable.

2.4 Multimodal Information Presentation

The application or system that use more than 2 modalities (i.e., Vision, Auditory, Gesture, Tactile, etc.) to present information is always refer to multimodal information presentation and also known as multimodal fission.

It can be classified on the basis of 3 criteria [19]: -

- Medium: refer to device used to deliver information. For example; Paper, computer display, speaker, mobile screen
- Presentation Mode (Information modality): refer to format of the message. For example; text, image
- Modality: refer to process information using human senses. For example; visual, auditory

Few researchers stated the guidelines for multimodal information presentation which are the grouping of information modalities ought to be minimized and only necessary to use it when there is a need to convey important information [20]. Furthermore, to improve the method of communication and transmission of information multiple information modalities can be combined in one presentation form [21].

Nevertheless, under a certain condition, combining multiple information modalities could provide significance support. However, it does not always give any benefit to the user and the system and sometimes create more burden to the user. Information modalities contain a really great expressive control as they can actually be way better than another at passing on certain information for certain condition. As an example, to display and giving out instruction or information when driving, sound command or speech is a better method. Whereas, the text is appropriate to display distance, temperature, level of measurements such as centimeter, meter and others.

3 Method

An experimental design needs to be done in order to conduct a study. The next subsection describes the experimental setup, followed by the method used to collect and analyzes the data. There are 3 main processes in conducting the experiment which are experimental procedures, data collection and data analysis. Details of these processes will be explained in details in the next section.

3.1 Experimental Procedures

Purpose. This purpose of this study is to investigate how information presentation is able to assist users in navigating and exploring the mobile AR content and to understand the roles of information presentation on user performance. Therefore, optimal combination of output modalities and its role will be proposed and identified.

Procedure. For the purpose of this study, five types of information modalities were selected which are text, image/icon, speech, sound and vibration. Two separate conditions are tested. The first condition is combination without haptic and sound feedback. The second condition is combination with haptic and sound feedback. Below are the 5 steps to ensure the experiment is properly conducted: -

- Before experiments begin: Participants were given an explanation about the study by the project leader.
- In the beginning of experiments: To familiarize with the mobile AR application, participants were given at least 5 min and they were asked if there are any question.
- During the experiment: Participants will then try the mobile AR application. Observation of the participant's reaction and interaction with the mobile AR application is recorded.
- At the end of experiment: Each participant was asked to answer a questionnaire and give any feedback that they have experienced.
- To test for second condition, step 3 and step 4 is repeated.

Participants. A total of 40 participants, with 20 males and 20 females volunteered in this study. The majority participants are between 20 to 28 years old. All the participants are familiar in using smartphone. By following the sample size rule, "sample size larger than 30 and less than 500 are appropriate for most research" [22]. Therefore, 40 sample is enough for this study.

3.2 Data Collection

Observation. Throughout the experimentation, a paper recording of the users' actions is taken. Hence, every action of participants that occurred during the study will be written and recorded to analyze the participant's feedback for reference.

Open-Ended Question. The open-ended questions are a non-structured way aimed to collect users' feedback on the application [23].

QUIS Questionnaire 5.5. A measurement apparatus designed to evaluate a user's subjective Satisfaction with the human-computer interface [24]. It contains a demographic questionnaire, a measure of overall system satisfaction, and a measure of specific interface factors such as screen visibility, terminology and system information, learning factors, and system capabilities.

3.3 Data Analysis

Comparison analysis was done between the first condition and second condition by testing on the response time and the score (user performance).

3.4 Mobile AR Apps

The mobile AR game interface is designed with a combination of 2D and 3D components. The 3D object consists of the brick wall, the bubbles, and the avatar. While for 2D object consists of the instructions, countdown timer, score panel and application control buttons which situated on planes floating above the 3D scene. The application was developed using Unity3D.

4 Results

A set of information modalities and the type of information to be conveyed need to be defined and categorized. In corresponding with cognitive theories, the modality set needed to include visual, auditory, verbal and non-verbal, haptic properties. Hence, in order to allow all combinations of these properties, five types of information modalities were selected which are text (visual, verbal), image/icon (visual, nonverbal), speech (auditory, verbal), sound (auditory, nonverbal) and vibration (haptic, nonverbal). The reason visual and auditory modalities were chosen is because it has been investigated the most in nearly all application domains.

A total of 40 participants were volunteered in this study. All the participants own a smartphone. Almost all of the participants make used audio interaction using their smartphone. All of the participants have tried at least one type of AR application and it shows that participants are familiar with AR technology.

Survey results were divided into 3 sections which are: - (i) Results from QUIS for First Condition; (ii) Results from QUIS for Second Condition; and (iii) Comparison between QUIS for first condition and second condition.

4.1 Results from QUIS for First Condition

In this result section, the first condition was on combinations of visual output modalities and auditory output modalities due to its natural uses in the mobile device. For visual output modalities, it consists of text, graphics and images. For auditory output modalities, only sound (background music) was available.

Results from the Overall Reactions to the Application. For Q1_A (Is it difficult or easy?), the majority (28 participants) find it difficult to use the interface of the application While for Q2_A (Is it frustrating or satisfying?), the majority (36 participants) respond it was frustrating. Q3_A (Is it dull or stimulating?) shows the majority (32 the participants) respond it was a dull application. However, the majority (28 participants) respond that the application is flexible on Q4_A.

4.2 Results from QUIS for Second Condition

In this result section, the second condition was on combinations of visual output modalities, auditory output modalities and haptic output modalities. For visual output modalities, it consists of text, graphics and images. For auditory output modalities, sound (background music and score sound) and speech were included together. For haptic output modalities, the vibration effect was added in the mobile AR application.

Results from the Overall Reactions to the Application. For Q1_B (Is it difficult or easy?), majority (30 participants) find it easy to use the interface of the application. While for Q2_B (Is it frustrating or satisfying?), the majority (31 participants) respond it was satisfying. Q3_A (Is it dull or stimulating?) shows majority (32 the participants) respond it was stimulating when using the application. Next, the majority (26 participants) respond that the application is flexible on Q4_B.

4.3 Comparison Analysis Between First Condition and Second Condition

Figure 1 shows the user performance based on response time. The result suggested that there was a significant difference in mean response time between the combination of with and without output modalities (sound and haptic feedback), with $Z = -6.742$; $p < .001$. Hence, it was concluded that combination with output modalities performs faster in terms of response time. Therefore, it was statistically confirmed that a combination with output modalities (Ct_HS) is able to improve user performance in mobile AR applications.

Figure 2 shows the user performance on the score. The combinations with output modalities have a greater effect on scores achieved by participants in this task-based performance due to its significance and higher median and mean scores compared to combinations without output modalities.

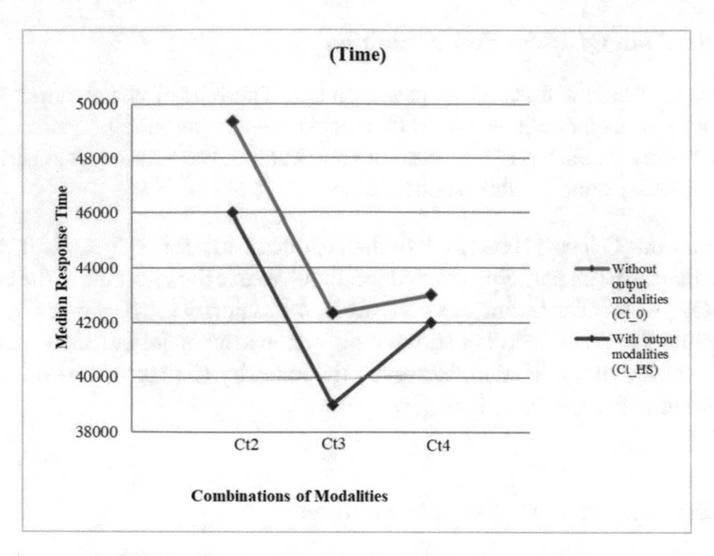

Fig. 1. User performance based on response time

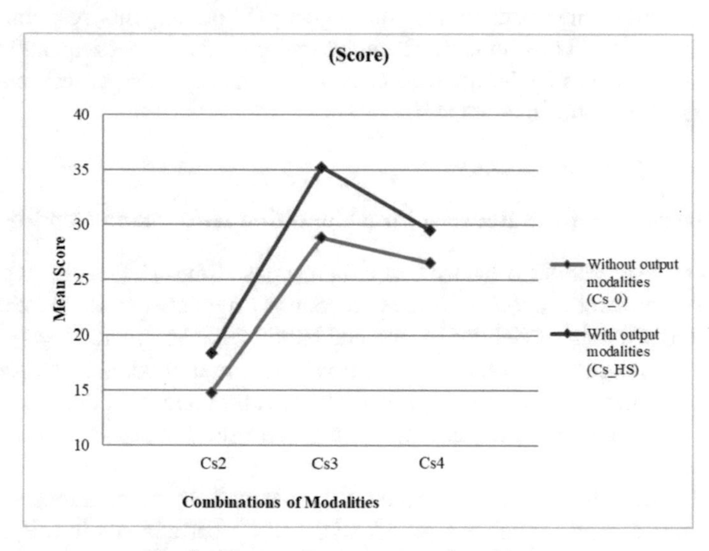

Fig. 2. User performance based on the score

5 Discussion

For the first condition, most of the participants gave a negative comment due to no additional information modalities being present in the first condition. In this mobile AR application, there are 3 interfaces, namely Main interface, Instruction interface and Game interface. In the main interface in the first condition, most of the participants found it was dull. In the Instruction interface, almost all participants' voice out that they found it was annoying when the speech modality (giving instruction) was present in the second condition. This was shown in negative reaction of Usability & UI part in survey result. Participants stated that it was not necessary to include the speech modality to give the instruction as they were able to read from the text given. Furthermore, it has created a privacy issue. In the Game interface for the first condition, the score and time (2D graphic) were positioned on the top left and right. While for 'HOME' and 'EXIT' button is on the bottom left and right of the mobile device screen. This has created a distraction and dissatisfaction as participants were not able to view other objects properly in the virtual scene. Moreover, as there were no sound modality and haptic modality available, participants mentioned that something felt missing. Furthermore, participants mentioned they were confused to interact with AR application when the environment around them was too bright or too dark. They also mentioned that the color of the avatar and other 3D object was small and almost the same as the image of AR marker.

For the second condition, most of the participants gave a positive comment, especially when sound modality and haptic modality was included together. Participants were aware of their surrounding in the virtual scene, when these two information modalities being present where participants getting a point, bonus point or clicking a button. In the Main interface, participants found it was exciting when there is a sound and vibration produced when they click 'PLAY' button. This has made them be ready for next interface. In the Instruction interface, participants stated they were able to read the instruction easily from the text given as they make used of zoom in and zoom out from the mobile device without any additional speech aid (adjusting and positioning the camera view). Participants also stated that the image of 'HOME' and 'EXIT' button was easy to be understood and both buttons were in the center of their view. Furthermore, the sound of clicking and vibration has made the participant to get ready to play the game as soon as the interface changed.

In the Game interface, participants mentioned that they were aware with the surrounding in the virtual environment due to the support from sound and haptic modality being present. Moreover, in the second condition, the score and time board were inside the virtual environment which did not block the view of the Game interface.

5.1 Implementation Concerns for Information Presentation in Mobile AR

There are 2 factors that become a concern when implementing information presentation in mobile AR which are the environment factor and user factor. These factors did affect the roles of information presentation in AR applications.

Environment Factor. Environmental factors that need to be considered are making sure the gesture recognition is possible through better lighting and brightness of screen display. Furthermore, able to adapt noisy condition and able to identify the user's hand motion. It also should be able to give the user the distribution of force, and pressure based on certain conditions.

User Factor. One of the user factors is user preferences which can be interchangeable to suit with the user choices. User preferences consist of familiarity with the application, interest in other interaction mechanisms and error avoidance. Another user factor that needs to be considered is user satisfaction which consists of comfortableness, being in control and easy to use.

6 Conclusion

This research has reached the aim of examine the roles and optimal combination of information presentation to support user performance in mobile AR application. It was found that to support visual modality of information presentation in mobile AR, the use of sound and haptic feedback is needed by providing feedback in response to interaction between user and virtual object. However, certain condition needs to be considered such as the condition of real environment (brightness, noises and etc.)

In conclusion based on results above, (i) it was not necessary to include the speech modality to give the instruction as they were able to read from the text given as it created a privacy issue, (ii) Too many icons create disturbance for the user and create confusions; (iii) With additional output feedback, it will instill awareness in virtual scene, (iv) Sound feedback and haptic feedback is the optimal combination of information modalities based on user preferences.

However, it is worth mentioning, that the use of information modalities is sometimes influenced by the user preferences and user perceptions to environment or surrounding. This can be classified as environment and user factor that will affect the user performance and user satisfaction towards the mobile AR application. Therefore, there is a need to conduct a further study that will combine information modalities with interaction modalities to find more empirical evidence and optimal combination to support the effectiveness of user performance.

References

1. Jaziar, R., Tim, A.M., Jennifer, F., Isabell, W.: A systematic review of immersive virtual reality applications for higher education: design elements, lessons learned, and research agenda. Comput. Educ. **147**, 103778 (2020)
2. Miller, M.R, Jun, H., Herrera, F., Yu, V.J., Welch, G., Bailenson, J.N.: Social interaction in augmented reality. PLoS ONE **14**(5), e0216290 (2019)
3. Doukianou, S., Daylamani-Zad, D., O'Loingsigh, K.: Implementing an augmented reality and animated infographics application for presentations: effect on audience engagement and efficacy of communication. Multimed. Tools Appl. **80**, 30969–30991 (2021)
4. Lee, G.A., et al.: Freeze-set-go interaction method for handheld mobile augmented reality environments. In: Paper Presented at the Proceedings of the 16th ACM Symposium on Virtual Reality Software and Technology, pp. 143–146 (2009)

5. Sun, M., Ren, X., Cao, X.: Effects of multimodal error feedback on human performance in steering tasks. Inf. Media Technol. **6**(1), 193–201 (2011)
6. Koelsch, M., Bane, R., Hoellerer, T., Turk, M.: Multimodal interaction with a wearable augmented reality system. IEEE Comput. Graph. Appl. **3**, 62–71 (2006)
7. Sarter, N.B.: Multimodal information presentation: design guidance and research challenges. Int. J. Ind. Ergon. **36**(5), 439–445 (2006)
8. MobiDev Homepage. https://mobidev.biz/blog/augmented-reality-development-guide. Accessed 21 Nov 2021
9. Mohring, M., Lessig, C., Bimber, O.: Video see-through ar on consumer cell-phones. In: Paper presented at the Proceedings of the 3rd IEEE/ACM International Symposium on Mixed and Augmented Reality, pp. 252–253 (2004)
10. Schall, G., et al.: Global pose estimation using multi-sensor fusion for outdoor augmented reality. In: 8th IEEE International Symposium on Paper presented at the Mixed and Augmented Reality, 2009. ISMAR 2009, pp. 153–162 (2009)
11. Interaction Design Foundation. https://www.interaction-design.org/literature/book/the-encyclopedia-of-human-computer-interaction-2nd-ed/3d-user-interfaces. Accessed 21 Nov 2021
12. Hornbæk, K., Hertzum, M.: The notion of overview in information visualization. Int. J. Hum Comput Stud. **69**(7), 509–525 (2011)
13. Bell, B., Feiner, S., Höllerer, T.: View management for virtual and augmented reality. In: Paper presented at the Proceedings of the 14th annual ACM symposium on User interface software and technology, pp. 101-110 (2001)
14. Bordegoni, M., et al.: A standard reference model for intelligent multimedia presentation systems. Comput. Stand. Interfaces **18**(6), 477–496 (1997)
15. Card, S.K., Mackinlay, J.D., Shneiderman, B.: Readings in Information Visualization: Using Vision to Think. Morgan Kaufmann, (1999)
16. Tegegne, T.H., Mincheol, K.: Mobile Augmented reality in electronic commerce: investigating user perception and purchase intent amongst educated young adults. Sustainability **12**, 9185 (2020)
17. Tobias, M.: Challenges in representing information with augmented reality to support manual procedural tasks. AIMS Electron. Electr. Eng. **3**(1), 71–97 (2019)
18. Lombard, M., Ditton, T.: At the heart of it all: the concept of presence. J. Comput. Media. Commun. **3**(2), JCMC321 (1997)
19. Reeves, L.M., et al.: Guidelines for multimodal user interface design. Commun. ACM **47**(1), 57–59 (2004)
20. Held, R.M., Durlach, N.I.: Telepresence. Presence: Teleoperators and Virtual Environments 1992 vol. 1, pp. 109–112 (1992)
21. Sarter, N.B.: Multimodal information presentation in support of human-automation communication and coordination. Adv. Hum. Perform. Cogn. Eng. Res. **2**, 13–36 (2002)
22. Sekaran U.: Research Method for Business: A Skill Building Approach. John Wiley & Sons (2003)
23. Nielsen, J.: Usability Engineering: Elsevier, Amsterdam (1994)
24. Chin, J.P., Diehl, V.A., Norman, K.L.: Development of an instrument measuring user satisfaction of the human-computer interface. In: Paper presented at the Proceedings of the SIGCHI conference on Human factors in computing systems, pp. 213–218 (1988)

Relevance Judgment of Argument Quality and Online Review Adoption During Information Search in e-Commerce Review Platform

Nur Syadhila Che Lah[1](✉), Ab Razak Che Hussin[2], Norazira A. Jalil[1], and Nor Fatiha Subri[1]

[1] Universiti Tunku Abdul Rahman, Kampar Perak, Malaysia
{syadhila,noraziraj,fatihas}@utar.edu.my
[2] Universiti Teknologi Malaysia, Skudai Johor, Malaysia
abrazak@utm.my

Abstract. The landscape of e-Commerce review platforms can be assumed to be in a state of constant growth due to the viral nature of web content. Furthermore, the leading features of these platform has been acclaimed to be among the influential factors in shaping the behavior of online consumer. Even so, in this regard, if the platform presents too many reviews in non-relevant manner, this may be time-consuming and cumbersome to be understand. Hence, awareness on identifying valuable content of online reviews during information searching process has become important part for online businesses. This study purposely aims to develop a model to understand consumer adoption of online reviews based on dynamics relevance judgment of argument quality in e-Commerce review platform. Elaboration Likelihood Model (ELM) is used in developing the research model to find the potential effects of consumer relevance judgment from information retrieval perspective, which include perceived informative and affective relevance. A quantitative research method has been applied to test and validate the proposed research model. Total of 238 valid respondents has been analyzed using the Partial Least Square Structural Modelling (PLS-SEM) technique. From the research findings, the study found that, content novelty, content topicality, content similarity, content tangibility and content sentimentality could positively influence perception of argument quality which led to information adoption behavior. To be concluded, the importance of information relevancy was also highlighted in this study, which reveals some appropriate features that can be utilized by e-Commerce practitioners to better refine their information search criteria in online review platforms.

Keywords: Online behavior · Information retrieval · Informative relevance · Affective relevance · ELM · PLS-SEM technique

1 Introduction

Online reviews can be described as any judgment posted by previous buyers to describe about the product, the services or the brand published on the websites. The accessibility

F. Saeed et al. (Eds.): IRICT 2021, LNDECT 127, pp. 604–615, 2022.
https://doi.org/10.1007/978-3-030-98741-1_50

of online reviews permits a consumer to make an alternative comparison adjusting to their need during information seeking process. The influence of this information roles is assumed to reach beyond any other marketing strategy and advertising campaign [1]. Many studies have been done to investigate the contribution factors of information quality. However, the results have shown inconsistent conclusions as to how this quality assessment could affect the adoption of online reviews [15]. Additionally, previous studies tend to focus the investigations on the single outcome of argument quality [3]. On the other side, information relevance is proved as one of the most salient subjective quality [4], but still few scholars applied this dimension to represent argument quality perceptions. Hence, the nature of information relevance is worth to be explored as valuable clues in online review platform [2]. Limited studies in testing the multidimensional constructs of argument quality and lack of knowledge on subjective influence towards information adoption behavior are the main identified problems that this study seeks to address. The adoption of IS theories can be made in this research model to test on the relationships of the proposed constructs. Based on this concern, the main research question to be answer is "How can a model be developed to improve argument quality perceptions in the adoption of online reviews across e-Commerce review platforms?".

2 Theoretical Background and Model Development

Dual-process theory of Elaboration Likelihood Model (ELM) designed by Petty and Cacioppo (1980), has been selected most as the research framework to study about argument quality perceptions. ELM posits that, the individual 's attitude change will be caused through the central and peripheral routes [16]. In the context of online review platform, when consumer take a central route, they are assumed to take the maximum effort in evaluating the quality of the received information [11]. Since the focus of this study is to enhance relevance filter of text recommendations, it is assumed that online consumer is more willing and highly motivated to process the pertinent content of review message. Hence, this study proposes that, online consumer will be more likely to use the central route, which involves the relevance judgment of quality dimension of review arguments. In general, the central route encompasses the higher level of information processing within an online communication context. At this stage, online consumer is assumed to critically analyze the message's contents rather than read in casually. Moreover, a consumer is likely to invest in inspecting the credible features of information content, hence the focus is attributed to the strength of message arguments. From literature review done by this study, the nature of information relevance is always perceptual in delivering the most valuable clues of information in a review platform which can be proved from the study by [2] that shows, perceived review relevancy was found to be the strongest predictors towards information diagnosticity, in both of their research sample in 2011 and 2016.

2.1 Factors Derivations

Based on ELM and the representation of argument quality as the central route, a theoretical model is proposed for this study. Since this study is concerned on how to assess the value of information content from informational and persuasive viewpoint, thus perceived informative relevance (informational value) and perceived affective relevance (motivational value) was selected in predicting consumer judgment of argument quality in online review platform. Both relevance dimensions are adopted from the previous research framework proposed by [6]. In the research framework, some relevance criteria have been confirmed that suit with informative and affective dimensions. The element of scope has been rejected from the research framework due the insignificant impact towards information relevance judgment. Thus, the study will adopt the element of novelty, topicality, reliability and understandability (readability) in the process of developing the research model for this study. In addition, a modification on previous framework from [7] are made with the extension on some relevance criteria concerning on argument quality dimensions. In performing this process, the next review analysis from previous studies is conducted related to information relevance judgment and their effect towards online behavior intention. From here, the study proposed the factors of informative relevance based on content novelty, topicality, reliability and similarity, while factors of affective relevance based on content tangibility, readability and sentimentality.

2.2 Research Hypothesis

According to [17], content novelty is defined as the degree, to which the information within the existing background knowledge of a consumer is perceived to be new. A unique experience with particular product knowledge may represent unforeseen product attributes that could activate the level of surprise amongst consumers. The level of surprise could be based on the variation of new and previous product consumptions. The novelties seeking behavior is assumed to lead the user judgment on informational value of online review credibility.

H1: Content novelty has a positive effect on the perceived informative relevance of online reviews.

Perceived content topicality refers to topical relatedness or 'about-ness' of received information towards a user's queries, which is viewed as a return towards informational value searching behavior [7]. The fundamental design of a system relevance from topicality conception is such a search engine, which should return a document that is assumed to be within the frame of the user's interests [18]. The topicalities seeking behavior is assumed to lead a user's judgment on informational and persuasive values of online review credibility.

H2: Content topicality has a positive effect on the perceived informative relevance (2a) and perceived affective relevance (2b) of online reviews.

Content reliability refers to the perceptions of information truthfulness in accordance with informational value seeking behavior. Concerning on this situation, this study assumed that, if the review system could be designed to filter informational cues based on information familiarities from one's background, and is assumed to well-fit with someone's knowledge, the readers may pay more attention towards the argument in the online reviews. The reliability seeking behavior is assumed to lead a user's judgment on the informational value of the online review credibility.

H3: Content reliability has a positive effect on the perceived informative relevance of online reviews.

Similarity cues may assist individuals to transfer their positive feelings over to the other person, social group or product and services [3]. In the context of online communication, [5] suggested that similarity cues could be obtained from personal and usage characteristics in an online review. Following these logics, this study assumed that, if the review platform could be designed to filter these similarity cues shared between the focal consumer, the informational and persuasive value of information could be created. These similarities seeking behavior thus could be used to predict the adoption of text recommendation in the online review platform.

H4: Content similarity has a positive effect on the perceived informative relevance (4a) and perceived affective relevance (4b) of online reviews.

Content readability is defined as the extent to which a user perceives a received document's information as easy to be read and understood [7]. [18] showed that, the reviews that are written with lesser content abstractness and highly comprehensive, tend to return much higher perceptions of review helpfulness. On the other hand, with certain levels of information relevance, documents that are difficult to read may causes fatigue and make a user less happy. Text readership is assumed to lead a user's judgment on the persuasive value of text recommendations.

H5: Content readability has a positive effect on the perceived affective relevance of online reviews.

Content tangibility can be defined as the extent to which information provided is assumed to be real, definite, proven and consists of tangible issues [20]. In addition, the essence of mental intangibility is defined as to whether the consumers could interpret the evaluation cues to ensure a clear representation of the object, and mentally make a visualization of the intangibilities [21]. Thc tangibility seeking behavior is assumed to lead a user's judgment on persuasive and the informational value of an online review's credibility.

H6: Content tangibility has a positive effect on the perceived informative relevance (6a) and perceived affective relevance (6b) of online reviews.

Perceived content sentimentality refers to the degree of affective response towards the given information [22]. In the context of online review platforms, the reviews with high levels of positive sentiments are the review's title, which would encourage more readership, while opinions with neutral polarity in the text recommendations are perceived to be more helpful [23]. This sentiment seeking behavior is assumed to lead a user's judgment on the persuasive value of a review's credibility.

H7: Content sentimentality has a positive effect on the perceived affective relevance of online reviews.

Perceived informative relevance or cognitive relevance judgment refers to the pragmatic values obtained from information content for the purpose of user problem solving [24]. This type of relevant judgment can be referred to as the degree of information enlightenment information content, which brings a user and can be judged as perceived knowledge enrichment by the user [7]. This process shows that, information recipients might undergo significant intellectual effort during an argument's evaluation when they have sufficient ability and cognitive resources. Based on these concerns, this study therefore expects that, the perceived informative relevance of content reviews might be achieved by identifying informational cues from text recommendations in the online review platform.

H8: Perceived informative relevance has a positive effect on the argument quality.

Affective relevance is defined as one's affective reaction, such as enjoyment or sadness, as the results from the activity consumption of a document [7]. In the context of online review platforms, past research works have shown that, the perceived high argument quality might be imposed through relevant judgment related to the strength of persuasive arguments embedded in the review content, which further predicts consumer behavior intentions [3]. Thus, this study assumed that the perceived affective relevance of review content can be activated by recognizing these emotional values and intrinsic motivation cues from text recommendations.

H9: Perceived affective relevance has a positive effect on the argument quality.

Argument quality is defined as the perceptions of strong and convincing messages, rather than weak and unreal ones [25]. In the context of online decision-making, information quality is defined as helpfulness of available information regarding product attributes, which could assist consumers in evaluating the quality of the product [26].

H10: Argument quality has a positive effect on the review helpfulness.

Perceived review helpfulness can be defined as an individual's perception related to the performance enhancement upon consumption of a new technology. The proposed concept of argument quality, which is defined based on the consumer's judgment of review relevancy, will be used to predict the consumer's perceptions towards information helpfulness.

H11: Review helpfulness has a positive effect on the review adoption.

3 Research Method

A survey method as a common research methodology for quantitative research approach was selected for this study. Through the survey method, the data collection phase can be conducted by gathering the valuable responses, which can be further used in testing the proposed research model and identifying the relationship amongst key factors. For that reason, a questionnaire was designed based on the developed research model and was distributed amongst respondents across two phases. The first phase involved a pilot testing of the questionnaire (confirming its reliability and validity) and the second phase (main study) was about the decision evaluation on the acceptance or rejection of the research hypothesis. Finally, the last phase involving the steps in validating the relationships in the proposed research model.

3.1 Data Collection

The questionnaire consisted of five sections. Section A was about the screening question on consumer's validity for participating in the survey. A respondent needs to answer about their experiences in reading the online product reviews. The subsequent sections B, C and D of the questionnaires, reflected the core element of this research. In total, 45 questions were put forth. Section B was about accessing the level of the consumer's agreement concerning the content characteristics of argument in the online reviews, and section C was related to the consumer's responses on the relevant judgment of argument quality embedded in the online reviews. Section D was developed to find the relationship between the consumer's relevant judgment of argument quality and information adoption behavior. In the last section, E, information on the respondent's demographic profile was gathered. In total, the questionnaire consisted of 59 questions. The respondents were asked to respond to each of the questions, by choosing one of five alternatives given, ranging from "strongly agree" to "strongly disagree", (5-point Likert scale) as proposed by (Likert, 1932). The final step in designing the appropriate survey instrument include the process of checking the validity and reliability of the survey content. The survey questions were then evaluated by five experts in the field of Information System (IS), Universiti Teknologi Malaysia, to check the item's relevancy with reference to each contrasting definition. From the results, some items did not perfectly pass the required threshold, which can be referred to its convergent validity, AVE. Design constructs of novelty, topicality, reliability and readability are those having AVE scores below 0.5. Thus, four items based on the outer loading achievement were removed to increase the AVE score, which were, NOV4, TOP1, REL2 and READ4. Consequently, a refined measurement items was generated, which can be used in the subsequent analysis.

4 Research Result

4.1 Assessment of Measurement Model

The internal consistency, convergent and discriminant validity analysis will be used to access those the reflective constructs. This was done by accessing the criteria from factor of outer loading, average variance extracted (AVE), Cross-factor loading and Fornell-Lacker test. On the other hand, the minimum value recorded for composite reliability test is 0.79 and all the values for the constructs are below than 0.95. The results show that, all the constructs have achieved the acceptable internal consistency reliability hence proved that all the constructs' indicators are reliable. The test from convergent validity, the results of outer loading (Table 1) for all the indicators have exceeded the suggested threshold, except for three indicators (REL2, TAN2, and TOP3), which the item's loading were less than the recommended value. Next, the three indicators that were identified for scale removal need to be deleted one by one to check if the AVE value could be changed after that.

Table 1. The results of convergent validity analysis

Construct		Convergent validity		
Construct Name	Construct Code	AVE (>0.5)	Outer Loading (>0.7)	
Argument Quality	ARQ	0.632	ARQ1	0.748
			ARQ2	0.870
			ARQ3	0.749
			ARQ4	0.808
Informative Relevance	PINR	0.764	PINR1	0.879
			PINR2	0.890
			PINR3	0.869
			PINR4	0.858
Affective Relevance	PAFR	0.647	PAFR1	0.797
			PAFR2	0.806
			PAFR3	0.806
			PAFR4	0.810
Novelty	NOV	0.584	NOV1	0.798
			NOV2	0.701
			NOV3	0.789
Readability	READ	0.554	READ1	0.751
			READ2	0.754
			READ3	0.727
Reliability	REL	0.532 After Item Deletion (0.595)	REL1	0.761
			REL2	**0.675**
			REL3	0.749
			REL4	0.728
Review Adoption	RADP	0.655	RADP1	0.812
			RADP2	0.850
			RADP3	0.825
			RADP4	0.748
Review Helpfulness	RHEP	0.699	RHEP1	0.786

(*continued*)

Table 1. (*continued*)

Construct		Convergent validity		
Construct Name	Construct Code	AVE (>0.5)	Outer Loading (>0.7)	
			RHEP2	0.853
			RHEP3	0.880
			RHEP4	0.822
Sentimentality	SENT	0.676	SENT1	0.817
			SENT2	0.834
			SENT3	0.779
			SENT4	0.856
Similarity	SIM	0.645	SIM1	0.766
			SIM2	0.878
			SIM3	0.781
			SIM4	0.784
Tangibility	TAN	0.506 After Item Deletion (0.596)	TAN1	0.710
			TAN2	**0.642**
			TAN3	0.744
			TAN4	0.744
Topicality	TOP	0.515 After Item Deletion (0.584)	TOP1	0.705
			TOP2	0.775
			TOP3	**0.680**
			TOP4	0.708

4.2 Assessment of Structural Model

This stage involves the step in examining the predictive capabilities of the model, together with their construct's relationships. The first step in this stage is to conduct the collinearity assessment, which can be done by obtaining the value of VIF test. From Table 2, the results for t value and p value for all hypotheses are acceptable, except for H3 and H7, which exceed the threshold value, thus, these two hypotheses, need to be rejected from the research model. Next, the assessment of coefficient of determination of R2 value need to be conducted. This was performed to measure the predictive power of the model. Therefore, the path coefficient representing the amount of variance for dependent constructs explained by all the independent constructs associating to it. The result shows that, all the five constructs have the moderate level of predictive power. From all data analysis results, the final research model for this study is visualized in Fig. 1.

Table 2. Evaluation of research hypothesis

Path	t values	p values	Significant level
Argument Quality - > Review Helpfulness	18.986	0.000	***
Informative Relevance - > Argument Quality	2.916	0.002	***
Affective Relevance - > Argument Quality	8.809	0.000	***
Novelty - > Informative Relevance	1.295	0.098	*
Readability - > Affective Relevance	0.991	0.161	NS
Reliability - > Informative Relevance	1.191	0.117	NS
Review Helpfulness - > Review Adoption	9.105	0.000	***
Sentimentality - > Affective Relevance	4.378	0.000	***
Similarity - > Informative Relevance	5.224	0.000	***
Similarity - > Affective Relevance	1.628	0.052	*
Tangibility - > Informative Relevance	2.660	0.004	***
Tangibility - > Affective Relevance	2.779	0.003	***
Topicality - > Informative Relevance	1.369	0.086	*
Topicality - > Affective Relevance	1.847	0.032	**

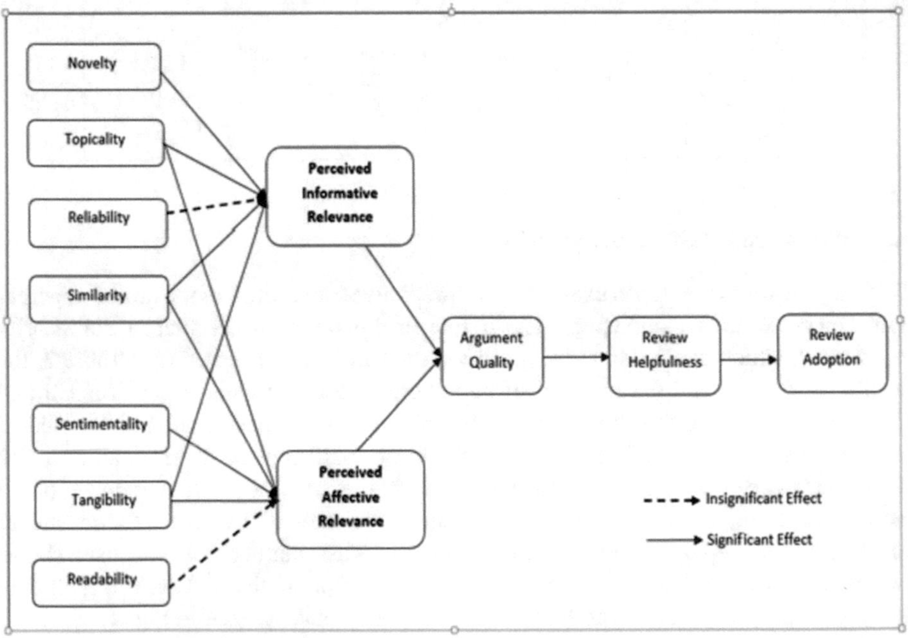

Fig. 1. A model of review adoption in e-Commerce review platform

5 Discussion and Conclusions

In this study, dimension of argument quality is classified into two relevant judgments of online information which are perceived informativeness and perceived persuasiveness. The model was drawn based on the studies of theory of information adoption, argument quality dimensions, theory of elaboration likelihood model and information retrieval perspective. The model tested by using a field survey data from the sample of users who are deemed to have the good experiences in online purchasing especially in reading online reviews from e-Commerce platforms such as Lazada.com, shopee.com.my and Carousell.com. The results show that, nine out of eleven proposed hypotheses were relatively significant which illustrated that, the proposed factors of content novelty, topicality, similarity, tangibility, and sentimentality have the positive influence on argument quality perception, which then contributes towards the adoption of online reviews in e-Commerce websites. The other two factors of argument quality, content reliability and readability, appeared to be the non-significant factors towards the perception of review helpfulness, which then effect the adoption of online reviews. Additionally, the predictors explained 44.8% of the variance of argument quality, which reflected a significant and appropriate result for the prediction of online review's adoption in e-Commerce websites.

5.1 Practical Contribution

The research model provides a contextualization on how to offer a preferred information search in e-Commerce review platform. The results shown that, by providing high quality review, the sales team will have the best strategy in terms of convincing the potential online consumers. The results from the first dimension of the research model suggested that modern e-Commerce should focus on designing a review filter, which could attract emotional attention from the information receivers. For example, the enhancement could be done by placing the online reviews in the prominent filters with such a visible or tangible content. This includes the attachment of useful and interesting external links, the attractive image or graphics, the organized form of a review's summary, and providing the advanced technology, which assumed to increase the probability of motivational values received by the online consumers. The results also revealed that, the review platform must be designed to provide the information filter based on the appropriate sentiment classifications. A tractable information cue based on emotional expressions from past experiences of the users could encourage the active engagement of a user's intentions and contribute to the consumer's decision quality. Therefore, the awareness of such matters on e-Commerce websites deserves continuous attention for practical considerations. The second dimensions of the research model provide the remarkable role of informational values specific to content novelty, content topicality and content similarity which assumed to strongly eliminate the information gaps amongst the knowledge seekers. For example, the review platforms can be supported with such a noticeable filter on the topicality search field.

5.2 Theoretical Contribution

Against the previous studies background, based on subjective measures of argument quality and taking the view of relevant judgment from information retrieval perspective, this study explores an additional path alongside the cognitive path of perceived credibility of online reviews. Since perceived content relevancy is amongst the heart of argument strength prediction as confirmed by [3], neglecting the effect and associated factors seems to be excluded in the case of an online review adoption. Hence, this study is amongst the first few to have investigated the subjective measure of argument quality to predict a better adoption of online revies. Consistent with the previous research results by [4], the findings from the study suggest that argument quality was the most influential stimulus provoking perceived helpfulness of online reviews. The first contribution can be seen from the delivery of the research model through the lens of Elaboration Likelihood Model (ELM), information adoption model and information retrieval perspectives. The study offers empirically validated factors pertaining to the information adoption behavior in e-Commerce review platform. Following the extensive research review and analysis, the study has demonstrated the promised factors according to two important dimensions of argument quality, which include perceived informative relevance (i.e., content novelty, content topicality, and content similarity) and perceived affective relevance (i.e., content tangibility and content sentimentality). These factors have shown the significant impacts on argument quality perceptions and subsequently effects the process of review adoption. Therefore, the future research for improving the conceptualization of argument quality perceptions should put extra considerations with regards to these factors, which are assumed to further offer better predictions for the consumer behavior in the e-Commerce websites.

References

1. 2018 ReviewTrackers Online Reviews Survey. (n.d.). https://www.reviewtrackers.com/online-reviews-survey. Accessed 5 March 2019
2. Filieri, R., Hofacker, C.F., Alguezaui, S.: What makes information in online consumer reviews diagnostic over time? the role of review relevancy, factuality, currency, source credibility and ranking score. Comput. Hum. Behav. **80**, 122–131 (2018)
3. Zhang, K.Z., Zhao, S.J., Cheung, C.M., Lee, M.K.: Examining the influence of online reviews on consumers' decision-making: a heuristic–systematic model. Decis. Support Syst. **67**, 78–89 (2014)
4. Watts, S., Shankaranarayanan, G., Even, A.: Data quality assessment in context: a cognitive perspective. Decis. Support Syst. **48**(1), 202–211 (2009)
5. O'Reilly, K., MacMillan, A., Mumuni, A.G., Lancendorfer, K.M.: Extending our understanding of eWOM impact: the role of source credibility and message relevance. J. Internet Commerce **15**(2), 77–96 (2016)
6. Xu, Y.: Relevance judgment in epistemic and hedonic information searches. J. Am. Soc. Inform. Sci. Technol. **58**(2), 179–189 (2007)
7. Xu, Y., Chen, Z.: Relevance judgment: what do information users consider beyond topicality? J. Am. Soc. Inform. Sci. Technol. **57**(7), 961–973 (2006)
8. Saracevic, T.: Relevance reconsidered. In: Proceedings of the Second Conference on Conceptions of Library and Information Science (CoLIS 2), pp. 201–218. ACM, New York, October 1996

9. Bhattacherjee, A., Sanford, C.: Influence processes for information technology acceptance: an elaboration likelihood model. MIS Q. 805–825 (2006)
10. Ahn, T., Ryu, S., Han, I.: The impact of Web quality and playfulness on user acceptance of online retailing. Inf. Manage. **44**(3), 263–275 (2007)
11. Meng, B., Choi, K.: Tourists' intention to use location-based services (LBS): converging the theory of planned behavior (TPB) and the elaboration likelihood model (ELM). Int. J. Contemporary Hospitality Manage. (2019)
12. Hair, F.J., Jr., Sarstedt, M., Hopkins, L., Kuppelwieser, G., V.: Partial least squares structural equation modeling (PLS-SEM) an emerging tool in business research. Eur. Bus. Rev. **26**(2), 106–121 (2014)
13. Huang, Y.F., Kuo, F.Y.: An eye-tracking investigation of internet consumers' decision deliberateness. Internet Res. **21**(5), 541–561 (2011)
14. Park, D.H., Lee, J., Han, I.: The effect of on-line consumer reviews on consumer purchasing intention: the moderating role of involvement. Int. J. Electron. Commer. **11**(4), 125–148 (2007)
15. Hong, H., Xu, D., Wang, G.A., Fan, W.: Understanding the determinants of online review helpfulness: a meta-analytic investigation. Decis. Support Syst. **102**, 1–11 (2017)
16. Le, T.D., Dobele, A.R., Robinson, L. J.: WOM source characteristics and message quality: the receiver perspective. Market. Intell. Plan. (2018)
17. Chen, Y.C., Shang, R.A., Li, M.J.: The effects of perceived relevance of travel blogs' content on the behavioral intention to visit a tourist destination. Comput. Hum. Behav. **30**, 787–799 (2014)
18. Foster, A., Rafferty, P. (Eds.): Innovations in information retrieval: perspectives for theory and practice. Facet Publishing (2011)
19. Li, M., Huang, L., Tan, C.H., Wei, K.K.: Helpfulness of online product reviews as seen by consumers: source and content features. Int. J. Electron. Commer. **17**(4), 101–136 (2013)
20. Balatsoukas, P., Ruthven, I.: An eye-tracking approach to the analysis of relevance judgments on the Web: the case of Google search engine. J. Am. Soc. Inform. Sci. Technol. **63**(9), 1728–1746 (2012)
21. Mazaheri, E., Richard, M.O., Laroche, M., Ueltschy, L.C.: The influence of culture, emotions, intangibility, and atmospheric cues on online behavior. J. Bus. Res. **67**(3), 253–259 (2014)
22. Bruza, P., Chang, V.: Perceptions of document relevance. Front. Psychol. **5**, 612 (2014)
23. Salehan, M., Kim, D.J.: Predicting the performance of online consumer reviews: a sentiment mining approach to big data analytics. Decis. Support Syst. **81**, 30–40 (2016)
24. Wang, X., Hong, Z., Xu, Y., Zhang, C., Ling, H.: Relevance judgments of mobile commercial information. J. Am. Soc. Inf. Sci. **65**(7), 1335–1348 (2014)
25. Petty, R.E., Briñol, P.: Emotion and persuasion: cognitive and meta-cognitive processes impact attitudes. Cogn. Emot. **29**(1), 1–26 (2015)

An Exploratory Study on the Use of Social Companion Robot for Adults with Motor Disabilities

Sofianiza Abd Malik[1], Linah Aburahmah[1], and Muna Azuddin[2](✉)

[1] Prince Sultan University, Riyadh, Saudi Arabia
sabdmalik@psu.edu.sa
[2] International Islamic University Malaysia, Kuala Lumpur, Malaysia
munaazuddin@iium.edu.my

Abstract. Assistive technology has been a significant topic in both the research and manufacturing industry for the past decades focusing on improving social interaction, supporting health care, business, education, and daily activities. There are different types of assistive technologies such as wearable devices, mobile applications, automated home appliances, and robots. There is lack of study conducted to investigate the use of robots among disabled users, such as adult users with motor disabilities. The aim of this study is to explore the use of a companion robot called Zenbo in assisting motor disability users in Saudi community. This paper presented a preliminary work on Zenbo's design evaluation in terms of functionality, acceptability, and effectiveness. The study used a mixed method such as observation (hands-on), interview, and survey questions to evaluate the purpose of the study. The findings showed positive acceptance of Zenbo as a companion robot due to the physical design. However, the interaction of Zenbo to notify the users through user interface and wheel light, and processing voice command were found ineffective and require more improvement.

Keywords: Adults with motor disabilities · Assistive technology · Companion robot · Zenbo robot

1 Introduction

Robots are machines programed by a computer to simulate humans, interact with them, and perform complex actions. The use of robots in the industry has been ages. However, started in year 2005, most of the previous studies regarding robots were discussed in the domain assisted technology (robotics) for health care and educational [1]. The context of these studies was, the use of robotics for elderly people and learning disability users (autism) [1], which the robots able to support them in their daily life and reducing the load on the caregivers. To date, there is a lack of studies discussed the use of robots among adults with motor disabilities to support them in their daily activities.

The aim of this study is to explore the feasibility of using social companion robot (Zenbo) in obstacle detection among adults with motor disabilities. The robot was used

F. Saeed et al. (Eds.): IRICT 2021, LNDECT 127, pp. 616–629, 2022.
https://doi.org/10.1007/978-3-030-98741-1_51

to assist their movement and to help them be more independent. The paper presented a preliminary study that discussed issues and challenges of using companion robot by adults with motor disabilities. The use of Zenbo as the companion robot in the research is due to the robot's various capabilities which is discussed in the related work. The findings may add knowledge to developers and researchers to improve the design of assisted technology such as robots which the utilization of the robots can be gained more effectively by the users. In addition, the findings also can assist the designers and researchers to specifically understand Zenbo's detection capabilities; issues and challenges, which may be important for later designing.

2 Related Work

2.1 Disabled People and Assistive Technologies

Around 1.1 billion people have some disability as reported by the World Health Organization and the World Bank [2]. About 110 million to 190 million of the disabled people are adults, which showed that they are the majority group of the disabled people. A total of 30.6 million out of them suffer from physical disabilities such as difficulty in walking [3]. People with physical disabilities need assistance from other people in their daily lives, such as to perform simple task – turn on lights, they need help from people in their surroundings. Therefore, ignoring disabled people creates a significant impact on society.

In Saudi Arabia, 3.73% of the population are people with functional disabilities such as physical, visual, and mental [4]. A total of 74.2% from this category group of people (3.73%) needed high attention from the caregivers [4].

Physical disabilities are defined as "the result of a condition affecting mobility, upper limb disorders or motor coordination in terms of fine and gross motor skills, diagnosed by a consultant which has an impact on lifestyle, work, movement, and independence." [5]. Different types of physical disabilities are either caused by a disease or an accident to result in temporary or permanent physical disability.

This study focused on adults with movement difficulties. Movement disorders are defined as severely compromising the person's ability to perform motor skills as ordinary people. These skills are such as walking, writing, turning around, or transferring in and out of bed [6]. People with Parkinson Disease suffered from different disorders such as Bradykinesia, Akinesia, and Episodes of freezing. Each disorder has its effect on the person's movement. Bradykinesia reduced the speed and the amplitude of motion. Akinesia caused difficulty in initiating movements. Episodes of freezing block the user movement suddenly while executing a movement sequence [6].

Functional disabled people need caregivers to support them on their daily tasks. There are different types of disabilities such as physical, mental, hearing, etc. The most frequent causes of physical impairments are a result of deficiencies to the muscles or the neurons [7].

The main major challenges that have been highlighted in many research papers are related to the movement they faced, such as having difficulties to move inside and outside their homes. They also have a lot of health issues as they are moving less, or not moving at all. Therefore, their health condition is worse than the ordinary adults of the same age

[21]. To minimize the efforts that caregivers provide to the disabled people, there are lots of assistive technologies have been developed in recent years [8–11] (Table 1).

Table 1. Assistive technologies for disabled people.

Technologies	Descriptions
Brain Computer Interface (BCI)	It is one of the technologies that enable the physically disabled adults to control a mobile robot through brain signals [5, 12]
Virtual Reality (VR)	It has been utilized in the educational aspects where they have a simulation on the real environment in 3D view [24]
Internet of Things (IoT)	It has many technologies that support disabled people. Automated home appliances are a common example of the internet of things that are controlled by disabled people through voice commands. Also, some devices have sensors and actuators that can detect incidents at home. This feature is very helpful in emergency cases [9, 13, 14]
Wearable Devices	Necklace and bracelet are examples of wearable devices that can detect the fallen behavior of a disabled person and notify caregivers, family members, or the responsible healthcare institutes [15, 16]
Robots	It is one of the technologies that are used heavily in the recent research studies. There are two main types of robots that are used to serve physically disabled people which are physically assistive robots and socially assistive robots. Some robots can be both socially and physically supportive. The physically assistive robots are usually used in therapy [17], feeding [18], or in moving the person from one place to another by acting as a wheelchair [18]

Social assistive robots are also called companion robots. This type of robot can mimic human behavior [19]. The companion robots have been used in social interactions which the disabled people use it to communicate with other people, as a daily reminder, as a fitness coach, respond to inquiries (through voice commands), and as entertainer (play games) [20–22].

Currently there are lack of research that investigate the use of assisted technology such as robots to assist the physically disabled people, in the context of adult with motor disabilities. To date, there are none of research studies in this domain, conducted in Saudi population. Thus, this study uses Zenbo robot which is designed to fit the use of adult with motor disability, which to support their movement and emotion.

2.2 Zenbo Robot as the Assistive Technology for Disabled People

Zenbo robot is a ready-made platform that can be customized to fit the different needs of the users. ASUS developed it with an Android operating system and launched it in 2017.

Zenbo is considered a family robot that is full of energy. The robot is lovely, polite, and respectful; and always takes the initiative to assist people. Zenbo expresses his emotions through his agile body and his facial expressions. There are 24 emotions that Zenbo can possess such as happy, proud, shocked, and tired. There are guidelines related to the use of Zenbo's emotion such as maintaining a ratio of 80% and 20% of positive and negative emotions respectively. Other than the emotions, the robot has high capabilities that allow developers, business teams, and system integrators to deploy different solutions and to engage the users compellingly.

Zenbo robot has a lot of built-in movements and functions to perform numerous tasks such as; i) Zenbo can follow any person by recognizing his face using a built-in camera, ii) Zenbo can be configured to understand the layout of the user's house so it can provide more assistance, iii) Zenbo can be used as a reminder and an alarm, iv) Zenbo can control home appliances by interacting with connected devices, and v) Zenbo can recognize the voices and therefore respond to the requests or the spoken questions.

Moreover, Zenbo could be linked with a mobile app and can allow the user to perform basic configurations. The most important feature that made Zenbo more convenient for people with movement disabilities is the voice command. Zenbo can receive voice command in long distance compared to average smartphones or tablets, and this may ease the disabled people to perform tasks.

For health purposes, Zenbo can help to remind users about their medications. It can also be used as a recording tool to track the health status of users. For example, the user can record the blood pressure and sugar concentration daily. In case any of the measurements are high, Zenbo will notify the responsible doctor or inform the family members through messages sent to their home. Moreover, Zenbo allows the doctor to follow up with patients remotely by using the video call feature. Zenbo can provide instructions to users to perform workouts or rehabilitation exercises.

In a study, Lee et al. [15] presented seven out of eleven emotions of Zenbo. The emotions were captured from students' emotion during different scenarios, and the study was conducted in Taiwan and Japan. The aim of the study was to assess the students' performance and obtain their feedback about learning systems. Zenbo was used in the developed module to present the emotions of students using the students' brainwaves and transformed it into physiological indices.

Lee and Shin [22] reviewed different companion robots in terms of their ability to support elderly. Zenbo was included in the review due to the Zenbo features such as moving around the home, controlling home appliances and doors, shopping online and searching for recipes through voice commands. Another powerful features that Zenbo has is the ability to detect human fall and notify family members. For this state of condition, older people need to wear a wearable device (bracelet) that sent signals to Zenbo.

Another study conducted by Chien et al. [23] focused on understanding older people's attitude towards robots as the robots have been increasingly used as assistants to the older people. The participants were given a self-rated questionnaire to evaluate their attitudes before and after their interaction with robot. The researchers prepared a set of tasks that participants need to perform while using the robot through utilizing the built-in commands. Some of the commands used were "Hey! Zenbo!", "what can you do?", "date is tomorrow?", "Follow me", "Tell me a story". Participants whose age ranged between 59–86 years old showed positive reaction of using the robot.

Meanwhile in the research context of disabilities, Kean [23] used Zenbo to interact with visually impaired people. The study was conducted among Taiwanese participants who had different levels of visual impairment ranging from mild to severe and different demographic backgrounds (12–19 years old). The participants used two robots, Alpha 2 and Zenbo. The results showed that both robots are humanoid and there was no difference highlighted during the interaction; other than the Chit Chat feature that was developed and deployed on Zenbo. The feature resulted in Zenbo being more empathetic while chatting.

All research papers that were discussed earlier involved Zenbo, by utilizing Zenbo's capabilities in recording videos, notifying, and calling family members, expressing different emotions, to support older people, students, or visually impaired people. To date, there were none previous studies has been reported to use Zenbo as the companion robot among adult with motor disabilities, in Saudi population. The use of Zenbo in the study will add another contribution for different range of users - to assist adult with motor disability to detect obstacle.

3 The Preliminary Study

The preliminary study consists of two phases: 1) the user requirements phase, and 2) the design phase. The first phase focuses heavily on the users (adult with motor disabilities) and their needs. The second phase, the requirements gathered from the first phase were transformed to low-fidelity prototype, which will be tested before implementing the solutions in Zenbo. The paper will focus only on Zenbo's evaluation among the participants.

It was found (phase 1) that an obstacle detection is needed to check for objects on the floor to provide users some safety measurement while moving from one location to another. This is vital to the users because they cannot inspect the path due to their condition. The following section discussed the embedded obstacle detection solution in Zenbo and findings of the evaluation. To develop the solution, the voice recognition feature of Zenbo was utilized to allow participants to communicate with it through a voice command to check for objects and obstacles on the floor.

4 Methodology

4.1 Participants

Five participants (2 males and 3 females); adults who have motor disabilities were recruited through the mobile phone and WhatsApp. The participants' age range was between 18–50 years old. Four of the participants have a bachelor's degree while one of them has a master's degree. All the participants were Saudis and their disability was since birth except one whose disability was due to a car accident. The five participants with motor impairments had different types of disabilities (one was diagnosed with Osteogenesis Imperfecta, two were diagnosed with Cerebral Palsy and two were diagnosed with Spinal Cord Injury). The participants had experiences with technology as they use smart phones and computer tablets daily to check on social media and communicate with others.

4.2 Setting

The study was conducted at five different coffee shops according to participants' time availability. The area of the movement was limited because the study was conducted in a coffee shop, Zenbo moved 600 cm from point A to point B. The obstacle was placed 300 cm away from the starting point. The obstacle used was a box that is 140 cm length, 125 cm width, and 50 cm height. The box was placed horizontally on the floor.

4.3 Materials

Zenbo Application. Zenbo is an android apps and has four types of sensors which are Sonar Sensor, Drop IR Sensor, Touch Sensor Area, and Auto Recharge Sensor. In this study, only the Sonar Sensor was activated. Zenbo has three sensors located at the front of its body that were used in measuring the distance between Zenbo and its surroundings. The built-in emotions (Confident and Shocked) were selected because they were the most understandable facial expressions among the 24 emotions that Zenbo have. Moreover, the wheel lights (red and green) were utilized for notification purposes after processing the command "Clear the way". Below is a description of how Zenbo reacts to the above-mentioned command:

- If the path is clear, Zenbo will move forward with confidence and the wheels lighten in green
- If an obstacle is found on the way, Zenbo activates the shocked face and the wheels lightens in red

Questionnaires. Table 2 explains the questionnaires and hands-on methods use in the study.

Table 2. Methods used in the study.

Methods	Descriptions
Demographic and background questionnaires	Demographic and background questionnaires were used to know about the participants demographics, daily activities and challenges, the recommended technologies that can overcome their challenges, and their experience with assistive technologies

(continued)

Table 2. (*continued*)

Methods	Descriptions
Tasks and Usability Measures	Participants performed two tasks: • Task 1: Activate Zenbo by saying "Hello Zenbo" • Task 2: Use Zenbo to guide you to check the path by saying "Hey Zenbo, clear the way" To evaluate Zenbo's obstacle detection ability, multiple measures were collected: • Time taken to complete task 1 and task 2. Time taken to complete task 1 was the time of giving the command by the participant, plus the time of processing the command by Zenbo, plus the time of giving a voice response by Zenbo. For task 2, the task time was the time of giving the command by the user, plus the time of processing the command by Zenbo, plus the time of Zenbo to move in the specified path to detect the obstacle and show the emotional and wheel light response • The task success rate of task 1 and task 2 was observed and collected. The task performance was classified using three categories: 1) performed with ease, 2) performed with difficulty, 3) failure to perform the task • The number of times the participants repeated the voice command until Zenbo reacts • The time in seconds the participant waited to say the command again when Zenbo did not detect it at the first time
Think-aloud Protocol and Observations	Participants were asked to think aloud while they were performing the above-mentioned tasks. Observations have been gathered as notes when the participants verbalize their cognitive thinking of doing the tasks and express. the users' facial expression when interacting with Zenbo
Post-test questionnaire	The post-test questionnaire is a 5-point Likert scale to evaluate the reliability, usefulness, and satisfaction of Zenbo. The scale is to measure Zenbo's capabilities and design, and acceptability of Zenbo's as companion

(*continued*)

Table 2. (*continued*)

Methods	Descriptions
Post-Test Interview	To understand participants' experiences interacting with Zenbo, usefulness, suggestions that help to make Zenbo more effective for navigational needs, and preferences to have Zenbo as their companion

Procedures. Table 3 explains the data collection procedures.

Table 3. Procedures phase.

No	Phase	Description
1	Before the evaluation	Before the testing began, the purpose and instructions of the session were explained to the participants
2	During the evaluation	The participants were explained on how to interact with Zenbo, so they can use it alone to perform the given tasks. Then, participants were asked to perform task 1 and task 2
3	After the evaluation	Post-Test Questionnaire and the post-test interview were conducted

5 Results and Discussions

5.1 Time Taken to Complete the Task

Table 4 shows the average time taken by the participants to complete Task 1 and Task 2. Zenbo spent more time completing task 2 than task 1. This is expected as task 2 requires Zenbo to move between two points to check if there are obstacles in the way. On the other hand, task 1 is to activate Zenbo by saying "Hello Zenbo", which requires less time.

Table 4. Mean of time on task.

Task #	Mean	Standard deviation
Task 1	22 s	16 s
Task 2	76 s	27 s

5.2 Task Success Rate

Figure 1 shows the success rate of the participants as "Completed with ease", "Completed with difficulty", or "Failed to complete". Zenbo completed 20% of task 1 commands with ease. Eighty percent of the task 1 and task 2 commands were completed with difficulty. Zenbo failed to perform 20% of task 2 commands. Sometimes Zenbo detected task 2 commands incorrectly. For example, Zenbo processed the command as "Close the way" instead of the right command "Clear the way". Participants had to repeat the command to Zenbo multiple times as demonstrated in Table 5.

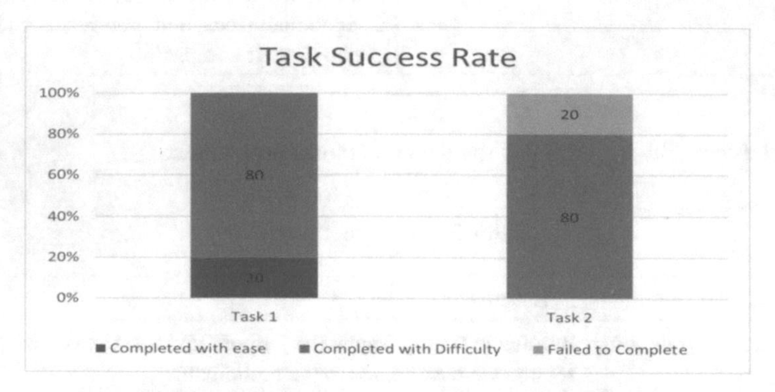

Fig. 1. Success distribution for task 1 and task 2.

Table 5. Frequency of repeating task 1 and task 2 commands by users

Users/Tasks	User 1	User 2	User 3	User 4	User 5
Task 1	3 times	5 times	2 times	7 times	3 times
Task 2	3 times	10 times	5 times	4 times	3 times

Participants waited between 8–12 s for Zenbo to perform the tasks before they repeated their command. Participants seemed worried when Zenbo was not performing their commands.

Based on the observation, there are some factors have affected the ability of Zenbo's to detect the voice commands: 1) the noise during the experimental (coffee shops were noisy), 2) not pronouncing the command loud enough for Zenbo to detect it, 3) the commands are in Arabic accent.

5.3 Zenbo's Design and Capabilities

Figure 2 shows the participant's evaluation of Zenbo's physical and aesthetic design as well as its functional capabilities. Moreover, the observation and interview data were analyzed to explain the participants' rating.

The results showed that participants were happy with Zenbo's physical appeal. When they saw Zenbo, they showed enthusiasm to interact with it. Participants rated the emotions expressions of Zenbo at 4.5. They loved the humanized face of Zenbo because it visualizes different emotions. This was mostly observed when they met Zenbo for the first time during the training session before the experiment. The height of Zenbo

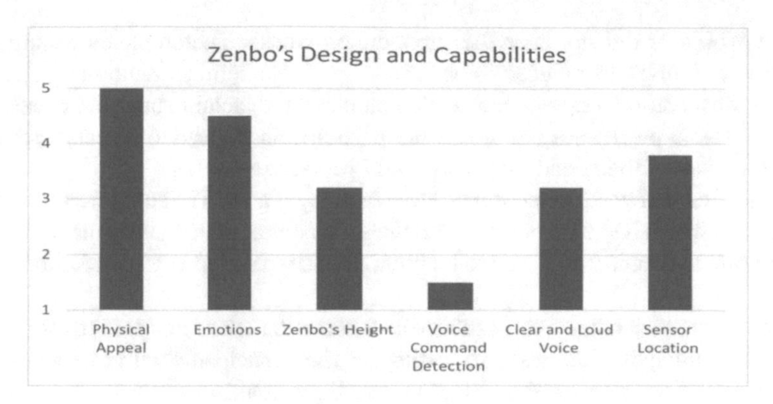

Fig. 2. Zenbo's design and capabilities

was convenient for the participants whose disability is not very severe because they can move their head to see what is close to them. One the other hand, the participants who have severe disabilities preferred Zenbo to be taller because they cannot move their body easily, therefore they have difficulty to see Zenbo clearly when it is near them.

5.4 Acceptability of Zenbo as Companion

All participants showed high acceptance for Zenbo as a companion (Fig. 3). Based on the interview, they would love to use Zenbo to perform other tasks such as controlling home appliances, which they do not have accessibility to. Furthermore, participants suggested improving Zenbo's intelligence to be able to carry conversations as a human being with users. This shows the willingness of the participants to have Zenbo as a companion.

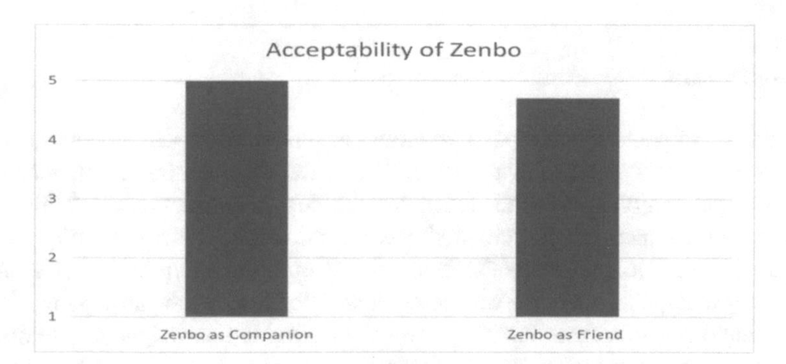

Fig. 3. Acceptability of Zenbo.

5.5 Solution Effectiveness

The worst rating for the solution effectiveness was 1.7 which is for the accuracy of voice detection (Fig. 4). Participants were frustrated as Zenbo failed to accurately detect different words or did not hear the pronounced words. Therefore, the rating for the reliability of Zenbo was reduced to be 2.5.

As an observational note, when Zenbo changed his facial expression because there was an obstacle on the way, none of the participants noticed it because Zenbo was walking in front of them, and they only could just see its back.

The accuracy of voice detection reduces in noisy places. The study was conducted at coffee shops which had a lot of noise and therefore impacted the performance of Zenbo. Furthermore, the command needs to be pronounced with loud voice for Zenbo to detect it.

Some participants had to raise their voices more than their normal tone for Zenbo to detect the commands. This was exhausting for the participants with motor disabilities as their muscles are weak or they cannot move them at all.

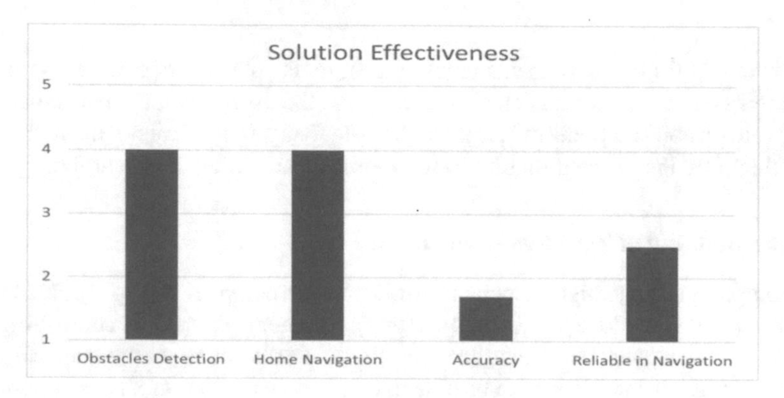

Fig. 4. Solution effectiveness

6 Conclusion

In general, participants showed positive emotions - likability to Zenbo and how Zenbo expressed itself through facial expression. They also showed high acceptance to have Zenbo as a companion and friend. However, the design instruction of Zenbo was not effective enough to meet the participants' needs. First, Zenbo was not reacting accurately to the participants' voice commands. Second, the emotional expression of Zenbo that notified the participants about the obstacles cannot be seen by the participants. This was because Zenbo position (user interface) was not facing the participants. The drawback of this interaction is because the participants were not able to see the notification of obstacle on the user interface (Zenbo's screen). The other notification of Zenbo - the flashing wheels may be effective for some users; however, it was not effective for others with severe motor disabilities. Users with severe motor impairments were not able to move their head down to notice the notifications. Moreover, they were not able to increase their voice tone for Zenbo to detect the voice command.

There have been many limitations and challenges encountered during some stages in this study. First, difficulties were experienced in recruiting people with motor disabilities for the study due to their non-availability and willingness to participate. Second is finding an accessible and quiet place to conduct the study was challenging. Third, Zenbo can understand English and Chinese languages only, so finding adults with motor disabilities who can speak English was great challenge.

In terms of Zenbo robot limitations, to program the movement of Zenbo in scanning the ground, Zenbo master app needed to be downloaded on the mobile phone. The app was in Chinese language and an effort was made to find the English version. Then to bind the robot with the app, an admin account of Zenbo needs to be used. In order to register the admin account, two verification methods were used, voice encoding and facial detection. The voice encoding was happening by saying the sentence that Zenbo showed three times. The main struggle was the sentence was in Chinese. This took a few days until a solution was found. A live translator app was used to say the sentence in Chinese. Moreover, Since the robot is relatively new in the market, there were not many documentations available in forums that can help in the development and troubleshooting. Furthermore, the ability of Zenbo to detect the voices was not efficient.

There are few suggestion for future work: 1) replicate the study with different cultures and wider population, 2) improve Zenbo's language setting – include Arabic language to be more accessible for Saudi community, and 3) improve Zenbo functions to notify family members through a phone call and to remove the obstacles and scan the paths between rooms in a site.

Acknowledgement. This research is funded by the Human Computer Interaction Research Group; Prince Sultan University, Riyadh, Saudi Arabia [RG-CCIS-2017–06-01].

References

1. Al-Razgan, M., AlFallaj, L.F., AlSarhani, L.S., Alomair, H.W.: Systematic Review of Robotics Use Since 2005. International Journal of Mechanical Engineering and Robotics Research **5**(2), 129–132 (2016)
2. Faroom, S., Ali, M.N., Yousaf, S., Deen, S.U.: Literature review on home automation system for physically disabled peoples. In: International Conference on Computing, Mathematics and Engineering Technologies (Icomet), Sukkur, pp. 1–5 (2018)
3. Dolbow, D., Figoni, S.: Accommodation of Wheelchair-Reliant Individuals by Community Fitness Facilities. Spinal Cord **53**(7), 515–519 (2015)
4. Kbar, G., Aly, S.: Smart workplace for persons with disabilities (Smartdisable). In: International Conference on Multimedia Computing and Systems (Icmcs), Marrakech, pp. 996–1001 (2014)
5. Schalock, R.I., Kiernan, W.E.: Habilitation planning for adults with disabilities. Springer Science & Business Media, 8 & 46 (2012)

6. Morris, M.: Movement Disorders in People with Parkinson Disease: A Model for Physical Therapy. Phys. Ther. **80**(6), 578–597 (2000)
7. Kassah, A.: Community-Based Rehabilitation and Stigma Management by Physically Disabled People in Ghana. Disabil. Rehabil. **20**(2), 66–73 (1998)
8. Gopinath, E.: Controlling A Human Computer Interface (Hci) Using Electro-Oculography (Eog) Signal. International Journal of Computing Communication and Information System (Ijccis) **6**, 55–59 (2014)
9. Freitas, D.J., Marcondes, T.B., Nakamura, L.H.V., Ueyama, J., Gomes P.H., Meneguette, R.I.: Combining cell phones and Wsns for preventing accidents in smart-homes with disabled people. In: 7th International Conference on New Technologies, Mobility and Security (Ntms), Paris, pp. 1–5 (2015)
10. Solórzano, S., Rojas-Ortiz, M., López-Molia, R., Clairand, J., Pozo-Espín, D.: Home Teleassistance system for elderly or disabled people in rural areas. In: International Conference on Edemocracy & Egovernment (Icedeg), Ambato, pp. 380–385 (2018)
11. Molteni, F., Gasperini, G., Cannaviello, G., Guanziroli, E., Exoskeleton et al.: End-effector robots for upper and lower limbs rehabilitation. Narrative Rev. **10**(2), 174–188 (2018)
12. Pasqualotto, E.: Usability and Workload of Access Technology for People with Severe Motor Impairment: A Comparison of Brain-Computer Interfacing and Eye Tracking. Neurorehabil Neural Repair **29**(10), 950–957 (2015)
13. Padhmaavathi, A., Nandhini, G., Keerthika, S.: Handsfree home automation for disabled people. J. Global Res. Comput. Sci. Technol. (2015)
14. Saunders, J., Syrdal, D.S., Koay, K.L., Burke, N., Dautenhahn, K.: Teach Me–Show Me—End-User Personalization of a Smart Home and Companion Robot. IEEE Transactions on Human-Machine Systems **46**(1), 27–40 (2016)
15. Qushem, U.B., Ahmad Dahlan, A.R., Ghani, A.S.B.M.: My emergency assistant device: a conceptual solution in enhancing the quality of life for the disabled and elderly. In: 6th International Conference on Information and Communication Technology for the Muslim World (Ict4m), Jakarta, pp. 82–87 (2016)
16. Lee, C.: Intelligent agent for real-world applications on robotic edutainment and humanized co-learning. J. Am. Intell. Humanized Comput. **11**, 1–19 (2019)
17. Chavarriaga, R.: Multidisciplinary design of suitable assistive technologies for motor disabilities in Colombia. In: IEEE Global Humanitarian Technology Conference (Ghtc 2014), San Jose California, pp. 386–391 (2014)
18. Lee, Y., Chiu, C., Jhang, L., Santiago, C.: A Self-reliance assistive tool for disable people. In: 3rd International Conference on Control and Robotics Engineering (Iccre), Nagoya, pp. 26–30 (2018)
19. Weinrich, C.: Estimation of human upper body orientation for mobile robotics using an Svm decision tree on monocular images. In: Intelligent Robots and Systems Conference (Iros), Portugal, pp. 2147–2152 (2012)
20. Torturella, V.C.: Analysis of the use of a robot to improve social skills in children with Autism spectrum disorder. Res. Biomed. Eng. **32**(2), 161–175 (2016)
21. Mavadati, S.M., Feng, H., Salvador, M., Silver, S., Gutierrez, A., Mahoor, M.H.: Robot-based therapeutic protocol for training children with Autism. In: 25th IEEE International Symposium on Robot and Human Interactive Communication (Ro-Man), New York, pp. 855–860 (2016)

22. Saturnino, M.: Fallen People Detection Capabilities Using Assistive Robot. Electronics **8**, 915 (2018)
23. Tan, E.: Impact of visual impairment and demographic factors in social participation with service robots. Ph.D. thesis, Asia (2018)
24. Sobota, B., Korečko, S., Jacho, L., Pastornický, P., Hudák, M., Sivý, M.: Virtual-reality technologies and smart environments in the process of disabled people education. In: 15th International Conference on Emerging Elearning Technologies and Applications (Iceta), Stary Smokovec, pp. 1–6 (2017)

A Comparison of Block-Based Programming Platforms for Learning Programming and Creating Simple Application

Umar AbdulSamad(✉) and Rohaida Romli

School of Computing, Universiti Utara Malaysia, 06010 Sintok, Kedah, Malaysia
s.abdullah097@yahoo.com, aida@uum.edu.my

Abstract. Among the several programming paradigms, block-based visual programming has become widespread in recent years. Visual programming language is any programming language which enables developers to design programs graphically, manipulating rather than by textually defining program elements. Since the first attempts in the 1970s, visual programming has come a long way, but it still has an aura of promises that had not been accomplished. Block-based programming avoid the occurrence of syntactic errors. In the current literatures, there have not much empirical evidence showing and revealing the usage and utilization of the available block-based programming platforms and how these platforms would offer programming environment that able to engage, motivate and provide satisfaction to novice learners. Thus, it is significant to analyze the block-based programming approach to determine the most effective block-based solutions. Thus, a suggestion on the most effective block-based programming platform(s) that enables novice learners to develop applications easily can be made. This paper provides a comparison among different block-based programming platforms that are currently available, in identifying those that support effective learning in programming as well as providing ability to speed up the process of writing codes.

Keywords: Block-based programming · Visual programming language · Learning programming · Novice programmers

1 Introduction

Inside today's computing landscape, there are several programming paradigms which can be used for programming. Some common programming paradigms include imperative models which can be object-oriented, procedural and many others; declarative models which includes functional, logical programming; and block-based programming or visual programming [1, 2].

Learning programming via traditional methods and text-based are regarded as quite difficult [3]. According to the Higher Education Statistics Agency HESA [4], degrees in Computer Science (CS) have the largest number of students who drop out. The most recent figures available from HESA, covering the year 2016/17, indicate that before finishing their degree, 9.8% of CS undergraduates dropped out. The most common

F. Saeed et al. (Eds.): IRICT 2021, LNDECT 127, pp. 630–640, 2022.
https://doi.org/10.1007/978-3-030-98741-1_52

explanation when it comes to why people quit degree courses across disciplines was because almost half (49%) said that they did not like it, and 33% said it was too complicated [4]. With this significant drop in the learners' or programmers' motivations to innovate, it is very important for programmers to have a high motivation and satisfaction [5]. Hence, an increase in satisfaction of programming approach may boost the morale of programmers or developers. As compared to other programming paradigms, visual programming makes the learning process simpler and more comprehendible for both children and programming novices [6].

There are different platforms that adapt block-based programming (that is based on Visual Programming Language - VPL), such platforms include Scratch, Blockly, App Inventor, Alice, Snap!, Code.org, Tynker many others [7]. Nowadays, block-based programming has been utilized by many potential learners or programmers ranging from young to adults as a steppingstone to learn programming as well as developing small scale-size applications. This block-based programming paradigm has been shown to make programming easier and more comprehendible [6]. Thus, it is crucial to ensure that this block-based programming paradigm provides a platform which can be used to develop and learn simple application as well as easy to use. For learners to stay motivated, it is very important to know any available block-based programming platforms that are satisfactory and fun to use [8].

As there have been not much published empirical evidence showing and revealing the usage and utilization of the available block-based programming platforms and how these platforms would offer programming environment that able to engage, motivate and provide satisfaction to novice learners or programmers to write codes, hence, it is significant enough to venture in this context of research. In our study, a suggestion on the most effective block-based programming platform (s) that novice learners or programmers can use to learn and develop small scale-based applications can be drawn. Also, this would be beneficial to them as block-based programming paradigm able to provide a better environment to speed up programming effort as well as easily absorb problem solving skills. However, in this paper, we are merely focusing on a conceptual analysis and comparison among the identified block-based programming platforms. After conceptually compared these platforms, three of them were selected to be analyzed further in providing a suggestion on the most effective block-based programming platform (s) that able to support in developing some simple application among the novice learners.

This article is arranged as follows: In Sect. 2, some fundamental concepts of among the available block-based programming are addressed. Section 3 provides the analysis and comparison result of all the block-based programming platforms explained in Sect. 2. Finally, Sect. 4 concludes of this paper.

2 Block-Based Programming Platforms

Nowadays, there are a lot of different kind of programming platforms which utilize the block-based programming that based on VPL. Some of these platforms include Scratch, Snap!, Blockly, Tynker, Code.org, Alice and many others, and they're designed to teach kids how to create games and programs, and rather than writing the code, users visually drag and snaps together blocks of code [9]. Like text-based programming, platforms that implements block-based programming paradigms can support imperative programming models or declarative models or both, for example, an extension to Scratch that was initially called BYOB which stands for Build your Own Blocks was developed by Harvey and Monig, this extension could implement the Object-Oriented Programming (OOP) paradigm of imperative models [10].

The sub-sequence paragraphs provide conceptual explanations related the identified block-based programming platforms. Figures 1, 2, 3, 4, 5, 6 and 7 visualize all the platforms.

Scratch: As discussed by [11], Scratch is a visual and multimedia programming that is a Squeak-based. It aims to construct animated sequences in an easy and effective manner for learning computer programming. Scratch has an interface that is intuitive, quick and comprehensible, so that novices can learn without much difficulty. users can work with pictures, photographs, music, create sketches, alter appearance, make objects communicate with each other and with the user, and make programming fully visual. Scratch's programming language and environment work together to create a framework that is extremely easy to understand. By having an interface which has a single-window, multipaned architecture, which keeps vital subcomponents accessible at all times, which thrives to make navigation as easy as possible, a liveness and tinker ability feature which means there is no need distinction between compilation and edit/run phase and allows users to play with commands and code fragments in the same way as mechanical or electronic components are tinkered with. Scratch also gives you visual cues on how well your program is working. And user cannot encounter error message using this platform. Scratch transforms variables into tangible objects in which users can see and operate, as well as allowing them to be better understood through experimenting and perusing. As Blocks snapped together in Scratch represents programming expressions, statements, or control structures which forms Scratch scripts, and there have been four basic types of blocks to pick from. which includes, function, command, control structure, and trigger blocks. Scratch also has three first-class data types which includes Number, String and Boolean. However, Scratch is an object-based, not an Object-Oriented Programming (OOP) language, since it lacks classes and inheritance. Thus, they do not have procedures or concurrency (multi-threading). There have been no straightforward methods for concurrency control, such as locks, monitors, and semaphores in scratch that are common in other programming languages. Instead, it adds concurrency control into its threading model in such a manner that almost all racing conditions are avoided. The description of scratch above was based on the study conducted by [12].

Blockly: Blockly was created especially for kids and novices. It was designed to allow this audience without a teacher to use the setting, as its educational mechanics were designed to be self-taught. With Blockly, the user receives instructions from a set of educational constructs and after completion users are supposed to be able to use the traditional text-based languages [11]. Blockly is still in its early stages of production, so it's only good for writing short scripts for the time being [13]. Blockly is written in JavaScript and is meant to be used in a web page [13]. It can also create code that can be executed independently. It can be modified to enable end users to program web apps since it can be embedded in a web page and is written in JavaScript [13].

App Inventor: App Inventor is described as a visual and intuitive programming environment that is designed to create completely functional applications for smartphones and tablets for all types of users including kids and novices [14]. The environment offers an intuitive metaphor for programming and consists of two parts: a designer that allows the users to pick application components and a block editor to specify the application's behaviours [11].

Alice: This is a block-based platform which allows making of animations, interactive storylines, and simple 3D games simple for novice [9]. It was created in 1994 at the University of Virginia. The environment is appealing to novice learners because it contains many 3D model elements such as objects, animals, and vehicles that can be animated by the user [11]. Alice comes with a number of built-in action commands. Alice's functions (procedures) are provided by the Python programming language. Functions are primarily used in Alice to implement recursion and looping, as well as to implement interactions through events [15]. Alice error messages, like many other languages, can be cryptic at times, which means it is possible to make errors in Alice [15].

Snap!: This is a free, block-based educational VPL and online community that enables users to learn about mathematical and computational concepts while experimenting with, or developing, games, interactive animations, stories, and more. One of the core ideas behind Snap! is that it allows programmers to expand the framework by creating blocks that look and function just like the ones that come pre-installed [16]. Snap! and Scratch are similar in terms of user interface, events and live parallel blocks. But despite being inspired from Scratch, Snap! has a lot of advanced functionality [16]. For-example, Snap! borrows the concept of first class heterogenous lists as the only essential complex data structure from the Scheme programming language, which we can use to create any other kind of data structure we might think of. As a result, enables the assignment of these type of lists to variables, to be used as parameters/dimension in blocks, return them from procedures, transmitted and received as message [16]. Some unique features of Snap! is its closures and first class procedures. Programming constructs which enable users to treat code like data are called closures. It records the context in which they were formed, as well as variable values in their scope [16].

Code.org: This is a website which hosts graphical programming courses [17]. its environment has been very successful since its release and is available in a variety of languages, making it accessible to people all over the world [17]. Novices can learn algorithms and logic, 'if' conditions, variables, loops, and functions by programming with building blocks (drag-and-drop blocks), which is provided by code.org [18]. According to [18], tutoring computer programming to fourth grade students on the code.org platform did not enhance their problem-solving abilities; however, the students formed a positive attitude toward programming.

Tynker: Tynker is a type of block-based programming platform like Scratch. The graphic design and concepts, like Hopscotch and Snap!, are based on the free Scratch programming language. Tynker is built on JavaScript and HTML5 and it can be used in the browser, and from smartphones and tablets too, without the need for plugins [19]. Tynker is an open source software that is more advanced than Scratch and ScratchJr. It is better used when user have been exposed to more simple apps or have had other programming experiences. Although Hutchison noted that it is not meant for novices, Tynker makes understanding coding easier because it does so by using games like Minecraft and Hour of Code to educate them [20].

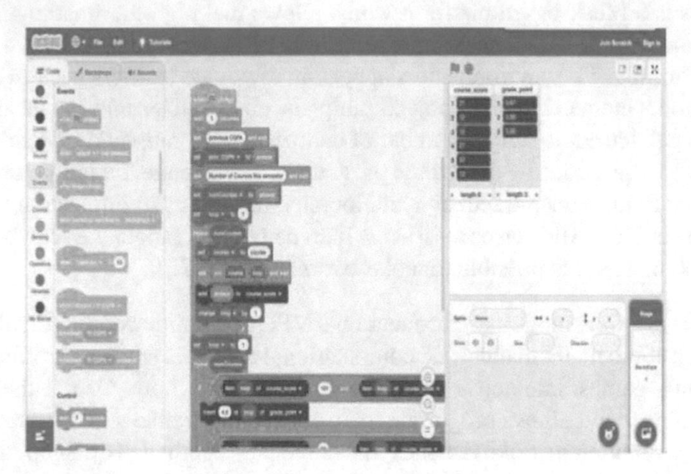

Fig. 1. Scratch user interface

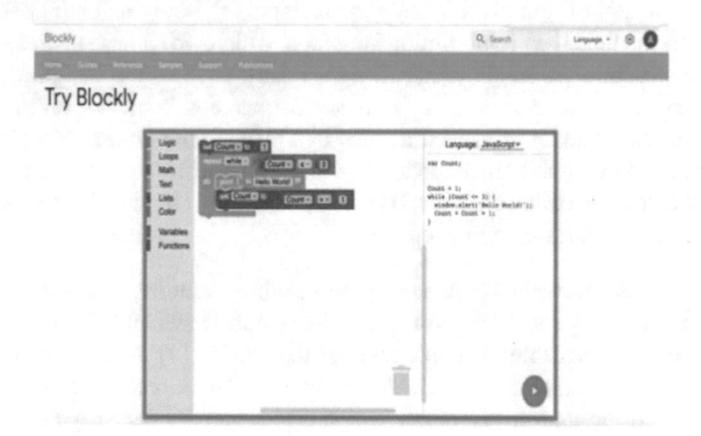

Fig. 2. Blockly user interface

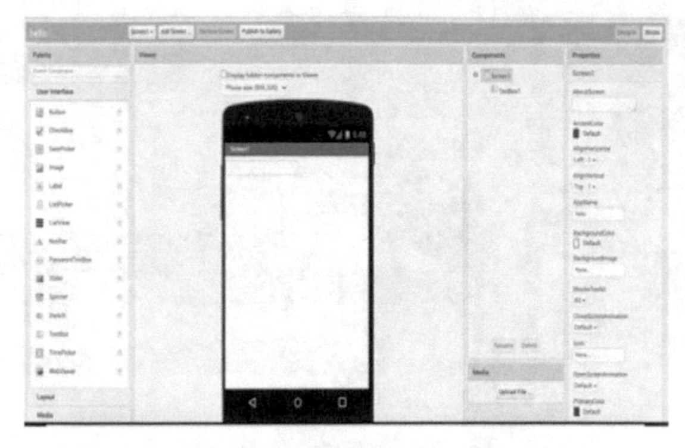

Fig. 3. Design section of app inventor interface

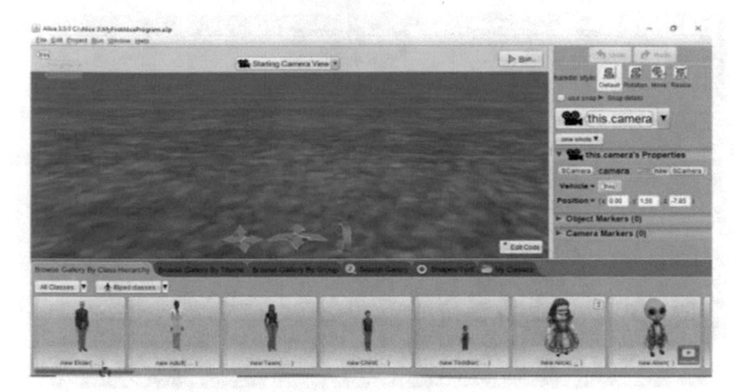

Fig. 4. Alice 3.5 interface

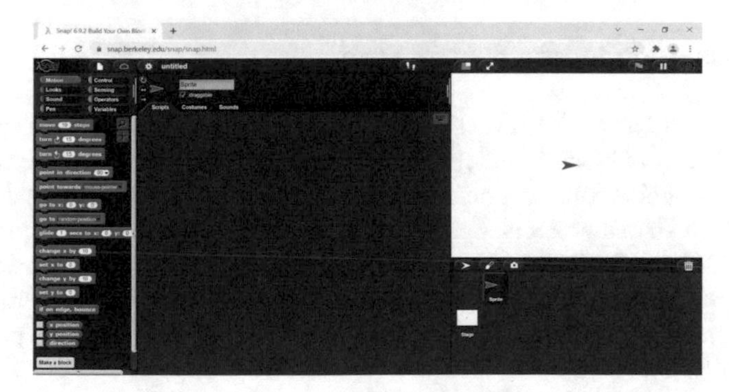

Fig. 5. Snap interface

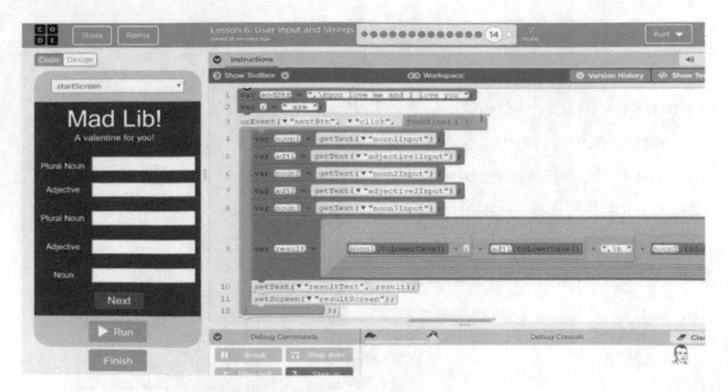

Fig. 6. Code.org interface

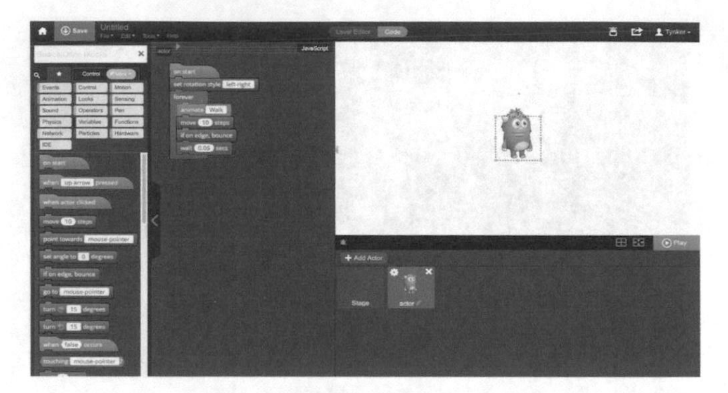

Fig. 7. Tynker interface

3 Analysis and Comparison Result

There are tremendous advantages of block-based programming. One of these common benefits is that any of block-based programming platform has served as an environment to welcome learners into the programming world. Since, the launch of Scratch, there have been 40 million shared projects. Scratch aims to provide a development platform with adequate scaffolding for inexperienced programmers to begin programming with almost no formal instruction, while also supporting complex programs [21]. Furthermore, it was crucial that it provides support for a variety number of programs and programmers as well as offering programmers with a platform to engage and express their art in a larger programming culture. Block-based programming platforms have motivational potentials features which have tremendous impact to programmers and can also lead to better productivity [10]. Also, block-based programming has been used widely in different domains over the years. Among of the domains are examples of where some types of these block-based programming have been used are sensor-controlled music, image processing, animations etc. Most types of block-based programming languages are highly portable, with desktop implementations already in place (Macintosh, Windows, BeOS, Acorn, Linux/Unix) as described by [22].

Table 1 shows the result of analysis and comparison among all the block-based programming platforms as explained in prior section in terms of their differences and similarities related to features offered by each platform. In terms of pedagogical characteristics, all of these platforms specialized on problem-driven learning and computational thinking [10]. In current practice, the three most prominent block-based programming platforms include Scratch, Blockly and App Inventor. Further discussion on these three platforms are also available in the sub-sequence paragraphs. Table 1. shows the similarities and differences in feature between the block-based programming platforms.

Scratch has a more attractive user interface among the three platforms, and it is mostly used as a benchmark for other block-based platforms. Scratch is a pioneer block-based platform, it has been so successful that there has been other application that has been developed based on scratch. Although some applications are an extension of Scratch, they lack Scratch's glamour. When using Scratch to develop applications or learn programming, it is a useful tool for novice programmers, and one of its most interesting features is the availability of its user community for codes sharing and it is an open-source (free) software which can be downloadable on PC. Most of the available block-based programming platforms are based on Scratch. Scratch was chosen because of its features, popularity and acceptance worldwide. Based on Table 1, it can be noticed that Snap!, Alice, Tynker and Code.org is similar to Scratch in terms of features. In fact, the platforms were designed based on Scratch [19].

Blockly is also a good tool for novice programmer to develop applications. Blockly is unique because it allows users to create custom blocks and blockly applications can be translated into other text-based languages like PHP, JavaScript, Python, Dart and many other languages. Blockly is also great for complex and abstract programs development and can put a coding environment on your webpage. Blockly app has a simple interface which is divided into 3 sections. The first section is where the blocks can be selected and the blocks in Blockly are divided into 8 categories which include Logic, Loops, Math, Texts, Lists, Color, Variables and Functions. The second section is the canvas where the programs can be formed. Blocks that has been dragged can be snapped together on the canvas. A section which is a unique feature that has been included only in Blockly, where it translates the program on the canvas into a selected text-based language of the user's

Table 1. Similarities and differences in features between block-based programming platforms

Features	Scratch	App inventor	Blockly	Alice	Snap!	Tynker	Code.org
Allow users to create custom blocks	No	Yes	Yes	No	Yes	No	Yes
Make syntax errors impossible	Yes	Yes	Yes	No	Yes	Yes	No
User community for code sharing	Yes	No	No	Yes	Yes	Yes	Yes

(*continued*)

Table 1. (*continued*)

Features	Scratch	App inventor	Blockly	Alice	Snap!	Tynker	Code.org
Downloadable on pc	No	Yes	No	Yes	No	No	No
Usable on browsers	Yes	Yes	Yes	No	Yes	Yes	Yes
Sharing sprites	Yes	No	Yes	No	Yes	Yes	Yes
Procedures	No	Yes	Yes	Yes	Yes	No	Yes
Recursion	No	Yes	Yes	Yes	Yes	No	Yes
Lists	No	Yes	Yes	Yes	Yes	No	Yes
Databases	No	Yes	No	No	No	No	Yes
Multi-threading	Yes	Yes	No	Yes	Yes	Yes	No
Inheritance	No	No	No	Yes	Yes	No	No

choice. Blockly has more programming functions like lists, recursion, custom blocks, procedures/functions etc., so it will be logical to select Blockly over Alice, Tynker or Snap!.

App Inventor is the most unique feature about App Inventor is that only App Inventor can be used to develop a mobile application. According to Park and Shin [23], App Inventor has the most numbers of blocks. For example, it has 204 event type blocks while Scratch only has 7 types of event type blocks [23]. Although custom blocks can be defined in Scratch but in App Inventor only custom procedures can be defined. The app Inventor has a palette tab which consists of items that can be used to design an application. For example, the textbox, listpicker, and password textbox are all included in the palette and next is the viewer where users can see a live feedback of how the application interface looks like. And then the Components tab which comprises of the list of all the contents of all the item that has been used in the application being developed. App inventor also has properties features where the properties of the application components can be modified. For example, the background color of a text button can be modified in the properties tab. In the blocks screen, App Inventor has a tab where blocks can be selected and dragged on to the canvas. The blocks are divided into 9 categories which include Control, Logic, Math, Text, Lists, Dictionaries, Colors, Variables, and Procedures. App Inventor was selected over Code.org because it would be diverse to have to choose a platform that is not based on only Scratch.

As mentioned earlier, in our study, an experimental evaluation was conducted to compare and analyze these three platforms by getting involved some novice learners in programming to experience using all the platforms. Based on the analysis of the collected responses from these learners, then a suggestion was made on deciding the most preferrable block-based programming platform that able to support in developing some simple application among the novice learners.

4 Conclusion

In summary, based on the analysis and comparison done among the block-based programming platforms, all three shortlisted are very good and recommended for novices. Scratch is ranked higher in terms of satisfaction, engagement and motivation and it is also preferred by the novices because they believed it is easier to use. Blockly is a great application with assortment of features. App Inventor is unique because of its ability to enables novices develop mobile app conveniently and easily. There are certain limitations encountered in this study as the usability and other factors of this platforms could not be measured. Also, further works can be done to reveal the usage and utilization of the available block-based programming platforms and how these platforms would offer programming environment that are able to engage, motivate and provide satisfaction to novice learners or programmers to write codes, hence, it is significant enough to venture in this context of research. And evaluate to what extend the identified block-based programming platforms achieved users' engagement, motivation and satisfaction.

References

1. Krishnamurthi, S., Fisler, K.: Programming paradigms and beyond. Cambridge Handb. Comput. Educ. Res. **37** (2019)
2. Pichler, P., Weber, B., Zugal, S., Pinggera, J., Mendling, J., Reijers, H.A.: Imperative versus declarative process modeling languages: an empirical investigation. In: Daniel, F., Barkaoui, K., Dustdar, S. (eds.) BPM 2011. LNBIP, vol. 99, pp. 383–394. Springer, Heidelberg (2012). https://doi.org/10.1007/978-3-642-28108-2_37
3. Kalelioğlu, F., Gülbahar, Y.: The effects of teaching programming via scratch on problem solving skills. **13**(1), 33–50 (2014)
4. Flinders, K.: Computer science undergraduates most likely to drop out. ComputeWeekly.Com. https://www.computerweekly.com/news/252467745/Computerscience-undergraduates-most-likely-to-drop-out. Accessed 1 Aug 2019
5. LeDuc, A.L.: Motivation of programmers. ACM SIGMIS Database **11**(4), 4–12 (1980). https://doi.org/10.1145/1113469.1113470
6. Williams, C., Alafghani, E., Daley Jr., A., Gregory, K., Rydzewski, M.: Teaching programming concepts to elementary students. In: 2015 Frontiers in Education Conference Proceedings (FIE 2015), pp. 706–714 (2015)
7. Resnick, M., et al.: Scratch: programming for all. Commun. ACM **52**(11), 60–67 (2009). https://doi.org/10.1145/1592761.1592779
8. João, P., Nuno, D., Fábio, S.F., Ana, P.: A cross-analysis of block-based and visual programming apps with computer science student-teachers. Educ. Sci. **9**(3) (2019). https://doi.org/10.3390/educsci9030181
9. Jenkins, T.: The motivation of students of programming. In: Proceedings of the Conference on Integrating Technology into Computer Science Education, ITiCSE, pp. 53–56 (2001). https://doi.org/10.1145/507758.377472
10. Papadakis, S., Kalogiannakis, M., Zaranis, N., Orfanakis, V.: Using scratch and app inventor for teaching introductory programming in secondary education. A case study. Int. J. Technol. Enhanced Learn. **8**(3–4), 217–233 (2016). https://doi.org/10.1504/IJTEL.2016.082317
11. Carlos Begosso, L., Ricardo Begosso, L., Aragao Christ, N.: An analysis of block-based programming environments for CS1. In: Proceedings - Frontiers in Education Conference, FIE, 2020-Octob (2020). https://doi.org/10.1109/FIE44824.2020.9273982

12. Maloney, J., Resnick, M., Rusk, N., Silverman, B., Eastmond, E.: The scratch programming language and environment. ACM Trans. Comput. Educ. **10**(4), 1–15 (2010). https://doi.org/10.1145/1868358.1868363
13. Lucy Black, Google Blockly - A Graphical Language with a Difference. https://www.iprogrammer.info/news/98-languages/4357-google-blockly-a-graphical-language-with-adifference.html. 12 June 2012
14. García Peñalvo, F.J., et al.: Evaluation of existing resources (study/analysis) (2016)
15. Pausch, R., Dann, W.: ALICE: a 3-D tool for introductory programming concepts. J. Comput. Sci. Coll. **15**(5), 107–116 (2017)
16. Romagosa, B.: The snap! Programming system. In: Tatnall, A. (ed.) Encyclopedia of Education and Information Technologies. Springer, Cham (2019). https://doi.org/10.1007/978-3-319-60013-0_28-2
17. Lambić, D., Đorić, B., Ivakić, S.: Investigating the effect of the use of code.org on younger elementary school students' attitudes towards programming. Behav. Inf. Technol. 1–12 (2020). https://doi.org/10.1080/0144929X.2020.1781931
18. Kalelioğlu, F.: A new way of teaching programming skills to K-12 students: Code.org. Comput. Hum. Behav. **52**, 200–210 (2015)
19. Rees, A.M., García-Peñalvo, F.J., Toivonen, T., Hughes, J., Jormanainen, I., Vermeersh, J.: A survey of resources for introducing coding into schools (2016)
20. Hutchison, A., Nadolny, L., Estapa, A.: Using coding apps to support literacy instruction and develop coding literacy. Read. Teach. **69**(5), 493–503 (2016)
21. Weintrop, D.: Block-based programming in computer science education. Commun. ACM **62**(8), 22–25 (2019). https://doi.org/10.1145/3341221
22. Burd, L., Kafai, Y., Rusk, N., Silverman, B., Resnick, M.: Scratch: a sneak preview [education]. In: Proceedings of Second International Conference on Creating, Connecting and Collaborating Through Computing, pp. 104–109 (2004). http://ieeexplore.ieee.org/xpls/abs_all.jsp?arnumber=1314376%5Cnpapers2://publication/uuid/556FB3A7-C6C7-47F5-BE7D-353071E9CCE1
23. Park, Y., Shin, Y.: Comparing the effectiveness of scratch and app inventor with regard to learning computational thinking concepts. Electron. (Switzerland) **8**(11) (2019). https://doi.org/10.3390/electronics8111269

Information Security Policy Compliance: An Exploration of User Behaviour and Organizational Factors

Angraini[1,3](✉), Rose Alinda Alias[2], and Okfalisa[3]

[1] School of Computing, Faculty Engineering, University Technology Malaysia, 81310 Johor, Malaysia
angraini@uin-suska.ac.id
[2] Department of Information System, Azman Hashim International Business School, University Technology Malaysia, 81310 Johor, Malaysia
[3] Department of Informatic Engineering, Faculty Science and Technology, Universitas Islam Negeri Sultan Syarif Kasim, Pekanbaru, Riau, Indonesia

Abstract. Organizations are adopting security policies to protect critical information, despite the fact that IT users frequently violate these standards. Numerous factors affecting user compliance have been identified in previous research, but few research findings have addressed human and organizational factors. The purpose of this study is to ascertain the human and organizational factors that influence user adherence to policies. The variables examined included leadership, organizational commitment, rewards, awareness, behavioral intentions, and habits, all of which were gender-related. This is a quantitative study that includes offline and online surveys of university users in Indonesia. The findings indicated that the awareness variable had the greatest effect, while the reward variable had no effect. This research is expected to contribute to an understanding of how to comply with information security policies.

Keywords: Information security · Compliance · User behaviour · Moderating variabel · Gender

1 Introduction

Cybercrime continues to grow in number as the use of information technology grows. For example, between January and September 2020, Indonesia experienced the highest level of online fraud in ASEAN and is the country hardest hit by ransomware attacks, with 1.3 million victims [1]. To minimize information security incidents, the organization has developed an information security policy and enforces compliance by employees [2–4]. The information security policy (ISP) is intended to ensure the safety of information and information technology assets in support of organizational goals and objectives [5]. There are still many users who do not comply with information security policies so that finding of internal violations [6, 7] and if this continues, individuals will disrupt organizational activities [8, 9].

F. Saeed et al. (Eds.): IRICT 2021, LNDECT 127, pp. 641–650, 2022.
https://doi.org/10.1007/978-3-030-98741-1_53

Numerous studies have been conducted on the ISP compliance model, utilizing a variety of theories, including the theory of planned behavior, the theory of protective motivation, and those that examine the variables affecting ISP compliance [2, 3, 10–15]. However, there have been few empirical investigations into combining factors from user behaviour and organization factors. Furthermore, it is necessary to develop a model that focuses on the variables required by the organization rather than on a particular theory to ensure that it only uses variables relevant to the organization. This study will conduct a survey of active information technology users in Indonesian universities to determine their compliance behavior with information security policies. This study aims to develop a compliance model by incorporating variables such as leadership, organizational commitment, reward, awareness, behavior intention, and habit with gender as moderating variables. This model is expected to be used by organizations to evaluate user compliance with information security policies.

This paper is structured as follows: an introduction, a theory explaining the study's variables, and a research model. Furthermore, the research approach and data processing was explained. The paper is followed by a presentation of the findings and a discussion of them. Finally, this paper concludes.

2 Literature Review

Leadership is a collaborative influence process when a group of people chooses someone as their leader to accomplish a common goal [16]. In the context of information security policy, leadership is a critical factor that influences employee compliance with ISP standards and, as a result, the protection of corporate resources [10, 17]. According to Humaidi and Balakrishnan (2015), Leaders play a critical role in ensuring that employees are aware of and adhere to the organization's information security policy [18]. Avey (2010) assert that leaders must serve as role models in developing governance frameworks that ensure proper information security. By fostering a trusting relationship, ethical leadership may boost employees' compliance intentions [19]. Organizational commitment is a term that relates to the degree to which employees identify with and participate in the organization for which they work [20]. Due to its prominence in understanding the relationship between employees and their organizational behavior, significant research efforts have focussed on organizational commitment as a significant antecedent of diverse workplace behaviors [21]. According to Herath and Rao (2009), organizational commitment is a strong determinant of employee compliance with ISPs [22]. Rewarding users for perceived compliance benefits has a considerable effect on their perceptions of the importance of adhering to security measures [10].

Although their findings varied, Moody (2018) discovered that rewards had no meaningful effect on intentions to follow information security policies [2]. This view is backed up by Siponen (2014), who assert that the incentive for adhering to information security policies is negligible [23]. This research will study the direct effect of reward on user compliance to information security policy. The term "habit" can be interpreted as "the degree to which humans perform behaviors automatically while interacting with information systems as a result of their experience [24]. Practice habits are essential because they suggest and support an individual's repeated engagement with IS.

Individual variables can affect behavioral intentions to adhere to security policies and their overall security behavior (directly or indirectly) [25]. Numerous models have been created based on General Detterance Theory (GDT) [26–29] in order to research, analyze, and predict the effect of perceived punishment components on behavioral compliance intents. In addition, compliance with the Information Security Policy (ISP) is influenced by various other elements within the company [30]. Therefore, this research incorporates various variables into its analysis of behavioral intention. Security awareness can be defined as "workers' total knowledge and comprehension of potential information security risks and their repercussions" [10]. Awareness, defined as the security professional's overall knowledge and awareness of practices, methods, systems, and their repercussions, is oriented toward planning, monitoring, strategizing, and executing incident management duties [31]. Employees' levels of awareness are the most predictive of their intention to follow the organization's information security policy [32].

This research will incorporate the gender variable as a moderator to enhance the information security policy compliance model. Variables from earlier research are used to construct a compliance model for information security policies, as illustrated in Fig. 1.

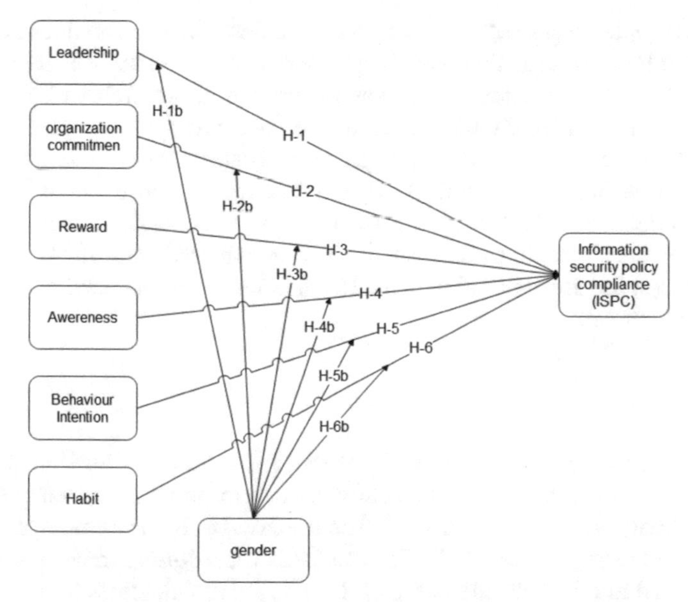

Fig. 1. Purpose model of information security policy compliance

The hypothesis for this research is as follows:

H-1: leadership have a significant effect on information security policy compliance (ISPC)
H-1b: Gender will positively moderate the influence of leadership to comply with information security policy (ISPC)
H-2: Organization commitment has a significant effect on ISPC.

H-2b: Gender will positively moderate the influence of Organization commitment to comply with information security policy (ISPC)
H-3: reward has a significant effect on ISPC
H-3b: Gender will positively moderate the influence of reward to comply with information security policy (ISPC)
H-4: awareness has a significant effect on ISPC
H-4b: Gender will positively moderate the influence of awareness to comply with information security policy (ISPC)
H-5: Behavior Intention has a significant effect on ISPC
H-5b: Gender will positively moderate the influence of Behavior Intention to comply with information security policy (ISPC)
H-6: Habit has a significant effect on ISPC
H-6b: Gender will positively moderate the influence of habit to comply with information security policy (ISPC)

3 Method

This research applies a case study approach to examine public universities in Indonesia. The participants are information technology users from a variety of Indonesian public universities. The questionnaire was adapted from earlier research with modifications to account for the unique circumstances of the case study. We circulated the online questionnaire via email invitations and group messages. There were a total of 1153 requests, however only 246 were responded to. The low response rate online is a result of the high sample size. Additionally, respondents were contacted directly via surveys. Three hundred questionnaires were issued; 196 were returned, indicating a response rate of 65 percent for the direct questionnaire. The data was then evaluated with Smart-PLS to validate the model.

4 Result

This research examines the data using the Partial Least Squares (PLS) method and the smartPLS software. PLS-SEM is frequently used in information systems research for model complexity and formative metrics. Additionally, PLS can be employed with small sample sizes and irregular data [33]. The standards for reporting the results of the PLS analysis utilized in this study are based on Hair's (2019) guidelines for evaluating formative measurement and structural models. The convergent validity, indicator collinearity, statistical significance, and relevant indicator weight of the formative measurement model are all analyzed [34]. The reliability of the variable items research instrument was determined using the loading factor value. Based on the value of the loading factor, the item can be used in research. When the loading factor is between 0.60 and 0.70, the item is considered "suitable" for exploratory study. Between 0.70 and 0.90 indicates that the item is "acceptable to good" [35]. On this research all variabel has value more than 0.60 so it can be use continue.

Discriminant validity is used to verify that each thought associated with a latent variable differs from other variables. If the loading value of each latent variable indicator is

Table 1. The discriminant validity test

	AW	Behavior Intention	HA	ISPC	Leader-ship	Organization Commitment	Reward	gender
AW	0.92							
Behavior Inten-tion	0.611	0.975						
HA	0.598	0.419	0.957					
ISPC	0.637	0.544	0.512	0.831				
Leadership	-0.056	0.123	0.106	0.154	0.942			
Organization Commitment	0.716	0.56	0.549	0.662	0.169	0.893		
Reward	0.055	0.064	0.1	0.077	0.041	0.045	0.794	
gender	-0.042	0.002	-0.054	-0.031	0.106	-0.006	0.07	1.000

more significant than the loading values of other latent variables, the model has excellent discriminant validity. The discriminant validity test results are shown in Table 1.

As illustrated in Table 2, multiple loading factor values for each indicator of each latent variable do not equal the loading value when coupled with other latent variables. Thus, this score indicates that each latent variable has a high discriminant validity, despite some hidden variables lacking a highly correlated gauge with other constructs.

Additionally, the reliability value of a construct and the Average Variance Extracted (AVE) value of each construct provides insight into the validity and reliability requirements. For example, the build is reliable if the value is more significant than 0.70 and the AVE is greater than 0.50. The Composite Reliability and Average Value of All Variables data will be provided in Table 2.

Table 2. The composite reliability and average value

	Cronbach's alpha	Composite reliability	Average Variance Extracted (AVE)
AW	0.963	0.971	0.846
Behaviour intention	0.983	0.987	0.951
HA	0.982	0.985	0.916
ISPC	0.848	0.899	0.69
Leadership	0.976	0.979	0.887
Organization commitment	0.936	0.952	0.797
Reward	0.861	0.895	0.63

According to the average Average Variance Extracted (AVE) results, each variable had a value greater than 0.50, and the composite reliabilities of the individual measurements ranged between 0.76 and 0.95, exceeding the prescribed value of 0.70. After a satisfactory evaluation of the measurement model, the SEM-PLS model is structurally evaluated.

Changes in the value of R-Squares can be used to explain the effect of certain exogenous latent factors on endogenous latent variables, regardless of whether the exogenous latent variables have a substantial effect. For instance, R-Squares values of 0.75 indicate a substantial value, 0.50 indicates a moderate, and 0.25 indicates a weak [36].

The R squared value 0.534 indicates the variance in each endogenous construct and the model's explanatory power [37]. R square values greater than 0.10 indicate that this research model can proceed to the hypothesis testing step.

The following step is to test each hypothesized association using simulation statistically. the SMART-PLS approach is applied to the sample using the bootstrap method. The purpose of bootstrap testing is to mitigate the issue of aberrant research data. Additionally, the predicted significant factors shed light on the link between the studied variables. Two of the thirteen beta coefficient paths had negative values, notably moderating gender with ISPC and moderating behavior intention with ISPC. Table 3 contains detailed information about the beta coefficient path and p-value.

Table 3. The result of hyphotesis

		confidence interval		T Statis-tics	P Values	result
	β value	2.50%	97.50%			
AW -> ISPC	0.233	0.113	0.354	3.796	0	Significant
AW x Gender -> ISPC	0.003	-0.128	0.127	0.044	0.965	not Significant
BIN x gender -> ISPC	-0.052	-0.148	0.043	1.045	0.296	not Significant
Behaviour Intention -> ISPC	0.153	0.07	0.239	3.568	0	Significant
HA -> ISPC	0.119	0.03	0.207	2.647	0.008	Significant
HA x gender -> ISPC	0.083	0.002	0.165	1.997	0.046	Significant
LD x gender -> ISPC	0.005	-0.064	0.078	0.133	0.894	not Significant
Leadership -> ISPC	0.081	0.02	0.152	2.325	0.02	Significant
OC x gender -> ISPC	0.002	-0.112	0.119	0.034	0.973	not Significant
Organization Commit-ment -> ISPC	0.331	0.212	0.435	5.851	0	Significant
Reward -> ISPC	0.026	-0.067	0.101	0.651	0.515	not Significant
Rw x Gender -> ISPC	0.023	-0.056	0.091	0.609	0.543	not Significant

The table above summarizes the findings of hypothesis testing by determining the p-value for each path coefficient, which can be one- or two-way depending on the previous researcher's knowledge of directions and coefficients that connected (Kock,

2015b). A two-sided type test with a p-value of 0.05 and a confidence interval of 97.5 percent was used in this study. Half of the twelve hypotheses offered in this study were not significant, with a p-value > 0.05. detail for each hypothesis descript below:

H-1: t-value of 2.325 > t-table 1.967 and the association between the leadership variable and ISPC, it is established that leadership has a significant influence on ISPC.
H-2: The relationship between Organization commitment and ISPC has a t-value of 5.851 > 1.967 and a p-value of 0.000 0.05. It may be inferred that organizational commitment has a significant effect on ISPC.
H-3: The reward variable's connection with ISPC has a t-value of 0.651 t-table 1.967 and a p-value of 0.515 > 0.05. Thus, it may be argued that incentive has a negligible effect on ISPC.
H-4: The relationship between awareness and ISPC has a t-value of 3.796 > t table 1.967 and a p-value of 0.000 0.05. It can be stated that awareness and ISPC have a significant influence.
H-5: The association between the variables Behavior Intention and ISPC has a t-value of 3.568 > t table 1.967 and a p-value of 0.000 0.05, indicating that Behavior Intention and ISPC have a significant influence.
H-6: The association between Habit and ISPC has a t-value of 2.647 > t table 1.967 and a p-value of 0.008 0.05, indicating that habit substantially affects behavior intention.

Additionally, the beta path coefficient with statistical significance for moderating factors (interacting) is non-significant for almost all hypotheses, with only one positive hypothesis being identified.

H-1b: When gender is controlled, leadership has no influence on improving ISPC
H-2b: gender had no effect on the interaction between organizational commitment factors and ISPC
H-3b: reward has no effect on improving ISPC when gender is controlled
H-4b: gender has no effect on the interaction between awareness and ISPC
H-5b: regardless of gender, behavior intention had no effect on ISPC
H-6b: Habit plays a beneficial function in improving ISPC, with gender having a moderating effect.

5 Discussion

Information security should be a primary strategic objective because this study discovered that leadership affected user compliance regardless of gender. This conclusion is consistent with Koohang's (2020) finding that leadership predicts employee compliance with information security policies [32]. Furthermore, commitment from leaders enables successful enforcement of ISP compliance within organizations [38], emphasizing the critical nature of transformational leadership because it directly impacts employee behavior levels [39].

The organizational commitment variable has a substantial effect on compliance with information security policies; Sharma (2018) supports this finding by stating that organizational commitment will be felt more strongly by employees when it comes to complying with ISPs [40]. Nevertheless, contrary to what Liu (2020) discovered, organizational commitment will erode self-efficacy regarding user compliance [41].

The hypothesis that reward can promote compliance was not established in this study. This study did not uncover an effect of reward that was either direct or mediated by gender. Moody (2018) discovered the same thing [2]. This data corroborates Bulgurcu's (2010) conclusion that reward do not significantly contribute to compliance with security policies [10]. Despite benefits for fulfilling security policy compliance objectives [42]. The outcomes of this study explicitly imply that user awareness matters, as earlier research has established that staff opinions also influence information security compliance attitudes [10]. Additionally, those who understand computers and are knowledgeable about computer security have a decreased interest in exploiting information technology.

The findings of this research contrast with Sommestad (2017) discovered that habits had no significant effect on behavioral intentions to adhere to information security standards [11]. However, it is consistent with Moody's (2018), which claims that habits, in addition to role ideals and anxiety, influence behavioral intentions [2]. However, earlier research relied on behavior intention as a moderator, demonstrating that habit directly affected compliance with information security standards.

6 Conclusion

The purpose of this research is to conduct a broad examination of the factors that influence user compliance with information security regulations, with a focus on gender. There are three organizational variables to consider: leadership, organizational commitment, and reward, as well as three behavioral variables to consider: awareness, behavior intention, and habit. Gender was chosen as a moderator due to its perceived ability to influence user compliance. The findings established categorically that gender had no effect on user compliance. Similarly, additional hypothesis revealed the same thing. Only one of the six presented hypotheses moderated by gender had an effect on adherence. As a result, additional research into the use of moderator factors is warranted. Additionally, the use of mediating variables to ascertain the relationship between more complicated variables should be included. This study's distribution of questionnaires and responders is limited. However, due to this survey's wide range of respondents, the response rate is relatively near to the ground. Additionally, this research should be developed from the variable selection process with complex theory.

References

1. Interpol (2021): Asean cyberthreat assessment 2021
2. Moody, G.D., Siponen, M., Pahnila, S.: Toward a unified model of information security policy compliance. MIS Q. **42**, 285–311 (2018)

3. Pahnila, S., Siponen, M., Mahmood, A.: Employees' behavior towards IS security policy compliance. In: Proceedings of the Annual Hawaii International Conference on System Sciences, pp. 1–10 (2007)
4. Manjula, R., Bagchi, K., Ramesh, S., Baskaran, A.: Policy compliance in information security. Int. J. Pharm. Technol. **8**, 22330–22340 (2016)
5. Doherty, N.F., Fulford, H.: Aligning the information security policy with the strategic information systems plan. Comput. Secur. **25**, 55–63 (2006)
6. Höne, K., Eloff, J.H.P.: What makes an effective information security policy? Netw. Secur. **2002**, 14–16 (2002)
7. Wiant, T.L.: Information security policy's impact on reporting security incidents. Comput. Secur. **24**, 448–459 (2005)
8. Sohrabi Safa, N., Von Solms, R., Furnell, S.: Information security policy compliance model in organizations. Comput. Secur. **56**, 1–13 (2016)
9. Furnell, S.: Malicious or misinformed? Exploring a contributor to the insider threat Comput. Fraud Secur. **2006**, 8–12 (2006)
10. Bulgurcu, B., Cavusoglu, H., Benbasat, I.: Information security policy compliance: an empirical study of rationality-based beliefs and information security awareness. MIS Q. **34**, 523–548 (2010)
11. Sommestad, T., Karlzén, H., Hallberg, J.: The theory of planned behavior and information security policy compliance. J. Comput. Inf. Syst. 1–10 (2017)
12. D'Arcy, J., Lowry, P.B.: Cognitive-affective drivers of employees' daily compliance with information security policies: a multilevel, longitudinal study. Inf. Syst. J. 1–27 (2017)
13. Alotaibi, M., Furnell, S., Clarke, N.: Information security policies : a review of challenges and influencing factors. In: 11th International Conference for Internet Technology and Secured Transactions, pp. 352–358 (2016)
14. Ifinedo, P.: Information systems security policy compliance: an empirical study of the effects of socialisation, influence, and cognition. Inf. Manag. **51**, 69–79 (2014)
15. Safa, N.S., Von, S.R., Furnell, S.: Information security policy compliance model in organizations. Comput. Secur. (2015). https://doi.org/10.1016/j.cose.2015.10.006
16. Silva, A.C.: What is Leadership? (2016)
17. Siponen, M., Willison, R.: Information security management standards: problems and solutions. Inf. Manag. **46**, 267–270 (2009)
18. Humaidi, N., Balakrishnan, V.: Leadership styles and information security compliance behavior: the mediator effect of information security awareness. Int. J. Inf. Educ. Technol. **5**, 311–318 (2015)
19. Avey, J.B., Palanski, M.E., Walumbwa, F.O.: When leadership goes unnoticed: the moderating role of follower self-esteem on the relationship between ethical leadership and follower behavior. J. Bus. Ethics **98**, 573–582 (2011)
20. Mowday, R.T.: Reflections on the study and relevance of organizational commitment. Hum. Resour. Manag. Rev. **8**, 387–401 (1998)
21. Lowry, P.B., Posey, C., Bennett, R.B.J., Roberts, T.L.: Leveraging fairness and reactance theories to deter reactive computer abuse following enhanced organisational information security policies: an empirical study of the influence of counterfactual reasoning and organisational trust. Inf. Syst. J. **25**, 193–273 (2015)
22. Herath, T., Rao, H.R.: Encouraging information security behaviors in organizations: role of penalties, pressures and perceived effectiveness. Decis. Support Syst. **47**, 154–165 (2009)
23. Siponen, M., Adam Mahmood, M., Pahnila, S.: Employees' adherence to information security policies: an exploratory field study. Inf. Manag. **51**, 217–224 (2014)
24. Limayem, M., Hirt, S.G., Cheung, C.M.K.: Research article how habit limits the predictive power of intention: the case of information. MIS Q. **31**, 705–737 (2007)

25. Consolvo, S., Langheinrich, M.: Identifying factors that influence employees' security behavior for enhancing ISP compliance. In: Fischer-Hübner, S., Lambrinoudakis, C., López, J. (eds.) Trust, Privacy and Security in Digital Business. TrustBus 2015. LNCS, vol. 9264., pp. 8–23 Springer, Cham (2015). https://doi.org/10.1007/978-3-319-22906-5_13
26. Lebek, B., Uffen, J., Neumann, M., Hohler, B., Breitner, M.H.: Information security awareness and behavior: a theory-based literature review. Manag. Res. Rev. **37**, 1049–1092 (2014)
27. Puhakainen, S.: Improving employees' compliance through information systems security training: an action research study. MIS Q. **34**, 757 (2010)
28. Abed, J., Dhillon, G., Ozkan, S.: Investigating continuous security compliance behavior : insights from information systems continuance model. In: Twenty-second Americas Conference on Information Systems San Diego, pp. 1–10 (2016)
29. Herath, T., Rao, H.R.: Protection motivation and deterrence: a framework for security policy compliance in organisations. Eur. J. Inf. Syst. **18**, 106–125 (2009)
30. Sharma, S., Warkentin, M.: Do i really belong?: Impact of employment status on information security policy compliance. Comput. Secur. **87**, 101397 (2019)
31. Thangavelu, M., Krishnaswamy, V., Sharma, M.: Impact of comprehensive information security awareness and cognitive characteristics on security incident management–an empirical study. Comput. Secur. **109**, 102401 (2021)
32. Koohang, A., Nowak, A., Paliszkiewicz, J., Nord, J.H.: Information security policy compliance: leadership, trust, role values, and awareness. J. Comput. Inf. Syst. **60**, 1–8 (2020)
33. Hair, J.F., Hult, G.T.M., Ringle, C.M., Sarstedt, M.: A Primer on Partial Least Squares Structural Equation Modeling (PLS-SEM), p. 165. Sage, Thousand Oaks (2013)
34. Hair, J.F., Risher, J.J., Sarstedt, M., Ringle, C.M.: When to use and how to report the results of PLS-SEM. Eur. Bus. Rev. **31**, 2–24 (2019)
35. Hair Jr, J.F., Sarstedt, M., Hopkins, L., Kuppelwieser, V.G.: Partial least squares structural equation modeling (PLS-SEM). Eur. Bus. Rev. **26**, 106–121 (2014)
36. Hair Jr, J.F., Black, W.C., Babin, B.J., Anderson, R.E.: Multivariate data Analysis (2018). https://doi.org/10.1002/9781119409137.ch4
37. Henseler, J., Sarstedt, M.: Goodness-of-fit indices for partial least squares path modeling, pp. 565–580 (2013)
38. Safa, N.S., Von Solms, R.: An information security knowledge sharing model in organizations. Comput. Hum. Behav. **57**, 442–451 (2016)
39. Guhr, N., Lebek, B., Breitner, M.H.: The impact of leadership on employees' intended information security behaviour: an examination of the full-range leadership theory. Inf. Syst. J. **29**, 340–362 (2019)
40. Sharma, S., Warkentin, M.: Do i really belong?: Impact of employment status on information security policy compliance. Comput. Secur. (2018). https://doi.org/10.1016/j.cose.2018.09.005
41. Liu, C., Wang, N., Liang, H.: Motivating information security policy compliance: the critical role of supervisor-subordinate guanxi and organizational commitment. Int. J. Inf. Manag. **54**, 02152 (2020)
42. Gerber, N., McDermott, R., Volkamer, M., Vogt, J.: Understanding information security compliance - why goal setting and rewards might be a bad idea. In: International Symposium on Human Aspects of Information Security & Assurance (HAISA 2016), vol. 10, pp. 145–155 (2016)

Understanding Wearable Device Adoption: Review on Adoption Factors and Directions for Further Research in Smart Healthcare

Md Ismail Hossain[1], Ahmad Fadhil Yusof[1](✉), and Mohana Shanmugam[2]

[1] School of Computing, Faculty of Engineering, Universiti Teknologi Malaysia, Skudai, Johor, Malaysia
ahmadfadhil@utm.my

[2] Department of Informatics, College of Computing and Informatics, Universiti Tenaga Nasional, Selangor, Malaysia
mohana@uniten.edu.my

Abstract. This paper analyses prior literature that identify adoption model for smart wearable healthcare devices. This assessment aims to contribute and identify factors that enable users to adopt wearable devices in the Internet of Things (IoT) based healthcare to monitor blood glucose measuring. This study has set off in quest of research in IoT smart healthcare focusing on blood glucose monitoring based on previous studies on wearable devices for smart healthcare. The key aim of this paper is to provide a summary of published articles and to find the current factors leading to the adoption of wearable devices for smart healthcare. The authors guided a systematic review of wearable devices in smart healthcare to explore the factors of adopting smart healthcare devices. 55 studies were analyzed where 21 studies directly address wearable devices, adoption models, and also IoT systems. Most of the studies covered a few factors; namely Interpersonal Influence, Self-efficiency, Individual Innovativeness, Attitude toward wearable devices, Self-interest, Perceived Expensiveness, and Perceived Usefulness in a wearable fitness tracker or monitoring. Findings show that the effect of trustworthiness has a very extensive potential to be explored to improve the model prediction to measure the adoption of IoT wearable devices in smart healthcare as well as blood glucose monitoring.

Keywords: Smart healthcare adoption · Wearable healthcare device · Adoption factors · Trustworthiness

1 Introduction

In this modern time, people wish to have a relaxed life with the creation of smart technologies. IoT is a buzzword that changes our daily lives and it also works by sensor to sensor (S2S) with a cloud-based application. IoT is an association of internet-linked objects which can gather and swap data. According to Fotiadis [1], a wearable healthcare device can be autonomous, non-invasive, and can carry out health functions namely to monitor and maintain health status over some time.

F. Saeed et al. (Eds.): IRICT 2021, LNDECT 127, pp. 651–662, 2022.
https://doi.org/10.1007/978-3-030-98741-1_54

Here, the authors identified some recent papers which discussed the adoption of wearable devices but were limited to smart healthcare-related devices especially on IoT devices (Table 2). In this paper, trustworthiness is also identified as an important factor to adopt a smart healthcare device for blood glucose monitoring whereas the other papers addressed trust and privacy concerns on other technology devices only. To complete this paper, the authors identified the influencing factors for smart healthcare devices especially on CGMs devices which is a new dimension in the domain of IoT healthcare devices.

Wearable technology is one of the gifted terms of IoT. As time goes by, many inventions came out in the area of wearable healthcare devices from the 13th to 20th century. The majority of people intend to have smart devices that can be used easily through sensor-based communication. IoT has made all the desires possible, giving the same opportunity and advantages to aged people and serious patients.

Wearable devices in healthcare start from different famous fitness trackers (Fitbit, Apple Watch, Samsung Gear) to more refined wearable healthcare devices [2, 3]. IoT healthcare offers a lot of opportunities and benefits however the level of adoption of wearable devices for blood glucose monitoring is still low compared to other wearable devices like fitness trackers. To accomplish the key objective of this study, we intend to address two key questions which will give an obvious idea to the readers by answering these questions:

RQ1. What are the factors influencing the adoption of wearable devices in smart healthcare?
RQ2. What are the limitations and gaps in the current research of wearable devices in smart healthcare?
RQ3. How trustworthiness can influence the adoption of smart healthcare devices?

The contribution of this study can be divided into two segments. Firstly, through the analysis of previous papers, comprehension of the existing models for wearable devices like fitness trackers will be easily gained. Secondly, readers can understand the most common and effective factors for wearable devices adoption through blood glucose measuring in smart healthcare. The residue of this study is as follows: Sect. 2 gives ideas for the surroundings of wearable devices and adoption model; Sect. 3 explains the adoption model for the adoption of wearable devices in smart healthcare to monitor blood glucose measuring; Sect. 4 discloses the literature review results; Sect. 5 informs the outcome of all the research quest, and lastly Sects. 8 and 9 sets up the discussion and conclusion.

2 Background

This division provides an outline of wearable devices, summarizes the core definition of wearable devices and, the adoption model of wearable devices in terms of smart healthcare.

2.1 Wearable Devices: An Overview

IoT is one of the fast-growing and dynamic areas in this technological era. Wearable devices are the main term regarding IoT as all the wearable devices work through sensor-based data transfer like S2S [4]. In IoT, there are different areas such as smart city, smart healthcare, smart agriculture. Currently, smart healthcare is a significant sector because people now wish to have more relaxation infused into their usual lifestyle [5]. That is why they wish to adopt wearable healthcare devices to save time. One of the smart healthcare applications named open APS Glucose monitoring device is used by Pharma as its connected system to help diabetes patients. Devices that are used during cancer treatment, ingestible sensors, connected contact lenses, arthritis, connected inhalers, wearable smart asthma monitoring, smart drill, wearable fitness tracker, wearable smartwatch, and so on are considered wearable devices. [3, 6]. Various definitions were provided by various researchers representing their understanding and contexts as shown in Table 1.

Table 1. Some wearable device definitions from previous studies

No	Definition	References
1	The new technologies which are based on sensor and internet connectivity are called smart wearable devices	[2]
2	Devices that are attached to our body externally as a fashion accessory or set in clothes are considered as smear wearable devices	[7]
3	Mobile technologies have headed to the rise of wearable devices which are smart and much popular	[8]
4	Smart devices are embedded with portable computers and electronics that are wearable on the body. These also allow for interactions between users and a smart environment anytime, anywhere	[3]

Definition 2 fits to our text as IoT devices work with sensor as well as continuous internet connectivity through wearable smart devices. Definition 4 also matches with the smart healthcare system where connectivity between users and systems is continuous, anytime and anywhere. This shows a combination of sensor connectivity, continuous use the of Internet and interactions with wearable devices.

2.2 Research in Wearable Device Adoption

According to the previous studies, several research has been conducted on IoT-based smart healthcare focusing on different wearable devices. Based on the existing literature, there is a lack of theoretical model on smart healthcare. In addition, the factors that explain the uses of wearable blood glucose monitoring devices, endure a significant strength for the developers of blood glucose monitoring devices [2, 9, 10]. Moreover, the adoption model delivers some significant factors that can identify users' intention to adopt smart healthcare devices [11–13].

Authors from past research have identified multiple factors indicating wearable smart healthcare device adoption intentions [14–17]. In another study, the researchers proposed a model to examine the factors affecting the intention to use wearable devices. The model was tested on smartwatches, one of the most prevalent wearable devices [18]. For Wearable Fitness Technology, TAM and SEM are implemented for the successful result of adopting a device [19]. Most of the previous research involved had empirical analysis to measure the intention to adopt wearable devices. This study shows the context of healthcare wearable device adoption especially on CGMs devices, that is yet needed to be explored. In line with Table 2, several studies were conducted by researchers on wearable device adoption. This study further identifies the model and constructs used in the adoption of wearable devices.

Table 2. Previous studies on wearable device adoption

No	Constructs	Sources
1	Perceived motivation, privacy, reliability	[20]
2	Self-efficacy, interpersonal influence, health interest, perceived expensiveness	[21]
3	Task scope, expert support, data sharing	[22]
4	Personal innovativeness, self-efficacy, satisfaction	[23]
5	Perceived value, perceived risk	[7]
6	Trust, satisfaction, resemblance	[8]
7	System quality, usability	[24]
8	The continuous intention, health ology	[25]
9	Adoption intention, ease of use, attitude toward using	[26]
10	Perceived ease of use, subjective norm, attitude toward using	[19]
11	Health concern, privacy concern, extended use	[27]
12	Functional, patient benefit	[28]
13	Privacy concern, trust, risk	[18]
14	Perceived usefulness, health belief	[29]
15	Intention to purchase, value, performance	[5]
16	Perceived usefulness, perceived risk, attitude toward using	[30]
17	Self-care, social support, security, privacy	[31]
18	Consumer satisfaction, trust towards doctor	[32]
19	Social influence, personality	[33]
20	Perceived usefulness, social influence	[34]
21	Interpersonal influence, personal innovativeness, health interest, attitude, trustworthiness	[10]

3 Research Methodology

For the completion of this paper, numerous steps were undertaken. The Authors downloaded journal articles, conference proceedings from various database: IEEE, Scopus, Science Direct, Springer Link and Atlantis press. Most articles cited here range from the year 2006 to 2021 because these all articles are similar to this paper context. During the searching and selecting process, authors used different keywords such as: "Wearable device", "Internet of Things", "Smart Healthcare", "Adoption model", Trustworthiness factor", "Blood Glucose Monitoring". After the research papers were downloaded, they were classified into different sections: 1) adoption model for wearable devices, 2) factors of adopting a wearable device and 3) smart healthcare system. Subsequently, when the classifying process was completed, the authors proceeded with the reviewing process.

In addition to reviewing journal papers, various adoption models for wearable devices that were mostly on smart healthcare devices through IoT were focused on. As this study focuses on the adoption model factors, the utmost priority was finding out which factor has a bigger influence on users' decision to use wearable devices for blood glucose monitoring. To respond to the above research questions, this study uses an organized review approach. Organized review is the combination of some processes like; identifying, evaluating, and interpreting all available researches that are relevant to the research questions, area of study, or rising phenomenon of interest [35]. For completion of this procedure, Mendeley desktop had been used as a tool in order to all of these research papers based on the keywords. Figure 1 illustrates the whole process of Research Methodology used to write this paper.

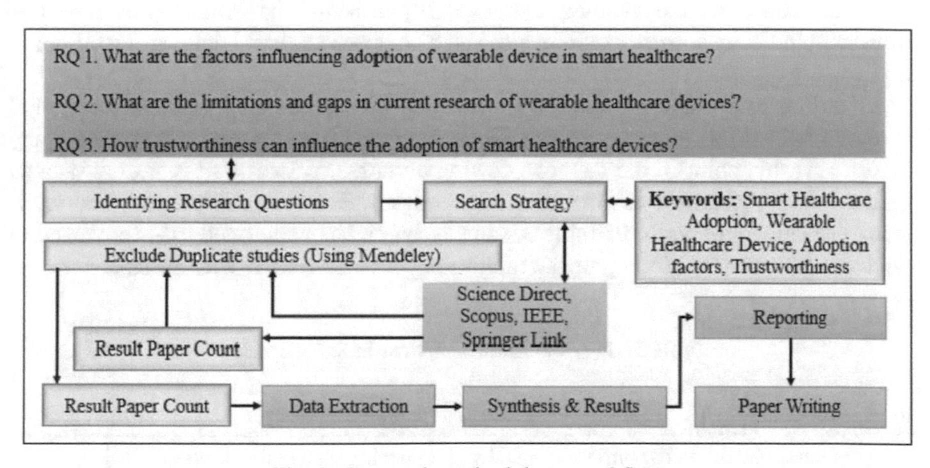

Fig. 1. Research methodology workflow

In the stage of Data Extraction & Synthesis, we recorded all the information in Microsoft Excel carefully by reading all the papers from Mendeley. However, in this paper few things were considered: research theme, source, publication time. These items were selected in alignment with the research questions for writing this paper.

4 Trustworthiness in IoT Adoption

The future phase of internet is IoT where machines talk with other machines [36]. Mobile technologies and computer are critical in our lives nowadays [37–39]. Wearable technologies have come forward following the growing fame of mobile technologies [40]. As wearable healthcare devices are the current trends, the systems need to be protected and assured to monitor users' healthcare daily [8, 41–43]. Health consciousness people would adopt a healthcare device if they find the devices trustworthy as it concerns their state of health [44]. Trust is a positive and important predictor for users' intention to adopt new healthcare devices [45]. Based on the findings, it is clearly shown that trustworthiness is one of the most important factors to be considered in measuring users' intention to adopt wearable healthcare devices.

5 Previous Study on Trustworthiness

Trustworthiness would have been mentioned several times considering that the majority of the publications talked about the factors for the adoption of wearable fitness trackers. One publication highlighted that trust is one of the most vital influencers of users' acceptance of new automated technologies [2]. The barrier to users' acceptance of healthcare devices is consumers' lack of trust in technologies [2]. Recently, consumers' concern regarding health has been increasing due to data accuracy and security [20, 27]. Accordingly, if users can get the authentic sources to consume wearable healthcare devices for monitoring their health status then they would positively consider it. In contrast, if they sense hesitation about the accuracy and reliability of health data obtained from healthcare wearable devices, they would evaluate it as a threat to their health and well-being [27].

According to previous studies [18], trust can be seen as an important factor that influences behavioral intention to use technology and has a strong effect on privacy concerns. At this point in the paper reviewing process, trustworthiness is only seen as a factor to adopt wearable devices in a fitness tracker. However, this proposed outset, it requires advanced research. In Table 3, some research has mentioned trust for wearable device adoption where blood glucose monitoring devices were not mentioned.

Table 3. Previous studies on trust-based adoption

No	Area	Year	Identified context	References
1	Purchase intention for online product	2018	Organic private label food	[46]
2	Adoption of cloud-based SCM	2013	Supply chain management	[47]
3	Perceptions of wearable fitness device impact	2018	Wearable fitness device	[48]

(continued)

Table 3. (*continued*)

No	Area	Year	Identified context	References
4	Role of initial trust for automated vehicles acceptance	2018	Vehicle automation	[45]
5	Consumer's online merchant's selection process: role of trust expectation	2015	E-commerce	[49]
6	Doctor's communication of trust care: breast cancer	2004	Healthcare	[50]
7	Subjective norms on user's truest intention to adopt cloud technology	2017	Cloud technology	[51]
8	Factors influencing health data sharing	2017	Healthcare	[14]
9	A Trustworthy system for patient sensitive information	2018	Healthcare	[8]
10	The effect of doctor-consumer interaction	2018	Social media, health	[52]
11	A model for wearable IoT device using intention in workplace	2018	IoT	[18]
12	Trustworthiness of medical devices	2014	Medical devices	[53]
13	Data trustworthiness in the internet of things	2018	IoT	[41]
14	Factors influencing adoption of CGMs device	2021	IoT healthcare device	[10]

The above table shows information regarding trust as a construct. In these 14 articles, we found trust as a strong construct for users' intention to use a device. Unfortunately, none of the papers discussed wearable healthcare device adoption specifically on blood glucose monitoring systems for smart healthcare. Along with this, it is essential to explore users' intention to adopt wearable blood glucose devices in smart healthcare.

6 Trustworthiness in Blood Glucose Monitoring

As stated in the previous studies, many publications addressed the various types of wearable devices in smart healthcare; but none can be found on the trustworthiness factor in blood glucose monitoring. Based on the reviewed papers, it is noticeable that trustworthiness is an important factor to influence users' intention to adopt healthcare-related devices. In a smart IoT healthcare system, it is crucial to have or maintain reliable and accurate data since all the systems work through sensors so that users can trust the wearable devices better. By the previous studies on different sectors like intention to have wearable device for fitness tracker authors also mentioned about the security and privacy issue which indicate trustworthiness to have a wearable device in blood glucose monitoring [10].

Most of the previous papers discussed smart fitness trackers and some factors for the adoption of wearable technologies. Trustworthiness can also be a major factor for sensing the glucose level devices as well as the adoption of the smart devices. Testing own blood glucose manually with devices is now an old trend like it had been for more than 50 years. Most recently continuous glucose monitoring is a new term that is now quite popular for diabetic patients [54]. To an extent that, the importance of trustworthiness is visibly highlighted in the related perspective. Thus it is relevant to see the impact of trustworthiness in measuring the user's intention to adopt IoT wearable healthcare devices.

7 Research Questions Outcomes

RQ1. What are the factors influencing the adoption of wearable devices in smart healthcare?

In Sect. 2.2 and Table 2, it is shown that several factors influence the user's intention to adopt wearable devices. In there, seven studies directly addressed some factors in the context of the smart healthcare sector where personal innovativeness, self-efficacy, interpersonal influence, health concern, privacy concern, attitude toward using wearable devices show significant influence on user's adoption intention to use wearable smart healthcare devices.

RQ2. What are the limitations and gaps in the current research of wearable devices in smart healthcare?

To continue this paper, we had gone through many articles where only 7 articles mentioned smart healthcare adoption intention, barriers of adoption. Most of the studies discussed only fitness trackers and automated devices that are wearable. As CGMs device is wearable and a smart solution for blood glucose monitoring, some researches can be done to give a proper recommendation to the user to adopt smart healthcare-related devices.

RQ3. How trustworthiness can influence the adoption of smart healthcare devices?

As mentioned in Table 3, trust is a significant construct to measure users' intention to adopt smart healthcare devices. In there, 14 studies mentioned trust-based model for adoption where only one study directly talked about the significance of trust to adopt smart healthcare devices. If the data from the wearable device is reliable and confirmed with experts, then users feel safe to use healthcare devices. Trustworthiness is a very sensitive term as the device is used for disease management and is also related to patient's health safety.

8 Discussion

This study delivers an overview of wearable healthcare devices. To answer the research questions, here authors have identified several factors for the adoption of wearable devices where trust was less highlighted compared to the other constructs. To adopt smart healthcare wearable devices, users should focus on some factors that have been discussed and decide the most decisive factors among all of them. As in IoT smart healthcare devices, all system works through the sensor to sensor communication, so it needs to assure the end-user about the trustworthiness of the data and devices accurately to the end-user who will use the system. It is generally accepted in consumer behavior research that source trustworthiness in health information is an important factor, and associated with belief [2].

Trust in caregivers and technology vendors may be the critical factors that disturb the users' adoption of healthcare information technology [34]. As blood glucose monitoring is a sensitive issue, it is very important to make sure of the data accuracy on a real-time basis to create user's satisfaction on trustworthiness. To adopt wearable devices for blood glucose monitoring, some factors may influence the users. Among all the aforementioned factors, trustworthiness plays a vital role in users' intention to adopt wearable devices for smart healthcare and blood glucose monitoring. A study on testing the relationship of trustworthiness through IoT device adoption should be conducted [55].

To identify the research gap, this study presents an overview of wearable device definition (Table 1). Furthermore, this study addresses also the existing factors of wearable device adoption including wearable fitness trackers, cloud technology. In a few papers, the authors mentioned the overview and benefits of using wearable CGMs devices where those studies did not describe anything clearly about the adoption factors for blood glucose monitoring devices. Here, the authors raise the issue of those points and also gave a preview of the existing articles providing directions for further researches on wearable CGMs devices that can be useful for the service providers of those devices and also the users as well.

9 Conclusion

In conclusion, by reviewing the previous studies on wearable devices, smart healthcare, blood glucose monitoring, and adoption model, we consider this effort could be valuable for the end-user of the smart healthcare wearable devices especially for the diabetic patients while service giver can find out the complete model for blood glucose monitoring device adoption. Trustworthiness can also be a smart solution to make the user's intention to adopt a wearable device easily.

As wearable device adoption in IoT healthcare is a new term so the finding shows that the factors for adoption of the devices will help the users as well as the service providers to help patients in many ways. By referring to this study, service providers of the smart healthcare systems can also get a proper initial idea on which of the factors could attract more users to adopt a wearable device for blood glucose monitoring. After examining the previous studies, it will be easier to find out the way to have a smart healthcare device for measuring blood glucose because wearable devices for fitness tracking apply the same concept as blood glucose monitoring devices.

References

1. Fotiadis, D.I., Glaros, C., Likas, A.: Wearable medical devices. Wiley Encycl. Biomed. Eng. (2006)
2. Kim, S., Kim, S.: User preference for an IoT healthcare application for lifestyle disease management. Telecomm. Policy **42**(4), 304–314 (2018)
3. Casselman, J., Onopa, N., Khansa, L.: Wearable healthcare: lessons from the past and a peek into the future. Telemat. Inform. **34**(7), 1011–1023 (2017)
4. Mahdavinejad, M.S., Rezvan, M., Barekatain, M., Adibi, P., Barnaghi, P., Sheth, A.P.: Machine learning for internet of things data analysis: a survey. Digit. Commun. Netw. **4**(3), 161–175 (2018)
5. Hsiao, K.L., Chen, C.C.: What drives smartwatch purchase intention? Perspectives from hardware, software, design, and value. Telemat. Inform. **35**(1), 103–113 (2018)
6. Aslani, P., et al.: Consumer opinions on adverse events associated with medical devices. Res. Soc. Adm. Pharm. **15**(5), 568–574 (2019)
7. Yang, H., Yu, J., Zo, H., Choi, M.: User acceptance of wearable devices: an extended perspective of perceived value. Telemat. Inform. **33**(2), 256–269 (2016)
8. Yachana, N.K., Sood, S.K.: A trustworthy system for secure access to patient centric sensitive information. Telemat. Inform. **35**(4), 790–800 (2018)
9. Buenaflor, C., Kim, H.C.: Six human factors to acceptability of wearable computers. Int. J. Multimed. Ubiquitous Eng. **8**(3), 103–114 (2013)
10. Hossain, M.I., Yusof, A.F., Hussin, A.R.C., lahad, N.A., Sadiq, A.S.: Factors influencing adoption model of continuous glucose monitoring devices for internet of things healthcare. Internet Things **15**, 100353 (2021)
11. Lin, D., Lee, C.K.M., Tai, W.C.: Application of interpretive structural modelling for analyzing the factors of IoT adoption on supply chains in the Chinese agricultural industry. In: IEEE International Conference on Industrial Engineering and Engineering Management, vol. 2017-Decem, pp. 1347–1351 (2018)
12. Gajanayake, R., Iannella, R., Sahama, T.: An insight into the adoption of Accountable-eHealth systems – an empirical research model based on the Australian context. IRBM **37**(4), 219–231 (2016)
13. Lee, S.Y.: Examining the factors that influence early adopters' smartphone adoption: the case of college students. Telemat. Inform. **31**(2), 308–318 (2014)
14. Moon, L.A.: Factors influencing health data sharing preferences of consumers: a critical review. Heal. Policy Technol. **6**(2), 169–187 (2017)
15. Haque, M.M., Ahlan, A.R., Mohamed Razi, M.J.: Factors affecting knowledge sharing on innovation in the higher education institutions (HEis). ARPN J. Eng. Appl. Sci. **10**(23), 18200–18210 (2015)
16. Gücin, N.Ö., Berk, Ö.S.: Technology acceptance in health care: an integrative review of predictive factors and intervention programs. Procedia Soc. Behav. Sci. **195**, 1698–1704 (2015)
17. Canhoto, A.I., Arp, S.: Exploring the factors that support adoption and sustained use of health and fitness wearables. J. Mark. Manag. **33**(1–2), 32–60 (2017)
18. Yildirim, H., Ali-Eldin, A.M.T.: A model for predicting user intention to use wearable IoT devices at the workplace. J. King Saud Univ. Comput. Inf. Sci. 1–9 (2018)
19. Lunney, A., Cunningham, N.R., Eastin, M.S.: Wearable fitness technology: a structural investigation into acceptance and perceived fitness outcomes. Comput. Human Behav. **65**, 114–120 (2016)
20. Rupp, M.A., Michaelis, J.R., McConnell, D.S., Smither, J.A.: The role of individual differences on perceptions of wearable fitness device trust, usability, and motivational impact. Appl. Ergon. **70**(April 2017), 77–87 (2018)

21. Lee, S.Y., Lee, K.: Factors that influence an individual's intention to adopt a wearable healthcare device: the case of a wearable fitness tracker. Technol. Forecast. Soc. Change **129**(December 2017), 154–163 (2018)
22. Dehghani, M., Kim, K.J., Dangelico, R.M.: Will smartwatches last? Factors contributing to intention to keep using smart wearable technology. Telemat. Inform. **35**(2), 480–490 (2018)
23. Martínez-Caro, E., Cegarra-Navarro, J.G., García-Pérez, A., Fait, M.: Healthcare service evolution towards the internet of things: an end-user perspective. Technol. Forecast. Soc. Change **136**(March), 268–276 (2018)
24. Keikhosrokiani, P., Mustaffa, N., Zakaria, N.: Success factors in developing iHeart as a patient-centric healthcare system: a multi-group analysis. Telemat. Inform. **35**(4), 753–775 (2018)
25. Dehghani, M., Joon, K., Maria, R.: Telematics and informatics will smartwatches last? Factors contributing to intention to keep using smart wearable technology. Telemat. Inform. **35**(2), 480–490 (2020)
26. Chuah, S.H.W., Rauschnabel, P.A., Krey, N., Nguyen, B., Ramayah, T., Lade, S.: Wearable technologies: the role of usefulness and visibility in smartwatch adoption. Comput. Human Behav. **65**, 276–284 (2016)
27. Marakhimov, A., Joo, J.: Consumer adaptation and infusion of wearable devices for healthcare. Comput. Human Behav. **76**, 135–148 (2017)
28. Hatz, M.H.M., Sonnenschein, T., Blankart, C.R.: The PMA scale: a measure of physicians' motivation to adopt medical devices. Value Heal. **20**(4), 533–541 (2017)
29. Li, J., Zhang, C., Li, X., Zhang, C.: Patients' emotional bonding with MHealth apps: an attachment perspective on patients' use of MHealth applications. Int. J. Inf. Manag. (March), 102054 (2019)
30. Nasir, S., Yurder, Y.: Consumers' and physicians' perceptions about high tech wearable health products. Procedia Soc. Behav. Sci. **195**, 1261–1267 (2015)
31. Anwar, M., Joshi, J., Tan, J.: Anytime, anywhere access to secure, privacy-aware healthcare services: Issues, approaches and challenges. Heal. Policy Technol. **4**(4), 299–311 (2015)
32. Wu, T., Deng, Z., Zhang, D., Buchanan, P.R., Zha, D., Wang, R.: International journal of medical informatics seeking and using intention of health information from doctors in social media : the effect of doctor-consumer interaction. Int. J. Med. Inform. **115**(April), 106–113 (2018)
33. Yee-Loong Chong, A., Liu, M.J., Luo, J., Keng-Boon, O.: Predicting RFID adoption in healthcare supply chain from the perspectives of users. Int. J. Prod. Econ. **159**, 66–75 (2015)
34. Holden, R.J., Karsh, B.-T.: The technology acceptance model: its past and its future in health care. J. Biomed. Inform. **43**(1), 159–172 (2010)
35. Asrar-ul-Haq, M., Anwar, S.: A systematic review of knowledge management and knowledge sharing: trends, issues, and challenges. Cogent Bus. Manag. **3**(1), 1–17 (2016)
36. Gubbi, J., Buyya, R., Marusic, S., Palaniswami, M.: Internet of things (IoT): a vision, architectural elements, and future directions. Futur. Gener. Comput. Syst. **29**(7), 1645–1660 (2013)
37. Jebaseeli, T.J., Durai, C.A.D., Peter, J.D.: IOT based sustainable diabetic retinopathy diagnosis system. Sustain. Comput. Inform. Syst. (2018). Elsevier Inc.
38. Byrne, J.R., O'Sullivan, K., Sullivan, K.: An IoT and wearable technology Hackathon for promoting careers in computer science. IEEE Trans. Educ. **60**(1), 50–58 (2017)
39. Ahmad, N.A., Drus, S.M., Kasim, H., Othman, M.M.: Assessing content validity of enterprise architecture adoption questionnaire (EAAQ) among content experts. In: 2019 IEEE 9th Symposium on Computer Applications and Industrial Electronics, pp. 160–165 (2019)
40. Balapour, A., Reychav, I., Sabherwal, R., Azuri, J.: Mobile technology identity and self-efficacy: implications for the adoption of clinically supported mobile health apps. Int. J. Inf. Manag. **49**(October 2018), 58–68 (2019)

41. Haron, N., Jaafar, J., Aziz, I.A., Hassan, M.H., Shapiai, M.I.: Data trustworthiness in internet of things: a taxonomy and future directions. In: 2017 IEEE Conference on Big Data Analysis, ICBDA 2017, vol. 2018-Janua, pp. 25–30 (2018)
42. Hennemann, S., Beutel, M.E., Zwerenz, R.: Ready for eHealth? Health professionals' acceptance and adoption of eHealth interventions in inpatient routine care. J. Health Commun. **22**(3), 274–284 (2017)
43. Lassar, W.M., Manolis, C., Lassar, S.S.: The relationship between consumer innovativeness, personal characteristics, and online banking adoption, 23(2) (2005)
44. Ayeh, J.K., Au, N., Law, R.: Predicting the intention to use consumer-generated media for travel planning. Tour. Manag. **35**, 132–143 (2013)
45. Zhang, T., Tao, D., Qu, X., Zhang, X., Lin, R., Zhang, W.: The roles of initial trust and perceived risk in public's acceptance of automated vehicles. Transp. Res. Part C Emerg. Technol. **98**(June 2018), 207–220 (2019)
46. Konuk, F.A.: The role of store image, perceived quality, trust and perceived value in predicting consumers' purchase intentions towards organic private label food. J. Retail. Consum. Serv. **43**(March), 304–310 (2018)
47. Liu, X., Li, Q., Lai, I.K.W.: A trust model for the adoption of cloud-based supply chain management systems: a conceptual framework. In: ICEMSI 2013 - 2013 International Conference on Engineering, Management Science and Innovation, pp. 1–4 (2013)
48. Rupp, M.A., Michaelis, J.R., McConnell, D.S., Smither, J.A.: The role of individual differences on perceptions of wearable fitness device trust, usability, and motivational impact. Appl. Ergon. **70**, 77–87 (2018)
49. Hong, I.B.: Understanding the consumer's online merchant selection process: the roles of product involvement, perceived risk, and trust expectation. Int. J. Inf. Manag. **35**(3), 322–336 (2015)
50. Wright, E.B., Holcombe, C., Salmon, P.: Doctors' communication of trust, care, and respect in breast cancer: qualitative study. Br. Med. J. **328**(7444), 864–867 (2004)
51. Ho, S.M., Ocasio-Velázquez, M., Booth, C.: Trust or consequences? Causal effects of perceived risk and subjective norms on cloud technology adoption. Comput. Secur. **70**, 581–595 (2017)
52. Wu, T., Deng, Z., Zhang, D., Buchanan, P.R., Zha, D., Wang, R.: Seeking and using intention of health information from doctors in social media: the effect of doctor-consumer interaction. Int. J. Med. Inform. **115**(April), 106–113 (2018)
53. Zhang, B.M., Raghunathan, A., Jha, N.K.: Trustworthiness of medical devices and body area networks, **102**(8) (2014)
54. Olczuk, D., Priefer, R.: A history of continuous glucose monitors (CGMs) in self-monitoring of diabetes mellitus. Diabetes Metab. Syndr. Clin. Res. Rev. **12**(2), 181–187 (2018)
55. Hossain, M.I., Yusof, A.F., Hussin, A.R.C., Billah, M., Shanmugam, M.: The content and construct development of CGMs device adoption model. In: Siconian 2019, vol. 172 (2020)

Factors Contributing to an Effective E- Government Adoption in Palestine

Tareq Obaid[1(✉)], Bilal Eneizan[2], Samy S. Abu Naser[1], Ghaith Alsheikh[3], Ahmed Ali Atieh Ali[4], Hussein Mohammed Esmail Abualrejal[4], and Nadhmi A. Gazem[5]

[1] Faculty of Engineering and IT, Alazhar University, Gaza, Palestine
tareq.obaid@alazhar.edu.ps
[2] Business School, Jadara University, Irbid, Jordan
[3] Human Resources Department, Faculty of Business, Amman Arab University, Amman, Jordan
[4] School of Technology Management and Logistic, College of Business, Universiti Utara Malaysia, 06010 Sintok, Kedah, Malaysia
abualrejal@uum.edu.my
[5] Management Information Systems Department, College of Business Administration-Yanbu, Taibah University, Medina, Saudi Arabia

Abstract. Despite the fact that the success of e-government adoption is dependent on individuals' willingness to utilize it, little attention has been paid to citizens' perspectives on e-government adoption. However, it appears that worldwide e-Government adoption has fallen short of predictions, but some countries are performing better than others. As a result, it is critical to improve residents' understanding of the reasons for and techniques of using government websites, as well as their attitudes about e-Government. This article addresses the issue by proposing a conceptual model for e-Government adoption that emphasizes the role of users in the implementation of e-Government. By adapting and tailoring the measurement scale from prior studies, the questionnaire approach was used to collect data. On 250 prospective respondents, a systematic convenience sampling approach was used. The finding of this study technical, personal, and dependability factors influence the intention to use e-Government, they have a significant impact on the actual adoption of e-Government services in Palestine. The government should develop a comprehensive e-government planning model based on demographic factors.

Keywords: Intention to use · Perceived-E readiness · e-Government · Adoption · Palestine

1 Introduction

The electronic government or e-Government employs information and communication technology (ICT) to successfully deliver government services and information to residents, other government organisations, and businesses (Rose et al. 2015). It is clear

F. Saeed et al. (Eds.): IRICT 2021, LNDECT 127, pp. 663–676, 2022.
https://doi.org/10.1007/978-3-030-98741-1_55

that the traditional public service provided through the new ICT systems or the addition of new online service delivery channel is not the main focus of e-Government, but it emphasizes on strengthening the transparency, governance, and accountability of the public sector services for the improvement in government effectiveness and development of new public value for businesses and residents (Wang 2014). Higher public involvement in e-Government facilities is important to fulfil these goals.

Although the efforts made in this domain are present, the low rate of adoption via the residents is a significant concern to the governments worldwide (Rana and Dwivedi 2015). Therefore, research attention is essential on this matter as effective employment of e-Government is greatly affected by the residents as well as the employment of such services (Panagiotopoulos et al. 2012). This situation illustrates that grasping the multi-faceted elements impacting the citizens' adoption of e-Government services is important. Despite the fact that an extensive research of technology adoption from the user's perspective has been conducted, in the e-commerce and Internet contexts (Al-Debei and Al-Lozi 2014), The number of studies on residents' adoption of e-Government services is limited. (Beldad et al. 2011).

In comparison to the critical adoption and implementation of a wide range of information technology in private businesses, the residents' adoption of e-Government services frequently takes place in unstable socio-political environments, including the changing budget reduction and political leadership. In this scenario, the adoption of e-government facilities should not be studied solely from a technological point of view, but a thorough and integrative method, which incorporates the cultural, political, and social views is required to obtain further knowledge in this subject (Carter et al. 2011). Notably, the lack of concrete comprehension of the elements of the residents' adoption of its services would disrupt the government from making informed strategic decisions for the improvement in e-Government adoption (Carter et al. 2011).

The previous investigation on the adoption of e-government primarily emphasised on the developed nations. As a result, there was a minor focus on the investigation on the adoption of e-government in developing nations, specifically the Arab nations. This is a large research problem due to the notable difference between these nations and the Western nations in the aspects of the social and cultural features (Olasina and Mutula 2015). Therefore, it could be predicted that the essential elements impacting people's acquirement of technologies in Arab nations might be different from the elements associated with the industrialised Western nations, including the nations from North America and Western Europe (Al-Gahtani 2004).

Palestine is among the nations in the Middle East, which has been dedicated to ICT-related actions and quality governance. It was illustrated in the recent literature that Palestine has exhibited a positive degree of electronic transformation in the aspect of political determination although the application of e-government in this nation is still in its infancy. However, some challenges are present in the e-Government implementation, which mainly include geopolitical phenomenon, inadequate legislation, decision-making processes, low consciousness and preparedness of residents to accept the recent digital evolution towards the true digital government, and policies (Shat et al. 2013).

A low degree of cooperation for e-Government actions is present among the ministries due to anxiety and trust issues regarding data control with other national organisations and ministries (Abu-Jaber 2011). As a result, the government ministries are confronted by the obstacles to the distribution of electronic information and insufficient safety of service for the users. This phenomenon distorts the users' reliance on the government's capability of employing e-government and ultimate results in ineffective e-Government actions (Ayyash et al. 2013).

The application of e-Government in Palestine possibly develops solutions to the issues about communication with government institutions and access to government services. Taking the notable distribution of the Palestine residents and Israel domination over the area into account, the development and implementation of an authentic electronic Government possibly results in the capability of the government to fulfil its role and perform the electronic distribution of public services to the Palestine residents and other stakeholders. Besides, the residents will be capable of performing two-way communication with the government. Notably, effective e-Government services in Palestine would enhance the efficacy of the Palestinian authority's potential in providing support for public institutions and catering to individuals and corporations. Accordingly, improving the comprehension of the elements impacting the residents' adoption is highly crucial. It would facilitate the policymakers in designing the service and assist the public institutions in delivering it to strengthen the service adoption among the residents.

2 Literature Review

The application of electronic Government involves the users' attempt for interaction and engagement with e-Government systems (Rana et al. 2015). It could also be identified as the users' preparedness to employ e-Government facilities and systems (Carter et al. 2016). During the previous years, the adoption of e-Government among the residents brought increasing attention among scholars. It was highlighted by (Kumar et al. 2007) that attempt and preparedness to use these systems indicate a dimension of the measurement of e-Government adoption, which does not only involve the use of electronic services and systems, but it also considers the frequency of the users' attempt of using and accepting the systems, what impacts their point of view, experiences and predictions, the elements influencing the adoption, and how this adoption and preparedness of using the systems could be adjusted (Athmay et al. 2016; Enas et al. 2019). Furthermore, users' predictions and needs are emphasised in this adoption to make a contribution to their attempt of using electronic government services. Moreover, a speech by the prime minister of the United Kingdom addressed the transformational government and emphasised that technology is essential to make a better decision regarding the public sector services for citizens (King and Cotterill 2007). It was also stressed that these services should be based on what is needed by the users instead of the suppliers (Linders et al. 2018).

Low adoption rate may result in an ineffective e-Government system. It was highlighted by (Anthopoulos et al. 2016; Nofal et al. 2021) that that ineffective adoption of the e-Government projects remains and may go from an incomplete to a total failure. It was also claimed that this failure would occur when the actual business needs, users' expectations, and preparedness for adoption and implementation are not fulfilled. Moreover, (Janssen and Estevez 2013) emphasised that various high transformation projects, such as e-Government, do not lead to the targeted project results when they are not adopted by the stakeholders. The ineffective e-Government project was classified into two types by (Anthopoulos et al. 2016), namely pre- or post-execution, and failed execution. Specifically, the first failure involved either the neglect of the project upon the implementation stage, which lead to total failure.

In a study by (Huang et al. 2013), the UTAUT was combined with dependence on citizens' conduct in the adoption and distribution of e-Government in Greece. It was found that effort and performance prediction, reliance on the government and the internet, and social impact are the elements influencing the user's attempt. As for the e-Government use, it was indicated from the analysis that 'facilitating conditions' was a notable indicator of the e-Government use (Rokhman 2011). The Diffusion of Innovation and perceived characteristics of innovating theories were used to examine e-Government adoption among Indonesian residents. In this research, four features were investigated, namely image, relative advantage, image, efficient use, and compatibility on the attempt of using e-Government services. It was noted from the results that the comparative advantages and compatibility had a notable impact on the attempt to employ e-Government facilities. It was also revealed that efficient use and image were not the ideal determinants of the attempts to employ the e-government facilities, and this result was consistent with the findings of a number of earlier investigations. (Belanger et al. 2005). Furthermore, Al Hujran et al. (2013) combined the Technology Acceptance Model constructs with new constructs, including reliability, service quality, and residents' satisfaction to develop a model of elements impacting the residents' employment of e-Government facilities in Jordan. It was found that residents' satisfaction, PEOU, PU, and reliability were the notable determinants of usage intention, which constituted 54.6% of the variation of the residents' attempt to using e-Government facilities. It was also demonstrated that the residents' attempt to use e-Government services was primarily impacted by the users' satisfaction. In a study by Azam et al. (2013), a combination of the model was created using UTAUT and initial reliance, while the elements proving the adoption of e-Government facilities in Pakistan were outlined. The analysis illustrated that performance prediction, social impact, and initial reliance positively affected the behavioural attempt of using e-Government services. A current study by Alomari (2014) examined the effect of word of mouth (WOM), avoidance to development, and favoritism on e-Government adoption in Jordan. This study emphasised that taking the cooperation of the Jordanian population into account was crucial when the elements influencing the e-Government adoption were examined.

Despite the existence of important literature on the factors influencing citizens' adoption in various developing and developed countries, few works of research highlighted the adoption of e-Government facilities in Palestine.

3 Conceptual Model

In analysing the e-Government adoption, a model was formulated. It was also among the main contributions of this study, which would be applied for the investigation and analysis of the elements with a considerable influence on various adoption and degrees of e-Government adoption among the users. Furthermore, the formulation of the model was according to a substantial analysis of the literature regarding the acceptance of technology and the understanding achieved from examining some theories or models. These aspects were normally employed to analyse the use and acceptance to technologies, namely the (UTAUT), the (DOI), the (TAM), and the (TRA) (Dwivedi et al. 2019; Enas et al. 2019; Nofal et al. Nofal et al. 2021). This research aimed to determine, examine, and perform an analysis of the effect of fundamental elements influencing the adoption rate of e-Government from the residents' belief. As a result, improved comprehension would be developed regarding various elements contributing to the strong effectiveness of the systems.

The theory of reasoned action (TRA) is a model, which was properly investigated and shown to effectively elaborate on the intention and actions in diverse domains. It was highlighted by Lean et al. (2009) that TRA was among the theories investigating the individuals' actions towards the acquirement of computers. Davis also highlighted that TRA was suitable in the investigation of the indicators of computer use conduct, and it was employed as the root for the development of the TAM model, which was also commonly applied to gain comprehension on the users' acceptance of technology (Davis 1986; Enas et al. 2019). Furthermore, the TRA was used in some research with a purpose to develop insights about the adoption and acceptance of systems led by the information and communication technologies (ICT), including the acquirement of online systems (Enas et al. 2019; Rehman et al. 2016). Nevertheless, the TRA comprised inadequate constructs, which should be addressed to examine and analyse the adoption of complex and major systems, including the e-Government. The constructs, which are not highlighted, refer to the quality of the system, the impact of consciousness, the simplicity of the information system, and the impact of reliance. Despite the important involvement of two constructs in TRA, namely the subjective norms and attitude towards behaviour, they were not adequate for a thorough comprehension of the adoption of the e-Government systems. It was highlighted by Davis (1986) that the least comprehension revolves around the subjective norm. Furthermore, it is possible for the subjective norm (SN) construct to indirectly affect behavioural intention (BI) through the perception towards behaviour (A) construct. This impact would lead to challenges in distinguishing the direct impact of SN on BI and the indirect impact of SN on BI through A. For this reason, increased comprehension of the model is important for the adoption of the use and e-Government analysis.

The TAM is a model applied in some research in the literature on the employment and acceptance of the technology. This model was used in several studies to examine the employment of e-Government systems (Al Hujran et al. 2013; Nofal et al. Nofal et al. 2021). In a study by Benbasat and Barki (2007), although the adoption and acceptance towards TAM were found to be the most significant in the literature in various areas, such as information systems, business, and management, several factors with a high association with technology adoption and acceptance were omitted. To give an example, this study did not consider the impact of social norms as outlined in the Theory of Reasoned Action (TRA), such as the impact of previous technology adoption, quality standard, and awareness of the attempt to use technology. The relationship between perceived ease of use (PEU), perceived usefulness (PU), and the attempt to employ technology is not entirely explained by one's attitude toward it (Ramayah and Ignatius 2005). TAM, on the other hand, did not conduct a detailed examination into the external factors that were identified as having an impact on PEU and PU (Nofal et al. Nofal et al. 2021; Sang et al. 2009). Additionally, Al-Shafi and Weerakkody (2010) emphasised that TAM omitted several crucial variance resources and other essential elements, which could avoid the users from employing the information systems, including time and financial restrictions.

One of the most recent frameworks in the literature on technology acceptance and use is the Unified Theory of Acceptance and Use of Technology (UTAUT). This framework is also more commonly applied in this area compared to other models and theories. For example, it is involved in the analysis of the use of social media in public-relations practitioners' engagement with the public. Furthermore, Curtis et al. (2010) aimed to investigate the elements influencing the attempt of using the advanced mobile services, while Carlsson et al. (2006) attempted to perform an analysis and gain an understanding of the application of online banking (Martins et al. 2014). The UTAUT was used in various studies for the analysis of the adoption of e-Government services and systems (Weerakkody et al. 2013). Although UTAUT was widely applied in many researches of various disciplines, the limitations of it were present in the analysis of technology adoption, especially in the e-Government area. However, the UTAUT highlights several highly crucial elements and constructs, including identified service standard and consciousness despite the high possibility of these elements to have a strong impact on the attempt of employing and implementing technology. Furthermore, it did not emphasise on the constructs associated with the elements of reliability, including management, reliance, privacy, and security. The UTAUT also did not emphasise on the influence of culture on the employment of technologies. Although UTAUT took the impact of specific personal demographic elements into accounts, including age and gender, the essential demographic elements were not highlighted, such as the user's academic degree and salary, which would possibly affect the adoption rate. It was stated by Huang et al. (2013) that the categorisation of elements in the UTAUT became a concern due to the integration of various disparate elements to form a single construct.

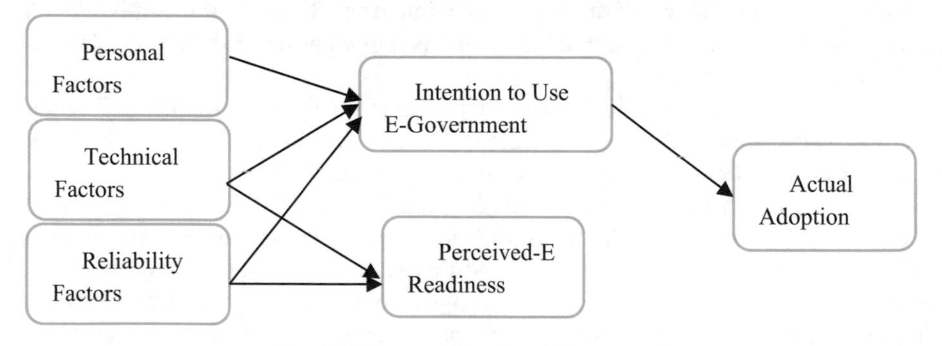

Fig. 1. Conceptual model of the research

Figure 1 illustrates the e-Government adoption model. The independent elements positioned on the left part of the model are personal factors (PF), technical factors (TF) and reliability factors (RF), which indicate the factor groupings.

Personnel factors (PF) is a crucial element in the model. It was indicated from the research that users' gender, academic level, age, salary, income, and computer literacy degree are the elements to be examined when the e-Government adoption is analysed. However, these elements were not considered by the majority of the previous adoption models, including TAM and DOI models, while several models, such as UTAUT, identified these elements as moderators instead of the primary factors. However, it was added by several works of research in the e-Government adoption literature that users' characteristics might be the significant elements influencing the employment of e-Government. To illustrate, it was proposed by Sciadas (2002) that older users often had a positive correlation with e-Government as more access was available to technology. However, this phenomenon did not remain in the current years nor represent the phenomenon in Palestine, which was the setting of this research. Overall, this situation indicated the importance of including personal factors when the technology implementation was performed in e-Government. The Personal Factors (PF) in the model of this study consisted of four primary elements, namely users' gender, age, location, and academic level.

Technical Factors (TF) is another crucial element in the model. Technical elements are present in any interactive information system, which should be highlighted to gain the results from the application of the systems. E-Government is among the information systems, in which more emphasis should be placed on the technical aspect due to the high number of users. There is a high possibility for the implementation degree of these users to be influenced by the technical problems of the systems.

4 Research Method

The data for this study was collected using a self-administered questionnaire, which took a quantitative approach. A thorough literature research was conducted in order to identify items that would be used to assess the actual adoption and intent to use the e-government construct. The research methodology involved e-government users. The items were adapted and modified to suit this study. Several items have been modified in order to suit the needs of the research. The 5 Likert-scale ranging from 1 (strongly disagree) to 5 (strongly agree) with the statement were used to measures the responses. A convenience sample of 250 e-government users from the West Bank and Gaza Strip was chosen for data collection and given the self-administered questionnaire.

5 Data Analysis

We used partial least squares (PLS) modeling using the SmartPLS 3.3.2 version. The study employed a two stages approached in testing the hypothesis of the study. The first stage consist of measurement model, which consist of the convergent and discriminant validity. Once the validities has been confirm, the study will proceed to the hypothesis testing, or the structural model.

The first is convergent validity, which determines if a given item measures the latent variable it claims to measure (Hair et al. 2017) (Fig. 2).

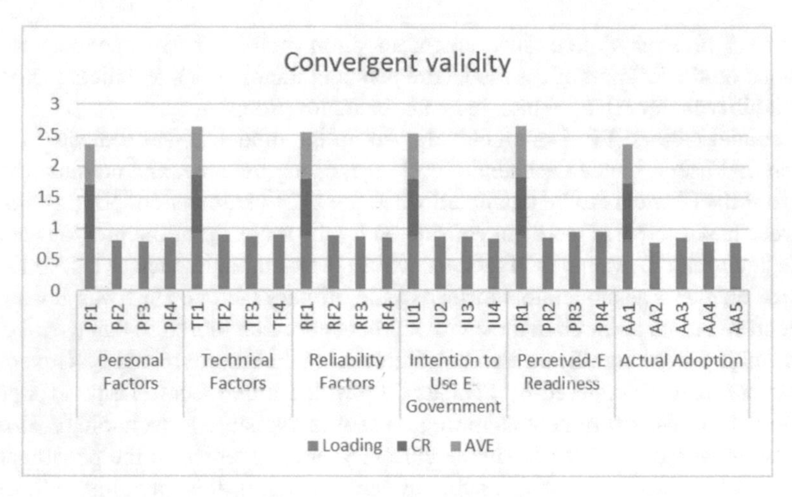

Fig. 2. Convergent validity

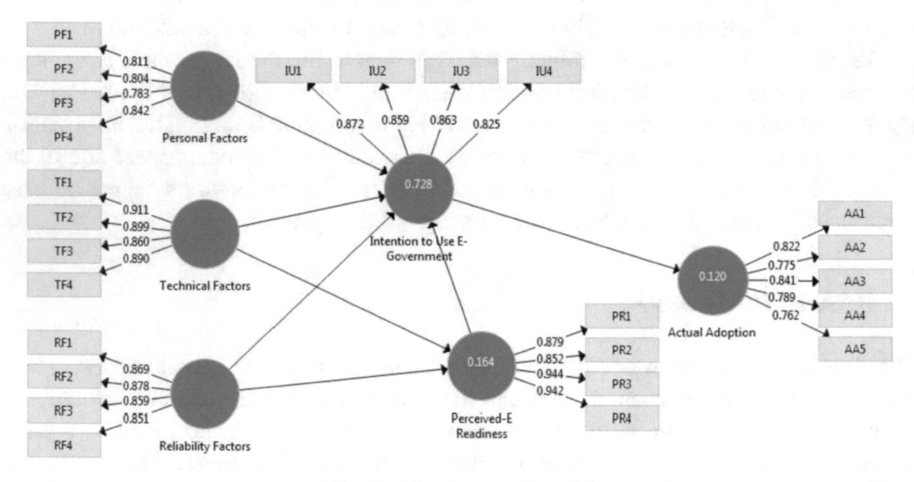

Fig. 3. Measurement model

According to (Fornell and Larcker 1981), the square root of AVE for each construct should be bigger than the correlation coefficient of the constructs included in the model, as shown in Fig. 3. This requirement has been met, as indicated in Fig. 3.

5.1 Structural Model

To produce t-values bootstrapping was also performed, Fig. 4 illustrates the outcomes of the hypotheses examining of direct relationships. The results of the study indicated that personal factors, Reliability Factors and Technical Factors effect positively and significantly on Intention to Use E-Government and Perceived-E Readiness. Perceived-E

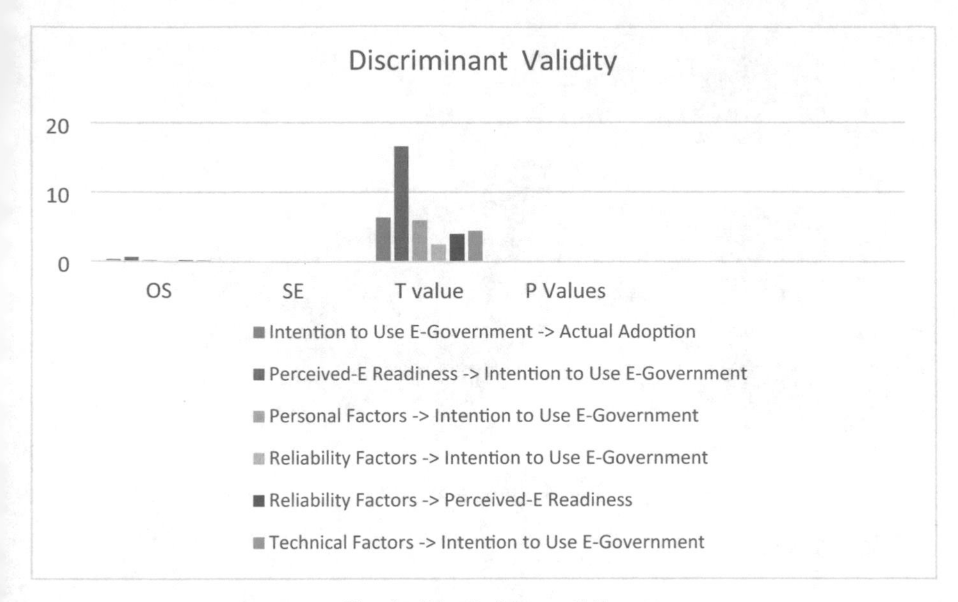

Fig. 4. Discriminant validity

Readiness effect positively and significantly on Intention to Use E-Government. Intention to Use E-Government effect positively and significantly on Actual Adoption (Figs. 5 and 6).

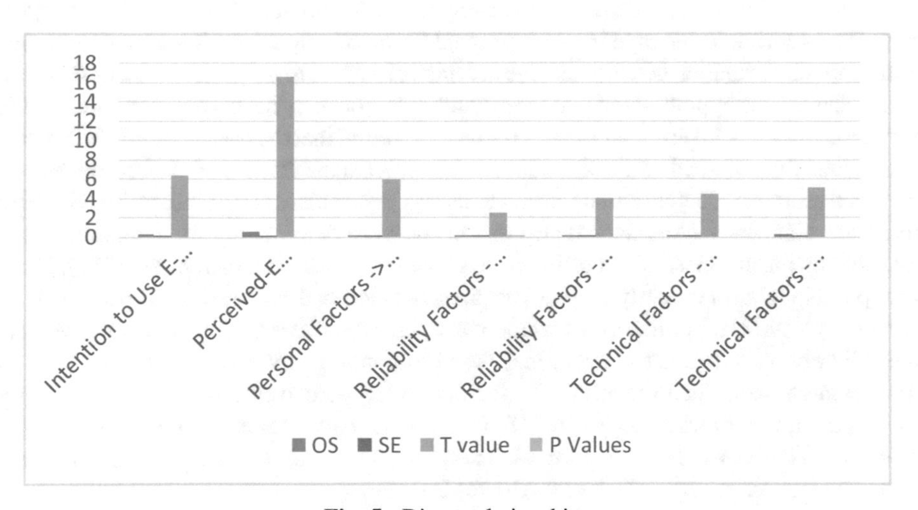

Fig. 5. Direct relationships

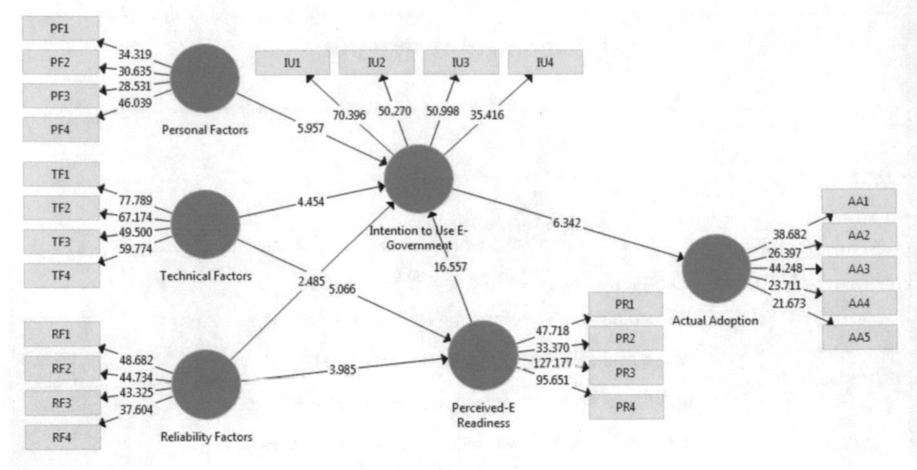

Fig. 6. Structural model

6 Discussion

In this study personal factors has been identified to have positive influence on intention to use e-Government in Palestine. The hypothesized association was determined to be statistically significant at 95% confidence interval ($\beta = 0.215$, t-value = 5.957, p-values = 0.000) significance at $p < 0.01$, indicating support for H1. This result is consistent with previous studies the examined intention to use e-Government (Mensah et al. 2017). Personal Factors must believe that the government has the management and technical resources needed to put these mechanisms in place and secure them. Citizens must have the intention to "engage in e-government," which includes the intentions to receive and supply information through on-line channels, in order to use e-government services. Also; The H2 has hypothesized that the reliability factors may have a positive effect on the intention to use e-Government in Palestine. It was found that the p-value was 0.013 which is less than the assumed value of 0.05 level. Thus, it can be concluded that the difference between reliability factors and intention to use e-Government is significant. This implies that the reliability factors does really matter much in determining the intention to use e-Government in Palestine according to (Ayyash et al. 2013; Obaid et al. 2020), For a few participants, the quality of e-government service had no bearing on people' trust since they would not utilize e-government service even if the quality was great because they did not trust internet systems in general to conduct any financial transactions. In this research, examined the reliability factors on the perceived e-readiness. According to the result, the direct effect β is 0.218, whereas the (p-values = 0.000) significance at $p < 0.01$. Hence, the H3 is supported. Therefore, the result of this study is consistent with several recent studies (Ali and Alrayes 2014).

7 Conclusion

The crucial elements impacting the users' attempt of using the system in Palestine were determined in this study, and a model was formed as a remarkable instrument, which facilitated the employment of e-Government in developing nations. The novelty of this study would lead to knowledge representation, while the research suggestions would be important for researchers and decision/policymakers who have the willingness for changes.

It was also believed that this study could be the basis of future research on the residents' employment of e-Government services in Palestine. Therefore, e-Government institutions would be presented with the information associated with the elements affecting the users' employment of e-Government facilities in Palestine. Subsequently, the government would be capable of focusing on every element and make developments. The primary role of researchers is to determine the main aspects, which would assist the policymakers from the e-Government authority in identifying the benefits of e-Government in future actions by the government. This study would also assist future studies in enhancing the implementation of e-Government.

8 Limitations and Future Studies

This research has formulated an integrated model to create a systematic method of understanding the implementation of e-Government services among users.

Future studies are recommended for the actual application of e-Government services rather than the dependent elements to evaluate e-Government employment (Shih and Venkatesh 2004). The effectiveness of the findings could be enhanced with the use of an observed variable rather than a construct for an online system measurement.

This study was performed according to some elements formulated from previous literature for the measurement of e-Government facilities in Palestine. However, an analysis of similar topics could be performed in future studies through the expansion of the research model and the incorporation of more elements. To illustrate, the identified risk is among the elements, which could be incorporated in future studies due to its notable impact on online purchase attempt (Featherman and Pavlou 2003). The factor of compatibility could also be taken into account as the extent to which a transformation is regarded to be in line with the current values, previous experience, and the possible adopters' needs. Additionally, the increasing use of the target technology by the users enhanced the suitability of the technology with the change, which impacted the compound responses via PU and EOU.

It was believed that these research findings would assist Palestine and other nations with the same features across the primary elements in the e-Government implementation. Accordingly, comparative research could be performed to make a comparison between the results of this research and those from other developing nations, particularly the nations with a similar vision as the Palestinian government. Through similar research in other nations, particularly the nations with similar features with Palestine, a comparison might take place between this study and other studies in terms of results, followed by their affirmation or extension.

References

Abu-Jaber, N.O.Y.: Strategic analysis and development of electronic government strategies for the palestinian municipalities (2011)

Al-Debei, M.M., Al-Lozi, E.: Explaining and predicting the adoption intention of mobile data services: a value-based approach. Comput. Hum. Behav. **35**, 326–338 (2014)

Al-Gahtani, S.S.: Computer technology acceptance success factors in Saudi Arabia: an exploratory study. J. Glob. Inf. Technol. Manag. **7**(1), 5–29 (2004)

Al-Shafi, S., Weerakkody, V.: Factors affecting e-government adoption in the state of Qatar (2010)

Al Hujran, O., Aloudat, A., Altarawneh, I.: Factors influencing citizen adoption of e-government in developing countries: the case of Jordan. Int. J. Technol. Hum. Interact. (IJTHI) **9**(2), 1–19 (2013)

Ali, H., Alrayes, A.: An empirical investigation of the effect of e-readiness factors on adoption of e-procurement in kingdom of Bahrain. Int. J. Bus. Manag. **9**(12), 220 (2014)

Alomari, M.K.: Discovering citizens reaction toward e-government: factors in e-government adoption. JISTEM-J. Inf. Syst. Technol. Manag. **11**(1), 5–20 (2014)

Anthopoulos, L., Reddick, C.G., Giannakidou, I., Mavridis, N.: Why e-government projects fail? An analysis of the Healthcare .gov website. Gov. Inf. Q. **33**(1), 161–173 (2016)

Athmay, A.A.A.A., Fantazy, K., Kumar, V.: E-government adoption and user's satisfaction: an empirical investigation. EuroMed J. Bus. (2016)

Ayyash, M.M., Ahmad, K., Singh, D.: Investigating the effect of information systems factors on trust in e-government initiative adoption in Palestinian public sector. Res. J. Appl. Sci. Eng. Technol. **5**(15), 3865–3875 (2013)

Azam, A., Qiang, F., Abdullah, M.I.: Determinants of e-government services adoption in Pakistan: an integrated model. Electron. Gov. Int. J. **10**(2), 105–124 (2013)

Belanger, F., Carter, L.D., Schaupp, L.C.: U-government: a framework for the evolution of e-government. Electron. Gov. Int. J. **2**(4), 426–445 (2005)

Beldad, A., De Jong, M., Steehouder, M.: I trust not therefore it must be risky: determinants of the perceived risks of disclosing personal data for e-government transactions. Comput. Hum. Behav. **27**(6), 2233–2242 (2011)

Benbasat, I., Barki, H.: Quo vadis TAM? J. Assoc. Inf. Syst. **8**, 7 (2007)

Carlsson, C., Carlsson, J., Hyvonen, K., Puhakainen, J., Walden, P.: Adoption of mobile devices/services-searching for answers with the UTAUT. Paper presented at the Proceedings of the 39th Annual Hawaii International Conference on System Sciences (HICSS 2006) (2006)

Carter, L., Shaupp, L.C., Hobbs, J., Campbell, R.: The role of security and trust in the adoption of online tax filing. Transform. Gov. People Process Policy (2011)

Carter, L., Weerakkody, V., Phillips, B., Dwivedi, Y.K.: Citizen adoption of e-government services: exploring citizen perceptions of online services in the United States and United Kingdom. Inf. Syst. Manag. **33**(2), 124–140 (2016)

Curtis, L., et al.: Adoption of social media for public relations by nonprofit organizations. Publ. Relat. Rev. **36**(1), 90–92 (2010)

Davis, F.D.: A technology acceptance model for empirically testing new end-user information systems, Cambridge, MA (1986)

Dwivedi, Y.K., Rana, N.P., Jeyaraj, A., Clement, M., Williams, M.D.: Re-examining the unified theory of acceptance and use of technology (UTAUT): towards a revised theoretical model. Inf. Syst. Front. **21**(3), 719–734 (2019)

Enas, A., Ghaith, A., Abdulllah, A.A., Tambi, A.M.b.A.: Review of the impact of service quality and subjective norms in TAM among telecommunication customers in Jordan. Int. J. Ethics Syst. (2019)

Featherman, M.S., Pavlou, P.A.: Predicting e-services adoption: a perceived risk facets perspective. Int. J. Hum. Comput. Stud. **59**(4), 451–474 (2003)

Fornell, C., Larcker, D.F.: Evaluating structural equation models with unobservable variables and measurement error. J. Mark. Res. **18**(1), 39–50 (1981)

Hair, J.F., Hult, G.T.M., Ringle, C.M., Sarstedt, M., Thiele, K.O.: Mirror, mirror on the wall: a comparative evaluation of composite-based structural equation modeling methods. J. Acad. Mark. Sci. **45**(5), 616–632 (2017)
Huang, W.-H.D., Hood, D.W., Yoo, S.J.: Gender divide and acceptance of collaborative Web 2.0 applications for learning in higher education. Internet High. Educ. **16**, 57–65 (2013)
Janssen, M., Estevez, E.: Lean government and platform-based governance—doing more with less. Gov. Inf. Q. **30**, S1–S8 (2013)
King, S., Cotterill, S.: Transformational government? The role of information technology in delivering citizen-centric local public services. Local Gov. Stud. **33**(3), 333–354 (2007)
Kumar, V., Mukerji, B., Butt, I., Persaud, A.: Factors for successful e-government adoption: a conceptual framework. Electron. J. E-Gov. **5**(1) (2007)
Lean, O.K., Zailani, S., Ramayah, T., Fernando, Y.: Factors influencing intention to use e-government services among citizens in Malaysia. Int. J. Inf. Manag. **29**(6), 458–475 (2009)
Linders, D., Liao, C.Z.-P., Wang, C.-M.: Proactive e-governance: flipping the service delivery model from pull to push in Taiwan. Gov. Inf. Q. **35**(4), S68–S76 (2018)
Martins, C., Oliveira, T., Popovič, A.: Understanding the Internet banking adoption: a unified theory of acceptance and use of technology and perceived risk application. Int. J. Inf. Manag. **34**(1), 1–13 (2014)
Mensah, I.K., Jianing, M., Durrani, D.K.: Factors influencing citizens' intention to use e-government services: a case study of South Korean students in China. Int. J. Electron. Gov. Res. (IJEGR) **13**(1), 14–32 (2017)
Nofal, M.I., Al-Adwan, A.S., Yaseen, H., Alsheikh, G.A.A.: Factors for extending e-government adoption in Jordan. Periodicals Eng. Nat. Sci. (PEN) **9**(2), 471–490 (2021)
Obaid, T., Abu Mdallalah, S., Jouda, H., Abu Jarad, A.: Factors for successful e-government adoption in palestine: a conceptual framework. Haitham and Abu Jarad, Ali, factors for successful e-government adoption in Palestine: a conceptual framework, 25 July 2020 (2020)
Olasina, G., Mutula, S.: The influence of national culture on the performance expectancy of e-parliament adoption. Behav. Inf. Technol. **34**(5), 492–505 (2015)
Panagiotopoulos, P., Al-Debei, M.M., Fitzgerald, G., Elliman, T.: A business model perspective for ICTs in public engagement. Gov. Inf. Q. **29**(2), 192–202 (2012)
Ramayah, T., Ignatius, J.: Impact of perceived usefulness, perceived ease of use and perceived enjoyment on intention to shop online. ICFAI J. Syst. Manag. (IJSM) **3**(3), 36–51 (2005)
Rana, N.P., Dwivedi, Y.K.: Citizen's adoption of an e-government system: validating extended social cognitive theory (SCT). Gov. Inf. Q. **32**(2), 172–181 (2015)
Rana, N.P., Dwivedi, Y.K., Williams, M.D.: A meta-analysis of existing research on citizen adoption of e-government. Inf. Syst. Front. **17**(3), 547–563 (2015). https://doi.org/10.1007/s10796-013-9431-z
Rehman, M., Kamal, M.M., Esichaikul, V.: Adoption of e-government services in Pakistan: a comparative study between online and offline users. Inf. Syst. Manag. **33**(3), 248–267 (2016)
Rokhman, A.: e-Government adoption in developing countries; the case of Indonesia. J. Emerg. Trends Comput. Inf. Sci. **2**(5), 228–236 (2011)
Rose, J., Persson, J.S., Heeager, L.T., Irani, Z.: Managing e-government: value positions and relationships. Inf. Syst. J. **25**(5), 531–571 (2015)
Sang, S., Lee, J.D., Lee, J.: E-government adoption in ASEAN: the case of Cambodia. Internet Res. (2009)
Sciadas, G.: Unveiling the digital divide (2002)
Shat, F.J., Mousavi, A., Pimenidis, E.: Electronic government enactment in a small developing country–the Palestinian authority's policy and practice. Paper presented at the International Conference on e-Democracy (2013)
Shih, C.-F., Venkatesh, A.: Beyond adoption: development and application of a use-diffusion model. J. Mark. **68**(1), 59–72 (2004)

Wang, C.: Antecedents and consequences of perceived value in mobile government continuance use: an empirical research in China. Comput. Hum. Behav. **34**, 140–147 (2014)
Weerakkody, V., El-Haddadeh, R., Al-Sobhi, F., Shareef, M.A., Dwivedi, Y.K.: Examining the influence of intermediaries in facilitating e-government adoption: an empirical investigation. Int. J. Inf. Manag. **33**(5), 716–725 (2013)

Preliminary Investigation on Malaysian Office Workers' Sedentary Behaviour, Health Consequences, and Intervention Preferences: Towards Designing Anti Sedentary Behaviour Change Support Systems

Nur Fadziana Faisal Mohamed[1,2](✉) and Noorminshah A. Iahad[1]

[1] Universiti Teknologi Malaysia, Johor Bahru, Malaysia
fadziana@uum.edu.my, minshah@utm.my
[2] Universiti Utara Malaysia, UUM, Sintok, Malaysia

Abstract. Sedentary behaviour is a phrase that describes low-energy activities that are commonly coupled with long periods of sitting. Sedentary behaviour has been linked to a variety of negative health effects. Nonetheless, health experts say that the best approach to avoid this condition is to take regular breaks from prolonged sitting. The goals of this study were to find out about 1) sedentary time and patterns among office workers who mostly use computers, 2) health effects of extended sitting, and 3) awareness about sedentary behaviour health repercussions and intervention preferences. From March to May 2019, a poll was conducted in several Malaysian government agencies. The findings suggest that Malaysian office workers work long hours and spend a lot of time sitting. As a result, reducing occupational sitting time is an effective preventative measure. Environmental restructuring was identified as the most popular intervention by respondents, followed by the use of technology to convince people to take a break from sitting.

Keywords: Sedentary behaviour · Office workers · Health consequences · Intervention preferences · Behaviour change support systems

1 Introduction

1.1 Workplace Sedentary Behaviour

The large percentage of today's workforce working in office-based settings and long hours sitting at work has made sedentary behaviour a major public health concern (Radas et al. 2013; Suhaimi et al. 2021). Office workers spend an average of more than 8 h per day at work during the week. Office workers, who primarily utilise computers as their primary working tool, are the greatest occupational category at danger. A growing body of research demonstrates that long periods of sitting are linked to negative health consequences (Jamil et al. 2016). To avoid overuse damage, workers should organise

F. Saeed et al. (Eds.): IRICT 2021, LNDECT 127, pp. 677–687, 2022.
https://doi.org/10.1007/978-3-030-98741-1_56

their breaks and stretching exercises in between tasks (Mahmud et al. 2014). Many studies have indicated that encouraging regular breaks from prolonged sitting can help to reduce the above-mentioned issues (Brändström and Dueso 2013; Conn et al. 2009; Stach 2012).

To date, there anti-sedentary intervention studies that focusing on environment restructuring (Lakerveld et al. 2013; Mahmud et al. 2014; Mahmud et al. 2011; Zafir Mohamed Makhbul et al. 2007). However, there are few studies on self-regulatory sedentary behaviour change interventions. Surveys that have been conducted are still insufficient in determining office workers' preferences for taking breaks from prolonged sitting. Hence, to further understands this matter, a survey was conducted to learn more about office workers' sedentary behaviour, health implications, and solution preferences. This paper shows the findings of a survey conducted among office workers who primarily utilise computers as their primary working tool. The information was gathered from 319 respondents in Malaysia's public sector offices. This research is necessary in order to comprehend the issue that affects the target group. Thus, the goals of this research are to find out about 1) sedentary time and patterns among office workers who mostly use computers, 2) health effects of extended sitting, and 3) knowledge about sedentary behaviour health consequences and intervention preferences.

2 Methodology

2.1 Respondents

A survey was conducted in various public-sector offices in Malaysia comprising workers who were working with computers to perform daily tasks. An email invitation was sent to these organisations to forward to their personnel, and the survey was accessed online via an external internet web-link. Some organizations were approached by providing a paper version of the questionnaire. Individuals who wanted to join had to be employed, work in a desk-based environment with a computer as their primary working tool, and not be impaired. Prior to beginning the survey, all participants had given their approval, and all survey replies were anonymous. Between March and May of 2019, 319 questionnaires were received. This sample size is adequate for this research. Sudman (1976) suggested that a minimum of 100 elements is needed for each major group. The surveys were handed to respondents for a week to complete. Participation was entirely voluntary.

2.2 Questionnaire

The questionnaire consisted of items covering demographic profiles of respondents, occupational sitting time, and physical activities, as well as intervention preferences to break sedentary behavior.

Demographic Profiles of Respondents. Items in the demographic profile section consisted of age, gender, and current job.

Occupational Sitting Patterns. Questions regarding occupational sitting patterns were adopted from Workplace Sitting Breaks Questionnaire (SitBRQ). Items for occupational sitting patterns are mainly concerned with respondents' daily activities while working with the computer during working days. Respondents were asked about the number of working days per week, the number of hours using the computer at work per day, and the frequency of taking breaks. Sedentary hours were self-reported.

Knowledge on Sedentary Behaviour. Respondents were given an infographic showing the illustrations of the health effects of sedentary behavior. They were then asked to study infographics and answer a polar question of yes or no to whether they were aware of the effects of sedentary behavior on their body.

Intervention Preferences. Items for intervention preferences were based on previously researched interventions to break sedentary behaviour. Items covered were:

- environmental changes (e.g., active workstations)
- policies targeting reduced sedentary time (e.g., allowing employees regular desk breaks),
- changing norms surrounding prolonged sitting (e.g., standing meetings),
- using technology to remind or encourage them to move (e.g., apps or computer-based prompting to stand or move).

Each item was clearly defined and accompanied by examples. Respondents were instructed to rank based on the suitability of their nature of work and working environment. The ranking order of 1 to 4 was labelled with 1 being most preferred and 4 being less preferred.

3 Results and Analysis

The survey findings and an analysis of the main results are presented in this section. The purpose of the discussion is to bring to light the key issues raised by the responses. The responses, which were based on descriptive approach, were assessed using a basic statistical method.

3.1 Demographic Profile

The participants' ages ranged from 18 to 62. Females made up 70.5% of the participants, while men made up 29.5%. The majority of the participants were between the ages of 20 and 40. The majority of participants (24.1%) work in management, followed by IT/technical/programmer (19.1%), clerical workers (18.8%), teacher/lecturer (16.9%), and researchers (13.5%). Operators (5.3%) and others (2.2%) made up the balance of the participants. The demographic profile of the respondents is shown in Table 1.

Table 1. Demographic profiles of the respondents

		Gender		Total
		Male	Female	
Ages	<20 years	3	3	6
	20–30 years	12	99	111
	31–40 years	62	98	160
	41–50 years	14	25	39
	> 60 years	3	0	3
Total		94 (29.5%)	225 (70.5%)	319 (100%)
Job	Clerical	6	54	60
	Managerial	16	61	77
	Teacher/Lecturer	10	44	54
	Researcher	11	32	43
	IT/Technical/Programmer	40	21	61
	Operators	6	11	17
	Others	5	2	7
Total		94 (29.5%)	225 (70.5%)	319 (100%)

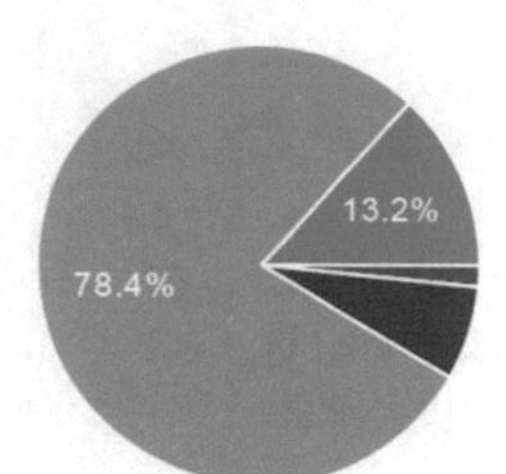

Days	Frequency	Percentage
1-2 days	5	1.6%
3-4 days	22	6.9%
5-6 days	250	78.4%
7 days	42	13.2%
Total	**319**	**100%**

Fig. 1. Number of working days spent per week.

3.2 Occupational Sitting Patterns

The number of working days spent per week was inquired of the responders. The vast majority of respondents (78.4%) worked 5–6 days a week (See Fig. 1). The range is still allowed by the Malaysian Employment Act (1955). Around 13.2% worked seven days each week, which was already more than the maximum of six days per week allowed. Only a small minority of those surveyed worked fewer than four days each week.

The respondents were then asked to estimate how much time they spent sitting during the course of a day at work. Figure 2 reveals that 87.2% of people sit for more than 4 h per day. This finding is in line with research showing that white-collar workers spend the majority of their working hours sitting, and that they do so in lengthy, uninterrupted periods (James Hopkin and Sarkar 2018). The majority of working persons in industrialised countries spend a significant amount of their waking hours at work (Chu et al. 2016). The current findings add to the growing body of research pointing to the workplace as a key location for high levels of sedentary behaviour.

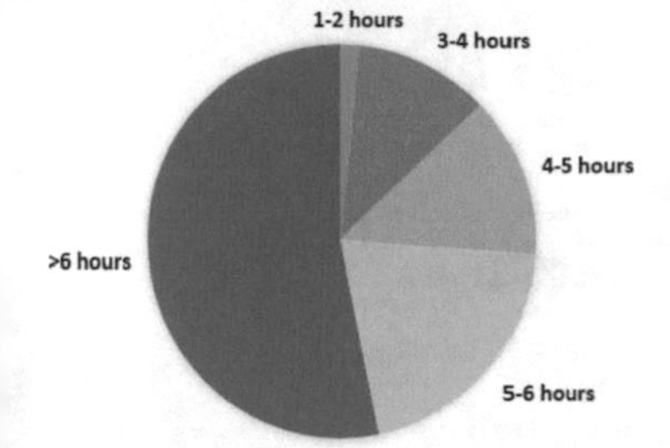

Time	Frequency	Percentage
1-2 hours	5	1.6%
3-4 hours	36	11.3%
4-5 hours	42	13.2%
5-6 hours	66	20.7%
>6 hours	170	53.3%
Total	**319**	**100%**

Fig. 2. Estimated amount of time spent sitting down as part of their work in a day.

Taking movement breaks every 30 min, according to experts, could lower mortality rates. Figure 3 shows only 6.3% of people took a break from prolonged sitting every 30 min. Every one hour, 15.7% takes a break, and every two hours, 23.5% takes a break. Half of the respondents sat for more than 3 h at a stretch. This conclusion indicates that the majority of respondents were at risk of a variety of negative health effects. Individuals who sit for more than 2 h at a time are more likely to develop diabetes, hypertension, and other metabolic risk factors. The result also shows, respondents were also at risk for lower back discomfort and other musculoskeletal issues.

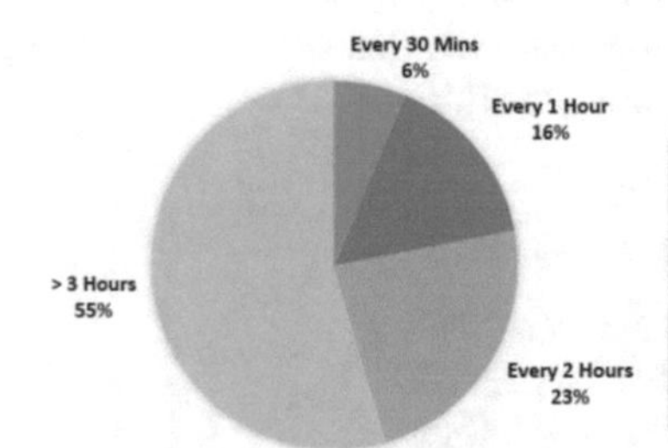

Time	Frequency	Percentage
Every 30 Mins	20	6.30%
Every 1 Hour	50	15.70%
Every 2 Hours	75	23.50%
> 3 Hours	174	55.10%
Total	319	100%

Fig. 3. Frequency of getting up or breaking from prolong sitting

In total, 90.6% of those surveyed felt that long periods of sitting were harmful to their health. Back pain (71.2%) and eye strain (51.4%) were the two most common health effects associated with prolonged sitting, especially when using a computer (See Fig. 4). Long periods of sitting have been linked by orthopaedic research to lumbar disc abnormalities. At the end of four hours of continuous sitting, lumbar 4–5 was dramatically decreased. Meanwhile, optometric research has found that extended computer use causes eye strain or tiredness, blurred vision, dry and irritated eyes, excessive tear secretion, double vision, headache, light or glare sensitivity, slowness in adjusting focus, and changes in colour perception.

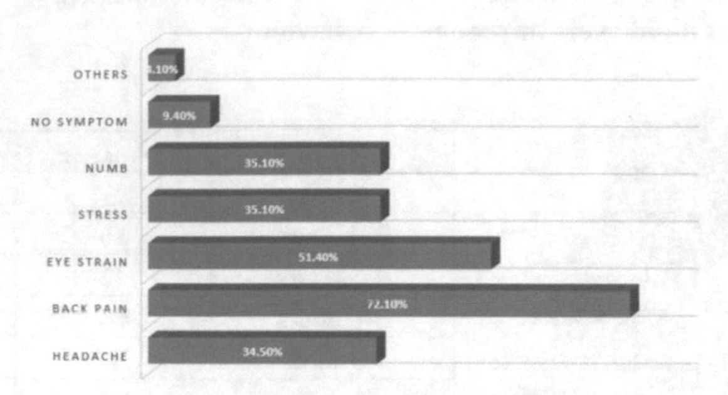

Fig. 4. Health consequences of prolong sitting.

3.3 Knowledge on Sedentary Behaviour

Only a small percentage of office workers were aware that sitting for long periods of time was a risk factor for hypertension (36.63%), type 2 diabetes (35%), cancer (21%), and premature mortality (12%), cardiovascular disease (30%) and obesity (25%) (See Fig. 5). Respondents, on the other hand, were well aware that sitting for lengthy periods of time was a risk factor for slipped discs (70%). Despite their extensive understanding of sedentary behaviour as a risk factor for slipped discs, the sedentary nature of their jobs prevents them from breaking free from long periods of sitting. In all, 67.2% of respondents said they were unaware that long periods of sitting are associated to the health problems indicated above. This information indicates that office workers were not adequately informed about the dangers of prolonged sitting.

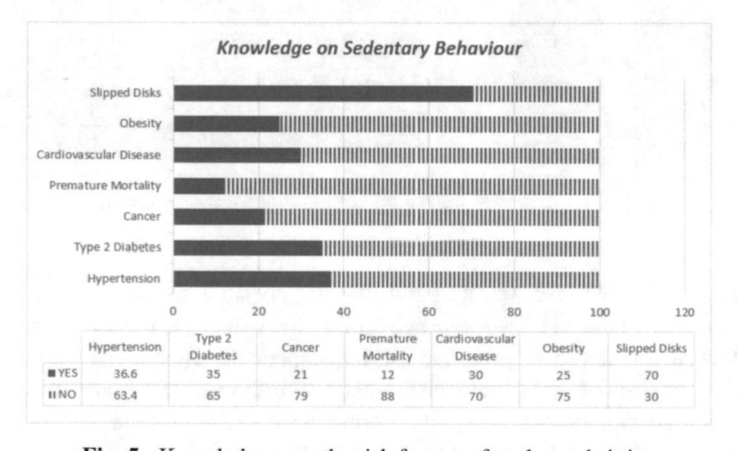

	Hypertension	Type 2 Diabetes	Cancer	Premature Mortality	Cardiovascular Disease	Obesity	Slipped Disks
YES	36.6	35	21	12	30	25	70
NO	63.4	65	79	88	70	75	30

Fig. 5. Knowledge over the risk factors of prolonged sitting

3.4 Intervention Preferences

The ranking order from 1 to 4 was used to conduct the analysis of intervention preferences. The results of the intervention preferences indicate the environmental restructuring came in first, followed by the use of technology to persuade a sitting break, according to the results of the intervention preferences. This finding is in line with (Gardner et al. 2015), which suggests that intervention based on environmental restructuring and persuasion is one of the most promising behaviour modification approaches. Policies aimed at reducing sedentary time and altering long-term seating standards were not as popular. The lowest ranking indicated that certain office workers may have difficulties and ambiguity in implementing this intervention. All four intervention preferences are ranked in Table 2.

Table 2. Intervention preferences by the respondents

Intervention preferences	Rank
Environmental restructuring	1
Technology to persuade sitting break	2
Policies targeting reduced sedentary time	3
Changing norms surrounding prolonged sitting	4

4 Discussion

Malaysian office workers work long hours and spend a lot of time sitting. As a result, reducing office sitting time is an important preventative measure. The respondents work five to six days a week. This is still within the bounds of the Malaysian Employment Act's (1955) permissible range. However, 90% of respondents said they sat for more than 4 h every day during work hours. This conclusion indicates that the majority of respondents were at risk of a variety of negative health effects. Individuals who sit for more than 4 h have a higher risk of diabetes, hypertension, and other metabolic risk factors, according to medical data. Respondents were also at risk for lower back discomfort and other musculoskeletal issues, according to this result.

Back pain and eye strain were the most common health problems reported as a result of prolonged sitting, particularly when using a computer (Gupta et al. 2015; Harman et al. 2014). Respondents were also at risk for lower back pain and other musculoskeletal issues, according to the findings. Continuous sitting should be limited to no more than 2 h over an 8-h workday, according to an ergonomic recommendation for static work postures. When it comes to the sitting interval, doctors advocate standing or moving every 30 min of sitting.

According to data on sedentary behaviour knowledge, office workers were not well exposed to the dangers of prolonged sitting. Poor health promotion programmes in public offices on sedentary behaviour can be attributed for a high percentage of people having a poor understanding of the risk factors for sedentary behaviour and its health consequences. Improved workplace health promotion, on the other hand, may lead to better lifestyle choices. Despite having a strong understanding of the dangers of prolonged sitting in terms of slipped discs and back discomfort, the nature of job and a lack of self-determination appear to be a barrier for the respondents, particularly when it comes to extended sitting at work.

The results on intervention preferences are consistent with (Stach 2012), with environmental restructuring and persuasion evaluated as particularly promising behaviour modification strategies. External surroundings and self-regulation, according to the intervention's creators, are two elements that can impact sedentary behaviour modification (Stach 2012). In the near term, reorganising the surroundings, such as giving sit-stand desks, has been shown to be effective in reducing inactive time. However, there is no certainty that it will have a long-term effect on behaviour. The usage of a sit-stand desk should be coupled by a reminder mechanism to stand at regular intervals, according to researchers (Carr et al. 2013). The disadvantage of reconstructing the exterior environment is that it necessitates the creation of new office settings and the replacement of furniture. All of this necessitates careful planning and training, as well as a significant financial investment. It's also limited to individual workstations and difficult to use in meeting rooms.

Persuasion intervention, on the other hand, does not have to be limited to rearranging workplace furniture and settings. Sedentary behaviour could be reduced across several environmental domains by focusing on strengthening persons' psychological capabilities (Mohamed et al. 2017). Changes in motivation and self-regulation, according to Social Cognitive Theory (SCT) (Bandura 1986), are at the basis of behaviour change. The core notion of SCT is self-efficacy, which is defined as "a person's belief in their ability to carry out a course of action successfully." Many health habits, particularly anti-sedentary behaviour and physical activity are influenced by self-efficacy. The motivational push and self-regulatory skills are required for self-management of health promotion (Gardner et al. 2015). This is in line with Bandura's claim that SCT incorporates both cognitive and motivational aspects of self-regulated behaviour. Self-regulatory mechanisms such as self-monitoring, social support, and goal planning influence health behaviour in both direct and indirect ways. In healthcare, the use of persuasion technology like as cellphones is fast rising. Various research have documented its capability and popularity. The majority of prior mobile phone research have used text messaging as part of a behaviour modification intervention, with motivating and informational text messages being received as one of the intervention components. Mobile apps as a behaviour change intervention have been shown to be convincing, low-cost, and result in significant reductions across multiple environmental domains (Rosenberger 2012).

5 Conclusion

The long hours of working and high sitting time exist in Malaysian office workers. Reducing workplace sitting time is therefore an important prevention strategy. The most preferred intervention strategies by office workers is environmental restructuring that is by providing sit stand desk to enable them to break prolonged sedentary sitting while working. The basic sit stand desk requires user to manually change the height of the table. The more sophisticated ones require mechanical controller to change the height. This intervention would be ideal to be implemented. However, the major drawback of sit stand desk lies in the high implementation cost (Chau et al. 2014). Having an adjustable desk height is meaningless if not equipped with a reminder system. Furthermore, it is limited to individual workstations and difficult to apply in meeting spaces. Researchers indicated that for a sit stand desk to be successful, it should be coupled by a reminder mechanism to stand at regular intervals (Radas et al. 2013). As an alternative, persuasive technology can be employed without requiring any changes to office furniture or environments.

Mobile apps have been reported in various behaviour change studies. Smartphones offer built-in tools for monitoring, reminding, providing feedback, instructing, informing, and recording data. Previous mobile phone research has used text messaging as part of a behaviour modification intervention, with motivating and informational text messages being one of the intervention components. Mobile apps as a behaviour modification intervention have been shown to be convincing, low-cost, and result in significant reductions across many environmental domains (Rosenberger 2012). Smartphones have the potential to support successful sedentary behaviour change techniques (Mohamed et al. 2017). Because of the popularity and mobility of smartphones, it is appropriate to provide person level support in addition to the technological capabilities they display. Smartphone apps are readily available for download at a minimal cost. Because of the prevalence of mobile technologies, a huge and growing number of people now hold smartphones, allowing interventions to reach a big number of people. Smartphones are an effective tool for encouraging people to improve their inactive habits on a personal level (Suhaimi et al. 2021). It is advised that intervention researchers look at persuasion technology to help people change their inactive habits.

6 Ethical Approval

Before the instrument was given out, each responder gave their informed consent. Everyone who took part in the survey was told that it was completely voluntary. The research data was kept private, and if necessary, a summary of the outcomes and findings was sent to the participants. There are no risks associated with the study just as there are no rewards or compensations for participating. This study has been carried out as a preliminary investigation for the Anti-Sedentary Behaviour Change Support Systems project.

References

Bandura, A.: Social Foundations of Thought and ACTION: A Social Cognitive Theory. Prentice-Hall Inc., New Jersey (1986)

Brändström, M., Dueso, A.: How to Encourage Stretching and Breaks at Work. Umea Universitet, Sweden (2013)

Carr, L.J., Karvinen, K., Peavler, M., Smith, R., Cangelosi, K.: Multicomponent intervention to reduce daily sedentary time: a randomised controlled trial. BMJ Open **3**(10), e003261 (2013). https://doi.org/10.1136/bmjopen-2013-003261

Chau, J.Y., et al.: The effectiveness of sit-stand workstations for changing office workers' sitting time: results from the Stand@Work randomized controlled trial pilot. Int. J. Behav. Nutr. Phys. Act. **11**, 127 (2014). https://doi.org/10.1186/s12966-014-0127-7

Chu, A.H.Y., Ng, S.H.X., Tan, C.S., Win, A.M., Koh, D., Müller-Riemenschneider, F.: A systematic review and meta-analysis of workplace intervention strategies to reduce sedentary time in white-collar workers. Obes. Rev. **17**(5), 467–481 (2016). https://doi.org/10.1111/obr.12388

Conn, V.S., Hafdahl, A.R., Cooper, P.S., Brown, L.M., Lusk, S.L.: Meta-analysis of workplace physical activity interventions. Am. J. Prev. Med. **37**(4), 330–339 (2009). https://doi.org/10.1016/j.amepre.2009.06.008

Gardner, B., Smith, L., Lorencatto, F., Hamer, M., Biddle, S.J.: How to reduce sitting time? A review of behaviour change strategies used in sedentary behaviour reduction interventions among adults. Health Psychol. Rev. **7199**(October), 1–24 (2015). https://doi.org/10.1080/17437199.2015.1082146

Gupta, N., Christiansen, C.S., Hallman, D.M., Korshøj, M., Carneiro, I.G., Holtermann, A.: Is objectively measured sitting time associated with low back pain? A cross-sectional investigation in the NOMAD study. PLoS ONE **10**(3), e0121159 (2015). https://doi.org/10.1371/journal.pone.0121159

Harman, K., Macrae, M., Vallis, M., Bassett, R.: Working with people to make changes: a behavioural change approach used in chronic low back pain rehabilitation. Physiotherapie Canada **66**(1), 82–90 (2014). https://doi.org/10.3138/ptc.2012-56BC

Jamil, A.T., Rosli, N.M., Ismail, A., Idris, I.B., Omar, A.: Prevalence and risk factors for sedentary behavior among Malaysian adults. Malaysian J. Publ. Health Med. **16**(3), 147–155 (2016). https://www.mjphm.org.my/mjphm/journals/2016

James Hopkin, T., Sarkar, S.: Cronicon Sedentary Behavior of White Collar Office Workers-Review (2018). https://www.ecronicon.com/ecnu/pdf/ECNU-03-0000102.pdf

Koepp, G.A., et al.: Treadmill desks: a 1-year prospective trial. Obesity **21**(4), 705–711 (2013). https://doi.org/10.1002/oby.20121

Lakerveld, J., Bot, S.D.M., Van der Ploeg, H.P., Nijpels, G.: The effects of a lifestyle intervention on leisure-time sedentary behaviors in adults at risk: the Hoorn Prevention Study, a randomized controlled trial. Prev. Med. **57**(4), 351–356 (2013). https://doi.org/10.1016/j.ypmed.2013.06.011

Lee, S., Wong, J., Shanita, S., Ismail, M., Deurenberg, P., Poh, B.: Daily physical activity and screen time, but not other sedentary activities, are associated with measures of obesity during childhood. Int. J. Environ. Res. Publ. Health **12**(1), 146–161 (2014). https://doi.org/10.3390/ijerph120100146

Mahmud, N., Bahari, S.F., Zainudin, N.F.: Psychosocial and ergonomics risk factors related to neck, shoulder and back complaints among Malaysia office workers. Int. J. Soc. Sci. Humanity **4**(4), 260–263 (2014). https://doi.org/10.7763/IJSSH.2014.V4.359

Mahmud, N., Kenny, D.T., Heard, R.: Office ergonomics awareness and prevalence of musculoskeletal disorders among office workers in the Universiti Teknologi Malaysia : a cross sectional study. Malaysian J. Med. Health Sci. (2011)

Matthews, C.E., et al.: Amount of time spent in sedentary behaviors in the United States, 2003–2004. Am. J. Epidemiol. **167**(7), 875–881 (2008). https://doi.org/10.1093/aje/kwm390

Mohamed, N.F.F., Rahman, A.A., Iahad, N.A.: Managing sedentary behavior with smartphone managing sedentary behavior with PACIS 2017 Proceedings (2017)

Radas, A., et al.: Evaluation of ergonomic and education interventions to reduce occupational sitting in office-based university workers: study protocol for a randomized controlled trial. Trials **14**, 330 (2013). https://doi.org/10.1186/1745-6215-14-330

Rosenberger, M.: Sedentary behavior: target for change, challenge to assess. Int. J. Obes. Suppl. **2**(Suppl 1), S26–S29 (2012). https://doi.org/10.1038/ijosup.2012.7

Stach, T.B.: Heart rate balancing for multiplayer exergames (2012). http://hdl.handle.net/1974/7525

Sudman, S.: Applied Sampling. Academic Press, New York (1976)

Suhaimi, S.A., Müller, A.M., Hafiz, E., Khoo, S.: Occupational sitting time, its determinants and intervention strategies in Malaysian office workers: a mixed-methods study. Health Promot. Int. (2021). https://doi.org/10.1093/heapro/daab149

Swartz, A.M., Squires, L., Strath, S.J.: Energy expenditure of interruptions to sedentary behavior. Int. J. Behav. Nutr. Phys. Act. **8**, 69 (2011). https://doi.org/10.1186/1479-5868-8-69

Tremblay, M.S., et al.: Sedentary behavior research network (SBRN) – terminology consensus project process and outcome. Int. J. Behav. Nutr. Phys. Act. **14**(1), 75 (2017). https://doi.org/10.1186/s12966-017-0525-8

Warburton, D.E.R., Nicol, C.W., Bredin, S.S.D.: Health benefits of physical activity: the evidence. CMAJ: Can. Med. Assoc. J. **174**(6), 801–809 (2006). https://doi.org/10.1503/cmaj.051351

Makhbul, Z.M., Idrus, D., Rani, M.R.A.: Ergonomics design on the work stress outcomes. Jurnal Kemanusiaan **9**, 50–61 (2007). http://myais.fsktm.um.edu.my/8343/

The National Industry 4.0 Policy Performance Review Based on Industry4WRD Readiness Assessment and Intervention Program

Zulhasni Abdul Rahim(✉), Nor Azian Abdul Rahman, and Muhamad Saqib Iqbal

Malaysia-Japan International Institute of Technology, Universiti Teknologi Malaysia, Kuala Lumpur, Malaysia
zulhasni@utm.my

Abstract. Industry growth has been accelerated by the discovery of emerging technology, from the early implementation of mechanical systems to support manufacturing processes to today's highly automated assembly lines, in order to be flexible and adaptable to today's changing consumer requirements and demands. As a result of the evolution of the industrial revolution, a variety of enabling technologies to have emerged. The manufacturing sector is vital to the development of smart and sustainable industries. As a result, Industry 4.0 aids in the shaping of smart future manufacturing through a variety of methods, one of which is the implementation of the Industry4WRD RA Program, which is influenced by the National Policy on Industry 4.0. The study depicts the performance of the National Industry 4.0 policy based on the SMEs Industry4WRD Readiness Assessment (RA) and intervention program. Analysis and discussion on the collective achievement of assessed Manufacturing and Manufacturing Related Services (MRS) companies for the year 2019 sorted primarily according to their respective Readiness Profiles will be presented in the following first application analysis before Readiness Profile achievement analysis, with suggestions to further improve the RA Program based on post assessment survey, and general observation and suggestions to assessed Manufacturing and MRS company.

Keywords: National Industry 4.0 policy · Industry4WRD · Readiness assessment · Intervention

1 Introduction of National Industry 4.0 Policy: Industry4WRD Program

1.1 The Initiation of Industry4WRD Program

Launched on the 31st October 2018, the Industry4WRD Policy underlines the concerted multi- ministerial strategy in realizing a 10-year vision to accelerate Malaysia's transformation into a smart and modern manufacturing system, with a threefold Attract-Create-Transform (ACT) objective of: increasing Malaysia's attractiveness as a preferred destination for high-tech manufacturing; creating the right ecosystem for Industry 4.0

F. Saeed et al. (Eds.): IRICT 2021, LNDECT 127, pp. 688–696, 2022.
https://doi.org/10.1007/978-3-030-98741-1_57

to be adopted; and, transform Malaysia's industry capabilities in both a holistic and an accelerated manner. Thus, at its core, the policy aims to facilitate Malaysian companies (especially SMEs) to embrace Industry 4.0 business model in a systematic and comprehensive manner, thus becoming smart, agile, and data-driven organizations powered by three Shift Factors: next-generation competent workers and leaders (people); next-generation product development and production methods (process); and next-generation Operation Technologies and IT Technologies (technology), showed in Fig. 1.

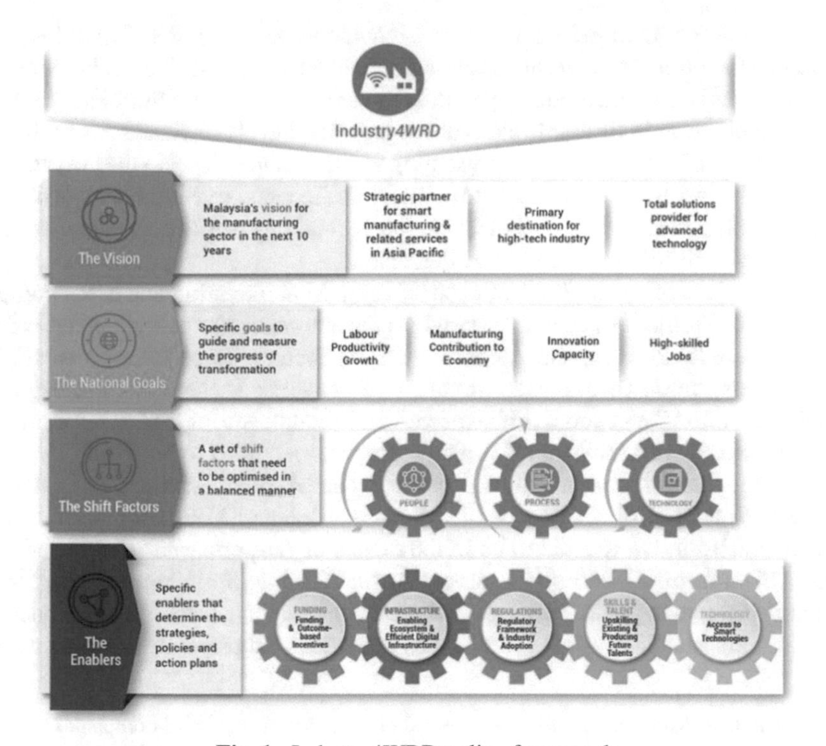

Fig. 1. Industry4WRD policy framework

Although the Industry4WRD Policy sets a 10-year vision for the Malaysian manufacturing and manufacturing related services sectors, it has also set up four National Goals (to be achieved by 2025) including: 30% productivity improvement; increased manufacturing sector Gross Domestic Product (GDP) contribution from RM254.7 billion to RM392 billion; improved innovation potential by achieving top 30 in the Global Innovation Index (GII)6; and improved sectoral skilled workers7 participation (from 18% to 35%). To achieve the National Goals, five Strategic Enablers (Funding, Infrastructure, Regulations, Skills and Talents, and Technology, or F.I.R.S.T) has been identified and this is further supported by thirteen Strategies, and thirty eight (38) Action Plans, showed in Fig. 1.

Among the many components to this Industry4WRD Policy Framework is Strategy R2, which supports the Regulations Strategic Enabler. This strategy highlights the need to create a platform and mechanism to help manufacturing firms, especially SMEs, assess and develop their Industry 4.0-ready (smart) capabilities, with the corresponding Action Plan stating the need to establish a National Readiness Program as a tool for conducting assessment, sharing global and local best practices, supporting the development of local firms, and identifying national Industry 4.0 priorities. This leads to the roll out of the Industry4WRD Readiness Assessment (RA) Program.

1.2 The Industry4WRD Readiness Assessment and Profile

There are nine RA Dimensions for each Manufacturing and MRS Technology Shift Factors, with a difference in terms of classification. Nevertheless, the Technology Shift Factor observes similar methodology with both People and Process Shift Factors, where each RA Dimension is further broken down into five Levels of Readiness with corresponding points of between 0 to 4 representing worst readiness level to the best readiness level respectively. Therefore, maximum point for the Technology Shift Factor is 45 points with an overall percentage of 50%. Hence, the Technology Shift Factor contributes the most to the overall Industry4WRD RA Percentage.

To classify the readiness level of each assessed Manufacturing and MRS company, its "Readiness Profile" is calculated based on the summation of the weighted percentage of the People, Process, and Technology Shift Factors. Table 1 shows each of the five Readiness Profile according to the range of percentage scored and corresponding general description. In general, it is expected that Manufacturing and MRS companies wanting to transform to Industry 4.0-ready (smart) operations to be within the ranges of "Newcomer" and "Learner" since they are expected to not have yet taken the steps to prepare for the transformation, while Manufacturing and MRS companies who has started to transform is expected to be in the ranges of "Experienced" and "Leader". In contrast, Manufacturing and MRS companies that fall into the "Conventional" Readiness Profile even though has low Overall RA Percentage scores, could still be interested in transforming to Industry 4.0-ready (smart) operations but presently lacking operation

Table 1. Readiness profile for assessed manufacturing and MRS companies

READINESS PROFILE	PERCENTAGE SCORED	GENERAL DESCRIPTION
Conventional	0 % to 20 %	Operation remains "as is" with no intention or initiative to move into Industry 4.0 adoption.
Newcomer	21 % to 40 %	Has interest to pursue Industry 4.0 but with none or very minimal efforts or initiatives.
Learner	41 % to 60 %	Has interest to pursue pilot line Industry 4.0 adoption in operation, with existence of planning and strategies, efforts or simple and patches of initiatives being implemented. Ready for some system adoption.
Experienced	61 % to 90 %	Has pursued small to medium scale Industry 4.0 adoption initiatives in operation, horizontal integration and ready for large scale system adoption.
Leader	91 % to 100 %	Has implemented large scale Industry 4.0 adoption initiatives (company-wide) and system integration.

strategy, organization, and technology mostly due to not having a management system in place. Thus, "Conventional" companies must be continuously guided in these areas until they are ready to transform into Industry 4.0-ready (smart) operations.

2 The Participation of Industry4WRD

2.1 The Industry4WRD Demographic of Participation by State

Out of the 452 Manufacturing and MRS companies receiving Government funding, highest concentration of committed participation is from Selangor (181 companies or 40.0%), Johor (68 companies or 15.0%), and Pulau Pinang (62 companies or 13.7%). This is to be expected since Selangor, Johor, and Pulau Pinang contributes highest to the (national) manufacturing sector GDP contribution in 201920 with RM95,942m (or 30.47% from total manufacturing sector GDP contribution), 21 also worth noting that in 2019, only Pulau Pinang is significantly dependent on manufacturing activity as the sector contributes to 43.2% to the state economy, as opposed to Selangor 22 RM40,125m (12.74%), and RM40,510m (12.86%) respectively, showed in Fig. 2.

However, it is (27.8%) and Johor (29.9%). In contrast, there are FIVE (5) States with less than 10 committed participations: Sabah (7), Terengganu (7), Pahang (5), Kelantan (3), and Perlis (0). This is to be expected from Kelantan and Perlis as in 2019, manufacturing activity contribution to state's total economic activity only accounted to RM1,300m (5.1% from state total) and RM470m (7.6%) 23 from state total) and RM12,767m (21.8%) respectively 25 respectively. However, when looking at Terengganu and Pahang (third and fourth lowest participation), manufacturing activity in these

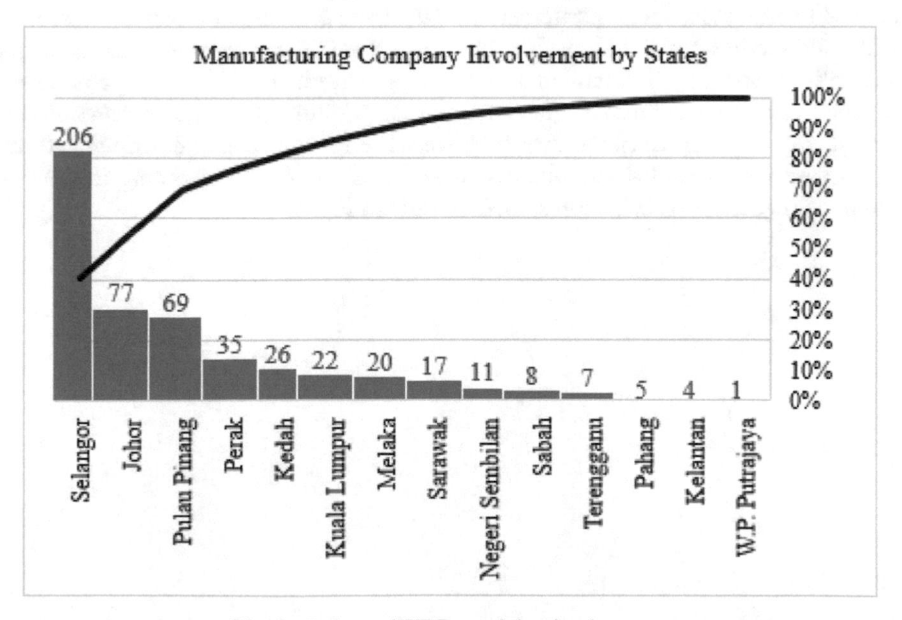

Fig. 2. Industry4WRD participation by states

states accounted to RM13,093m (37.5% 24. This is comparable to Perak (RM13,683m or 18.0% from state total) and Kedah (RM13,430m or 28.7%). But, unlike Perak and Kedah who has the fourth and fifth best committed participation to the RA Program, Terengganu and Pahang sits at the opposite end with committed participation contribution of only 1.6% and 1.1% (from total of 452) respectively. The final state with less than 10 committed participants is Sabah, but since the manufacturing activity only contributes to 7.6% (RM6,472m) to the total state economic activity, the low quantity of committed participants is expected.

2.2 The Industry4WRD Demographic of Participation by Manufacturing Sectors

In 2019, the manufacturing sector contributed to 22.3% to the Malaysian GDP. According to the 2008 Malaysia Standard Industrial Classification (MSIC 2008) Manufacturing organizations can be further classified into 24 Divisions. These Divisions are then further classified into 51 corresponding Classes and 241 Sub-Classes. For the RA Program in 2019, the 444 Manufacturing companies receiving Government funding was made up of committed Manufacturing companies performing activity across 23 out of the 24 Divisions. Out of the 23 Divisions with committed participation in the RA Program, Divisions 10 (Food products), 22 (Rubber and plastic products), and 25 (Fabricated metal products, except machinery and equipment) has committed participation with more than 60 Manufacturing companies each, showed in Fig. 3.

According to the Industry4WRD standard for MRS, there are sixteen MRS types with: eight types of services which supports activities in the Pre-Manufacturing stage; five types of services which supports activities in the Manufacturing stage38; and three types 39 of services which supports activities in the Post Manufacturing stage. For 2019, out of 20 MRS companies' participation, only 8 were committed participants: three in Logistic services; two in Manufacturing support services; one in Inspection, testing and quality control; one in Maintenance, repair, and overhaul of machinery equipment; and one in Environmental management services. Additionally, stage concentration of committed participation is spread evenly between Pre-Manufacturing and Manufacturing stages, with no committed participation from MRS companies operating in the Post Manufacturing stage. This is represented visually in Fig. 4.

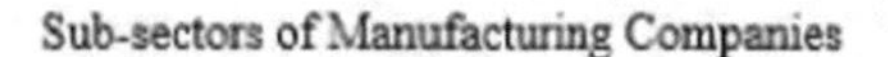

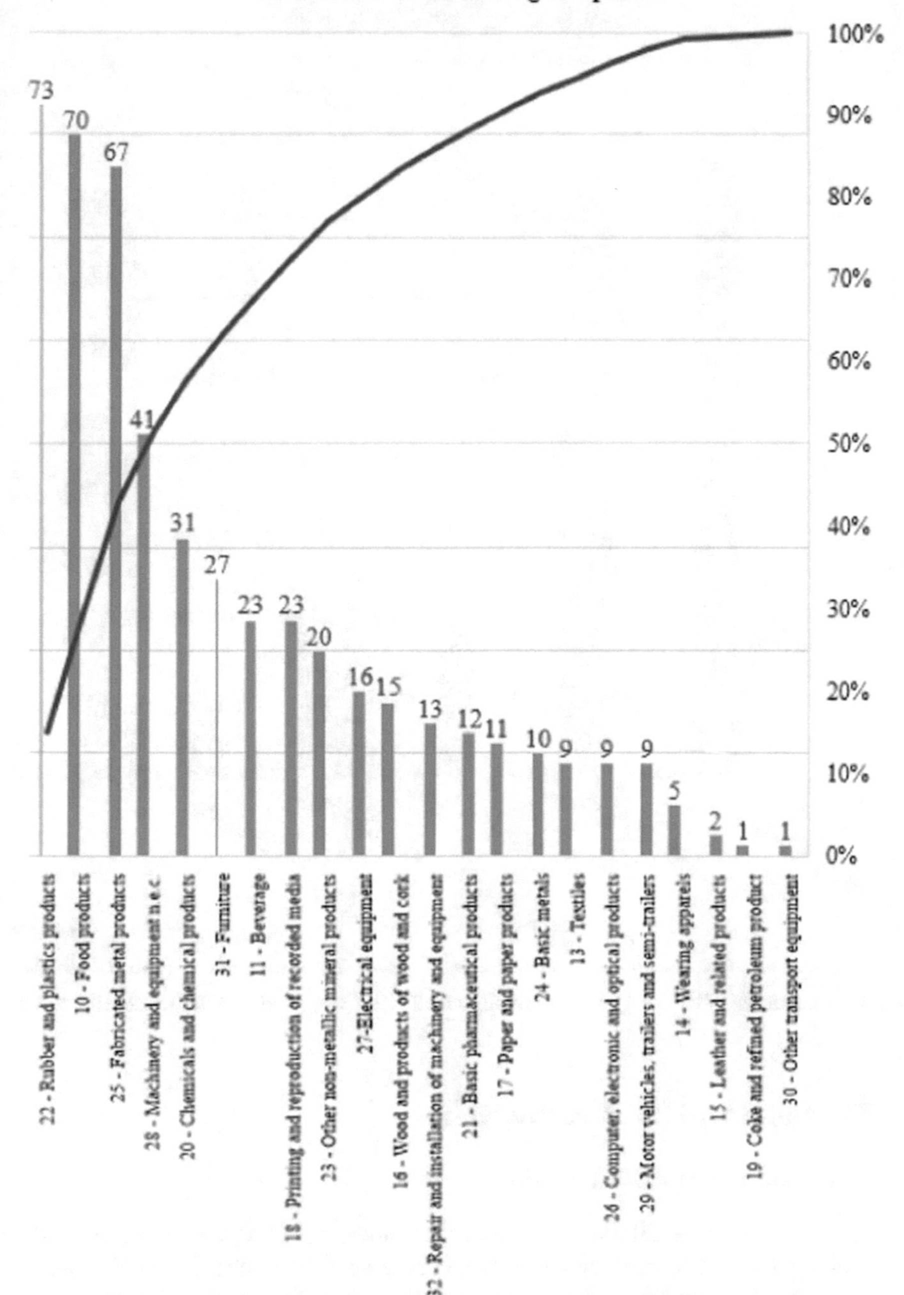

Fig. 3. Breakdown of RA Program participation for 2019 (Govt Funded, Manufacturing) according to MSIC Code 2008 Division

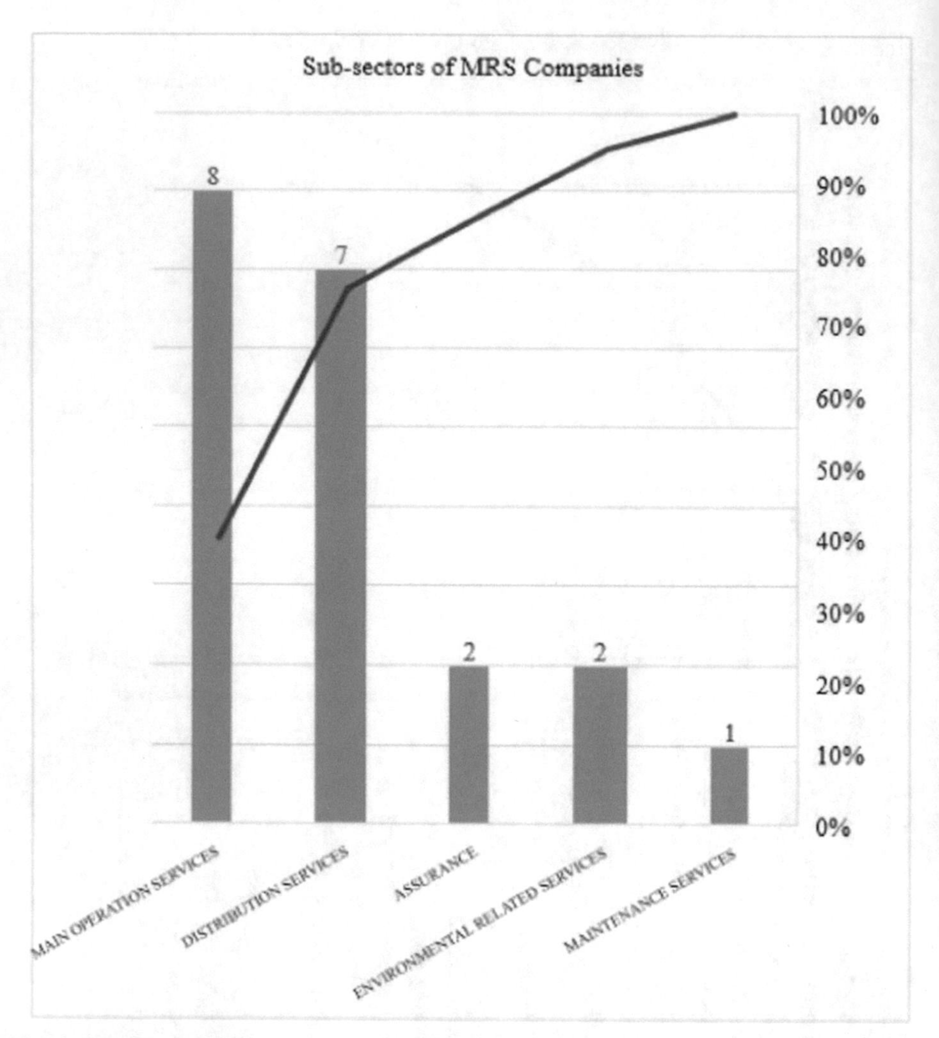

Fig. 4. Breakdown of RA Program participation for 2019 (Govt Funded, MRS) according to MRS Type

3 The Industry4WRD Performance

3.1 The Industry4WRD RA Profile

As previously described, there are five RA "Readiness Profiles" which are categorized based on the Overall RA Percentage score. For the year 2019, out of the 470 Manufacturing and MRS companies (Government funded and self-funded) that were assessed: 31 companies achieved an Overall RA Percentage score of between 0 to 20 and are categorized as "Conventional"; 398 categorized as "Newcomer" (21 to 40 overall score); 35 categorized as "Learner" (41 to 60 overall score); and 6 categorized as "Experienced" (61 to 90 overall score). No assessed company in 2019 managed to achieve Overall RA

Percentage score of between 91 and 100. This is shown in Fig. 5. Although the overall result skews to the left, this result is expected 43 and is in line with findings from Khazanah Research Institute.

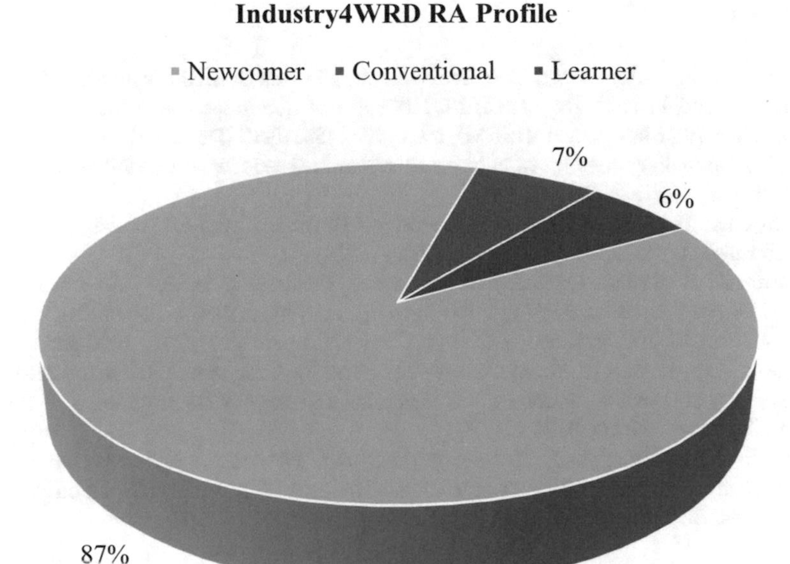

Fig. 5. Breakdown of Industry4WRD RA profiling

4 The Conclusion and Recommendations

The National Policy on Industry 4.0 is a critical policy that aims to change or transform the Manufacturing and MRS sectors through 13 strategies and 38 action plans. The policy outlines five national strategies with the aim of attracting stakeholders to Industry 4.0 technologies and processes while also increasing Malaysia's attractiveness as a preferred manufacturing location. To further strengthen this, the improvement should focus on developing a consolidated information platform on Industry4WRD awareness and solutions, innovation, recommended vendor list, forms, templates, application, reports, and status under a central platform should be explored. It is envisioned that the platform can help institutions and firms to update their knowledge base, allowing companies to identify the value of external information, assimilate it, and apply it to commercial purposes. Furthermore, developing an effectiveness assessment program to begin implementing the reorientation of various engineering and technical systems towards the digital economy, a long-term effectiveness assessment program on the RA Program considerations on the assessed Manufacturing and MRS companies should be considered.

Acknowledgement. This paper is sponsored by Ministry of Higher Education, under FUNDAMENTAL RESEARCH GRANT SCHEME (FRGS/1/2021/SS02/UTM/02/16).

References

1. Lin, W.D., Low, M.Y., Chong, Y.T., Teo, C.L.: Application of SIRI for industry 4.0 maturity assessment and analysis. In: 2019 IEEE International Conference on Industrial Engineering and Engineering Management (IEEM), pp. 1450–1454. IEEE (Dec 2019)
2. Man, J.C., Strandhagen, J.O.: An Industry 4.0 research agenda for sustainable business models. Procedia Cirp **63**, 721–726 (2017)
3. Karacay, G.: Talent development for Industry 4.0. In: Industry 4.0: Managing the Digital Transformation, pp. 123–136. Springer, Cham (2018)
4. Department of Statistics, Malaysia, Malaysia Standard Industrial Classification 2008 (MSIC 2008). Source: https://www.dosm.gov.my/v1/uploads/files/4_Portal%20Content/3_Methods%20%26%20Classifications/2_List%20of%20References/MSIC_2008.pdf
5. Zulhasni, A.R., Roslan, M.M., Syukri, W.W.M.: The Application of TRIZ in the development of readiness assessment model for the Malaysian Industry4WRD program. IOP Conf. Ser. Mater. Sci. Eng. **1051**(1), 012036 (2021)
6. Zulhasni, A.R., Kamaliah, J., Roslan, Y.M., Syukri, W.W.M.: A review of talent adaptive concept and conceptual framework of accelerated Industry4WRD talent adaptation in Malaysia. J. Adv. Res. Bus. Manage. Stud. **21**(1), 10–18 (2020)

Construction 4.0 Readiness and Challenges for Construction Skills Training Institutions in Malaysia

Muhammad Fariq Abdul Hamid[1](✉) and Zulhasni Abdul Rahim[2]

[1] Malaysia-Japan International Institute of Technology, Kuala Lumpur, Malaysia
fariqhamid79@gmail.com

[2] University of Technology Malaysia, Kuala Lumpur, Malaysia

Abstract. Rapid changes in technology application due to increment of market requirements have been a pushing factor to radical industry adoption and adaptation upon new technologies. The integration of emerging technologies associated with Industry 4.0 with construction delivery processes had founded the Construction 4.0 term which been emerging in the recent research corpus. The adoption of Construction 4.0, major changes in the construction process delivery stages, project structures and organization and ultimately integrate the known highly fragmented construction industry atmosphere including its work force. These changes will require another level of skill set for the construction personnel who involve in the construction project life cycle and its value chain. The current level of awareness on Construction 4.0, key challenges faced and technologies adoption readiness amongst construction skill training institutes in Malaysia upon changes associated with Construction 4.0 technologies need to be assessed and well understood. This will be the basis for construction lead body in Malaysia to mitigate the way forward for the construction skills training institutions of the nation. As there are still limited research and study conducted in understanding Construction 4.0 adoption clarity by the construction skills training institutions in Malaysia, this research will contribute to the enrichment of academic studies documentation related to the Construction 4.0 in specific and the Industry 4.0 generally for Malaysia context.

Keywords: Construction 4.0 · Construction · Skill training

1 Research Background

1.1 Introduction

The robust changes in technology applications in fulfilling the needs and demands of continuous increment of market requirements have been a pushing factor to radical industry adoption and adaptation upon new technologies. The Fourth Industrial Revolution (Industry 4.0) that was first mentioned by the executive chairman and the founder of the World Economic Forum (WEF), Klaus Schwab, in Davos-Klosters, Switzerland back in

F. Saeed et al. (Eds.): IRICT 2021, LNDECT 127, pp. 697–706, 2022.
https://doi.org/10.1007/978-3-030-98741-1_58

2016 had highlighted that, the integration of business and manufacturing processes as well as all players in the industry value chain is the profound concept of Industry 4.0 approach [1].

Industry 4.0 mainly focusing on range of advanced technologies adoption across all industries value chain. Automation, robotics, artificial intelligence, nanotechnology, quantum computing, biotechnology, industrial internet of things, decentralized consensus, fifth-generation (5G) wireless technologies, 3D printing, and fully autonomous vehicles are considered as the main emerging technologies that driving Industry 4.0 forward while at the same time creating both threats and opportunities to the conventional industries environment. Continuous increment of digital technology applications in the current conventional methods of delivering things especially in manufacturing industry which emphasizes in advanced communication and connectivity had driven the emergence of cyber-physical production systems (CPPS). In short, it is a result of coordination and integration between hardware, software and biological elements in enhancing traditional monitoring of physical processes, decisions making and troubleshooting towards cost reduction, increase productivity and control the risks during production stages.

In response to the needs and challenges arise in Industry 4.0 era, construction industry, as other industries, has been reacting in positive direction. Researchers in the construction industry had begun exploring the potential integration of Industry 4.0 technologies into construction thus the term 'Construction 4.0' recently emerged in the 21st century research corpus (Rastogi D. S., 2017, as cited in [2]). The Construction 4.0 term, according to the European Industry Construction Federation (FIEC), is coined to Architecture, Engineering & Construction (AEC) industry as part of Industry 4.0 and its mainly refers to the digitalization of the industry ([3], as cited in [2]).

According to Rastogi (2017), Construction 4.0 can be understood as a counterpart of Industry 4.0 in which, aims to digitalize the whole life cycle of construction project monitoring and with the aid of multiple technologies. Through the adoption of Construction 4.0, major changes in the construction process delivery stages, project structures and organization and ultimately integrate the known highly fragmented construction industry atmosphere. These changes will require another level of skill set for the construction personnel who involve in the construction project life cycle and its value chain. The required skill set may be acquired from construction skill training institutes available in a country which mostly governed by certain body under the local government or international conferring bodies. In order to produce construction personnel with the required skill sets related to Construction 4.0 technologies, it is crucial for the construction skill training institutes to realize on the changes involve. A sound understanding on the Construction 4.0 and the emerging technologies that may disrupt the current methods in developing the future skilled workforce for construction must be well acknowledged and anticipated towards successful adoption of the changes.

1.2 Issue Statement

Workforce readiness towards technological adoption to construction processes has been highlighted as one of domain enabler towards embracing the implementation of Construction 4.0. Involvement of construction skills institutions to equip and prepare the future workforce capabilities are highly crucial as highlighted in the Construction 4.0.

Malaysia had portrayed readiness in embracing new construction revolution, based on The Global Competitiveness Report 2019, Global Innovation Index (GII) 2019 and IMD World Competitiveness Ranking 2019 [4]. People (workforce) have been identified as one of four enablers that leads to the success of Construction 4.0 agenda and to be equipped and ready with new skills for the future workforce [5].

However, study has revealed that Malaysia's TVET lecturers are not really understand how to apply Industry 4.0 thus relatively present potential threat to the adoption of Construction 4.0 in the construction skill training programs [6]. Clarity on roles and necessity to change amongst construction skills training institutions are crucial to extensively understand their readiness in implementing Construction 4.0. A clear understanding on Construction 4.0 implementation and potential challenges to be faced by the construction skills training institutions will enhance their competitiveness level in adapting with changes.

Therefore, it is crucial to deep dive into understanding the current level of awareness on Construction 4.0 among the construction skill training provider in Malaysia and analyse the readiness for them to meet up with the new emerging technologies bundled in Construction 4.0. It is also essential to understand the anticipated challenges that may present barriers in Construction 4.0 adoption among the construction skill training institutes in Malaysia for feasible initiative to be proposed in the recent future.

1.3 Research Purpose

The purpose of this research is to develop a sound understanding on the current level of awareness upon Construction 4.0 and to analyze Construction 4.0 adoption readiness among of the construction skills training institutions in Malaysia. This research will also aim to analyze the collective anticipated challenges faced by the institutions in adopting Construction 4.0 technologies in the current training program for further strategic decision and initiatives formulation in the future.

1.4 Research Objectives and Questions

In response to the problem identified with regards to the adoption and readiness towards Construction 4.0 technologies changes by the construction skill institutions in Malaysia, this research is conducted to:

i. Assess the level of awareness on Construction 4.0 amongst the construction skills training institutions in Malaysia.
ii. Identify the key challenges faced by the construction skills training institutions in adopting Construction 4.0
iii. Assess the Construction 4.0 adoption readiness level by the construction skills training institutions in Malaysia.
iv. Propose the way forward for the construction industry lead body in Malaysia to undertake based on the construction skills training institutions current Construction 4.0 adoption readiness level

In order to streamline the research towards achieving the objectives set, these research questions are developed to understand the identified problem in depth as well as building further argumentative questions to verify research findings:

i. What are the critical elements of Construction 4.0 need to be aware by the construction skills training institutions in Malaysia?
ii. To what extend the construction skills training institutions in Malaysia are clear on their roles and scope in adopting the critical elements of Construction 4.0?
iii. What are the challenges faced by Malaysia construction skills training institutions in adopting the critical elements of Construction 4.0?
iv. What are the key elements to be measured and analyzed in understanding Malaysia construction skills training institutions current level of readiness in adopting Construction 4.0?
v. What are the feasible intervention initiatives can be undertaken by the construction industry lead body in Malaysia for the Construction 4.0 adoption readiness way forward?

1.5 Research Framework

A clear research framework is essential to lead a research processes and stages towards achieving its aims and objectives. According to Dickson Adom [22], a clear conceptual framework enables to guide a research path towards building a credible foundation for a good investigation. It is also mandatory requirement of a thesis or dissertation for a researcher to map their study flow comprehensively. In order to organize the flow and provide an overview on the entire contents of the research, the following conceptual framework is structured and outlined as shown at Fig. 1 below:

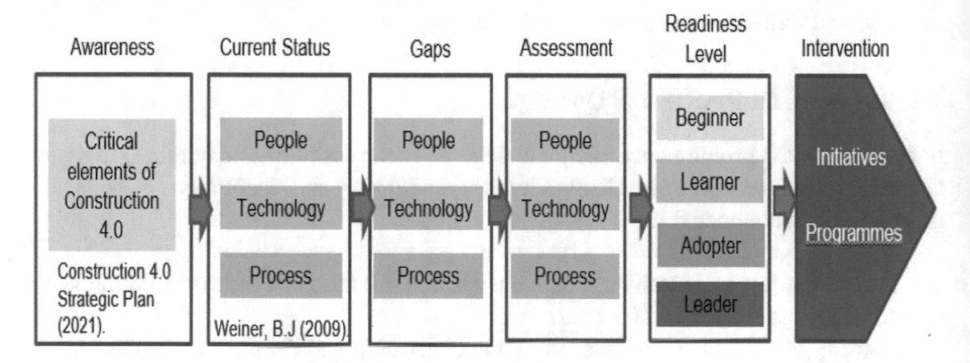

Fig. 1. Conceptual research framework

1.6 Research Limitation

This research is limited to construction skills training institutes in Malaysia and the findings shall not be treated to generalize upon all TVET institutes in Malaysia. However, it is believed that some issues are very much related and may present the same method of intervention as recommended for future way forwards.

2 Literature Review

2.1 Industry 4.0

A better understanding on Industry 4.0 is through the chronological events that lead to the birth of Industry 4.0 era. The industrial revolutions history is always related to certain discovery in manufacturing industry in the form of new innovative inventions.

The innovative ways in steam power engines usage for industrial purposes back in the 18th century had demarcated the beginning of the First Industrial Revolution. The fully man-powered weaving loom in textile industry had been mechanised and powered with steam engines, a real breakthrough that increase to eight times in volume of the same time in manual handling. In brief, the Industrial Revolution transforms the ways of goods and services being produced or delivered. It was also driven by large market demand of certain manufactured product with the advancement of technology leverage during that period of time [5].

The Second Industrial Revolution began in 1870's, whereby mass production systems were used with the introduction of electrical energy. It was also demarcated by an innovative method that Henry Ford had introduced in automobile production which had significantly altered the assembly processes to faster production at much lower cost.

The third industrial revolution began in the late 1950s, whereby manufacturers had slowly adopting the use of electronic machines and later the use of computer technology into their factories. The digital technology and automation with the aid of software programs for robotic tools became the shift from analogue and mechanical based tools. In the past few decades, the fourth industrial revolution has emerged, known as Industry 4.0. The digital technology from previous decades has been elevated to a whole new level with the help of interconnectivity through the Internet of Things (IoT), access to real-time data, and the introduction of cyber-physical systems (CPS).

A more comprehensive, interlinked, and holistic approach for manufacturing industry. Connection between physical with digital allows for better collaboration and accessibilities across internal and external parties. Industry 4.0 offers business owners much better control and accessibility to all aspect of their operation. It allows them to leverage and manipulate instant data to boost productivity, improve processes and project growth.

2.2 The New Technologies

The Fourth Industrial Revolution (Industry 4.0) that was first mentioned by the executive chairman and the founder of the World Economic Forum (WEF), Klaus Schwab, in Davos-Klosters, Switzerland back in 2016 had highlighted that, the integration of business and manufacturing processes as well as all players in the industry value chain is the fundamental concept of Industry 4.0 approach.

According to Klaus Schwab, (2016) the Fourth Industrial Revolution, will change not only what we do but finally also who we are. It will affect our identity and all the issues associated with it: our sense of privacy, our notions of ownership, our consumption patterns, the time we devote to work and leisure, and how we develop our careers, cultivate our skills, meet people, and nurture relationships [5].

In term of technologies associated with Industry 4.0, the so called emerging technologies being discussed around the world are merely new technology. The fact that these technologies are already in the market, however, the interaction and resulting convergence of these technologies is creating an unprecedented pace and breadth of impact [9].

2.3 Construction 4.0

According to Osunsanmi, T.O., Aigbavboa, C.O., Emmanuel Oke, A. and Liphadzi, M. [11], to drive focus of Industry 4.0 discussion towards construction, the term Construction 4.0 was coined from Industry 4.0 as a form of transformation that representing the digitalization of the construction industry. It is no doubt that the construction industry has also benefited from the progress brought by Industry 4.0 in which the term Construction 4.0 was mention by Roland Berger GMBH in Munich, Germany back in 2016.

Construction 4.0 was first mentioned as an awareness concept based on the digitization of the construction industry, promoting the construction industry players to adopt four elements in Industry 4.0 which were digital data, automation, connectivity, and digital access [12].

However, Construction 4.0 should be viewed and understood in a wider perspective as it is not just traditional construction with technological upgrades but a new way of understanding construction in light of innovation and increased productivity [13].

In a nutshell, the transition towards Construction 4.0 need to be strategically paved. A study by [2] had introduced a four-layer implementation plan through an abstruse review of commonly cited technologies of Construction 4.0 which are Building Information Modelling (BIM), Augmented Reality (AR), Virtual Reality (VR), robotics, 3D printing, Artificial Intelligence (AI), and drones. As the digitalization concept promoted in Construction 4.0 mostly is about integration, two level of integration efforts;

i. integration of a Construction 4.0 technology throughout the construction project lifecycle, and
ii. integration and connectivity of Construction 4.0 technologies;

were assessed and evaluated in the study. A roadmap of Construction 4.0 integration across a project life-cycle was proposed and parameters required for the implementation were also highlighted [2].

In Malaysia context, generally, the need to embrace Industry 4.0 technologies have been addressed in many national documents. Focusing into construction industry, a national strategic plan known as Construction 4.0 Strategic Plan 2021–2025 was published in 2020, by the Construction Industry Development Board (CIDB) Malaysia. According to YB Dato' Sri Haji Fadillah bin Haji Yusof, Senior Minister of Infrastructure, Minister of Works Malaysia, Construction 4.0 Strategic Plan is a roadmap for the

Malaysian Construction Industry to embrace the Fourth Industrial Revolution (IR 4.0) in ways that would transform its productivity and competitiveness. The Construction 4.0 is created to be aligned to the Shared Prosperity Vision 2030 (SPV 2030) and the implementation of the National Policy on Industry 4.0 (Industry4WRD). The strategic plan also supports and compliment the National Internet of Things (IoT) Strategic Roadmap, the Malaysia Smart City Framework and the Digital Economy Blueprint, among others. It covers twelve emerging technologies and its implementation plan within the short, medium and the long term [5].

2.4 Construction 4.0 Strategic Plan (2021–2025)

The Construction 4.0 Strategic Plan has been developed in collaboration with industry stakeholders with aim to elevate Malaysia construction industry in the era of technological revolution by embracing digital technologies across the construction supply chain. However, the document does not provide all answers to issues and challenges but rather a framework on how the Malaysian Construction Industry players should position their businesses and enhance their service deliveries with the aid of technologies offered in Industry 4.0.

With a vision to be the leading Construction 4.0 country in the South East Asian Region, the Strategic Plan is aimed to support digital transformation of Malaysia construction industry by leveraging the country's experience and the current digitalised ecosystem. While the Strategic Plan's mission is to transform the Malaysian construction industry by empowering smart construction concept for future society, whereby digital technologies and industrialised manufacturing techniques are utilised in full from the building design phase, construction phase until the building operation and maintenance phase. Through the smart construction concept, productivity can be enhanced, whole life-cycle cost of a building can be minimised while the sustainability of a building can be improved and users' benefits are maximised [15].

In brief, there are 12 "disruptive technologies" which are being focused in order to change the current Malaysia construction landscape towards the future; Building Information Modelling (BIM), pre-fabrication and modular construction, autonomous construction, augmented reality and virtualization, cloud and real time collaboration, 3D scanning and photogrammetry, big data and predictive analysis, internet of things, 3D printing and additive manufacturing, advanced building materials, block chain and artificial intelligence. There are four key enablers of the Strategic Plan are being highlighted in ensuring transition and adoption towards the industry's digital transformation are able to be achieved within 5 years of its implementation [8]. In relation to Enabler 1 identified in the Strategic Plan, under the Strategic Thrust 1 Building Capacity, has stated that "Preparing future workforce for Construction 4.0" is the Strategic Objectives No.1 as shown in Fig. 2 below:

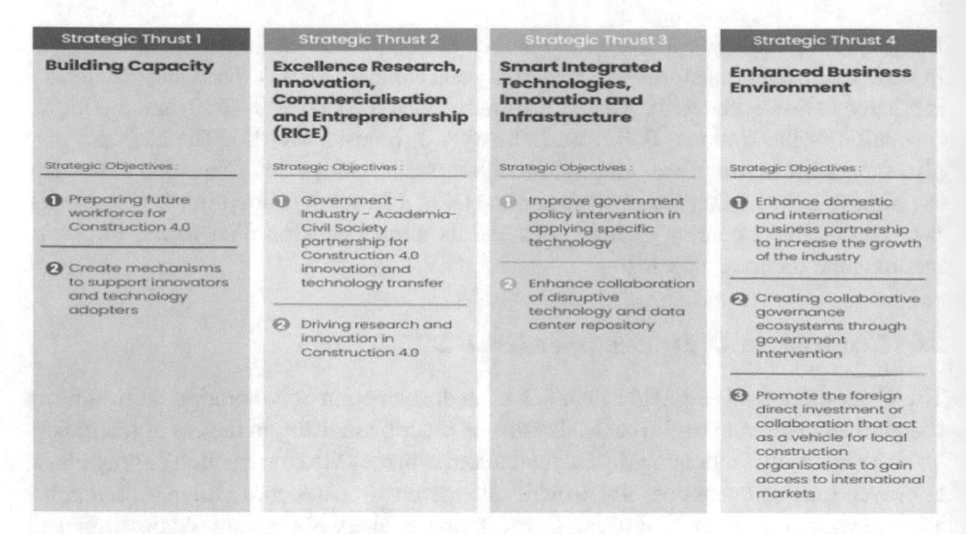

Fig. 2. The four strategic thrusts of construction 4.0 strategic plan 2021–2025 [8].

2.5 Construction Skills Training Institutions in Malaysia

Technical and vocational education and training (TVET) emphasized on the acquisition of knowledge and skills in the world of work. Broad definition on the term of TVET has been discussed in many years. The prominent term is within the context of UNESCO and according to the 2001 UNESCO Revised Recommendation concerning TVET which concluded that TVET refers all aspects of the educational process involving, in addition to general education, the study of technologies and related sciences, and the acquisition of practical skills, attitudes, understanding and knowledge relating to occupations in various sectors of economic and social life (Hollander A., Mar N.Y., 2009).

In the context of construction skills training in Malaysia, the Industry Lead Body (ILB) appointed by the Department of Skills Development (DSD), Ministry of Human Resources Malaysia (MOHR) is the Construction Industry Development Board Malaysia (CIDB) (MOHR Malaysia, 2020). Governed under the Lembaga Pembangunan Industri Pembinaan Malaysia Act 1994 (Act 520), CIDB has the power to accredit and certify skilled construction worker as stated in Sect. 33A (1) to those specified in the Third Schedule (Amendment 2017) and establish, promote and accredit training institutions as stated in Sect. 33B (a) under the same Act.

Basically, there are two main types of institution in relation to construction skills training centre accredited by CIDB;

i. Certified Competency Training Centre (CCTC)
ii. Certified Competency Assessment Centre (CCAC)

A CCTC is a certified training institution which has been accredited to conduct construction skills trainings for the skills trade listed in the Third Schedule of CIDB Act. There are three types of CCTC being accredited, governed and monitored by CIDB which are;

i. CCTC on Management, which offers training for construction executive, officer and manager level (level 5–6)
ii. CCTC on Supervisory, which offers training for construction site supervisor (level 4)
iii. CCTC on Skills, which offers training for skills trade for level 1–3 construction personnel (operator) (level 1–3)

While CCAC is referred to a certified assessment centre accredited by CIDB to conduct assessment for the skills trade assessment (level 1–3) construction personnel.

There are two types of CCAC which are;

i. Local CCAC for skills trade assessment
ii. Overseas CAC for skills trade assessment

2.6 Research Significance

Through the study, it is hoped that the level of awareness on Construction 4.0 among the construction skill training institutions in Malaysia can be understood and concluded. This will lead to further understanding on the level of readiness of construction skills training institutions in Malaysia in adopting Construction 4.0 technologies in delivering their training programs. Areas of concern in the Construction 4.0 adoption process can be highlighted, challenges can be anticipated and further interventions in mitigating problems can be strategized.

As there are still limited research and study conducted in understanding Construction 4.0 adoption clarity by the construction skills training institutions in Malaysia, it is belief this research will contribute to the enrichment of academic studies documentation related to the Construction 4.0 in specific and the Industry 4.0 generally for Malaysia context.

References

1. Muñoz-La Rivera, F., Mora-Serrano, J., Valero, I., Oñate, E.: Methodological-technological framework for construction 4.0. Arch. Comput. Methods Eng. **28**(2), 689–711 (2020). https://doi.org/10.1007/s11831-020-09455-9
2. El Jazzar, M., Urban H., Schranz, C., Nassereddine, H.: Construction 4.0: A Roadmap to Shaping the Future of Construction (2020)
3. García de Soto, B., Agustí-Juan, I., Joss, S., Hunhevicz, J.: Implications of Construction 4.0 to the workforce and organizational structures. Int. J. Constr. Manage., 1–13 (2019)
4. Malaysia's Performance in The Global Competitiveness Index 2019. World Economic Forum (WEF). https://www.mpc.gov.my/wp-content/uploads/2019/10/Malaysias-Performance-in-The-Global-Ccompetitiveness-Report-2019-Topline.pdf. Accessed 06 Sep 2021
5. CIDB Malaysia,: Construction 4.0 Strategic Plan 2021–2025, p. 47, https://www.cream.my/my/publication/construction-4-0-strategic-plan-2021-2025/construction-4-0-strategic-plan-2021-2025. Accessed 06 Dec 2021
6. Zulnaidi, H., et al.: J. Tech. Educ. Training **12**(3), 89–96 (2020). https://penerbit.uthm.edu.my/ojs/index.php/jtet. Accessed 06 Dec 2021

7. Wesam Salah Alaloul, M.S. Liew, Noor Amila Wan Abdullah Zawawi, Icke Baldwin Kennedy: Industrial Revolution 4.0 in the construction industry: Challenges and opportunities for stakeholders. Ain Shams Eng. J. **11**(1), 225–23 (2020)
8. CIDB Malaysia: Construction 4.0 Strategic Plan (2021–2025), Strategic Plan for Construction Industry: Gearing Up for the Fourth Industrial Revolution, p. 8 (2020)
9. MITI Malaysia: Industry 4WRD: National Policy On Industry 4.0, p. 16 (2018)
10. Maskuriy, R., Selamat, A., Ali, K., Maresova, P., Krejcar, O.: Industry 4.0 for the Construction Industry—How Ready Is the Industry? (2020). https://www.researchgate.net/publication/334488532_Industry_40_for_the_Construction. Accessed 17 June 2021
11. Osunsanmi, T.O., Aigbavboa, C.O., Emmanuel Oke, A., Liphadzi, M.: Appraisal of stakeholders' willingness to adopt construction 4.0 technologies for construction projects. Built Environ. Project Asset Manage. **10**(4), 547–565 (2020). https://www.emerald.com/insight/content/doi/https://doi.org/10.1108/BEPAM-12-2018-0159/full/html. Accessed 21 June 2021
12. Forcael, E., Ferrari, I., Opazo-Vega, A., Pulido-Arcas, J.A.: Construction 4.0: a literature review. Sustainability **12**(22), 9755. MDPI AG. (2020). Accessed 21 June 2021
13. Bock, T.: The future of construction automation: technological disruption and the upcoming ubiquity of robotics. Autom. Constr. **59**, 113–121 (2015)
14. CIDB Malaysia: Construction 4.0 strategic plan 2021–2025, p. 47, https://www.cream.my/my/publication/construction-4-0-strategic-plan-2021-2025/construction-4-0-strategic-plan-2021-2025. Accessed 12 June 2021
15. Construction Leadership Council 2018, Smart Construction - A Guide for Housing Clients, p. 3. https://www.constructionleadershipcouncil.co.uk/wp-content/uploads/2018/10/181010-CLC-Smart-Construction-Guide.pdf. Accessed 22 June 2021
16. Construction Skills Training and Competency Program, CIDB Malaysia. https://www.cidb.gov.my/en/construction-info/skills-training/construction-skills-training-competency-program. Accessed 22 June 2021
17. Construction Skills Training and Competency Program, CIDB Malaysia. https://www.cidb.gov.my/en/construction-info/skills-training/construction-skills-training-competency-program. Accessed 22 June 2021
18. Ying Yi, L.: The Edge Markets 'CIDB allocates RM70m for programmes to enhance construction industry' (2020). https://www.theedgemarkets.com/article/cidb-allocates-rm70m-programmes-enhance-construction-industry. Accessed 22 June 2021
19. Aspers, P., Corte, U.: What is qualitative in qualitative research. Qual. Sociol. **42**(2), 139–160 (2019). https://doi.org/10.1007/s11133-019-9413-7
20. William, P., Trochim, M.K.: (2021) https://conjointly.com/kb/qualitative-approaches/. Accessed 23 June 2021
21. Dickson, A., Emad, H., Joe, A-A.: Theoretical and conceptual framework: mandatory ingredients of a quality research. Int. J. Sci. Res. **7**, 438–441 (2018). https://www.researchgate.net/publication/322204158_Theoretical_And_Conceptual_Framework_Mandatory_Ingredients_Of_A_Quality_Research
22. Baškarada, S.: Qualitative case studies guidelines. The Qualitative Report **19**(40), 1–25 (2014). https://papers.ssrn.com/sol3/papers.cfm?abstract_id=2559424
23. Rashid, Y., Rashid, A., Warraich, M.A., Sabir, S.S., Waseem, A.: Case study method: a step-by-step guide for business researchers. Int. J. Qual Methods (2019). https://doi.org/10.1177/1609406919862424
24. DeJonckheere, M., Vaughn, L.M.: Semistructured interviewing in primary care research: a balance of relationship and rigour. Family Med. Commun. Health 2019 **7**, e000057 (2019). https://fmch.bmj.com/content/7/2/e000057
25. Guest, G., Namey, E., Mitchell, M.: Sampling in qualitative research. In: Collecting qualitative data, pp. 41–74. SAGE Publications, Ltd. (2013). https://doi.org/10.4135/9781506374680

A Conceptual Framework for Democratization of Big Data Analytics (BDA)

Nor Haslinda Ismail(✉) and Rose Alinda Alias

Azman Hashim International Business School, Universiti Teknologi Malaysia, Johor, Malaysia
nor78@graduate.utm.my

Abstract. Organizations implement Big Data Analytics (BDA) to help the organization to improve the efficiency and effectiveness of the business. However, the successful of the BDA implementation is not achieved because of lack communication and collaboration between the BDA stakeholders. As we know stakeholders for example a data scientist played an important role in BDA implementation. Therefore, democratization is introduced to address these issues. This paper introduces the concept of democratization in big data analytics (BDA) by applying the Technology Organization Environment Model (TOE) in a conceptual framework that is used in the process of BDA implementation.

Keywords: Big data analytics · Democratization · Technology Organizational Environment (TOE) model

1 Introduction

Big Data is now widely available for organization in different fields. Since the Big data had gained a significant impact for organization in achieving organizational vision and mission. Therefore, by adopting an advanced analytics technology, organizations can use big data for developing innovative insights, products, and services. Big data analytics (BDA) has recently been employed by organizations to speed up decision making, facilitate communication and respond quickly [1]. Therefore, a good communication and collaboration between the stakeholders who have a same understanding and know a clear mission and vision of the organization will make the implementation of Big Data Analytics is successful.

Organizations implement Big Data Analytics (BDA) to help them improve the efficiency and effectiveness of the business and for getting assistant in the decision-making process. However, the effectiveness of the BDA implementation is not achieved because of lack communication and collaboration between the BDA stakeholders. In order to make big data analytics implement successful this study introduce the concept of democratization in BDA.

This paper is aimed at further understanding the concept of democratization for Big Data Analytics in organizations. And this paper also provides an overview of democratization in big data analytics. The successful implementation of big data analytics influences by the factors that is related to the successful of BDA such as technology

F. Saeed et al. (Eds.): IRICT 2021, LNDECT 127, pp. 707–712, 2022.
https://doi.org/10.1007/978-3-030-98741-1_59

such as the technology readiness, unclear of project goals, lack of experience with technology. Secondly organization factors also will influence the democratization of BDA success for instance factors of demand for big data, senior leadership, trust in project team and management policies and procedures. Finally, the environmental factors such as government regulations also will give an impact in democratization of BDA success.

This paper is organized as follows: Sect. 2 discusses issues in democratization of BDA, Section 3 discusses the theoretical discussion on Technological Organization and Environmental (TOE) and stakeholder theories. Section 4 describes the proposed model in detail. Finally, Sect. 5 concludes this paper, along with the recommendation for future work.

2 Problem Statement

Big data analytic implementation is one of the challenges processes which is required a good communication and collaboration between the stakeholders involve in the implementation process. Furthermore, as a data scientist who play an important role in BDA implementation, he or she must full adopt their capabilities in making a decision [11]. The research starts with an approach of concept of democratization in big data analytics. The paper illustrates the use of democratization for BDA success in organization and shows the current gaps between the literature and the research aims to understand the concept of democratization in order to make BDA implementation successful.

3 Literature Review

3.1 Big Data and Big Data Analytics

Big Data is defined as "information assets characterized by such a high volume, velocity, and variety to require specific technology and analytical methods for its transformation into value" [2]. Big data is an abstract concept. There is no single description for it, and research researchers, scientific and technology firms, data analysts, and technical practitioners all have diverse perspectives on what it is [3] (Fig. 1).

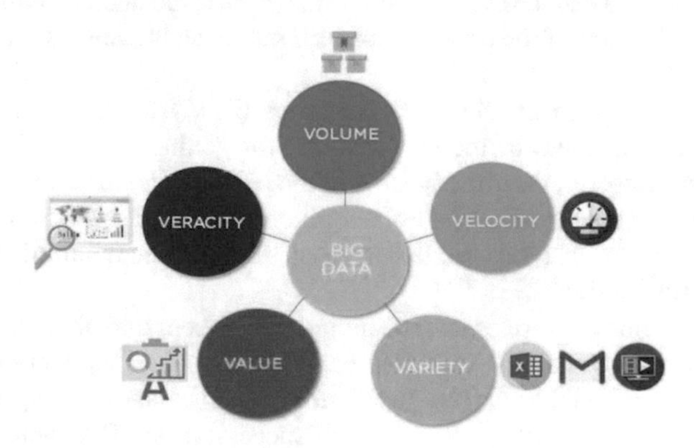

Fig. 1. The 5Vs of big data (www.quora.com)

The big data analytic topic has become a hot research topic in recent ten years. Thus, many organizations, both commercial and public, are concerned about implementing BDA because they expect insights from BDA to help them improve productivity, satisfy consumer requests, cut operational costs, and expand their businesses [4].

3.2 Democratization Definition from Previous Work

Data democratization has lately been discussed in many industry, with the suggestion that data should be democratized to make data analytics more accessible [5]. Additionally, with democratization stakeholders could readily draw on information across an organization which enables them to interact and communicate effectively among them. Below are the studies of the concept of democratization apply generally in a Big Data field:

- First the term of democratization of technology was introduced by [6] stated that technology that was once considered high-tech is now available to practically everyone. The technologies used by ordinary peoples are growing in the opposite way; they are developing later in industry than in everyday use[7].
- The democratization of data, which is defined as intra-organizational open data, allows employees to transition from data users to citizen data scientists who may give useful insight [8].
- Democratization is defined as an organizational culture that encourages information sharing and acceptance of diversity based on fresh knowledge [1].

3.3 The Importance of Technology Democratization

From what we have study from the past literature, democratization will help organization to articulate of strategies based on availability, accessibility, and usability of the information flow. Furthermore, democratization will allow data to transit from the non-technical to technical people within the organization.

4 Theoretical Framework

4.1 Technological Organizational Environmental (TOE) and Stakeholder Theories

The TOE framework was created by [9] which the technological, organizational, and environmental elements all have a role in how a technology innovation is embraced and deployed. All three aspects were utilized in this study since they have been found to be essential in the literature when evaluating BDA implementation democratization. In terms of technology, consider whether the organization's current technology and experience with it are compatible with the BDA deployment. The organizational aspect examines BDA demand, as well as a few other factors such as project team trust, organizational norms and procedures, and senior leadership. For the environmental aspect looks into the government regulations that will influence the democratization of BDA implementation success.

4.2 B. Definition of the Stakeholders?

A stakeholders can be anybody who can affect or affected by an organization, strategy, or project implementation. In other definitions suggest that stakeholders must be those who have the power to impact an organization or project. For example people or small groups with the power to respond to, negotiate with and change the strategic future of the organization [10].

However [11] defines a stakeholder as any group or individual who can affect or is affected by the achievement of the organization's objectives. For example, data scientist may not have a choice in the process of implementation of a Big Data Analytics but he or she will be the key factor in the long-term adoption of the project. If they do not fully adopt and use with full capabilities, then it will impact to the successful of BDA implementation. As a result, stakeholders must be identified, even if they look powerless at first. It is also being used in other domains where conflicting interests and management are important, such as operational research, political economy, and, of course, information systems research [12].

4.3 The Proposed Conceptual Framework

This paper provides a conceptual framework as indicated in Fig. 2 based on the theoretical discussion above and insights from the literature. It shows the relationship between the four dimensions of the study. Each dimension and its relationship with other construct as depicted in the model are discussed further in the remainder of the paper. From the proposed conceptual framework, four propositions are suggested as follows:

Proposition 1 (P1): From the technological perspective, adequate technology, with a clear project goal and have an experience using the technology will impact the democratization of BDA success in the organization.

Proposition 2 (P2): From the organizational perspective, the combination of strong senior leadership, trust in project team, adequate management policy and procedure and good demand for big data will impact the democratization of BDA implementation in the organization.

Proposition 3 (P3): From the environmental perspective, government regulation will impact the democratization of BDA implementation in the organization.

Proposition 4(P4): Stakeholders with good communication and collaboration during the process of implementation of BDA will strongly influence the successful of BDA in the organization.

We will evaluate the propositions qualitatively using data from the in-depth interviews with the stakeholders in the future study.

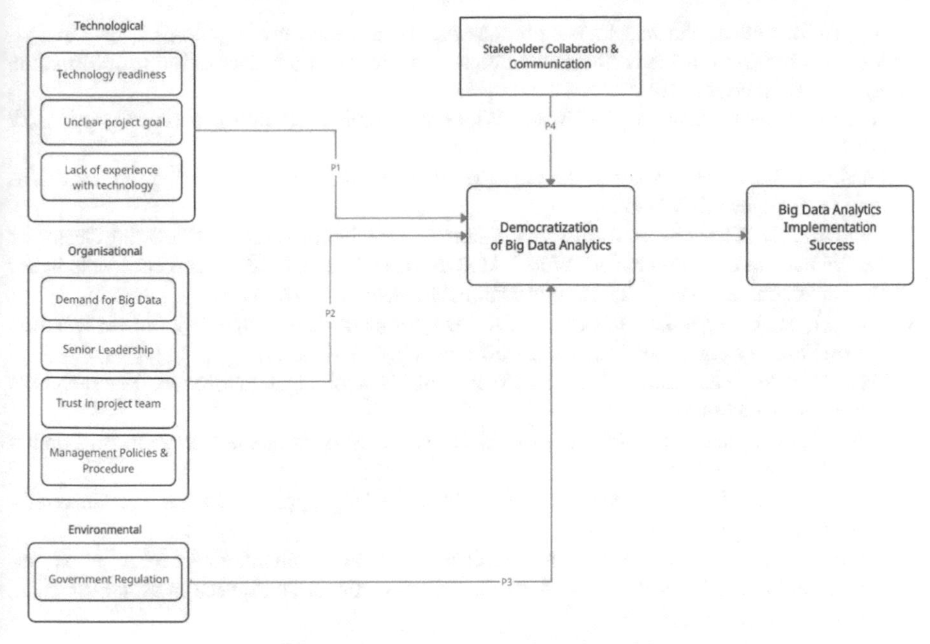

Fig. 2. Propose conceptual framework

5 Conclusion

This main aim of the study was to highlights the concept of democratization of BDA implementation success in the organization. From the literature reviewed, organizational, technological, environmental (TOE) factors and stakeholders will influence the democratization of BDA implementation success. This research was underpinned by TOE framework and eight BDA factors. Thus, future researchers will be able to extend the current of democratization of BDA using the proposed framework.

The authors express their gratitude to Universiti Teknologi Malaysia (UTM) for providing support to this work and, special thanks to all reviewers of an earlier version of this paper for their helpful.

References

1. Hyun, Y., Hosoya, R., Kamioka, T.: The moderating role of democratization culture: Improving agility through the use of big data analytics. In: Proceedings of the 23rd Pacific Asia Conference on Information System Security ICT Platform 4th Industry Revolution, PACIS 2019 (2019)
2. De Mauro, A., Greco, M., Grimaldi, M., Ritala, P.: In (Big) data we trust: value creation in knowledge organizations - introduction to the special issue. Inf. Process. Manag. **54**(5), 755–757 (2018)
3. Chen, M., Mao, S., Liu, Y.: Big data: a survey. Mob. Netw. Appl. **19**(2), 171–209 (2014). https://doi.org/10.1007/s11036-013-0489-0

4. Ijab, M.T., Salleh, ohdMa.M., Wahab, S.M.A., Bakar, A.A.: Investigating big data analytics readiness. In: 6th International Conference on Research and Innovation in Information Systems (ICRIIS) (2019)
5. Díaz, T., Rowshankish, A., Saleh, K.: Why data culture matters. Mckensey Q., pp. 1–17 (2018)
6. Friedman, T.L.: The Lexus and the Olive Tree: Understanding Globalization. Farrar, Straus and Giroux, New York (1999)
7. Karlovitz, T.J.: The democratization of technology – and its limitation. In: Managing Customer Experiences in an Omnichannel World: Melody of Online and Offline Environments in the Customer Journey, pp. 13–25. Emerald Publishing Limited (2020)
8. Awasthi, P., George, J.J., George, J.: A case for data democratization. In: Association Information System, AMCIS 2020 Proceedings, pp. 0–10 (2020)
9. Tornatzky, M., Fleischer, L.G.: The Process of Technological Innovation. Massachusets Lexington Books (1990)
10. Eden, C., Ackermann, F.: Making Strategy: The Journey of Strategic Management. London Sage Publications (1998)
11. Freeman, R.E.: Strategic Management: A Stakeholder Approach. Cambridge University Press, Cambridge (1984)
12. Pouloudi, A.: Aspects of the stakeholder concept and their implications for information systems development. In: Proceedings of the Hawaii International Conference on System Science, vol. 00, no. c, p. 254 (1999)

Construction 4.0 Intervention in Quality Assessment System in Construction's Implementation

Syed Muhammad Nazir Bin Syed Othman[1(✉)] and Zulhasni Abdul Rahim[2]

[1] Malaysia-Japan International Institute of Technology, Kuala Lumpur, Malaysia
syedmuhammadnazir@graduate.utm.my
[2] University of Technology Malaysia, Kuala Lumpur, Malaysia

Abstract. The quality of construction projects (buildings and infrastructure) is an important parameter in determining the maturity level of construction industry. The issues related to quality in construction projects is not relatively new and has been around for decades. To address this issue, Construction Industry Development Board (CIDB) Malaysia has introduced Quality Assessment System in Construction (QLASSIC) or also known as Construction Industry Standard 7 (CIS7) back in 2007 as a benchmark yardstick to rate the quality level of building projects specifically in the workmanship area. The association of Industry 4.0 concept with construction delivery process has resulted the Construction 4.0 concept. Through the adoption of Construction 4.0, the construction industry is expected to experience major changes in the entire project delivery process. These changes require further update on the existing CIS7 to suit the measurement methodology with the upcoming emerging technologies and new construction methods. The clarity of gaps between existing measurement parameters stated in CIS7 and the requirement of emerging technologies must be made clear and well-understood. This will be the foundation for CIDB Malaysia as sole construction leader in Malaysia to improvise CIS7 to a higher standard and ready for Industry 4.0 era. As there are limited study and research conducted in understanding the integration of Construction 4.0 in QLASSIC and limitation of CIS7, this study will contribute to the enrichment of academic studies documentation related to Construction 4.0 generally and QLASSIC in specific.

Keywords: Industry 4.0 · Construction 4.0 · QLASSIC · CIS7 · Quality-rated building · CIMP · CITP

1 Research Background

1.1 Introduction

The Fourth Industrial Revolution (Industry 4.0) that was first mentioned by the executive chairman and the founder of the World Economic Forum (WEF), Klaus Schwab, in Switzerland back in 2016. During his presentation, Klaus mentioned that the integration of business and manufacturing processes as well as all players in the industry value chain

F. Saeed et al. (Eds.): IRICT 2021, LNDECT 127, pp. 713–722, 2022.
https://doi.org/10.1007/978-3-030-98741-1_60

is the profound concept of Industry 4.0 approach [1]. The original concept of Industry 4.0 is mainly focusing on range of advanced technologies adoption across all industries value chain. Automation, robotics, artificial intelligence, nanotechnology, quantum computing, biotechnology, industrial internet of things, decentralized consensus, fifth generation (5G) wireless technologies, 3D printing, and fully autonomous vehicles are considered as the main emerging technologies that driving Industry 4.0 forward while at the same time creating both threats and opportunities to the conventional industries environment.

Following the Industry 4.0, industry experts and researchers has explored the integration of emerging technologies with construction process thus creating the new concept of Construction 4.0. Construction 4.0 can be understood as a counterpart of Industry 4.0 in which, aims to digitalize the whole life cycle of construction project monitoring and with the aid of multiple technologies [2]. Through the adoption of Construction 4.0, it is expected the major changes to take place in the construction process delivery stages, project structures and organization and ultimately integrate the highly known fragmented construction industry atmosphere. These changes will further require the major change on the entire component of construction industry such as standards for practices, personnel skills competency and numerous procedures in construction activities. From construction standards point of view, the existing standards should be updated with the consideration of the emerging Construction 4.0 technologies application in construction practices.

1.2 Issue Statement

Today, more and more countries have come forward to ensure they are left behind in becoming the best in adopting Industry 4.0 technologies. Malaysia has portrayed a serious commitment internationally to adopt and explore digital technologies into its economic value chain thus transforming businesses. Malaysia was ranked at 22nd position worldwide in Institute of Management Development (IMD) World Competitiveness Ranking 2019 and 26th position in World Competitiveness Yearbook (WCY) in 2019 based on the progress of technological infrastructure and the agility of its businesses. From construction perspective, the industry player must be made ready to drive the technological advancement from various angle including industry standards [3].

As the national document which referred daily by construction players in project implementation activities, it is crucial for CIS7 to be updated from time to time to suit the changes which will take place in construction industry. CIS7 was developed in 2007 and since that, it has undergone revision process once in 2014, where it was updated to incorporate the parameters enlisted in 8th Edition of CONQUAS. With upcoming revolution around the corner, it is crucial for CIS7 to be updated and equipped with measurement parameters which considered the implementation of new emerging technologies as suggested in Construction 4.0. To achieve this, it is utmost important to first understand the limitation of CIS7 and the requirement of emerging technologies to be implement in construction projects.

1.3 Research Purpose

The purpose of this research is to understand the limitation of CIS7 towards the adoption of Construction 4.0 technologies in construction practices. This research also will dive deep in understanding the implementation method of Construction 4.0 technologies in construction projects thus assisting the formulation of future CIS7 revision process.

1.4 Research Objectives and Questions

In response to the issue identified which related to the limitation of CIS7 in adoption of Construction 4.0 technologies change, this research is conducted to:

i. Identify the Construction 4.0 technologies implementation method in construction projects.
ii. Assess the feasibility of existing quality measurement methodology in CIS7 with Construction 4.0 technologies implementation method.
iii. Identify the new parameter required to support the requirement of Construction 4.0 technologies.
iv. Propose way forward for CIDB Malaysia to undertake the revision of CIS7 based on the Construction 4.0 technologies adoption gaps identified.

In order to streamline the research towards achieving the objectives set, the following research questions are developed to understand the identified problem in depth as well as building further argumentative questions to verify research findings:

i. How are the new Construction 4.0 technologies should be implemented in construction works?
ii. What are the critical elements in CIS7 which require urgent attention in accelerating Construction 4.0 technologies adoption?
iii. What would be the new parameter that has to be incorporated in CIS7 as Construction 4.0 technologies is implemented?

1.5 Research Framework

The development of theoretical and conceptual framework is important to provide an illustration pathway of research to support theoretical constructs. The objective of both framework is to ensure generalization, guide the research to a meaningful finding and aligned with theoretical constructs. Research without the theoretical or conceptual framework makes it difficult for readers in ascertaining the academic position and the underlying factors to the researcher?s assertions or hypotheses. This renders the research sloppy and not appreciable as contributing significantly to the advancement of the frontiers of knowledge [4].

In this research, the design and flow to provide the overview of the research content is developed by using RIBA Plan of Work 2020 and Construction Project Lifecycle [5]. The intervention of Construction 4.0 technologies will be analyzed throughout 5 construction phase that are conceptual stage, planning & design stage, procurement stage, construction stage and operation & maintenance stage. The overview of conceptual framework for this research as follows (Fig. 1):

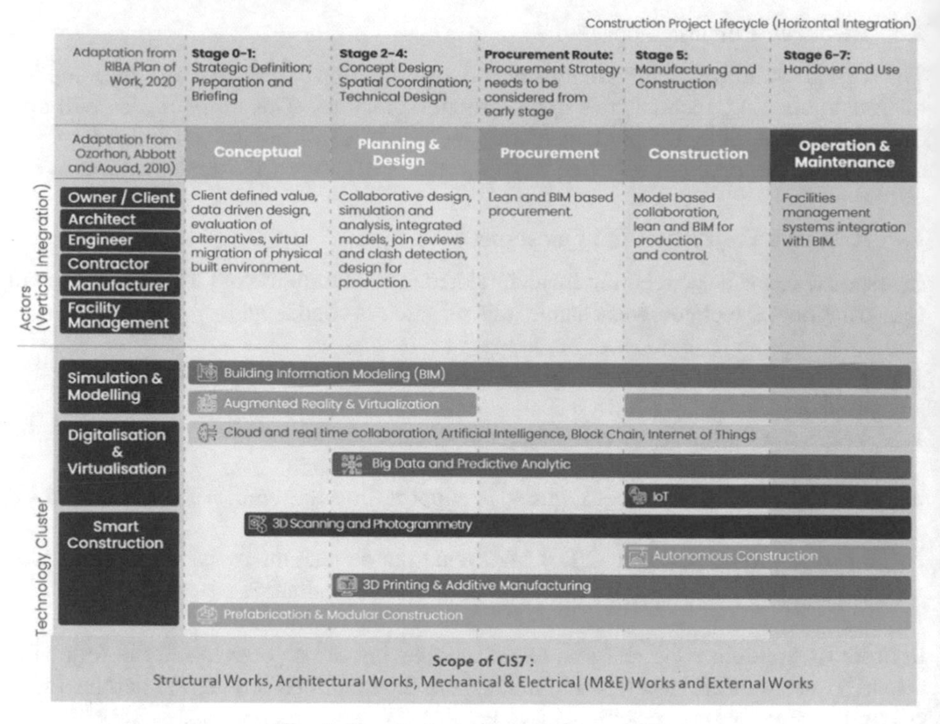

Fig. 1. Research conceptual framework

1.6 Research Limitation

This research is limited to Construction Industry Standard 7 (CIS7) implementation in Malaysia and the findings shall not be treated to generalize in other country. However, it is believed that some issues are very much related and may present the same method of intervention as recommended for future way forwards.

2 Literature Review

2.1 Overview of Malaysia Construction Industry

The construction industry has been a key economic engine in Malaysian economy ever since and play a significant role in driving the physical development of nation. From economy point of view, the construction industry possesses a strong composition with strong volume contribution in economy. In the past ten years, the total volume of construction projects executed by both public and private sectors remains above RM100 billion annually, peaking RM241 billion in 2016.

The construction industry is a unique industry because of its ability to create two-times multiplier economic effect and it is the only industry that have more than 120 other industries relying on for their growth and sustainability. In general, construction activities consume about 15% of total manufacturing output in Malaysia [6]. The construction industry act as a vital component of Malaysia?s Gross Domestic Product (GDP) with approximately 4% contribution in 2013 and continually improve annually and recorded peak at 5.9% in 2017 and decline to 0.4% in 2020 [2]. The growth of 5.9% in 2017 surpass the expectation set in Construction Industry Transformation Programme (CITP) which was 5% by 2020 to outpace Malaysia?s overall economy which is expected to grow at a steady rate of 5% - 6% per year.

Since March 2020, Malaysia construction industry was hit by global COVID-19 pandemic as the Movement Restriction Order (MCO) was enforce by government, all construction activities were put at hold. According to Senior Minister of Works and Infrastructure of Malaysia, the estimated lost in construction industry is RM42 billion during MCO period of March 2020 until September 2021. As Malaysia entering endemic stage, construction industry is expected to recover at 10.3% per year as the industry demonstrates strong correlation with economic development, with the construction share of GDP positively correlated with GDP per capita. As developing nation, there is a big necessity for more higher standard and quality, energy-efficient buildings, and infrastructures to improve people?s life quality. In the past 10-years, we have seen the demand is being delivered by government through series of mega projects such as Mass Rapid Transit (MRT), Light Rail Transit (LRT), Highways (Pan-Borneo, DUKE Phase 2 and Phase 3) etc. In future, more of such projects is required to match the demands and support national population growth headings should be numbered (Fig. 2).

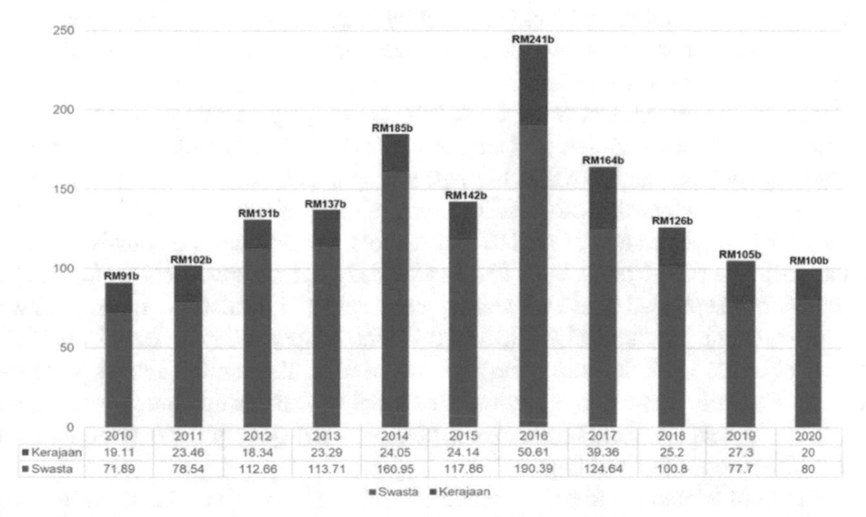

	2010	2011	2012	2013	2014	2015	2016	2017	2018	2019	2020
Kerajaan	19.11	23.46	18.34	23.29	24.05	24.14	50.61	39.36	25.2	27.3	20
Swasta	71.89	78.54	112.66	113.71	160.95	117.86	190.39	124.64	100.8	77.7	80

Fig. 2. Construction projects volume by cost from 2010 to 2020 (Source: Convince CIDB Malaysia)

2.2 Quality Assessment System in Construction (QLASSIC)

Conventionally, the quality of the management, operation and products of the organization is measured by using the standard management system derived from International

Organization of Standardization (ISO) 9000. Because of the nature of construction is different from other industries such as manufacturing, the implementation of ISO9000 in construction industry was founded very difficult. Due to this, the QLASSIC is introduced by CIDB for the use and benefits of the entire construction industry. QLASSIC is a simplified terminology for Quality Assessment System in Construction, developed by CIDB Malaysia in late 2005 with the main objectives to benchmark the level of quality of the construction industry in Malaysia and have a standard quality assessment system for quality of workmanship of building projects. QLASSIC is a system or method used to measure and assess the quality of construction work based on the Construction Industry Standard (CIS 7:2014), similar to guidelines used for construction projects in achieving quality outcomes [11].

Initially, QLASSIC was developed as CIS7:2006 through the adoption of 6th Edition of Construction Quality Assessment System (CONQUAS), a management system developed by Singapore?s Building & Construction Authority (BCA) [12]. QLASSIC was then updated in 2014 in accordance with CIS7:2014 and 8th Edition of CONQUAS [11]. The quality and reliability of CIS7:2006 was monitored and examined by a Technical Committee formed by CIDB which composed the representatives from various professional bodies and associations. To further enhance its adoption, QLASSIC initiatives was elevated to national agenda when it was incorporated in Construction Industry Master Plan 2006?2015 (CIMP) followed by Construction Industry Transformation Programme 2016 ? 2020 (CITP). Despite of various efforts done, QLASSIC adoption in on-ground projects is still low and not widely practiced by construction stakeholders. Due to this, it is significant for a study to be conducted to explore the critical issues and challenges faced by construction stakeholders in adopting QLASSIC in construction projects.

Currently, the assessment using QLASSIC are only applicable to building projects regardless the size of the project and are not applicable to benchmark the quality level of infrastructure projects such as roads, highways, seaport etc. Commonly, the assessment is being conducted on building projects including landed residential, stratified residential, building for public use such as offices and schools, in addition to distinctive buildings such as hospitals and airports, etc. [13]. In CIS 7:2014, the assessment methodology is created as four separated principal components that are i. Structural Works, ii. Architectural Works, iii. Mechanical & Electrical Works (M&E) and iv. External Works. The assessment of the workmanship is carried out based on the components as established under the standard where points are awarded if the workmanship complies to the standard. These points are then summarized, giving a total quality (TQ) score called the QLASSIC Score for the building [11].

The level of adoption and performance of QLASSIC give an indication of how deep the quality element is emphasize in construction project generally. The information of both adoption and performance can assessed through the reports published by CIDB Malaysia. To understand the implementation status in construction sector the information of data and statistics on the volume of project assessed using QLASSIC and total number of building projects and data on average QLASSIC score achieved was analyzed.

According to statistical data published in [14], from early year 2015 till 2020, there were 1,969 buildings projects completed the quality assessment by using QLASSIC. As comparison, the total buildings projects recorded for the same timeline is 22,495 projects.

This data shows there are only 8.7% of building projects in Malaysia were quality-rated using QLASSIC for the past 5 years. Based on this statistic, the QLASSIC adoption for the past 5 year is ranging between 6% to 15%. The adoption increased from 2015 to 2017 and peak at 15%. The adoption declined till 2019 at 6.4% before slightly increased in 2020 at 7.6%. In terms of QLASSIC performance, the statistic shows a nearly stagnant scoring from 2015 to 2020. All projects assessed with QLASSIC achieved an average QLASSIC score between 69% to 74% (Figs. 3, 4 and 5).

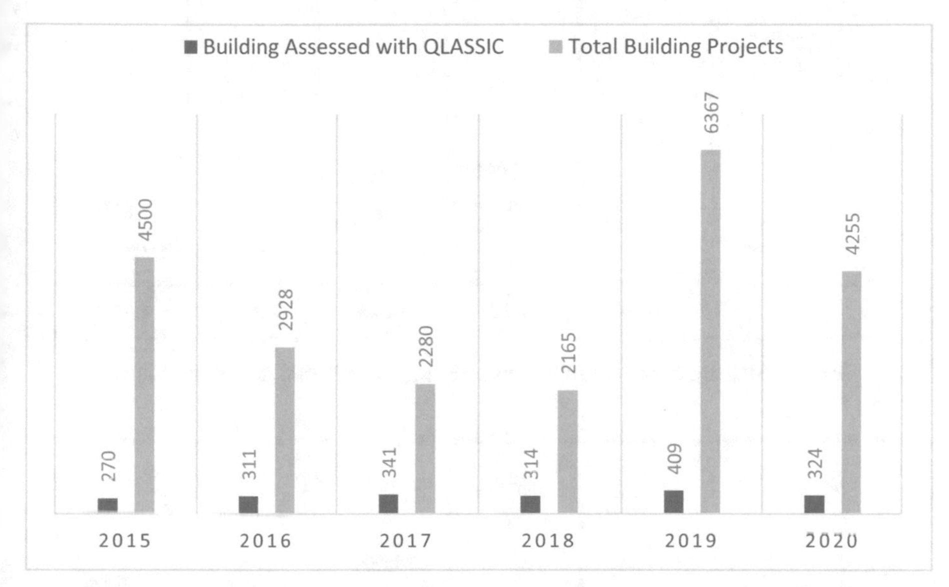

Fig. 3. Data on building assessed with QLASSIC and total number of building projects in Malaysia (from 2015 until 2020)

2.3 Construction 4.0 in Malaysia Landscape

The terminology Construction 4.0 was derived from the concept of Industry 4.0 where the bigger concept of Industry 4.0 was streamlined and focused on the needs and its intervention in construction industry. The main focus of Industry 4.0 is to encourage technology adoption across manufacturing industry in such modernizing industry, improving productivity and people?s life. Automation, robotics, artificial intelligence, nanotechnology, quantum computing, biotechnology, industrial internet of things, decentralized consensus, fifth generation (5G) wireless technologies, 3D printing, and fully autonomous vehicles are considered as the main emerging technologies that driving Industry 4.0 forward while at the same time creating both threats and opportunities to the conventional industries environment. Even though the idea of Industry 4.0 was originally focused on manufacturing industry, the idea of revolutionizing the industry was followed by other industries.

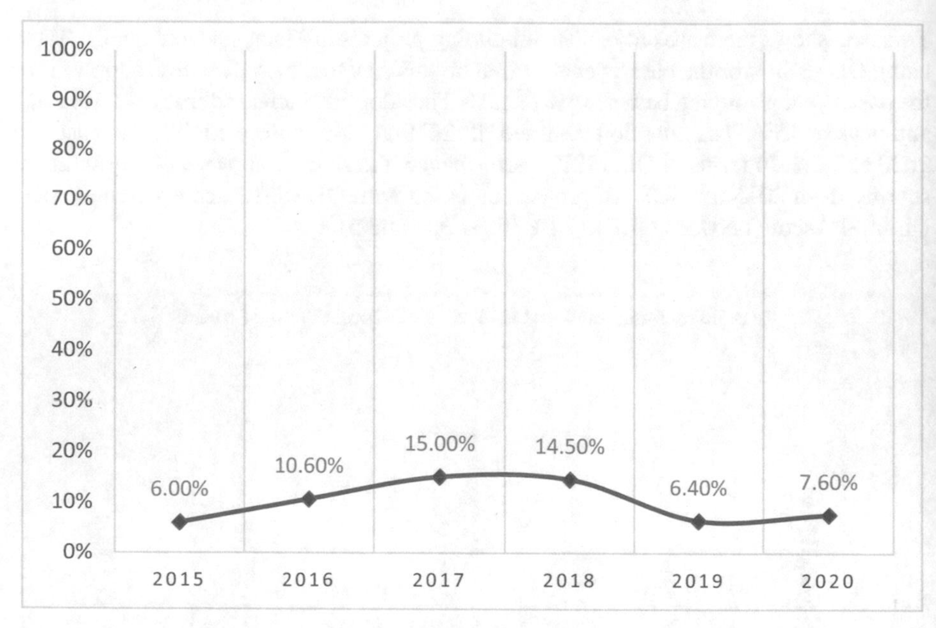

Fig. 4. Statistic on QLASSIC adoption in Malaysia (From 2015 until 2020)

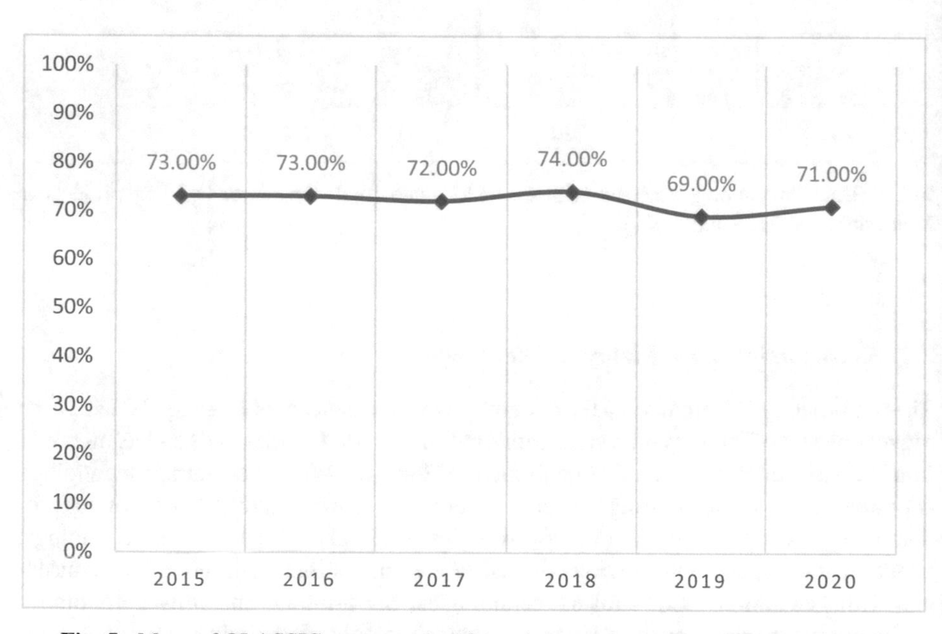

Fig. 5. Mean of QLASSIC score resulted from the assessment (From 2015 until 2020)

Just like other industries, construction industry has been moving towards the same direction. Industry experts and researchers has been actively participated in exploring the integration between the emerging technologies in Industry 4.0 into construction thus creating the term ?Construction 4.0? into research corpus [2]. Construction 4.0 can be understood as a counterpart of Industry 4.0 in which, aims to digitalize the whole life cycle of construction project monitoring and with the aid of multiple technologies. Via the adoption of Construction 4.0, the existing fragmented construction practices is expected to meet major changes as well as construction process delivery stages, project structures and organization. These changes will require the further elevation on the existing standards of practices to suit with the requirement of Construction 4.0 technologies implementation. In Malaysia context, the standards which refer to construction quality (CIS7) is govern by CIDB Malaysia. In order to ensure smooth technology adoption, it is vital for CIS7 to be updated at par with the requirement of Construction 4.0 technology.

In 2020, Malaysia government through Ministry of Works has launched Construction 4.0 Strategic Plan 2021?2025 (CR4.0). The document has been developed in collaboration with industry stakeholders with aim to elevate Malaysia construction industry in the era of technological revolution by embracing digital technologies across the construction supply chain. According to CR4.0, 12 disruptive technologies were identified to be focused on in order to change the current Malaysia construction landscape towards the future that are Building Information Modelling (BIM), pre-fabrication and modular construction, autonomous construction, augmented reality and virtualization, cloud and real time collaboration, 3D scanning and photogrammetry, big data and predictive analysis, internet of things, 3D printing and additive manufacturing, advanced building materials, block chain and artificial intelligence. The Construction 4.0 is created with aligned to the Shared Prosperity Vision 2030 (SPV 2030) and the implementation of the National Policy on Industry 4.0 (Indus-try4WRD). The strategic plan also supports and compliment the National Internet of Things (IoT) Strategic Roadmap, the Malaysia Smart City Framework, and the Digital Economy Blueprint, among others [5].

3 Conclusion

It is belief that through this study, the implementation method of Construction 4.0 technologies on real ground can be identified. A clear understanding on it will further assist the identification of the gap between existing CIS7 and the requirement of emerging technologies implementation in construction sector. The clarity within this area will then be an assist for future revision process of CIS7 in supporting the adoption of Construction 4.0 technologies by industry players.

As there are limited study and research conducted in understanding the integration of Construction 4.0 in QLASSIC and limitation of CIS7, it is hoped this study will contribute to the enrichment of academic studies documentation related to Construction 4.0 generally and QLASSIC in specific.

References

1. Muñoz-La Rivera, F., Mora-Serrano, J., Valero, I., Oñate, E.: Methodological-technological framework for construction 4.0. Arch. Comput. Methods Eng. **28**(2), 689?711 (2020). https://doi.org/10.1007/s11831-020-09455-9

2. El Jazzar M., Urban H., Schranz C., Nassereddine H.: Construction 4.0: a roadmap to shaping the future of construction. In: 2020 Proceedings of the 37th ISARC, Kitakyushu, Japan, pp. 1314-1321 (2020)
3. Malaysia?s Performance in The Global Competitiveness Index 2019. World Economic Forum (WEF). https://www.mpc.gov.my/wp-content/uploads/2019/10/Malaysias-Performance-in-The-Global-Ccompetitiveness-Report-2019-Topline.pdf
4. Abdul Rahman, H., Berawi, M.A., Berawi, A.R., Mohamed, O., Othman, M., Yahya, I.A.: Delay mitigation in the Malaysian construction industry. J. Constr. Eng. Manage. **132**(2), 125?133 (2006)
5. CIDB Malaysia: Construction 4.0 Strategic Plan 2021?2025, p. 47. https://www.cream.my/my/publication/construction-4-0-strategic-plan-2021-2025/costruction-4-0-strategic-plan-2021-2025
6. CIDB Malaysia, Construction Industry Transformation Programme 2016?2020 Public Document Pages 20, 44, 63?65 (2015)
7. Department of Statistics Malaysia (DOSM), Malaysia Economic Performance 2020. https://www.dosm.gov.my/v1/index.php?r=column/cthemeByCat&cat=100&bul_id=dUl6ZW5ZaTMycTV4bW51d0NlWWYzUT09&menu_id=TE5CRUZCblh4ZTZMODZIbmk2aWRRQT09. Accessed 25 Oct 2021
8. Abdul-Rahman, H., Wang, C., Wood, L., Khoo, Y.: Defects in affordable housing projects in Klang Valley, Malaysia. J. Perform. Constructed Facilities, in press (2012). https://doi.org/10.1061/(ASCE)CF.1943-5509.0000413
9. Sufian, A., Abdul-Rahman, R.: Quality housing: regulation and administrative framework in Malaysia. Int. J. Econ. Manage. **2**(1), 141?156 (2008)
10. Ali, A.S., Wen, K.H.: Building defects: possible solution for poor construction workmanship. J. Build. Perf. [S.l.], 2(1), (2012). ISSN 2180-2106. http://spaj.ukm.my/jsb/index.php/jbp/article/view/20. Accessed 25 Oct 2021
11. CIDB Malaysia. Construction Industry Standard, CIS7:2014, Quality Assessment System For Building Construction Works. CIDB Malaysia (2014)
12. Ali, M., Ismail, R., Kam, K.J., Dzulkalnine, N.: Preliminary findings on potential areas of improvement in QLASSIC. Elixir Proj. Qual. **76**, 28341?28349 (2014)
13. CIDB Malaysia. CIDB Technical Report Publication No: 206: Analysis Defect CIS 7 & QLASSIC Acceptable Score (2015?2018). CIDB Malaysia. Kuala Lumpur, Malaysia. ISBN: 978-967-0997-84-1 (2020)
14. CIDB Malaysia. Buletin QLASSIC (2020). https://www.cidb.gov.my/sites/default/files/202103/Buletin%20QLASSIC%202020%20-%20Final%20%28A4%29.pdf
15. Hairuddin, M., Hassan, P.F., Siti Khalijah, Y.: Construction Handbook Series Project Management, Construction Management & Site Management. Penerbitan UTHM, Johor, Malaysia (2018)

Gamification Elements in E-Library Services in Higher Education: A Systematic Review

Folashade Oyinlola Adedokun[1,2](✉), Norasnita Ahmad[2], and Suraya Miskon[2]

[1] The Federal Polytechnic, Ado-Ekiti, Nigeria
oyinlola@graduate.utm.my
[2] Universiti Teknologi Malaysia, 81300 Skudai, Johor Bahru, Malaysia

Abstract. E-libraries in higher education is to support teaching, learning, and research. Various services like online library services, e-reference services, e-SDI, and bibliographic services are rendered in the library to meet the users' information, education, and research needs. E-libraries in institutions of higher learning play vital roles, such as the provision of metadata to access e-resources and the introduction of plagiarism software into the course management system to promote good practice. Despite the relevance of the e-library services, the library management experiences low patronage by the prospective users. As a result, of not being aware of the e-library services within the academic community, the academic performance of the potential users is affected negatively. Based on this, there is a need to adopt gamification in e-library services in higher education to promote library services and improve the academic performance of library users. Gamification is an act of using game elements to engage and motivate learners in non-game contexts. The study aims to explore various game elements used in e-library services. Therefore, this study explores the Scopus database to identify, extract, and analyze various game elements used in e-library services. Articles were selected using PRISMA Statement for inclusion and exclusion criteria. Out of the 41 articles extracted, 29 were thoroughly read and analyzed. In addition, the study results show that rewards, points, feedback, badges, leaderboards, and prizes are significant elements used in e-library services to bring fun, engagement, and enthusiasm. This study will guide the library management in providing necessary facilities that will aid in the implementation of gamification in e-library services in higher education. Lastly, the study suggests future research.

Keywords: Gamification · Game elements · e-Library service · Higher education

1 Introduction

The advent of ICT has brought tremendous change to every facet of life. Libraries have benefitted immensely from technological advancement that has turned the entire world into a global village over time. Digital library is the result of the influence of technological development in the educational field and consequently has found its application in various libraries, like national, academic, special, school, research, and private [1]. The

F. Saeed et al. (Eds.): IRICT 2021, LNDECT 127, pp. 723–733, 2022.
https://doi.org/10.1007/978-3-030-98741-1_61

term digital library is synonymous with e-library, virtual or library without walls. Digital Library stores information in digital form or fulfils information needs from external information sources to users registered as specific customers and the community in general. The e-libraries found in the institutions of higher learning are to support teaching, learning, and research. Examples are Universities, Polytechnics, and Colleges of Education. Today, digital libraries offer online library services, e-reference services, e-selective dissemination of information (e-SDI), and bibliographic services [2, 3]. E-libraries provide vital roles in the institutions of higher learning. Such as integrating plagiarism software into e-learning/course management systems to promote good practice and provision of metadata that serves as an access point to the e-resources [4]. Despite the roles that e-libraries play by providing adequate e-resources and e-services for students in higher education, the libraries still recorded low patronage due to a lack of awareness of e-library services [5]. Studies revealed that gamification had been applied to various services in the e-library to motivate and engage the students in creating awareness of the services rendered [6, 7]. There is a need to explore the empirical studies covering gamification in e-library services in the context of higher education to understand various variables that have guided these studies.

Gamification has gained popularity in all the fields of human endeavour, with the library not an exception. The era of Information Communication Technology has made Gamification cuts across all areas of human work. Various gamification APPs and game elements are making it possible to adapt to all fields. Different scholars have defined gamification based on the broader study of the term. Gamification applies game design elements in non-game contexts to improve users' experiences and increase their engagements [8, 9]. In gamification, game elements are the potent tools used to inspire and motivate learners. Gamification is widely used in educational settings and other non-academic institutions to increase student engagement and motivation by incorporating game design elements outside a full-fledged game [9]. Points scoring, leaderboards, levels, badges, prizes, and feedback are examples of game elements. However, there could be other game elements yet to be identified. Therefore, this study aims to explore current literature related to gamification elements that could find their expressions in other areas of interest in e-library services in higher education. As a result, one research question is: what are the gamification elements that could be further explored within the e-library services in higher education? There are four sections in this study. Section two reviews the literature, section three describes the methodology, and section four analyzes the results and discusses the study. Lastly, we conclude and make suggestions for future research.

2 Literature Review

2.1 E-Libraries

The primary goal of the e-libraries in higher education is to help their parent institutions by acquiring relevant information materials, processing, organizing, and disseminating them to library users. It aims at improving the university community's learning, teaching, and research activities [1]. There are various resources in the e-library that could help students actualize their learning and improve their academic performance. Examples of information resources available in the e-libraries are; e-books, e-journal, e-articles, e-theses, e-newspapers, e-magazines, video, and audios. Some scholars identified e-library services as information literacy services, online internet search services, digitalization of local contents, and e-reference service. Others are CD-ROMs searching service, online inter-library services, technical training in ICT for staff and users, data management services, awareness and workshop services, e-mail services, data analysis services, and audio/video conferences [4, 10].

2.2 Gamification

Gamification refers to designing systems, services, organizations, and activities to create similar experiences and motivations to those experienced when playing games with the added educational goal of affecting user behaviour [9]. Studies have shown that gamification applies to many academic library services like library instruction, a compulsory course offered by all fresh students in institutions of higher learning. Gamification helps to improve skills needed in effective searching from various databases and exploring independently [11]. Since there are too many things contending for the attention of academic community members leading to information overload, the implementation of gamification in e-library services makes learning more exciting and engaging [12]. Gamification makes boring activities more interesting, thereby bringing about fun and enjoyment, making learning more enjoyable.

Most libraries have successfully moved their orientation program to online services using game elements. Some of these elements, sometimes described as components, are seen in most games nowadays, including Points scoring, leaderboards, levels, badges, prizes, and feedback [13]. Gamification is also used in orientation services to create awareness of e-library resources and services for first-year students [14]. The study showed that gamification was used in e- welcoming orientation activities and made positive connections with new students [15–17]. The Inclusion of Gamification into the academic library could prepare the users for academic work and entrepreneurship [18]. Studies have revealed that gamification increases learners' attention, motivation, engagement, performance, satisfaction, and knowledge retention [19–22]. Gamification could break procrastination habits and reinforce consistency in attaining attainable goals [23].

2.3 Gamification in e-library Services

Januszak and Koorie [7], in their survey at Leigh University, there was low attendance of library users based on a lack of awareness of the resources in the library. So, they decided to gamify the library orientation for first-year students, structured their courses in Moodle, and incentivized Moodle with lots of prizes, gifts, and digital badges. After the gamified orientation, the statistics showed that 1311 students collected badges, and the outcome was encouraging as the participants were enthusiastic. Since then, they accessed the resources in the library without imposition. Also, in State University Library, New York Buffalo, the librarians used a Photo-based Scavenger hunt called Goose Chase. For library tours of their new students. The librarian shared iPads among the students, which they used for the library instruction course. At the end of the library instruction course, the students have high engagement in learning and develop collaboration among themselves [6].

3 Methodology

The study will adopt the following methodology to explore articles regarding elements of gamification in relation to e-library services in higher education.

3.1 Research Design

The study adopted four-phase systematic review approach. Firstly, relevant articles were methodically acknowledged, after which the researchers grouped them. Thirdly, inclusion and exclusion activities took place in the third phase. Lastly, the relevant papers were examined using the research background - gamification elements in e-library services. The following subsections give details of the review process.

3.2 Database Search

The researchers searched Scopus, a reputable academic database, for the related literature from the identified research topic. The first keywords used to search in the database were gamification AND librar*, giving the results of 487. To narrow down the search, gamification AND digital librar* were used, which best described our research topic. We found one hundred thirty-eight (138) articles, conference papers, and review papers, excluding book chapters and book series. Figure 1 below illustrates our search process following the PRISMA Model [24].

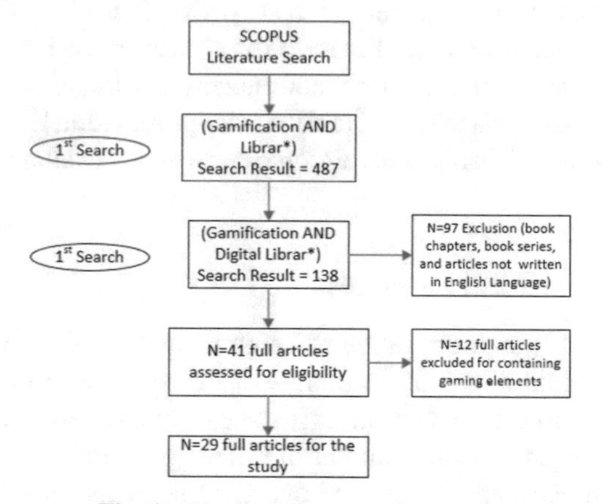

Fig. 1. The literature search process

3.3 Selection Criteria

The researchers checked abstracts to analyze and purify the articles in the review process, ensuring published academic literature quality and relevance. We only selected those articles written in the English Language while excluding the non-English Language articles. It spanned through 2013–2021. Forty-one (41) articles were assessed for eligibility. While going through the abstract, 12 full articles were finally excluded for not having information regarding the gaming elements that were relevant for the study. Therefore, the researchers eventually used twenty-nine (29) papers,

3.4 Data Extraction

Data from the selected studies were extracted and transferred into the worksheet planned for the evaluation. Articles and review papers with gamification elements in e-library services were brought together, while conference papers in e-library services were also grouped.

4 Results and Discussion

This section highlights the result and the discussion that the researchers generated from the papers under review.

4.1 Results

This section discussed the results emanated from the reviewed papers. The researchers grouped the results into statistical and literature classification. The distribution of the reviewed articles is of the following publication types: thirteen (13) journal articles, fifteen (15) conference papers, and one (1) reviewed paper. Under the statistical analysis, the researchers provided two charts to show the graphical representation of the reviewed documents, and one table was provided to illustrate various game elements used in gamifying e-library services. Lastly, the literature classification discussed in detail the results of the study.

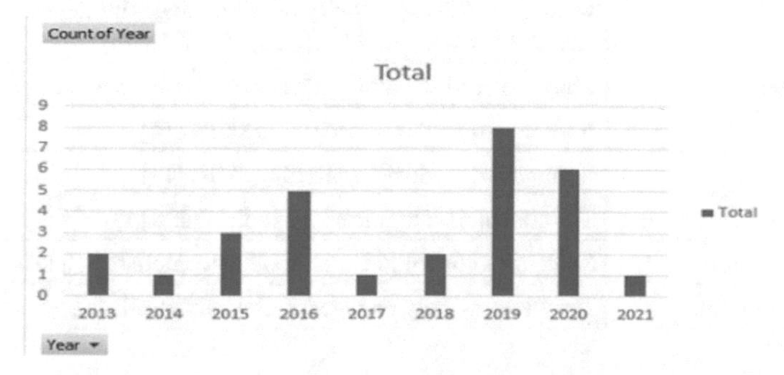

Fig. 2. Number of publications against the indicated years.

Figure 2 shows the years that the review covered. It also shows that 2019 has the highest publication in gamification in academic libraries, followed by 2020. While 2016 and 2015 have average publications compared to those years.

Table 1. Game elements used in e-library services and their outcomes

S/No.	Game elements	Outcomes
1	Feedback	It was used in library instruction, and students felt a sense of accomplishment when achieving a task [25–29]
2	Badges	Students could earn badges for completing specific tasks, such as learning how to use an online document delivery service [7, 11, 30, 31]
3	Teamwork	It was used in library orientation service and library instruction. Teamwork has been proven effective at engaging students in the learning process and helping students to retain information [7, 14]
4	Reward	It increased engagements among the students [25, 27, 32–36]
5	Avatar	It increased students' awareness and collaboration [32]
6	Leaderboard	Information retrieval service was gamified. Leaderboards produce user activity focused on the top-ranking members, with 97% of an action directed to the top 4 positions [11, 37, 38]
7	Challenge	It increased users' awareness of the library [32]
8	Not-specified	It increased users searching skills on various library databases [39, 40]
9	Competition	It increased students' enthusiasm. Students were engaged and involved in the process [38]
10	Storytelling	It helped the students to remain engaged in the game [11, 41]
11	Achievement	The Library web application service was gamified for better engagement [30]
12	Quest,	Students were encouraged to access the library and therefore increased students' engagement [27]
13	Point	Students could earn points for completing specific tasks, and users were given the opportunity of interacting with the website to enhance knowledge [11, 20, 28, 30–33]
14	Prizes	They are used to gamify library orientation services [7, 38, 42]
15	Fun	It improved students' searching skills [14]
16	Time out	It improved students' searching skills [14]
17	Flow enhancement	The students were immersed in the game [43]
18	Immersion	Students were enthusiastic about accomplishing a task [43]
19	Progression	They were deeply engaged in the game [43]

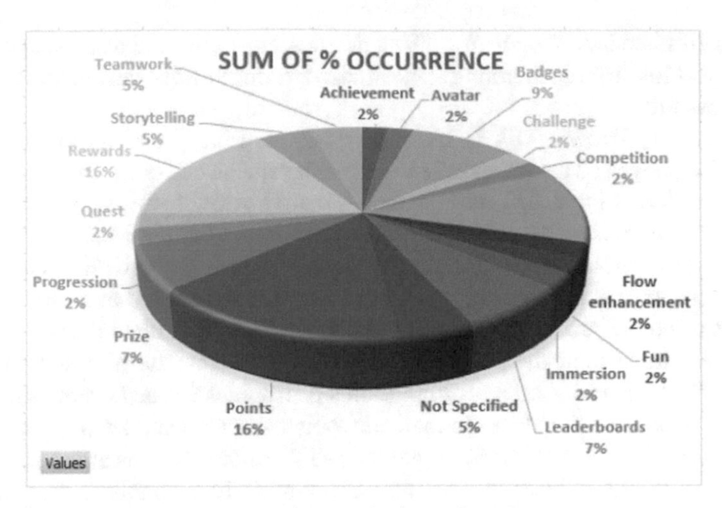

Fig. 3. Game elements in the reviewed papers

Figure 3 shows that reward, points, feedback and badges topped the game elements used in the reviewed works, followed by leaderboard and prizes with equivalent grades. The above result indicated that users are enjoying playing games based on the external reward.

4.2 Discussion

In this systematic literature review, we have investigated and reviewed the gamification elements in e-library services. Kaneko et al. [20] designed a motivational model called ARCS, consisting of four components that would motivate the learner throughout the process (attention, relevance, confidence, and satisfaction). It is deduced from Kaneko that the model itself must be motivational. That is, it must bring fun and enjoyment [11]. For better engagement, a librarian teaching the pharmacy students used competition mode. After each question, a live leaderboard was configured to show fictitious names to maintain user anonymity [38]. At the end, prizes like free food, coffee, library branded promotional items were shared for the participants. At the same time, the game-winner was awarded a grand prize. It indicated that the librarian motivated the learners with the prizes and the other gifts. When the trivia game ended, the student found the game fun and engaging. Many of the students cited the competitiveness of the ranking and prizes as being incentivized [38].

Most of the scholars in the reviewed work believed in "Hands-On" [14, 20, 29, 44]. Hands-on is when the user is fully involved in the game, which makes the users have the mastery of the subject and actively participate in the game. According to Adams et al. [45], hands-on was used to assess students' nurses' skills when there was a lack of engagement and a passive learning approach. A survey indicated that they the students were immersed in the gaming activity and full of a high level of confidence [45]. For students to get engaged with the instructional content, game-based learning can also motivate learners with fun and excitement [46, 47]. The game elements were categorized into seven (immersion, support for different roles, flow enhancement, visual enhancement, support for different learning stages and experience levels, design for interactivity, and progress [43].

According to Brown [48], in his survey outside library and information studies, observed that they used measures of learning achievement, self-efficacy, and motivation. And he also stressed that LIS professionals should borrow these variables from them. The essence is to make a case that gamification improves learning and promotes library services. Some scholars believe that one primary tool in Gamification is the reward. They divided the reward into four; the reward of glory, the reward of access, the reward of a facility, and the reward of sustenance [49, 50]. They described the reward of glory as having no impact on the gameplay itself but providing the player with status or achievement like leaderboards for high scores or trophies for achievements. A reward of sustenance permits the player to maintain their status quo and keep objects acquired until that point. Such as health packs, portions, and armour. The reward of access allows players to access new places or resources not previously available to them, like keys, passwords, or unique weapons. And the reward of the facility enables the player to do things they could not do once or enhance existing abilities [49, 50].

Some scholars supported teamwork as a tool that can generate motivation. Since playing the game alone can be tedious and cannot bring out the best in them. Gamification is about reaching a goal in a fun way and bringing internal satisfaction.

5 Conclusion

This study explored the numerous game elements gamification elements used in the delivery of e-library services. These are rewards, feedback, points, badges, leaderboards, prizes, storytelling, avatar, progression, immersion, flow enhancement, fun, achievement, competition, challenges, quest teamwork and others that could not be specified. The reviewed works showed that game elements like rewards, points, feedback, badges, leaderboard, and prizes are significant elements used in e-library services in higher education. Therefore, from the analysis above, gamification improves learning, increases usage of e-resources, and promotes library services. This study will guide the library management in providing necessary facilities that will aid the successful implementation of game elements in e-library services. It will also enhance the awareness of e-library services among library users. Therefore, future works should investigate the use of various apps in gamifying e-library services.

References

1. Perdana, I.A., Prasojo, L.D.: Digital Library Practice in University: advantages, challenges, and its position. In: International Conference on Educational Research and Innovation (ICERI 2019), pp. 44–48 (2020)
2. Ozohue, C.E., Yaya, J.A.: Provision of current awareness services and selective dissemination of information by medical librarians in technological era. Am. J. Inf. Sci. Comput. Eng. **2**(2), 8–14 (2016)
3. Unegbu, V., Otuza, C.E.: Use of Library and Information Resources: Library Use Education. Emaphine Reprographic Ltd, Lagos (2015)

4. Dahiru, S., Adamu, R.: Integration of e-Library Services and e-Learning Platforms: A New Approach to University Education in Digital Era, pp. 297–311. Ahmadu Bello University Press, Zaria (2021)
5. Bizi, M.K.: Exploring E-Library challenges in the North East of Nigeria Tertiary Institutions Library. Int. J. Sci. Eng. Appl. Sci. **7**(1), 137–145 (2021)
6. Foley, M., Bertel, K.: Hands-on instruction: the iPad self-guided library tour. Ref. Serv. Rev. **43**(2), 309–318 (2015). https://doi.org/10.1108/RSR-07-2014-0021
7. Januszak, A., Koorie, C.: Designing and deploying a virtual IT services orientation for first-year undergraduate students in Moodle. In: Proceedings of the 2018 ACM SIGUCCS Annual Conference, pp. 87–89 (2018)
8. Deterding, S., Dixon D., Khaled, R., Nacke, L.: From game design elements to gamefulness: defining gamification. In: Proceedings of the 15th International Academic MindTrek Conference: Envisioning Future Media Environments, MindTrek 2011, pp. 9–15 (2011). https://doi.org/10.1145/2181037.2181040
9. Dichev, C., Dicheva, D.: Gamifying education: what is known, what is believed and what remains uncertain: a critical review. Int. J. Educ. Technol. Higher Educ. **14**(1), 1–36 (2017)
10. Omeluzor, S.U., Akibu, A.A., Dika, S.I., Ukangwa, C.C.: Methods, effect and challenges of library instruction in academic libraries. Libr. Philos. Pract. **1465** (2017)
11. Brigham, T.J.: An introduction to gamification: adding game elements for engagement. Med. Ref. Serv. Q. **34**(4), 471–480 (2015). https://doi.org/10.1080/02763869.2015.1082385
12. Regalado, F., Costa, L.V., Veloso, A.I.: Online news and gamification habits in late adulthood: a Survey. In: Gao, Q., Zhou, J. (eds.) HCII 2021. LNCS, vol. 12786, pp. 405–419. Springer, Cham (2021). https://doi.org/10.1007/978-3-030-78108-8_30
13. Mohamad, S.N., Sazali, M.N.S.S., Salleh, M.A.M.: Gamification approach in education to increase learning engagement. Int. J. Humanity Arts Soc. Sci. **4**(1), 22–32 (2018)
14. Veach, C.C.: Breaking out to break through: re-imagining first-year orientations. Ref. Serv. Rev. **47**(4), 556–569 (2019). https://doi.org/10.1108/RSR-06-2019-0039
15. Wise, H., Lowe, J., Hill, A., Barnett, L., Barton, C.: Escape the welcome cliché: designing educational escape rooms to enhance students' learning experience. J. Inf. Lit. **12**(1), 86–96 (2018)
16. Vrbancic, E.K., Byerley, S.L.: High-touch, low-tech: investigating the value of an in-person library orientation game. Coll. Undergrad. Libr. **25**(1), 39–51 (2018). https://doi.org/10.1080/10691316.2017.1318429
17. Hottinger, P.R., Zagami-Lopez, N.M., Bryndzia, A.S.: FYI for FYE: 20-minute instruction for library orientation. Ref. Serv. Rev. **43**, 468–479 (2015)
18. Walsh, A.: The potential for using gamification in academic libraries in order to increase student engagement and achievement. Nord. J. Inf. Lit. High. Educ. **6**(1), 39–51 (2014). https://doi.org/10.15845/noril.v6i1.214
19. Alsawaier, R.S.: The effect of gamification on motivation and engagement. Int. J. Inf. Learn. Technol. **35**(1), 56–79 (2018). https://doi.org/10.1108/IJILT-02-2017-0009
20. Kaneko, K., Saito, Y., Nohara, Y., Kudo, E., Yamada, M.A.: A game-based learning environment using the ARCS model at a university library. In: 2015 IIAI 4th International Congress on Advanced Applied Informatics, pp. 403–408 (2015)
21. Subhash, S., Cudney, A.: Gamified learning in higher education: a systematic review of the literature. Comput. Human Behav. **87**, 192–206 (2018)
22. Woolwine, S., Romp, C.R., Jackson, B.: Game on: evaluating the impact of gamification in nursing orientation on motivation and knowledge retention. J. Nurses Prof. Dev. **35**(5), 255–260 (2019)
23. Bohyun, K.: Gamification in education and libraries. Libr. Technol. Rep. **51**(2), 20–28 (2015). http://search.ebscohost.com/login.aspx?direct=true&db=a9h&AN=101029551&lang=fr&site=ehost-live%0Afiles/498/2015

24. Page, M.J., et al.: The PRISMA 2020 statement: an updated guideline for reporting systematic reviews. BMJ **372**, 71 (2021)
25. Kaneko, K., Saito, Y., Nohara, Y., Kudo, E., Yamada, M.: A game-based learning environment using the ARCS model at a university library. In: Proceedings - 2015 IIAI 4th International Congress on Advanced Applied Informatics, IIAI-AAI 2015, pp. 403–408 (2016). https://doi.org/10.1109/IIAI-AAI.2015.285
26. Prandi, C., et al.: Gamifying cultural experiences across the urban environment. Multimedia Tools Appl. **78**(3), 3341–3364 (2018). https://doi.org/10.1007/s11042-018-6513-4
27. Bălutoiu, M.A., et al.: Libquest - revitalize libraries and reading through gamification. In: eLearning and Software for Education Conference, pp. 173–180 (2019). https://doi.org/10.12753/2066-026X-19-023
28. Colasanti, N., Fiori, V., Frondizi, R.: Promoting knowledge circulation in public libraries: the role of gamification. Libr. Manage. **41**(8/9), 669–676 (2020). https://doi.org/10.1108/LM-04-2020-0064
29. Shannon, C.: Engaging students in searching the literature. Med. Ref. Serv. Q. **38**(4), 326–338 (2019). https://doi.org/10.1080/02763869.2019.1657726
30. Laubersheime, J., Ryan, D., Champaign, J.: InfoSkills2Go: using badges and gamification to teach information literacy skills and concepts to college-bound high school students". J. Libr. Adm. **56**(8), 924–938 (2016)
31. Barr, M., Hopfgartner, F., Munro, K.: Increasing Engagement with the Library via Gamification Graduate Skills and Game-Based Learning View project News Recommendation Evaluation View project Increasing Engagement with the Library via Gamification (2016). http://ceur-ws.org
32. Raflesia, P.S., Surendro, K.: Designing gamified service towards user engagement and service quality improvement. In: 1st International Conference on Wireless and Telematics, pp. 1–4 (2015)
33. Shannon, C.: Engaging students in searching the literature. Med. Ref. Serv. Q. **38**(4), 326–338 (2019)
34. Bilandzic, M., Johnson, D.: Hybrid placemaking in the library: designing digital technology to enhance users' on-site experience. Aust. Libr. J. **62**(4), 258–271 (2013). https://doi.org/10.1080/00049670.2013.845073
35. Colasanti, N., Fiori, V., Frondizi, R.: Promoting knowledge circulation in public libraries: the role of gamification. Libr. Manage. **41**(8–9), 669–676 (2020). https://doi.org/10.1108/LM-04-2020-0064
36. Honeyman, D., Walker, D.: Evolving customer engagement: Using mobile technology and gamification to improve awareness of and access to library services. (2015). https://www.researchgate.net/publication/310771185
37. Biasini, M., Carmignani, V., Ferro, N., Filianos, P., Maistro, M., Nunzio, G.M.D.: FullBrain: a Social E-learning Platform. In: IRCDL, pp. 25–41 (2021)
38. Jones, E.P., Wisniewski, C.S.: Gamification of a mobile applications lecture in a pharmacy course. Med. Ref. Serv. Q. **38**(4), 339–346 (2019). https://doi.org/10.1080/02763869.2019.1657728
39. Bigdeli, Z., Haidari, G., Haji, A., Yakhchali, R., Jahromi, B.: Gamification in library websites based on motivational theories. Webology **13**(1), 1–12 (2016)
40. Prince, J.D.: Gamification. J. Electron. Resour. Med. Libr. **10**(3), 162–169 (2013). https://doi.org/10.1080/15424065.2013.820539
41. Clarke, S., Collins, B., Flynn, D., Arnab, S.: Gamifying the university library: using RPG maker to re-design library induction and online services. Proc. Eur. Conf. e-Learning ECEL **2018**, 721–725 (2018)

42. Honeyman, D., Walker, D.: Evolving customer engagement: using mobile technology and gamification to improve awareness of and access to library services. In: THETA 2015 At Gold Coast Convention and Exhibition Centre, Broadbeach, Gold Coast, Queensland, Australia (2015)
43. Schulz, R., Martinez, S., Hara, T.: Towards a game-design framework for evidence-based clinical procedure libraries. In: 2019 IEEE 7th *International Conference* on *Serious Games* and Applications for *Health* SeGAH 2019, no. November, pp. 1–8, (2019).https://doi.org/10.1109/SeGAH.2019.8882474
44. Brigham, T.J.: An introduction to gamification: adding game elements for engagement. Med. Ref. Serv. Q. **34**(4), 471–480 (2015)
45. Adams, V., Burger, S., Crawford, K., Setter, R.: Can you escape? Creating an escape room to facilitate active learning. J. Nurses Prof. Dev. **34**(2), E1–E5 (2018)
46. Smale, M.A.: Learning through quests and contests: Games in information literacy instruction. J. Lib. Innov. **2**, 36–55 (2011)
47. Strickland, H.P., Kaylor, S.K.: Bringing you a-game: Educational gaming for student success. Nurse Educ. Today **40**, 101–103 (2016)
48. Brown, R.T.: A literature review of how videogames are assessed in library and information science and beyond. J. Acad. Librariansh. **40**(5), 447–451 (2014)
49. Hallford, N., Hallford, J.: Swords and Circuitry: A Designer's Guide to Computer Role-Playing Games. Prima Publishing, Roseville (2001)
50. Salen, K., Zimmerman, E.: Rule of Play Game Design Fundamentals. MIT Press, Cambridge (2004)

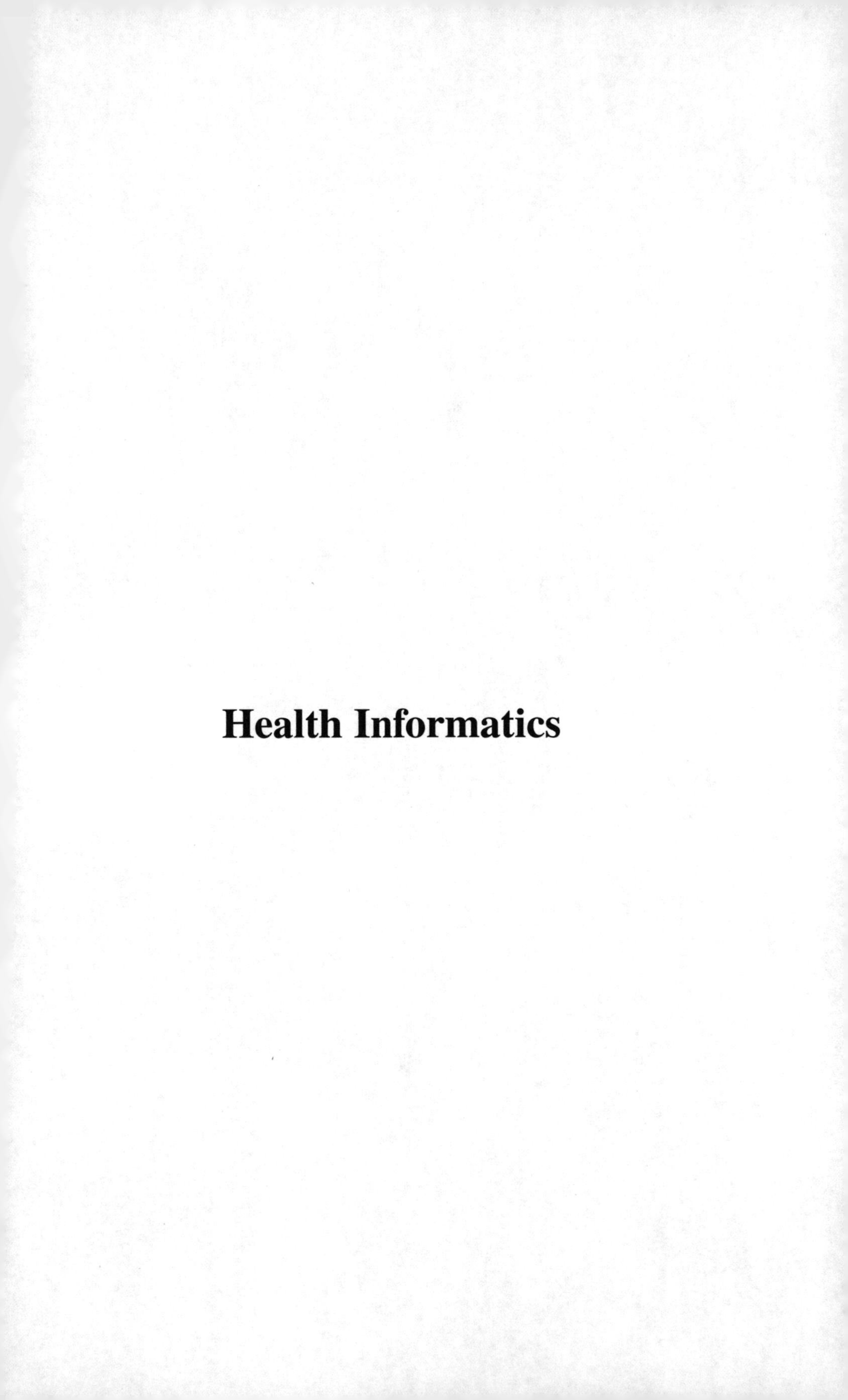

Health Informatics

Bayesian Model for Detecting Influence Directionality of Heart Related Diseases with Application in Multimorbidity Understanding

Faouzi Marzouki(✉) and Omar Bouattane

Laboratory of SSDIA, ENSET Mohammedia, Hassan II University of Casablanca, Casablanca, Morocco
faouzi8marzouki@gmail.com, o.bouattane@enset-media.ac.ma

Abstract. Multimorbidity is the existence of two or more than two diseases in the same patient at the same time. It is a major problem in the modern healthcare system and several studies have pointed out the association between the burden of multimorbidity and poor quality of life. It is quite intuitive to represent multimobid diseases as a weighted graph. We define comorbidity pattern detection of valvular heart diseases in a machine learning framework. We aim to investigate the directionality influence between comorbid valvular heart diseases by algorithmically extract this structural knowledge from real medical data. We investigate the performance of four well-known Bayesian network algorithms by comparative analysis methodology. First, we build a comparative baseline based on association strength estimation of all pairs of studied diseases. Then the four algorithms outcomes are compared against the baseline algorithm, and against each other. The results suggest that score based methods outcomes are the closest to baseline algorithm. Besides, Tabu search and Hill climbing algorithms with AIC criterion as objective function, are the most performing in terms of log-likelihood loss. Despite differences in algorithm directionality outcomes, it seems that the used approaches are comparable for learning graph skeleton.

Keywords: Multimorbidity · Comorbidity · Data science · Machine learning · Valvulopathy

1 Introduction

Researches in epidemiology indicate the high risk and prevalence of having multiple health conditions at the same time as age increases. Multimorbidity, i.e. the presence of two or more diseases in the same patient at the same time [1], is a significant health problem in modern medicine. There are several risk factors implicated in the development of Multimorbidity: environmental, genetic predisposition, lifestyle, the process of aging, pathophysiological process nature of the disease. These highly inter-related conditions make a further burden on patients in terms of polypharmacy and difficulties in their informal careers [2], which reduces considerably their quality of life.

F. Saeed et al. (Eds.): IRICT 2021, LNDECT 127, pp. 737–747, 2022.
https://doi.org/10.1007/978-3-030-98741-1_62

Unfortunately, health systems are still designed in a single disease paradigm rather than Multimorbidity. However, the transition from disease-centered care, to patient-centered care is ongoing [1]. In medical literature, several approaches were proposed to explore facets of Multimorbidity: statistical techniques (descriptive statistics, regression) and data analysis (segmentation and regressions) [3–5], probabilistic graphical models [6–8], network analysis based models [9, 10], machine learning based methods [11, 12]. Despite the important work done in literature, the Multimorbidity remains a challenging problem due to the multifactorial complexity aspects of this phenomenon. Recently, initiatives to exploit Big data techniques and the increasing amount of electronic health care data [13] to get insight about this phenomena.

Typically, data scientists find the right data, clean it up, transform it into the suitable format, and apply models and algorithms to extract the targeted knowledge from the original unstructured raw data. See Fig. 1. In this perspective, we contribute in exploring the use data science methods and machine learning techniques for multimorbidity modeling. We give a formal algorithm of the process of extracting Comorbidity Disease Network from real medical data. Then, we investigate the influence directionality between nodes/diseases in this network using Bayesian network learning algorithms.

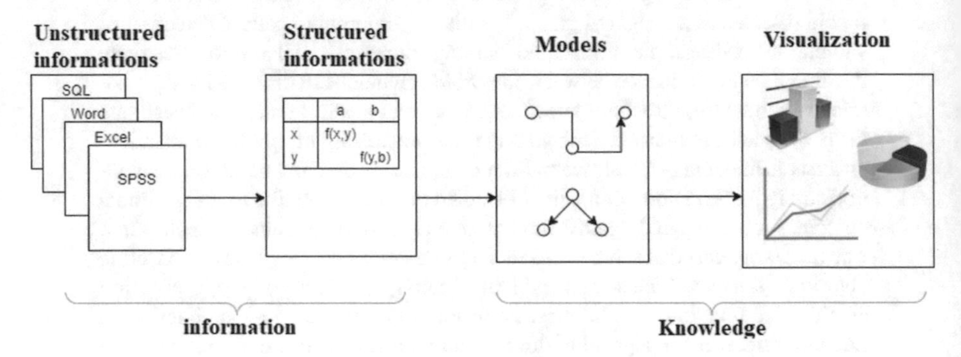

Fig. 1. General methodology for data science followed in this work.

When applying machine learning algorithms, the suitability of particular techniques for a particular domain of application is important to consider. Since these techniques are based on different concepts and assumptions, it is necessary to perform a comparative analysis in order to select the suitable model, according to that domain of interest. In this paper, we focus our study on analyzing structure and influence directionality of some valvular heart disease related diseases.

We organize this work in two phases. First, we implement a pairwise based approach to construct a comorbidity model as a weighted graph of a Comorbidity Disease Network (CDN). The edge weights are calculated using Multimorbidity Coefficient (MC) as association strength between two comorbid diseases. Then we compare the resulting CDN structure skeleton to outcomes of some well-known Bayesian network structure learning algorithms. Second, we execute these Bayesian network model learning algorithms to extract the dependence directionality of edges over nodes/diseases in the obtained graph skeleton.

The remainder of this paper is organized as follows: in Sect. 2 we review some related works to the multimorbidity modeling. Section 3 is devoted to data and methods used in this work. We present results in Sect. 4 before we conclude in Sect. 5.

2 Related Works

Recently, a growing number of studies have been conducted in the medical literature to address the burden of multimorbidity, examine risk factors for multimorbidity, its impact on quality of life, mortality, or the costs and utility of care medical [14]. Technically, the models and methods used differ either in data (cross-sectional or longitudinal) or whether the objective is to explain, explore, or predict.

Combinations of traditional data analysis and machine learning were proposed as promising multimorbidity research methods. The authors in [15] applied classification/regression trees and random forest to data of elderly patients to identify how the specific combinations of chronic conditions, functional limitations, and geriatric syndromes affect costs and inpatient utilization. In [16], the authors applied the k-means algorithm to a cross-sectional study using digital records of patients, aged between 45 and 64 years, to distinguish population groups from others. In [17], the author added fuzziness to k-means algorithm to create clusters of patients and their membership matrix. This later indicates the membership degree of a patient to a given cluster.

Other approaches used network science tools to draw insights about comorbidity disease networks. Hernández et al. [18] applied network analysis and association rules to study comorbidity patterns of some diseases in 6101 Irish adults aged >50 years. They perform Louvain algorithm to detect communities of diseases from the disease network. Standardized lift and confidence scores of the association rules was put as probabilistic measuring of how conditionally the diseases are related. In the study of [19], logistic regression models, adjusted by age and sex and odd ratio, were used to estimate the multimorbidity networks.

The aforementioned studies tried to construct weighted graphs based on the idea of association strength between diseases. Other approaches in the literature focused on the dependency idea under a probabilistic framework. For example Lappenschaar et al. [20] proposed a probabilistic framework to model these concepts using a causal Bayesian network. This model was extended with a time dimension in [12]. These authors proposed in [8] a Bayesian network structure learning method for modeling the risk factors interactions explaining co-occurrences of malignant tumors in the oncological domain.

In this work, we define comorbid valvular heart diseases pattern extraction in a machine learning framework. We investigate the performance of four well-known Bayesian network algorithms by comparative analysis methodology. First, we build a comparative baseline based on association strength estimation of all pairs of studied diseases. Then the four algorithms outcomes are compared against the baseline algorithm, and against each other.

3 Data and Methods

3.1 Problem Setting

Let $D = \{d_1, d_2, \ldots, d_{|D|}\}$ a finite set containing |D| number of diseases present in medical dataset, such that |S| denotes the number of elements of a given set S. Let $X = \{X_1, X_2, \ldots, X_{|X|}\}$ the set of all observations of patients such that: $X_i = (x_{1,i}, x_{2,i}, \ldots, x_{|Xi|,i})$ with $x_{j,i} \in D$ a tuple of observed diagnoses for the patient i. We assume that data X are governed by the same underlying Multimorbidity Mechanism, and X are independent and identically distributed (i.i.d) samples.

Let R consists of a binary relation over Cartesian product set $D \times D$. Two diseases d_1 and d_2 are related with the relation R if and only if they satisfy a predefined condition of interest. This relation R is usually estimated by a metric to measure its strength. In this work, we define the binary relation R using two concepts: association strength and dependence/independence concepts.

Association Strength Definition. Let d_1 and d_2 be two binary random variables for occurrence/absence of diseases 1 and 2 respectively. Let $P(d_i)$ stands for the occurrence probability of the disease $d_i \in D$. We use Van Den Akker et al.'s definition of cluster comorbidity [21]: if d_1 has occurred, then d_2 will be more likely to occur than what would be expected just by chance.

We consider that d_1 and d_2 are in positive comorbidity, if $P(d_1, d_2) > P(d_1)P(d_2)$. If $P(d_1)P(d_2) \approx P(d_1, d_2)$ we consider that the two diseases are in random co-occurence. The final case $P(d_1, d_2) < P(d_1)P(d_2)$ can be interpreted as d_1 and d_2 are in protective comorbidity (e.g. myopia may be protective against diabetic retinopathy [22]).

To measure how strongly disorders are linked, a Multimorbidity Coefficient (MC) is calculated. MC is a commonly used method for measuring pairwise association in medical research on multimorbidity [23]. MC is defined as the division of the observed rate of comorbidity (multimorbidity) by the rate which is expected under the null hypothesis of no association between the separate disorders. See table below.

		Disease 2		
		Occurrence	Absence	Total
Disease 1	Occurrence	a	b	a+b
	Absence	b	d	c+d
	Total	a+c	b+d	a+b+c+d=N

Taking into account the notation of table above, the Multimorbidity Coefficient (MC) score for Disease 1 and Disease 2 is as follows:

$$MC = \frac{\frac{a}{N}}{\frac{a+c}{N} * \frac{a+b}{N}} = \frac{aN}{(a+c) * (a+b)} \tag{1}$$

We use this pairwise approach to learn the weighted structure of CDN (See Algorithm 1). We will consider this pairwise approach as baseline to be compared to Bayesian network structure learning algorithms.

Dependence/Independence Definition. Another possible approach to model the structure of CDN is to measure how diseases are linked in term of dependences/independences rather than the association strength idea. This is can be done using several methods in Bayesian network literature, which we can be divided into score based methods, constraint based methods, and hybrid methods.

Let us consider the graph $G = (V, E)$, such that V is the set of nodes (diseases), E is the set of edges (association between diseases). To be able to use Bayesian dependence/independence concept to learn structure and directionality of CDN, we add the two hypotheses below:

- $G = (V, E)$ is a directed acyclic graph, in which vertices V are described by: $X = \{X_v | v \in V\}$ the set of binary random variables indexed by v.
- a joint probability distribution P(X) over X.

The tuple (G, X, P) is a Bayesian network, a graphical model where nodes represent random variables of the presence of diseases (we will use these two terms interchangeably), and arcs models probabilistic dependencies between them. The joint probability P can be factorized into smaller local probability distributions, as a product of the probability of each random variable, conditional on their parent variable:

$$P(x_1, x_2, \ldots, x_n) = \Pi_{i \in V} p\big(x_i | x_j \forall j \in \mathrm{Parent}(i)\big) \tag{2}$$

The diversity of possible techniques to learn the structure and the influence directionality of the CDN makes the choice of the suitable technique of the particular domain of Multimorbidity unclear. Therefore, we will conduct a comparative analysis between the approaches and techniques discussed in this section. The comparison will be against a set of diseases that exhibit a causal relationship. By this special methodology, we construct a ground truth to compare these techniques with each other. In this work we study the following algorithms: Incremental Association Markov Blanket (IAMB) and Grow Shrink for constraint based algorithms, Tabu search and Hill Climbing for score based approaches, Min Max Hill Climbing and (mmhc) rsmax2 for hybrid approaches.

3.2 Building Comorbidity Disease Network Algorithm

In this section we define the pairwise methodology for building Comorbidity Disease Network. Let N_{diag} denote number of diagnoses and N_{dis} number of diseases presented in the dataset, N the number of diseases. Let $D = \{d_1, d_2, d_3, \ldots, d_{N_{dis}}\}$ disease set. $M_k \subset D$ such that $k > 1$, is the subset of size k diseases from D. (*e.g.* M_2 is the subset of possible co-morbidities, M_3 represent the subset of possible tri-morbidities an so forth). Let $f : I \subset \mathbb{N} \rightarrow \{D_1, D_2, \ldots, D_{N_{diag}}\} \subset \mathcal{P}(\mathcal{D})$ be an application that maps every patient i to its recorded diagnoses $\{x_1^{<i>}, x_2^{<i>}, \ldots, x_{N_{diag}}^{<i>}\}$.

Algorithm 1 searches for $\frac{n!}{(n-2)!2!}$ potential combinations of comorbidity and estimates MC for each combination using MC definition presented in Sect. 3.1. this algorithm is easily generalizable to Multimorbidity. If the MC is higher than 1 then we consider that these two diseases are in comorbidity, and these two diseases are linked by an edge whose weight is equal to MC. If the MC is less than 1 then we say that these two diagnoses are in protective comorbidity. The bigger this number is, the stronger the association is considered. We are interested in this work by positive comorbidity.

Algorithm 1: Comorbidity Disease Network building

```
=========================================
Input: a patient – diagnosis function map f: I ⊂ ℕ → {D_1; D_2; ...; D_{N_diag}}
a disease set D,
Output: a Comorbidity Disease Network G = (V, E)
=========================================
Begin Program
For Each M2∈ 𝒫(D) do:
    W_expected ← ∏_{d∈M_2} Count_occ({d}, I)
    W_observed ← Count_occ(M_2, I)
    MC ← (W_observed * N_diag) / W_expected
If H0:"W_expected ≥ W_observed" is rejected at risk 0.001
then:
        E_{d_1,d_2} ← MC, such that {d_1, d_2} = M_2
    End If
End For
Procedure Count_occ (S: a set, I: a subset of integers )
    Initialize S_occurences ← ∅
    For each X ∈ S do:
        For each i ∈ I do:
          S_occurences ← S_occurences ∪ (X ∩ f(i))
        End For
    End For
    Return |S_occurences|
End Procedure
End Program
```

3.3 Data

The analysis was applied in a case study of a real medical dataset [24]. Each patient has a recorded diagnosis recorded by a unique distinct ICD 10 Code. The data contain 78451 patients (34639 males, and 43812 females). The maximum number of registered diagnoses per admission is 20. We choose a valvulopathy related set of diseases on which to apply Algorithm 1. This group consists of the following node diseases: Non-rheumatic mitral and tricuspid and aortic (valve) insufficiency (coded respectively in ICD10 as I34.0 and I36.1 and I35.1). Non-rheumatic aortic (valve) stenosis (I35.0). Rheumatic tricuspid insufficiency (I07.1). Rheumatic disorders of both mitral and tricuspid valves (I08.1). Combined rheumatic disorders of mitral, aortic and tri-cuspid valves (I08.3). Other pulmonary hypertension (I27.2). Other ill-defined heart diseases (I51.89). Several studies reveal causal relationships among these diseases [25, 26]. This is one of the reasons we choose these diseases for the comparative analysis.

3.4 Evaluation Metrics

Metrics. The learned models quality is compared based on Akaike's Information Criteria (AIC) and Bayesian Information Criteria (BIC). AIC and BIC are both penalized-likelihood criteria. BIC estimates the posterior probability of a model being true, assuming a Bayesian perspective, so that a lower BIC means that a model is considered more likely to be the true model. AIC, which is based on Kullback-Leiber information loss, estimates a constant plus the relative distance between the unknown true likelihood function of the data and the fitted likelihood function of the model, that is, a lower AIC means a model is closer to the truth-model.

$$\mathrm{AIC} = -2\log\left(\mathrm{Likelihood}\left(\ominus^{*}\right)\right) + 2\mathrm{k} \tag{3}$$

$$\mathrm{BIC} = -2\log\left(\mathrm{Likelihood}\left(\ominus^{*}\right)\right) + \log(\mathrm{n})\mathrm{k} \tag{4}$$

Where $\ominus^*$ is estimated parameters for $\ominus$ value and k corresponds to the number of estimated model parameters, n is the number of observations. Unlike the AIC, the BIC penalizes the model more in term of complexity, i.e. that more complex models in terms of parameters n, will be less likely to be selected.

Bayesian Network Structures Comparison. Structural Hamming Distance (SHD) is a metric widely used to quantify similarities and differences between Bayesian networks. SHD counts missing, additional and reversed arcs of the learned network compared to a reference network. To omit the directionality of arcs, either because are less important than the association between two variables or because of feedback relation, one can use SHD on Bayesian network without directionality: it ignores arc directions and compares the skeletons of the two networks.

4 Results and Discussion

We applied Algorithm 1 to the valvular heart diseases defined in Sect. 3.3, the weighted graph in Fig. 2 and Table 1 show the results of detected comorbidity disease network for males in older adulthood (>65 years). The thickness of edges reflects visually the differences of calculated MC weight on pairs of diseases. The absence of edges means either the association is random or not significant (the null hypothesis was not rejected at risk 0.01) or both, according to our data of application. Figure 2 shows for example that Non rheumatic tricuspid insufficiency (I36.1) co-occurs with non-rheumatic mitral insufficiency (I34.0) 20.8 times more than what would be expected just by chance. This high score can reflect a potential causal relationship, which can be due to functional abnormalities in heart functioning.

To detect potential influence directionality, we compared Bayesian network learning algorithms mentioned in Sect. 3.1 to select the best performing. We performed 10-fold

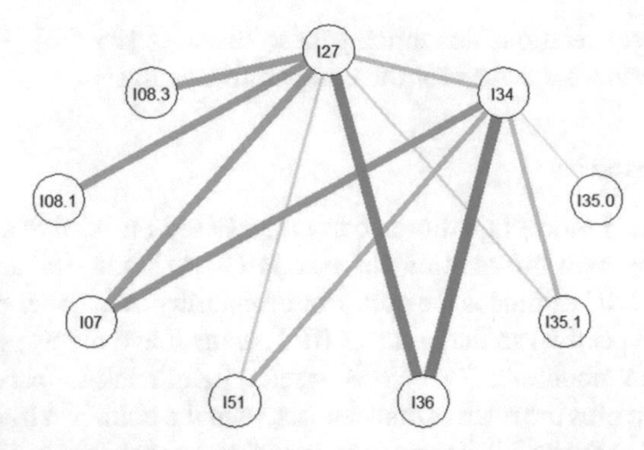

Fig. 2. Example of co-occurrence structure of some ICD 10 codded diseases for males in older adulthood (>65 years). The thickness of edges reflects the strength of MC score for pairs of diseases (see Table 1). This is the skeleton of the studied graph. For example, non rheumatic aortic stenosis (I35.0) co-occurs with non-rheumatic mitral insufficiency (I34.0) 3.17 times more than what would be expected just by chance. In this figure the disease codes are abbreviated. See Sect. 3.3 for more details.

Table 1. MC scores computed by Algorithm 1 (Sect. 3.2) for the structure of co-occurrence of Fig. 1. Since the built graph is undirected, the weight matrix is symmetric. Empty cases means that either the MC score is equal to one, or the null hypothesis is not rejected, or both.

	I27.2	I34.0	I35.0	I35.1	I36.1	I51.89	I07.1	I08.1	I08.3
I27.2									
I34.0	**7.70**								
I35.0	-	**3.17**							
I35.1	**4.54**	**7.97**	-						
I36.1	**19.07**	**20.8**	-	-					
I51.89	**5.03**	**9.42**	-	-	-				
I07.1	**14.21**	**16.13**	-	-	-	-			
I08.1	**15.07**	-	-	-	-	-	-		
I08.3	**13.42**	-	-	-	-	-	-	-	

cross-validation in which we set the negative expected log-likelihood of the test set for the Bayesian network fitted from the training set. Lower value is better. We repeated this procedure 100 times and averaged the results. For each algorithm performance, the average and standard deviation are calculated. Figure 3 suggests that hill climbing and tabu search algorithms (score based approaches) such that AIC criterion included as penalizing term of objective function, are the best performing. While constraint based approaches were the poorer performing algorithms. The presence of outliers may reflect the initialization and local minima problems. Hybrid algorithms had medium performance.

Further, we set manually two scenarios of the following directions in the skeleton of Fig. 2: from I34.0 to all its neighboring nodes, and I27.2 to all its neighboring nodes (first scenario). The second scenario is the reverse directions. These scenarios were the most performing model according to AIC and BIC. See Table 2. That is among the reasons to put it as a baseline for comparison to the studied Bayesian network learning algorithms. While the Algorithm 1 structure with the first scenario was the most performing in term of both AIC and BIC, it has comparable performance with other approaches in the reversed scenario.

While we conducted the comparison analysis, we noticed that constraint based methods (Iamb and grow shrink) failed to decide directions between diseases I27.2, I08.3, I08.1 in one hand, and between I51.89 to I35.1 in other hand. We set then, the directions manually, from I27.2 to I08.3, and I08.1, I51.89 to I35.1 which increased the AIC and BIC scores for the mentioned algorithms.

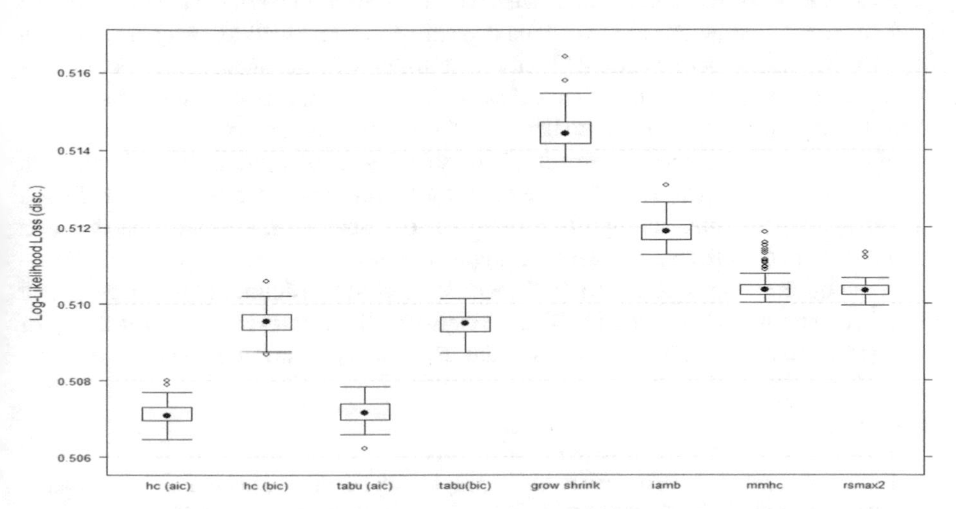

Fig. 3. Performance comparison between Bayesian network structure learning algorithms.

In consistence with results in Fig. 3, score based approaches had the lowest structural distance from the network reference in terms of hamming distance. However, still differences in performance according to directionality of arcs. For the reversed scenario (the second scenario) of directionality, score based approaches are the closest models for the graph of reference in terms of true positives, followed by hybrid methods. Hill climbing had the most performance on term of high precision (=0.92) and recall (=1) in reversed

Table 2. Comparison of the Algorithm 1, and some well-known algorithms.

	Constraint based		Score based		Hybrid		Algorithm 1
	iamb	Grow shrink	Hill climbing	Tabu search	Mmhc	Rsmax2	
Hamming distance	4	4	1	1	3	3	
BIC	−8220.19	−8220.19	−8169.61	−8169.61	−8184.07	−8184.07	−8866
AIC	−8124.27	−8124.27	−8066.02	−8066.02	−8107.34	−8107.34	−8221.03

scenario. Furthermore, false negative rate is the lowest among the other methods (=0) for reversed scenario.

5 Conclusion and Perspectives

In this work we tried to model multimorbidity of diseases as weighted graph such that weights represent strength between diseases (structure of Comorbidity Network Diseases measured by Multimorbidity Coefficient) and probability of observing a disease given another disease (directionality detection). We formulated CND detection as a machine learning task. We implemented a pairwise based approach to learn CND structure, and we compared the structure of the obtained graph with some well-known algorithms in Bayesian network structure learning literature. Further, we investigated the directionality of arcs using comparative analysis against AIC, BIC and negative expected log likelihood. The results suggest that score based methods outcomes are the closest to pairwise approaches for CND detection. Besides, Tabu search and Hill climbing algorithms with AIC criterion as objective function, are the most performing in terms of log-likelihood loss. Despite differences in algorithm directionality outcomes, it seems that the used approaches are comparable for learning graph skeleton.

We choose to use of AIC and BIC metrics, as well as Multimorbidity Coefficient to evaluate and build Comorbidity Disease Network. Therefore, the generalizability of these results to other empirical data and other metrics is envisaged in perspectives.

References

1. Rijken, M., et al.: How to improve care for people with multimorbidity in Europe? European Observatory on Health Systems and Policies, Copenhagen (Denmark) (2017)
2. Doyle, J., et al.: Addressing medication management for older people with multimorbidities: a multi-stakeholder approach. In: Proceedings of the 11th EAI International Conference on Pervasive Computing Technologies for Healthcare, pp. 78–87. Association for Computing Machinery, New York (2017)
3. Kirchberger, I., et al.: Patterns of multimorbidity in the aged population. Results from the KORA-Age study. PLoS One **7**, e30556 (2012). https://doi.org/10.1371/journal.pone.0030556
4. Fortin, M., Hudon, C., Haggerty, J., van den Akker, M., Almirall, J.: Prevalence estimates of multimorbidity: a comparative study of two sources. BMC Health Serv. Res. **10**, 111 (2010). https://doi.org/10.1186/1472-6963-10-111
5. Elhai, J.D., Calhoun, P.S., Ford, J.D.: Statistical procedures for analyzing mental health services data. Psychiatry Res. **160**, 129–136 (2008)
6. Lappenschaar, M., et al.: Multilevel temporal Bayesian networks can model longitudinal change in multimorbidity. J. Clin. Epidemiol. **66**, 1405–1416 (2013). https://doi.org/10.1016/j.jclinepi.2013.06.018
7. Lappenschaar, M., Hommersom, A., Lucas, P.J.: Probabilistic causal models of multimorbidity concepts. In: AMIA ... Annual Symposium Proceedings. AMIA Symposium, pp. 475–484 (2012)
8. Lappenschaar, M., Hommersom, A., Lagro, J., Lucas, P.J.F.: Understanding the co-occurrence of diseases using structure learning. In: Peek, N., Marín Morales, R., Peleg, M. (eds.) AIME 2013. LNCS (LNAI), vol. 7885, pp. 135–144. Springer, Heidelberg (2013). https://doi.org/10.1007/978-3-642-38326-7_21

9. Lai, Y.-H., Wang, T.-Y., Yang, H.-H.: Network-based analysis of comorbidities: case study of diabetes mellitus. In: Wang, L., Uesugi, S., Ting, I.-H., Okuhara, K., Wang, K. (eds.) MISNC 2015. CCIS, vol. 540, pp. 210–222. Springer, Heidelberg (2015). https://doi.org/10.1007/978-3-662-48319-0_17
10. Cramer, A.O.J., Waldorp, L.J., van der Maas, H.L.J., Borsboom, D.: Comorbidity: a network perspective. Behav Brain Sci. **33**, 137–150 (2010). https://doi.org/10.1017/S0140525X09991567
11. Faruqui, S.H.A., Alaeddini, A., Jaramillo, C.A., Potter, J.S., Pugh, M.J.: Mining patterns of comorbidity evolution in patients with multiple chronic conditions using unsupervised multi-level temporal Bayesian network. PLoS ONE **13**, e0199768 (2018). https://doi.org/10.1371/journal.pone.0199768
12. Guo, M., et al.: Analysis of disease comorbidity patterns in a large-scale China population. BMC Med. Genomics **12**(Suppl 12), 177 (2019)
13. Pastorino, R., et al.: Benefits and challenges of Big Data in healthcare: an overview of the European initiatives. Eur. J. Pub. Health **29**, 23–27 (2019)
14. Vetrano, D.L., et al.: Joint action ADVANTAGE WP4 group: frailty and multimorbidity: a systematic review and meta-analysis. J. Gerontol. A Biol. Sci. Med. Sci. **74**, 659–666 (2019). https://doi.org/10.1093/gerona/gly110
15. Schiltz, N.K., et al.: Identifying specific combinations of multimorbidity that contribute to health care resource utilization: an analytic approach. Med. Care **55**, 276–284 (2017)
16. Violán, C., et al.: Multimorbidity patterns with K-means nonhierarchical cluster analysis. BMC Fam. Pract. **19**, 108 (2018)
17. Marengoni, A., et al.: Patterns of multimorbidity in a population-based cohort of older people: sociodemographic, lifestyle, clinical, and functional differences. J. Gerontol. Ser. A **75**, 798–805 (2020). https://doi.org/10.1093/gerona/glz137
18. Hernández, B., Reilly, R.B., Kenny, R.A.: Investigation of multimorbidity and prevalent disease combinations in older Irish adults using network analysis and association rules. Sci Rep. **9**, 14567 (2019). https://doi.org/10.1038/s41598-019-51135-7
19. Aguado, A., Moratalla-Navarro, F., López-Simarro, F., Moreno, V.: MorbiNet: multimorbidity networks in adult general population. Analysis of type 2 diabetes mellitus comorbidity. Sci. Rep. **10**, 2416 (2020). https://doi.org/10.1038/s41598-020-59336-1
20. J.p.: Preface. In: Pearl, J. (ed.) Probabilistic Reasoning in Intelligent Systems, pp. vii–ix. Morgan Kaufmann, San Francisco (1988)
21. van den Akker, M., Buntinx, F., Metsemakers, J.F., Roos, S., Knottnerus, J.A.: Multimorbidity in general practice: prevalence, incidence, and determinants of co-occurring chronic and recurrent diseases. J. Clin. Epidemiol. **51**, 367–375 (1998). https://doi.org/10.1016/s0895-4356(97)00306-5
22. Lim, L.S., Lamoureux, E., Saw, S.M., Tay, W.T., Mitchell, P., Wong, T.Y.: Are myopic eyes less likely to have diabetic retinopathy? Ophthalmology **117**, 524–530 (2010). https://doi.org/10.1016/j.ophtha.2009.07.044
23. Barabási, A.-L., Gulbahce, N., Loscalzo, J.: Network medicine: a network-based approach to human disease. Nat. Rev. Genet. **12**, 56–68 (2011)
24. Bonis, J.: drbonis/CMBD_MAD_2016 (2019). Accessed 01 July 2021. https://github.com/drbonis/CMBD_MAD_2016
25. Tichelbäcker, T., et al.: Pulmonary hypertension and valvular heart disease. Herz **44**(6), 491–501 (2019). https://doi.org/10.1007/s00059-019-4823-6
26. Maeder, M.T., Weber, L., Rickli, H.: Pulmonary hypertension in aortic valve stenosis. Trends Cardiovasc. Med. **S1050–1738**(20), 30158–30164 (2020)

Data Science for Multimorbidity Modeling: Can Age and Sex Predict Multimorbidity Burden?

Faouzi Marzouki(✉) and Omar Bouattane

Laboratory of SSDIA, ENSET Mohammedia, Hassan II University of Casablanca, Casablanca, Morocco
faouzi8marzouki@gmail.com, o.bouattane@enset-media.ac.ma

Abstract. Age and sex are important biological factors that should be taken into account in each medical phenomenon. With the increasing amount of recorded data, data science methods became necessary tools for extracting useful knowledge. We propose in this work to investigate the role of age and sex in prediction of developing multimorbidity. In machine learning perspective, we formulate the problem of predicting multimorbidity count given a patient profile, and we compare some of regression based models on real data to estimate the significance of sex and age as predictors of multimorbidity count. Results show, in accordance with previous medical studies, that age is critical factor in developing multimorbidity, while sex has negligible contribution as predictor for multimorbidity according to our data of interest. Besides, third polynomial regressor was the best performing model for predicting averaged multimorbidity for male patients between one and 95 years old.

Keywords: Machine learning · Multimorbidity · Comorbidity · Data science

1 Introduction

Comorbidity is defined as "any distinct additional clinical entity that has existed or that may occur during the clinical course of a patient who has the index disease under study" [1]. It is a significant health problem in modern medicine, and the more conditions are (i.e. Multimorbidity), the more burdens is put on patient and healthcare systems. Unfortunately, health systems are still designed in a single disease paradigm rather than Multimorbidity. However, the transition from a disease-centered care, to a patient-centered care is ongoing [2].

In medical literature, several models were proposed to explore Multimorbidity: statistical techniques (descriptive statistics, regression) and data analysis (segmentation and regressions) [3–5], probabilistic graphical models [6–8], network analysis based models [9, 10], machine learning based methods [11, 12]. The multiplicity of models reflects the multi-facets by which we can approach and model multimorbidity. Therefore, studies results in discrepancies in prevalence rates and patterns of multimorbidity, which is also highly influenced by methodology (population and measures [13], heterogeneity in multimorbidity definitions and how chronic conditions are classified [14]). Most of

F. Saeed et al. (Eds.): IRICT 2021, LNDECT 127, pp. 748–758, 2022.
https://doi.org/10.1007/978-3-030-98741-1_63

the research on multimorbidity starts with modeling disease counts using count data model techniques and other generalized linear model [15, 16]. For instance, in recent study [16], researchers used generalized linear model regressions with a log link function and negative binomial distribution to estimate the association of age, gender, and language with the number of chronic diseases, as well as to predict length of stay per admission among inpatients in different departments. Several medical studies pointed out the importance of considering age and sex factors in multimorbidity burden understanding [17–19], which make these variables necessary to be considered in modeling multimorbidity.

Recently, initiatives to exploit Big data techniques and the increasing amount of electronic health care data [20] are taken to get an insight into this phenomenon. In this perspective, we contribute in filling the gap between data science researches and multimorbidity studies in medical area. We define multimorbidity count prediction using machine learning terminology; we explain how to make use of this terminology to draw conclusions about multimorbidity from real data.

Data science methodology consists of four steps in general: Collecting and transforming data of interest in a pertinent format; applying, visualizing and evaluating models. We focus in this work to model a predictive system that predicts average of diseases (disease counts) given a patient profile. A patient profile can be any statistical characteristics of a patient: age, gender, socio-demographic specificities and so on. We set a formal definition of this predictive task and we propose and assess a Meta-algorithm that searches models that fit data given the patient profile, with a focus in age and sex as predictor variables (patient profile), and generalized linear models as hypothesis space explored by the meta algorithm.

The rest of the paper is as follow: in the next section we present the methodology followed in this work. In Sect. 3 we present obtained results. We finish in Sect. 4 by main conclusions of our work.

2 Data and Methods

2.1 Problem Setting

In order to understand the potential relationship hidden in our data of interest, between gender, aging process and multimorbidity, we computed averages of distinct diagnosis in the data per age for both gender across our studied time period (2016). We put the research question in a machine learning framework, i.e. we algorithmically build from data, a functional relation of k-morbidity number (we denote it in the following by $Y_{<morb>}$) as function of sex and age.

Let $D = \{d_1, d_2, \ldots, d_{|D|}\}$ a finite set of diseases present in medical dataset. $X = \{X_1, X_2, \ldots, X_{|X|}\}$ the set of all observations of patients such that $X_i = (x_{(1,i)}, x_{(2,i)}, \ldots, x_{(|Xi|,i)})$ with $x_{j,i} \in D$ a tuple of observed health conditions for the patient i. Let X_v be the subset of patients with profile v (the profile can be any set of medical or socio-demographic characteristics). $X^v = \{X^v{}_1, X^v{}_2, \ldots, X^v{}_{|X^v|}\}$ is a finite subset of X indexed by v. We suppose that X are independent and identically distributed (i.i.d), i.e. that all samples from the datasets are generated from the same generative law, and that the generative process is assumed to have no memory of past generated samples. In other words, in this work we build our analysis on the important assumption that every patient sample consists of separate cases, and these cases are caused by a same underlying Multimorbidity Mechanism. Finally, we define the dependent variable $Y_{<morb>}$ distribution as follows:

$$\begin{aligned} Y_{<morb>} &= \text{average}\left(\left|X^{v}\right|\right) \\ &= \sum\nolimits_{i<|X^{v}|} \frac{\left|X_i^{v}\right|}{\left|X^{v}\right|} \text{ for all non negative integer i.} \end{aligned} \quad (1)$$

Let f be a statistical model such that $Y_{<morb>} = f(X; \theta)$ with parameters, that explains the observations X. We consider the hypothesis space $H = \{f \mid f: X \rightarrow Y_{<morb>}\}$. Technically, statistical models f are grouped as family of equations and H is framed based on assumptions underlying the problem of interest. We are interested in algorithmically building this statistical model. To do so we propose the following meta-algorithm:

```
Meta-Algorithm1
Input: observations X^v, Y_<morb> and hypothesis space H.
Output: a learned statistical model F: X^v→Y_<morb>.
Begin
   1- Observe the random vectors X^v and Y_<morb>.
   2- For each statistical model candidate h ∈ H,evaluate
      its predictive quality with a given quality metric.
   3- Select the optimal h*=f.
   4- Initialize the set of all predictors v_i∈V (explain-
      ing variables) in the model f.
   5- Iteratively eliminate non contributive predictors
      in explaining the model f outcomes.
   6- If the model f has a hyper-parameters k,then fine-
      tune k of f_k against a given Loss function L(.),
      such that f_k are the set of selected model f in-
      dexed by their hyper-parameters k.
Return F with parameter k=argmax L(f_k).
End
```

In this work we implemented this meta-algorithm with the following setting. First, we selected the raw data and we prepared it to be inputted to the algorithm. We precise the hypothesis space in the next section. The algorithm assesses the predictive quality of $h \in H$ using AIC, and BIC metrics. See Evaluation metrics section. The set of predictors are initialized by two predictors/profile characteristics $v = (a, b)$ such that gender $a \in \{\text{female, male}\}$ and age $b \in [1, 150]$ years. The algorithm eliminates non- contributive predictors by calculating R^2 and BIC metrics of all combinations of predictors (age only, sex only, age and sex in the same time) and selects the optimal combination. Finally, fine-tuning the hyper parameters will be based on BIC and adjust R^2. Adding more settings to this meta-algorithm will result in more informative outcomes.

2.2 Hypothesis Space H

We framed the hypothesis space H in a subset of generalized linear models (GLMs). GLMs describe the dependence of a scalar variable y_i ($i = 1, \ldots, n$) on a vector of regressors x_i [21]. The conditional distribution of yi |xi is a linear exponential family with probability density function:

$$p(y; \lambda, \varphi) = \exp(\frac{y \cdot \lambda - b(\lambda)}{\varphi} + c(y, \varphi)) \tag{2}$$

Where λ is the canonical parameter that depends on the regressors via a linear predictor and φ is a dispersion parameter that is often known. The functions $b(\cdot)$ and $c(\cdot)$ are known and determine which member of the family is used, e.g., the normal, binomial or Poisson distribution. Conditional mean and variance of y_i are given by $E[y_i \mid x_i] = \mu_i = b'(\lambda_i)$ and $VAR[y_i \mid x_i] = \varphi \cdot b''(\lambda_i)$, $b'(.)$ and $b''(.)$ are numerical functions. Thus, up to a scale or dispersion parameter φ, the distribution of y_i is determined by its mean. Its variance is proportional to $V(\mu) = b''(\lambda(\mu))$, also called variance function. The dependence of the conditional mean $E[y_i \mid x_i] = \mu_i$ on the regressors x_i is specified as:

$$g(\mu_i) = x_i^T \beta \tag{3}$$

where $g(\cdot)$ is a known link function and β is the vector of regression coefficients which are typically estimated by Maximum Likelihood (ML) using the iterative weighted least squares algorithm.

In this paper we restrict our analysis in polynomial and count data models. In count data models, $Y_{<morb>}$ is considered as discrete data with non-negative integer values which represent disease number. We propose to study Poisson, negative binomial and geometric distributions. They are defined respectively:

$$\text{Poisson: } p(y; \mu) = \frac{e^{-\mu}.\mu^y}{y!} \tag{4}$$

$$\text{Negative binomial: } p(y; \mu, \theta) = \frac{\Gamma(y + \theta)}{\Gamma(\theta) \cdot y!} \frac{\theta^\theta.\mu^y}{(\mu + \theta)^{y+\theta}} \tag{5}$$

With mean μ and shape parameter θ; $\Gamma(\cdot)$ is the gamma function. Geometric distribution is a special case of negative binomial such that $\theta = 1$.

2.3 Evaluation Metrics

Besides statistical measures like R^2 and Mean squared error, the learned models quality are compared based on Akaike's Information Criteria (AIC) and Bayesian Information Criteria (BIC) [22]. AIC and BIC are both penalized-likelihood criteria. BIC estimates the posterior probability of a model being true, assuming a Bayesian perspective, so that a lower BIC means that a model is considered more likely to be the true model. AIC estimates a constant plus the relative distance between the unknown true likelihood function of the data and the fitted likelihood function of the model, that is, a lower AIC means the model is closer to the truth-model.

$$AIC = -2\log(\text{Likelihood}(\Theta^*)) + 2k \quad (6)$$

$$BIC = -2\log(\text{Likelihood}(\Theta^*)) + \log(n)k \quad (7)$$

Where θ^* is estimated parameters for θ value and k corresponds to the number of estimated model parameters, n is the number of observations.

2.4 Data

Our work was applied in a case study of real medical dataset [23]. Each patient has a recorded diagnosis which is recorded by a unique distinct ICD 10 Code in a hospital inpatients' diagnosis dataset, taken originally from admissions in NHS hospitals (The National Health Service hospitals) of Madrid, Spain during 2016. The data contain 78451 patients (34639 males, and 43812 females). The diseases are encoded in 12763 unique ICD10 code (almost 1611 categories). The maximum number of registered diagnosis per admission is 20.

In the remainder of the paper, we analyze and discuss the outputs of the meta-algorithm proposed in the Sect. 2, alongside; we perform some exploratory analysis of our variable of interest.

3 Results and Discussion

3.1 Gender and k-morbidity Variables

Figure 1 shows prevalence of different morbidities by gender. In general, we observe that prevalence of patients tend to decrease as distinct recorded conditions per patient increase continually. It seems that there are differences according to gender. We conducted a Two-sample Kolmogorov-Smirnov test data to compare male and female distributions. We found $D = 0.2$, p-value $= 0.832$, therefore, we did not rejected the null hypothesis which suggests that there is not a significant distribution differences based on gender, for all patients in dataset. However, significant gender differences could be detected in some age ranges, for example, in elderly patients (>70 years), females have more potential to develop multimorbidity than man. We set the following hypothesis H_0^k: "females have less or equal proportions of k-distinct recorded diseases than males", and we applied Pearson's chi-squared test statistic and found that $\max_k(p_k - \text{value}) \ll 0.01$ *for* $k \in \{3, .., 9\}$. Thus, we rejected the null hypothesis in favor of the alternative H_1^k: "females have more proportions of k distinct recorded diseases than males" for $k \in \{3, .., 9\}$.

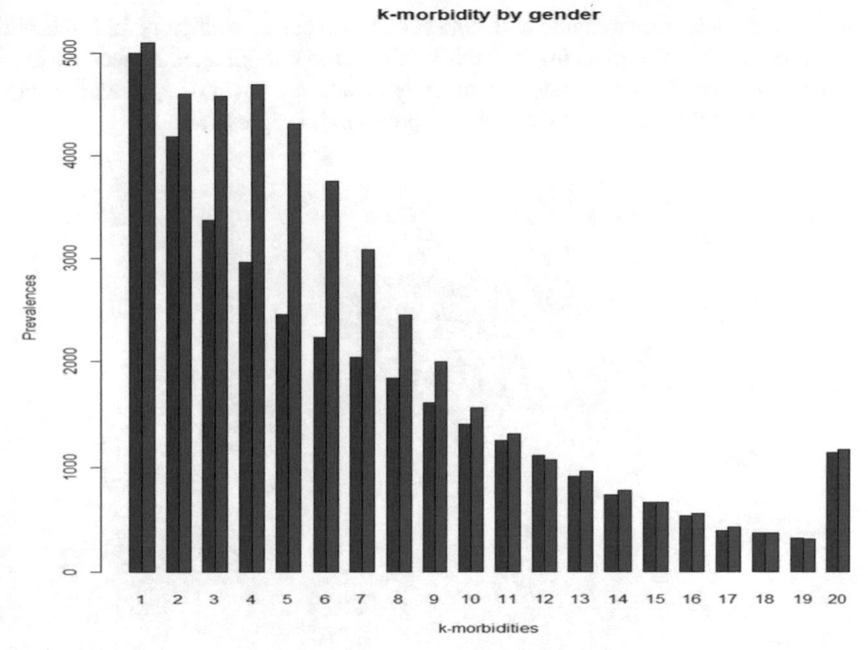

Fig. 1. Prevalence of k-morbidity by gender. Two-sample Kolmogorov-Smirnov test data was performed for male and female, we found D = 0.2 and p-value = 0.832.

3.2 Modeling Relationship of Age and Gender to Multimorbidity

In order to model the relationship between aging process and gender and multimorbidity, we computed averages of distinct diagnosis in the data per age for both gender. In this context we suppose that the number of distinct diagnosis recorded for the patient i is the number of multimorbid diseases (k-morbidity) for the patient i, for our studied time period (2016). The algorithm fitted Poisson, geometric, negative binomial, and a multi-linear model to data of interest. These models were evaluated by Akaike's Information Criteria (AIC) and Bayesian Information Criteria (BIC).

For all models, gender was not of significance in predicting number of conditions (all p-values of gender variable for the studied models are greater than 0.273), in contrary to age variable (all p-values were less than 0.001 with a standard error less than 0.002). This is in line with observation of researchers in [16]. Furthermore, geometric model and Poisson models were respectively the worst and the best count data model, and linear model was the best fitting data according to both AIC and BIC, with low standard errors (SE < 0.002).

To verify further the non-contribution of gender variable as predictor of average k-morbidity, the algorithm backward-eliminated the two variables (age and gender) based on AIC and adjusted R Squared (R^2). Figure 2 shows the results.

Figure 2 shows that Linear model with Gender only as selected predictor results in poor explained error variability $R^2 = 0.0039$ and poorer AIC score. Meanwhile, models with both age and gender selected (compared to age only selected) are quasi-equals ($R^2 \approx 86.07$). As a result, adding gender variable does not improve explained variability any further. Furthermore, linear model with both gender and age as predictors for k-morbidity is the highest AIC score, meaning that this model is too complicated unnecessarily.

In this step, gender is excluded from analysis and the form of age relationship to multimorbidity is further investigated with a polynomial regression.

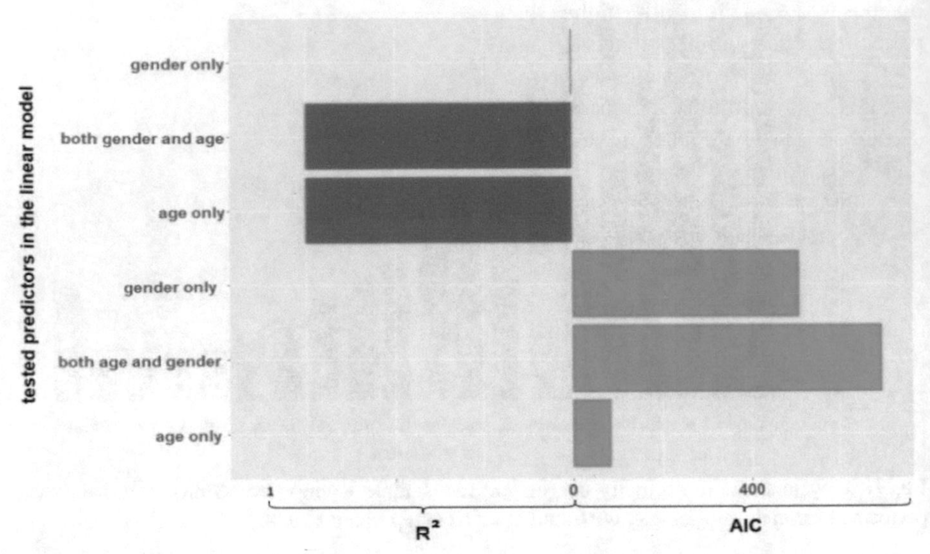

Fig. 2. AIC and adjusted R^2 for different variable combinations. Notice the difference in scale of x-axis: R squared is plotted in inverse direction for ease of visualization and comparison.

3.3 Age Relation to Multimorbidity Modeling

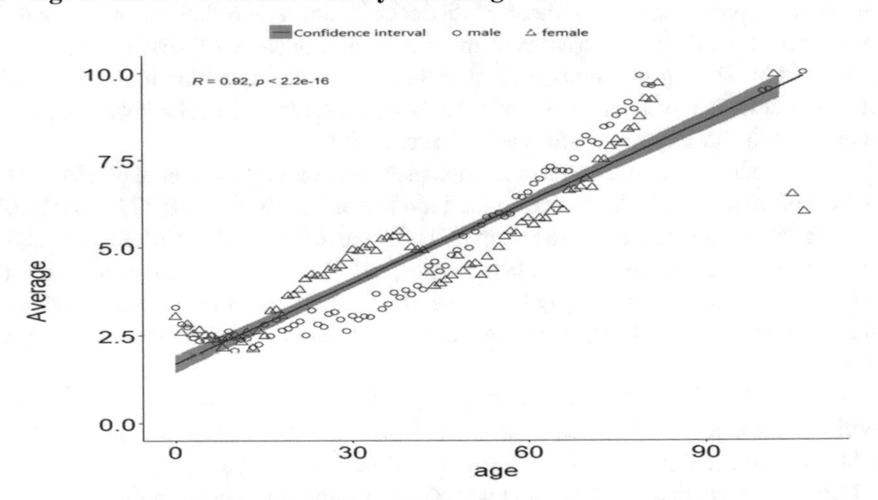

Fig. 3. Average k-morbidity by age for both genders.

Figure 3 describes distribution of average of total disease count per age for males and females. A linear regression was fitted to data point and reaches $R^2 = 0.92$ for females and $R^2 = 0.95$ for males, i.e. almost 90% of data could be explained by a linear relationship. We noticed that for female the interval between 18 and 45 years had significantly greater k-morbidity mean compared to males (p-value $\prec\prec 0.01$). Further, significant differences between genders was also detected ($p - value \prec 0.05$) in older adulthood, in which the proportion of women who was recorded with more than 11 diagnoses was significantly higher than males, and was less or equal proportions for patient recorded with less than 10 diagnoses.

These observations suggest one more time, in consistence with other studies [24–28], that multimorbidity increases significantly with age, potentiality to multimorbidity diseases depend on gender in young adulthood and older adulthood phase, with higher rank for females.

Although the linear regression explains 92% of variability of data showing a positively correlated tendency between age and multimorbidity, a residual analysis for males reveals a systematic pattern in residual points (curvature form, see Fig. 4), which suggest that a linear regression could be a simplifying assumptions for age-multimorbidity relationships. To investigate more the form of this relationship we increased complexity to the initial model by fitting polynomial regression, i.e. we fitted the model $f_h = Y = \beta_0 + \beta_1 X + \beta_2 X_2 + \ldots + \beta_h X^h + \epsilon$ such that $h = \{1, 2, 3, 4, 5, 6, 7\}$ and ϵ are respectively the degree of the polynomial and model error. A 10-fold cross validation was performed against AIC and adjusted R^2. Figure 5 shows that metrics start to stabilize by the third degree and the standard deviation of these metrics tend to very small quantities as degree increases.

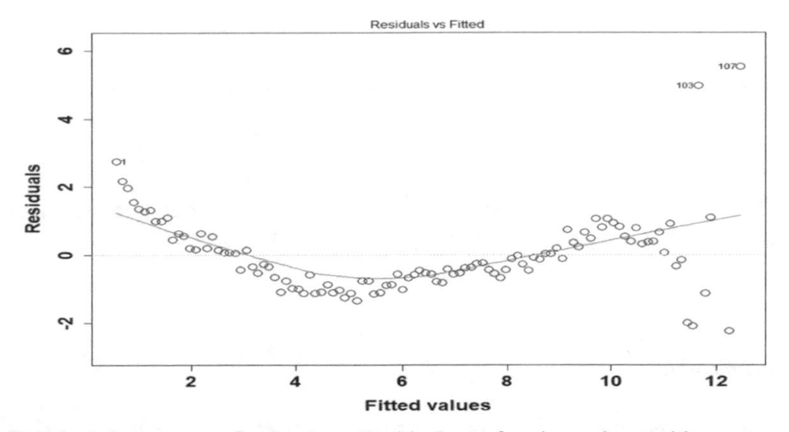

Fig. 4. Residuals in respect to fitted values. Residuals are forming a shape with curvature which suggests that simple linear regression is a simplistic assumption.

For data concerning males between one and 95 years the best describing model is

$$\begin{aligned} Y_{<morb>} &= \beta_0 + \beta_1.age + \beta_2.age^2 + \beta_3.age^3 \\ &= 5.64065 + 36.42487.age + 9.83039.age^2 + 1.27109..age^3 \end{aligned}$$

With variability explained adjusted $R^2 = 0.9565$ and overall p-value << 0.01 for the model. Further, all coefficients of the model β_k have significantly effects on the model output, with $\max_{(k<4)}\{\text{p-value of } \beta_k\} << 0.01$.

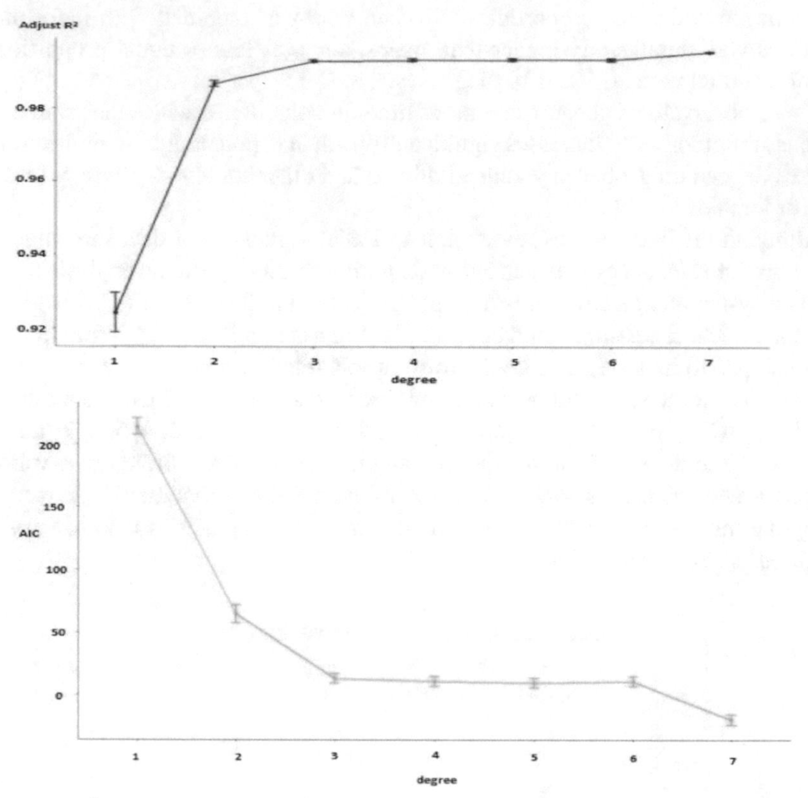

Fig. 5. AIC, R^2 and Means squared Error metrics computed for 10 fold cross validation. Averages and standard deviation are plotted for each hyper-parameter k of the model.

4 Conclusion

In this work we investigated relationship between three health related variables: age, gender and Multimorbidity. In a machine learning framework, we formulated the problem of modeling Multimorbidity as learning an optimal statistical function explaining average conditions based on age and gender. We found, consistently with epidemiological literature, that aging process influences significantly on developing Multimorbidity burden. Gender was not influencing as predictor according to our data of interest, but significant differences between genders was detected in some age intervals. The analysis was conducted by investigating two types of models: count data and polynomial regressors. Polynomial regression to model age and averaged k-morbidity was done after obtaining optimal results for linear model in comparison with count data models and the non-contribution of gender predictor. Most performing model was the third degree polynomial for males between one and 95 years old.

Further works are needed to investigate the generalizability of our conclusions in other real datasets. Second, our study started by investigating two predictors; further predictors will shed more lights on multimorbidity phenomena. Third, used models are based on assumptions which need to be more investigated.

References

1. Feinstein, A.R.: The pre-therapeutic classification of co-morbidity in chronic disease. J. Chronic Dis. **23**, 455–468 (1970). https://doi.org/10.1016/0021-9681(70)90054-8
2. Rijken, M., et al.: How to improve care for people with multimorbidity in Europe? European Observatory on Health Systems and Policies, Copenhagen (Denmark) (2017)
3. Kirchberger, I., et al.: Patterns of multimorbidity in the aged population. Results from the KORA-Age study. PLoS One **7**, e30556 (2012)
4. Fortin, M., Hudon, C., Haggerty, J., van den Akker, M., Almirall, J.: Prevalence estimates of multimorbidity: a comparative study of two sources. BMC Health Serv. Res. **10**, 111 (2010). https://doi.org/10.1186/1472-6963-10-111
5. Elhai, J.D., Calhoun, P.S., Ford, J.D.: Statistical procedures for analyzing mental health services data. Psychiatry Res. **160**, 129–136 (2008). https://doi.org/10.1016/j.psychres.2007.07.003
6. Lappenschaar, M., et al.: Multilevel temporal Bayesian networks can model longitudinal change in multimorbidity. J. Clin. Epidemiol. **66**, 1405–1416 (2013)
7. Lappenschaar, M., Hommersom, A., Lucas, P.J.: Probabilistic causal models of multimorbidity concepts. In: AMIA ... Annual Symposium proceedings. AMIA Symposium, pp. 475–484 (2012)
8. Lappenschaar, M., Hommersom, A., Lagro, J., Lucas, P.J.F.: Understanding the co-occurrence of diseases using structure learning. In: Peek, N., Marín Morales, R., Peleg, M. (eds.) AIME 2013. LNCS (LNAI), vol. 7885, pp. 135–144. Springer, Heidelberg (2013). https://doi.org/10.1007/978-3-642-38326-7_21
9. Lai, Y.-H., Wang, T.-Y., Yang, H.-H.: Network-based analysis of comorbidities: case study of diabetes mellitus. In: Wang, L., Uesugi, S., Ting, I.-H., Okuhara, K., Wang, K. (eds.) MISNC 2015. CCIS, vol. 540, pp. 210–222. Springer, Heidelberg (2015). https://doi.org/10.1007/978-3-662-48319-0_17
10. Cramer, A.O.J., Waldorp, L.J., van der Maas, H.L.J., Borsboom, D.: Comorbidity: a network perspective. Behav. Brain Sci. **33**, 137–150 (2010)
11. Faruqui, S.H.A., Alaeddini, A., Jaramillo, C.A., Potter, J.S., Pugh, M.J.: Mining patterns of comorbidity evolution in patients with multiple chronic conditions using unsupervised multi-level temporal Bayesian network. PLoS ONE **13**, e0199768 (2018). https://doi.org/10.1371/journal.pone.0199768
12. Guo, M., et al.: Analysis of disease comorbidity patterns in a large-scale China population. BMC Med. Genomics **12**(Suppl 12), 177 (2019). https://doi.org/10.1186/s12920-019-0629-x.PMID:31829182;PMCID:PMC6907122
13. Xu, X., Mishra, G.D., Jones, M.: Evidence on multimorbidity from definition to intervention: an overview of systematic reviews. Ageing Res. Rev. **37**, 53–68 (2017)
14. Diederichs, C., Berger, K., Bartels, D.B.: The measurement of multiple chronic diseases-a systematic review on existing multimorbidity indices. J. Gerontol. A Biol. Sci. Med. Sci. **66**, 301–311 (2011)

15. Uijen, A.A., van de Lisdonk, E.H.: Multimorbidity in primary care: prevalence and trend over the last 20 years. Eur. J. General Pract. **14**, 28–32 (2008). https://doi.org/10.1080/13814780802436093
16. Guerin, E., Bouattane, E.M., Joanisse, J., Prud'homme, D.: Bouattane Mostafa Clusters of multimorbidity across hospital services and by language groups. JHA **10**, 6 (2021)
17. Abad-Díez, J.M., et al.: Age and gender differences in the prevalence and patterns of multimorbidity in the older population. BMC Geriatr. **14**, 75 (2014)
18. Jin, L., et al.: Multimorbidity analysis according to sex and age towards cardiovascular diseases of adults in northeast China. Sci. Rep. **8**, 8607 (2018). https://doi.org/10.1038/s41598-018-25561-y
19. Broeiro-Gonçalves, P., Nogueira, P., Aguiar, P.: Multimorbidity and disease severity by age groups, in inpatients: cross-sectional study. PJP **37**, 1–9 (2019)
20. Pastorino, R., et al.: Benefits and challenges of Big Data in healthcare: an overview of the European initiatives. Eur. J. Pub. Health **29**, 23–27 (2019)
21. McCullagh, P., Nelder, J.A.: Generalized Linear Models (1989)
22. Burnham, K.P., Anderson, D.R.: Multimodel Inference: understanding AIC and BIC in model selection. Sociol. Methods Res. **33**, 261–304 (2004)
23. Bonis, J.: drbonis/CMBD_MAD_2016 (2019). https://github.com/drbonis/CMBD_MAD_2016. Accessed 01 July 2021
24. Ryan, B.L., et al.: Beyond the grey tsunami: a cross-sectional population-based study of multimorbidity in Ontario. Can. J. Public Health **109**(5–6), 845–854 (2018). https://doi.org/10.17269/s41997-018-0103-0
25. Makovski, T.T., Schmitz, S., Zeegers, M.P., Stranges, S., van den Akker, M.: Multimorbidity and quality of life: systematic literature review and meta-analysis. Age. Res. Rev. **53**, 100903 (2019)
26. Nunes, B.P., Flores, T.R., Mielke, G.I., Thumé, E., Facchini, L.A.: Multimorbidity and mortality in older adults: a systematic review and meta-analysis. Arch. Gerontol. Geriatr. **67**, 130–138 (2016)
27. Violán, C., et al.: Patrones de multimorbilidad en adultos jóvenes en Cataluña: un análisis de clústeres. Atención Primaria **48**, 479–492 (2016)
28. Koné Pefoyo, A.J., et al.: The increasing burden and complexity of multimorbidity. BMC Public Health **15**, 415 (2015)

Advanced Analytics for Medical Supply Chain Resilience in Healthcare Systems: An Infection Disease Case

Brenno Menezes[1(✉)], Robert Franzoi[1], Mohammed Yaqot[1], Mohammed Sawaly[1,2], and Antonio Sanfilippo[3]

[1] Division of Engineering Management and Decision Sciences, College of Science and Engineering, Hamad Bin Khalifa University, Qatar Foundation, Doha, Qatar
bmenezes@hbku.edu.qa
[2] Department of Supply Chain, Hamad Medical Corporation, Doha, Qatar
[3] Qatar Environment and Energy Research Institute, Hamad Bin Khalifa University, Qatar Foundation, Doha, Qatar

Abstract. The COVID-19 impacts go beyond healthcare systems as they also challenge global markets and society. A comprehensive knowledge involving the elements to contain the virus is fundamental for properly planning and implementing a quick response to the problems faced worldwide. Learning to coexist with the COVID-19 pandemic has become part of our daily life. Hence, the scientific community's capabilities to continuously provide solutions for pandemics are crucial to mitigate the spread of the pandemic. The main contribution of this work is to propose applications of advanced analytics (AA) in healthcare treatment networks that predict epidemiology curves and the distribution of patients' severity towards. These tools assist the optimization of such networks with innovative solutions aiming to increase the capacity, responsiveness, and preparedness of the infrastructure and management in healthcare systems. Such a decision-making environment can forecast the spread of the disease by utilizing given inputs such as social distance, out-of-stock of personal protective equipment (PPE) items, lockdown policies, environmental factors, etc. These forecasts are especially important to allow a) medical corporations to design and operate healthcare treatment systems and b) governments to develop policies aiming to maintain the balance between social progress and a sustainable economy.

Keywords: Advanced analytics · Medical supply chain resilience · COVID-19 · Optimization

1 Introduction

The COVID-19 cases have been imposing many challenges on the capacity, operation, and control of healthcare treatment systems, exhausting a lot of their resources in material, equipment, and personnel. COVID-19 is an infectious disease that spreads exponentially quicker than severe acute respiratory syndrome (SARS) or the Middle East

F. Saeed et al. (Eds.): IRICT 2021, LNDECT 127, pp. 759–768, 2022.
https://doi.org/10.1007/978-3-030-98741-1_64

respiratory syndrome (MERS). So far, such an unprecedented pandemic has proven to be extremely hard to contain and revealed that healthcare systems worldwide are unprepared to respond to the required changes effectively. Governments and healthcare systems must pursue enhanced capabilities to be better prepared for dealing with the multiple waves of COVID-19 and any future outbreaks.

The COVID-19 impacts surpassed healthcare systems by affecting educational processes, local and international markets, and global supply chains. Therefore, a resilient supply chain response should be as quick as the spread of the virus for properly containing it, whilst providing adequate care [1]. A detailed and robust understanding of the causes and consequences in markets, communities, and healthcare systems is necessary to be resilient by resisting (avoiding and containing) and recovering (stabilizing and returning) when planning and executing timely responses [2]. Despite the vaccination efforts made so far to provide immunization as quickly as possible, the vaccine distribution chain is challenging and is likely to delay the demise of COVID-19. Hence, the scientific community is fundamental to continuously study and investigate the pandemic's dynamic evolution aiming to enhance institutional preparedness with resistance and recovery capabilities.

This research focuses on the development of advanced analytics in healthcare treatment networks for predicting epidemiology curves and distribution of patients' severity. Healthcare networks can be properly optimized with innovative solutions towards increased capacity, responsiveness, and preparedness of healthcare systems infrastructure and management. In the proposed framework, a data-driven machine learning (ML) technique (predictive analytics) is firstly applied to identify epidemiology curves of future outcomes in terms of numbers of positive cases and their distribution among asymptomatic/mild, moderate, and severe stages. Second, the healthcare treatment networks' design, operation, and control (prescriptive analytics) are determined using the predictions on the epidemiology curves by integrating both predictive and prescriptive analytics. Then, sensitivity analysis is conducted by inserting disruptive inputs in the model to infer a sustainable economy with social progress in equilibrium with the healthcare treatment systems under evaluation.

The proposed research provides a platform embedded with ML and optimization algorithms configured by predictive and prescriptive analytics for the operation and coordination of the healthcare networks for disease treatment. This platform can predict disease outbreaks based on specified inputs such as social distance, out-of-stock personal protective equipment (PPE) supplies, lockdown policies, environmental parameters such as temperature and humidity, etc. Such projections enable a) medical corporations to build and execute healthcare treatment systems; and b) governments to establish regulations and policies based on the solution's feasibility assessment, with the goal of maintaining the balance between social progress and sustainable long-term economic viability.

2 Impacts of Infectious Diseases in the Medical Supply Chain

Pandemics and natural disasters create unanticipated operational shocks to healthcare and emergency response systems and organizations. The backbone to absorb and mitigate pandemic shock waves are hospitals, which are the most vulnerable and rarely ever prepared for large-scale crises. Hospitals all over the world were severely overwhelmed by the COVID-19 pandemic. These negative impacts could have been mitigated or even avoided had there been effective ways to optimize resources and operations. For instance, Italy experienced high infection rates amongst healthcare workers because of inadequate supply and access to PPE. One of the primary reactions was a frantic effort by individuals and medical staff to secure PPE, which was at odds with the concerns of supply chain personnel to limit waste and prioritize response.

Optimization of the distribution center stocks is vital to successfully respond to pandemic events. In many countries, there were far more COVID-19 positive and symptomatic people outside than inside hospitals due to lack of space, lack of utilization of bed capacity in hospitals, and operational inefficiencies. Such design obstacles indicate that many patients are not treated in time (or at all), which significantly increases the death rate. In times of crisis, the challenges are multi-layered, so that there is an urgent need to have enough qualified staff, expand treatment capacity, treat more patients and discharge them faster, allocate resources to those most required. All these challenges are faced simultaneously while facing a pandemic with multiple difficulties and uncertainties. During such a crisis, employees are in constant fear of being infected, working extremely long hours, confused, and tense. Fear, along with illness, are the two biggest factors that lead to workers absenteeism [3, 4]. Hence, scheduling of staff is vital to maintain workflow in hospitals where there are ever-changing demands. These dynamics and concomitant factors eventually strained the whole local supply chain of medical items locally and worldwide.

Several institutes worldwide have addressed models for the growing spread of the pandemic. For example, in March 2020, Qatar's Energy Environmental Research Institute (QEERI) proposed a data-driven estimation and forecasting approach of COVID-19 transmissions based on machine learning (ML) modeling of epidemiological, socioeconomic, environmental, and global health indicator data. QEERI's model currently targets only the prediction 7 days ahead of the expected COVID-19 cases per day. The forecasting horizon of the model can be increased to several weeks, in addition to providing forecasts for the statistical distribution of the symptomatic conditions of the infected population. For the confirmed COVID-19 cases per day, Fig. 1 gives a snapshot of the good correlation of the global aggregate value and the prediction of QEERI's model (R2 of 0.964). The plot at the top shows the prediction accuracy of the model when tested over an unseen portion of the dataset. The bottom figure depicts the overall model performance when considering the whole dataset (training and testing sets).

Some studies have tried to predict COVID-19 spread from 1–3 up to 6 days ahead using ML-based techniques. Ribeiro et al. [5] forecast cumulative cases of COVID-19 in Brazil using forecasting techniques of different time series such as support vector regression, autoregressive integrated moving average, ridge regression, random forest, cubist regression, and stacking-ensemble learning. Chimmula and Zhang [6] use a deep learning approach (long short-term memory networks) to forecast future COVID-19 cases in Canada, Italy, and the USA. A model for COVID-19 cases in a real-time prediction for France, Canada, India, South Korea, and the United Kingdom is developed by Chakraborty and Ghosh [7] based on a combination of the ARIMA algorithm and

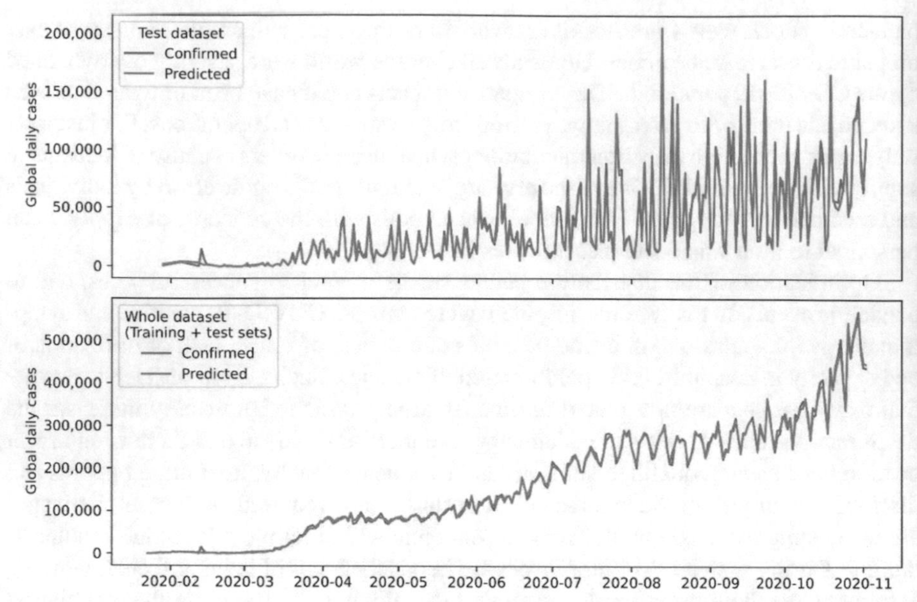

Fig. 1. Comparison between the confirmed and predicted COVID-19 daily cases at the global level.

wavelet-based forecasting techniques. Stübinger and Schneider [8] propose the forecast of the COVID-19 spread by utilizing the identified lead-lag effects among diverse countries with the help of the well-known dynamic time warping (DTW) used extensively in batch process monitoring and analysis.

In reference to bed capacity management, Alban et al. [9] developed a computer simulation model that uses a stochastic queuing model for ICU patients flow to determine the amount of positive and negative COVID-19 patients to be assisted in a limited ICU capacity. Their model considers beds that are reserved for COVID-19 patients, as well as beds for unplanned urgent cases. The conclusion is that the inclusion of both COVID and non-COVID patients in an ICU facility adds an operational constraint to ICU bed management. To optimize large-scale emergency preparedness, Lee et al. [10] developed a decision-making software called RealOpt, which optimizes a public healthcare system for a complete set of emergency responses. This framework can be used in areas of infectious disease outbreaks, radiological or biological terrorism, and national disaster resource planning. In addition, RealOpt can be configured for different inputs to get desired fast results through many what-if scenarios.

To manage resources during pandemic events, Garbey et al. [11] use data from the French Government during COVID-19 within a computational model that anticipates the patient moves to different care units and the amount of PPE required by these units, as well as other key measurements of the performance of the French healthcare system during the COVID-19 crisis. This model is meant to reproduce the hospital workflow during an epidemic, which in this case, admits a maximum of 50 patients per day. They use a Markov process to augment the workflow of patients and employ a statistical model to determine the lengths of stay of patients at each stage of their admission. The model helped senior medical directors to determine the number of beds needed and whether transferring of patients among facilities was required.

To the best of our knowledge, no work has been reported so far covering healthcare treatment systems' infrastructure (design), operation, and control for their planning, scheduling, and coordination over multiple stages of the disease. This is especially important for developing a performance model that minimizes the deviation from targets of healthcare, efficiency, service, etc., for an assessment of the balance between social progress and a sustainable economy. Thus, this work aims to propose a decision-making framework to address such an important topic and provide future research guidelines.

3 Proposed Framework

The proposed framework integrates a) machine learning predictive analytics for the epidemiology curves of COVID-19 positive cases (and their distribution in terms of severity) and b) optimization (or prescriptive analytics) to prescribe future design, operation, and control of healthcare treatment systems. Such methodology can be greatly useful to enhance the economy towards its sustainability and help governments and society cope with the unforeseen impacts in healthcare.

The spread of the new daily cases (referred to as epidemiology curve) can be predicted by a ML method based on data analytics (Step 1). Then, these predictions can be used for determining healthcare treatment systems' optimal design, operation, and control (Step 2) to assess a COVID-19 facility with specific reference to ICU units (for severe patients), In-Patient Clinics/tents (for mild-moderate patients), and Emergency ward (for symptomatic patients), and lastly other quarantine sites for asymptomatic positive patients. The combination of Steps 1 and 2 allows sensitivity analysis to assess the integration of social progress and sustainable economy using what-if cases or predicted epidemiology curves with respect to the spread of the disease. A summary of the steps is illustrated in Fig. 2.

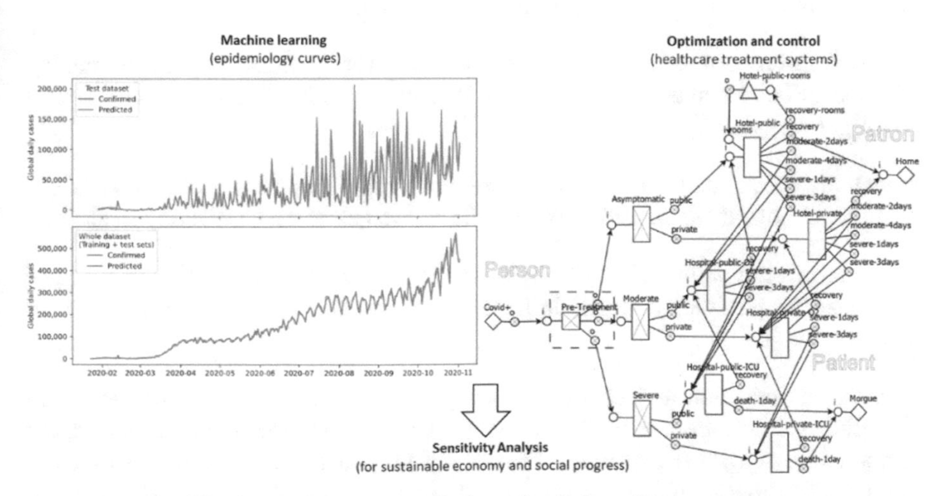

Fig. 2. Phases of the medical supply chain resilience study.

3.1 Epidemiology Curve Prediction

From the challenges faced by the medical corporations worldwide in the COVID-19 pandemic, it is fundamental to efficiently determine the disease spread to be better prepared for peaks in the number of patients within the healthcare treatment networks. When simulating or measuring the specific inputs (e.g., social distance, out-of-stock PPE supplies, climate, lockdown policies, etc.), epidemiology curve predictions have the ability to forecast the statistical distribution of the symptomatic conditions of the predicted infected population.

As an example, this can be based on Gradient Boosted Regression Tree (GBRT) models. GBRT is an additive stochastic model that combines multiple sequentially connected weak learners (regression trees). The new learners fit the residuals from the previous stage for optimizing the overall predictive performance. The models built using such methodology include nonlinear interactions and are sufficiently flexible, highly accurate, and robust to outliers or missing data. The dataset used for the forecasting approach can include lagged values of epidemiological, socioeconomic, environmental, and global health indicator factors [12]. The model is trained using a random part of the dataset, in which the remaining data points test the prediction accuracy to avoid any sort of biased behavior from the data. The hyperparameters in the model can be optimized based on a combination of grid-search and 5-fold cross-validation approaches to avoid overfitting and to reduce the variance erroring the error predictions.

3.2 Optimal Design, Operation and Control of the Medical Supply Chain

With the prediction of the epidemiology curve with respect to the defined inputs, and with the parameter of the rate of the PPE items for emergency, in-patient, and ICU COVID-19 treatments, decisions can properly determine the optimal design, operation, and control of a resilient medical supply chain. The decision variables for the medical resource supply chain resilience are categorized and described as follows:

Design. Capacity of the facilities in terms of patients as continuous variables, and type and number of different treatments (ICU, In-Patient, Operating Theatres, etc.) as discrete and integer variables.

Operation. Stocks and flows of resources (material, equipment, personnel) in each healthcare treatment site considering the different stages of the COVID-19 treatment.

Control: Level of supply chain services and PPE distribution/reposition in near real-time among the multiple sites to minimize deviation for standards or targets of healthcare, efficiency, service, etc.

In the optimization and control of healthcare treatment systems, the network in Fig. 3 shows a flowsheet of facilities and connections in the unit-operation-port-state superstructure (UOPSS) constructs from Kelly [13] that is built-in in the Industrial Modeling and Programming Language (IMPL) software [14]. The objects or shapes are: a) sources and sinks (◊), batch-processes (□), continuous-processes (⊠), and tanks or inventories (Δ) represented by unit-operations $\boldsymbol{m}$ and b) the connectivity of arrows (→),

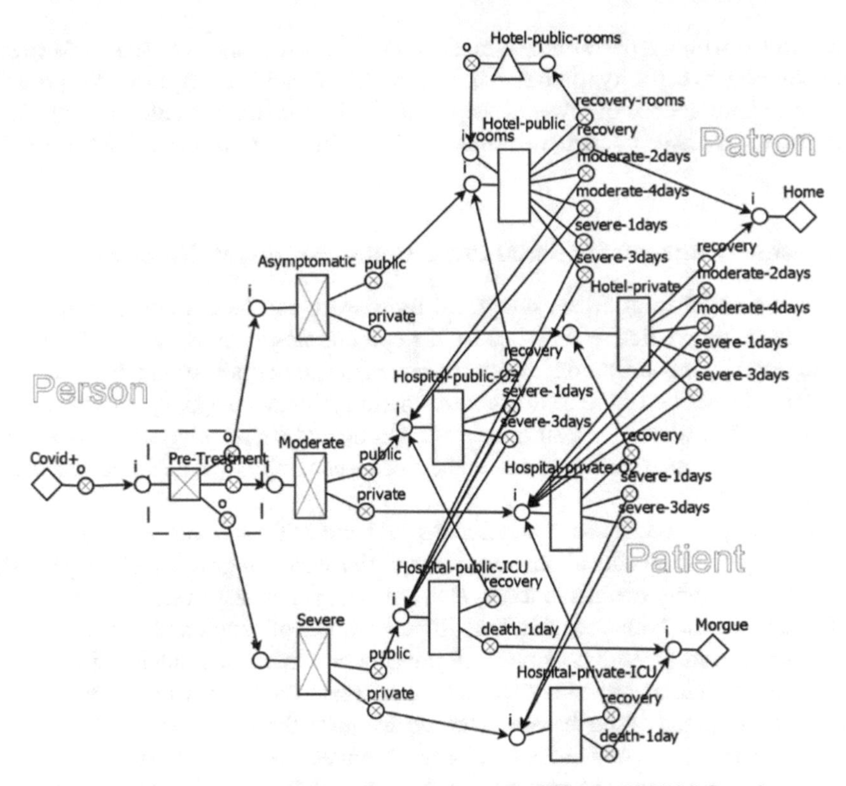

Fig. 3. Healthcare treatment system constructed within the UOPSS flowsheet.

inlet-ports ***i*** (○) and outlet-ports ***j*** (⊗). Both binary ***y*** and continuous ***x*** variables are defined for unit-operations and arrows and the ports represent process yields.

For the modeling of units, materials, tasks, etc., two approaches are usually used to represent production systems in the chemical engineering literature. They are known as state-task network (STN) [15, 16] and resource-task network (RTN) [17]. These models are originated from sequential batch-type production in which a sequence of tasks is performed on renewable (units) and/or non-renewable resources (states). However, as a superset of the STN and RTN superstructures, the UOPSS network gives an anywhere-to-anywhere connectivity usually referred to as a flowsheet, routing, mapping, topology, or block-diagram for its various objects, shapes, or structures that are needed to configure and construct the problem networks. Brunaud et al. [18] demonstrate that the UOPSS is computationally superior to STN and RTN in complex-scope scheduling problems using batch processes in the chemical production industry, solving large-scale problems within minutes to seconds instead of hours.

From such definition of design, operation, and control for the medical resource supply chain resilience to COVID-19 pandemic, a generalized performance model could potentially and efficiently minimize deviation from targets, standards, and policies. Such methodology needs to address uncertain information such the forthcoming number of positive case patients. Methodologies to determine the contagious curve can be estimated and employed within a performance model according to a) targets or standards (treated as soft bounds), b) capacity limitation for the treatment facilities, c) correlated processes considering hard bounds of lower and upper limits in decision variables, and d) penalty values for variables or constraints aiming to avoid infeasibilities (e.g., out of stock of PPE).

3.3 Sensitivity Analysis for Social Progress and Sustainable Economy

From such a novel solution, an integrated framework can be developed to include a) machine learning predictive analytics for the epidemiology curves of COVID-19 positive cases (and their distribution in terms of severity) and b) optimization (or prescriptive analytics) to prescribe future healthcare treatment systems' design, operation, and control. This can be utilized for a sustainable economy and social progress assessments to help governments and society cope with the unforeseen impacts in healthcare, economy, supply chains, etc.

Considering social distance restrictions that are still ongoing in some countries around workplaces and educational centers, and the sectors highly affected by COVID-19 damages in supply chains, tourism, etc., the companies and overall society need to handle the pandemic events considering a limited amount of people and resources. Therefore, learning to mitigate the COVID-19 impacts and achieving enhanced knowledge and experience under pandemic events is fundamental to continue with the resistance by a) avoiding the spread of the disease, when determining the targets of social distance, as an example, and b) its containment by better preparedness of the healthcare treatment networks to mitigate the consequences for those symptomatic patients both in moderate and severe stages.

In-deep studies to understand how to recover and re-establish previous stages of the economy and social livelihoods may be determined with such advanced analytics framework, whereby predictions of the near future epidemiology curves and prescription of the optimized healthcare treatment for the future responses, both detective and cognitive analytics [19], can be used to determine stabilization stages and moments of returning to past or new states of social and economic progress.

4 Conclusion

As we have witnessed, COVID-19 did not disappear after a few months, but has in fact developed and become a problem to persist over the years. With the aid of advancements in predictive and prescriptive, we can be able to predict epidemiology curves of the virus spreading to be well prepared to act accordingly. It is shown in this study that healthcare systems can be better designed and operated in anticipation of worst-case scenarios, through timely and efficient response mechanisms. Such modeling capabilities can be used in future crisis situations, whether they are other virus outbreaks or natural disasters. Hence, the scientific community is fundamental to continuously study and investigate the dynamic evolution of the pandemic aiming to enhance institutional preparedness with resistance and recovery capabilities.

It is evident from the COVID-19 events that the interconnection among countries is linked in a way that no one can escape the outreach of most matters, particularly virus outbreaks. Everyone's lives have been impacted, and many lives have been lost. Protecting the people lives entails that we need sufficient resources, allocated properly and efficiently. Further to this work, additional methodologies and strategies, such as procurement planning, can be developed and implemented to ensure that no stock-outs of PPE or medical equipment occur. Staff scheduling models can be employed to ensure proper treatment for everyone so that no sick person is left unattended. The design of whole healthcare networks can be enhanced to make sure that every bed space in a community is fully utilized. Quarantine and hotel facilities can be planned to be better utilized. The development of better epidemiology curves, showing the potentials of newer strains of viruses with newer causations can also be studied. Overall, many advanced analytic techniques can be developed, improved, and implemented to provide more efficient capabilities for handling emergency situations in the current and eventually future pandemic events.

References

1. Murthy, S., Gomersall, C.D., Fowler, R.A.: Care for critically ill patients with COVID-19. J. Am. Med. Assoc. **323**(15), 1499–1500 (2020)
2. Melnyk, S., Closs, D., Griffis, S., Zobel, C., Macdonald, J.: Understanding supply chain resilience. Supply Chain Manage. Rev. **18**(1), 34–41 (2014)
3. Itzwerth, R.L., MacIntyre, C.R., Shah, S., Plant, A.J.: Pandemic influenza and critical infrastructure dependencies. Med. J. Aust. **185**(10), 70 (2006)
4. Balicer, R.D., et al.: Characterizing hospital workers' willingness to report to duty in an influenza pandemic through threat- and efficacy-based assessment. BMC Public Health **436**(10), (2010)
5. Ribeiro, M.H.D.M., da Silva, R.G., Mariani, V.C., Coelho, L.C.: Short-term forecasting COVID-19 cumulative confirmed cases: Perspectives for Brazil. Chaos, Solitons & Fractals, pp. 109853 (2020)
6. Chimmula, V.K.R., Zhang, L.: Time series forecasting of COVID-19 transmission in Canada using LSTM networks. Chaos, Solitons & Fractals, p. 109864 (2020)
7. Chakraborty, T., Ghosh, I.: Real-time forecasts and risk assessment of novel coronavirus (COVID-19) cases: a data-driven analysis. Chaos, Solitons & Fractals, p. 109850 (2020)
8. Stubinger, J., Schneider, L.: Epidemiology of coronavirus COVID-19: forecasting the future incidence in different countries. Healthcare **8**(2), 99 (2020)
9. Alban, A., et al.: ICU capacity management during the COVID-19 pandemic using a stochastic process simulation. Intensive Care Med. **7**, 1–3 (2020)
10. Lee, E.K., Chen, C.H., Pietz, F., Benecke, B.: Modeling and optimizing the public-health infrastructure for emergency response. Interfaces **39**(5), 476–490 (2009)
11. Garbey, M., Joerger, G., Furr, S., Fikfak, V.: A model of workflow in the hospital during a pandemic to assist management. PLOS ONE **15**(11), e0242183 (2020)
12. Friedman, J.H.: Greedy function approximation: a gradient boosting machine. Annals of statistics, pp.1189–1232 (2001)
13. Kelly, J.D.: The unit-operation-stock superstructure (UOSS) and the quantity-logic-quality paradigm (QLQP) for production scheduling in the process industries. In: Multidisciplinary International Scheduling Conference Proceedings: New York, United States, pp. 327–333 (2005)

14. Kelly, J.D., Menezes, B.C.: Industrial Modeling and Programming Language (IMPL) for off- and on-line optimization and estimation applications. In: Fathi, M., Khakifirooz, M., Pardalos, P. (eds.) Optimization in Large Scale Problems. SOIA, vol. 152, pp. 75–96. Springer, Cham (2019). Doi: https://doi.org/10.1007/978-3-030-28565-4_13
15. Kondili, E., Pantelides, C.C., Sargent, R.W.H.: A general algorithm for short-term scheduling of batch operations – I MILP formulation. Comput. Chem. Eng. **17**, 211–227 (1993)
16. Shah, N., Pantelides, C.C., Sargent, R.W.H.: Optimal periodic scheduling of multipurpose batch plants. Ann. Oper. Res. **42**, 193 (1993)
17. Pantelides, C.C.: Unified frameworks for optimal process planning and scheduling. In: Foundations of Computer-Aided Process Operations. CACHE Publications, New York (1994)
18. Brunaud, B., Perez, H.D., Amaran, S., Bury, S., Grossman, I.E.: Batch scheduling with quality-based changeovers. Comput. Chem. Eng. **132**, 106617 (2020)
19. Menezes, B.C., Kelly, J.D., Leal, A.G., Le Roux, G.C.: Predictive, prescriptive and detective analytics for smart manufacturing in the information age. IFAC-PapersOnline **52**(1), 568–573 (2019)

Application of Temporal Network on Potential Disease Transmission: Hospital Case Study

Yaseen Alwesabi(✉), Dong Dinh, and Xilin Zhang

Department of Systems Science and Industrial Engineering, SUNY Binghamton University, Binghamton, NY 13902, USA
yalwesa1@binghamton.edu

Abstract. Early diagnosis of potential epidemic transmission of diseases such as influenza or coronavirus in hospitals where one-to-one contact occurs is central not only to save patients' life, but also to prevent disease propagation to staff, nurses, medical doctors, and other workers. This paper aims to predict the risk threshold of influenza disease transmission in a temporal network; the hospital's data in Lyon, France is taken as a case study. The network involves 46 health care workers and 29 patients. The Susceptible Infectious Recovered (SIR) model is used for the analysis. The SIR model is more fit for the influenza disease because a patient is not suspected to spread the disease after recovery. The results show that the disease propagation rate is lower in the temporal network compared with the corresponding aggregated network. It is found out that that the threshold of an epidemic occurs when the transmission percentage is 10%. Most importantly, it is found that the nurses and administrators are more likely to be infected than physicians or patients in this case study. The proposed model is applicable in hospitals, schools, or any work organization for epidemiologic control.

Keywords: Epidemic transmission of disease · Temporal network · Susceptible infectious recovered · Susceptible infectious susceptible

1 Introduction

Based on the recent statistics from World Health Organization in August 2020, more than three million influenza cases and up to half a million deaths worldwide [1]. Infection control is a vital approach to prevent some potential bacterial and viral transmissions [2–4]. Nurses or healthcare workers in hospitals have direct interaction with patients and colleagues. These interactions lead to a high risk of potential epidemic transmission of infectious diseases such as influenza and COVID-19. To monitor this phenomenon, wearable sensors were used to detect interactions between individuals [4]. The recorded data has 46 staff members (27 nurses, 11 physicians, and 8 administrative staff) as well as 29 patients. The data has been collected and analyzed by [4]. Three methods have been used to study disease transmission from a temporal network, time-slice networks, ongoing networks, and exponential-threshold networks [4]. The results indicated that exponential-threshold was able to capture the most relevant information while static or

F. Saeed et al. (Eds.): IRICT 2021, LNDECT 127, pp. 769–774, 2022.
https://doi.org/10.1007/978-3-030-98741-1_65

aggregated network performs poorly. However, the likelihood of an infectious disease outbreak using the SIR model for this case study has not been investigated in the literature according to the authors' best knowledge. Therefore, this study aims to extend the work of [4] by detecting the transmission rate using the SIR model, as well as providing a comparison between temporal and static networks.

Epidemic models on dynamic temporal-driven networks have been investigated by several researchers [5, 6]. Derived evidence from [6] shows that temporal networks can reduce the epidemic prevalence due to the time factor that is not active all the time. In this study, the behavior of disease propagation will be analyzed using the SIR model. The SIR model is established to measure disease transmission when the patient does not transfer the disease after recovery. The remains of the paper are organized as follows. Section 2 illustrates the literature review while the proposed approach or methodology is demonstrated in Sect. 3. Results, discussion, and conclusions are shown in Sects. 4, 5, and 6, respectively.

2 Related Work

A reliable estimation of the epidemic threshold of infectious disease is of utmost importance for the probability of disease contagion prediction, identifying the containment of the infectious disease epidemic and perhaps preventing disease propagation [7]. The typical models used to quantify the epidemic threshold are SIR and SIS models [8, 9]. The difference between the SIS model and the SIR model is that the infected individuals are susceptible again after recovery in the SIS model, while the infected individuals can recover with lifelong immunity or die in the SIR model.

In the literature, three commonly used theoretical methods are reported to predict epidemic thresholds, namely the mean-field-like (MFL) method, the dynamical message passing (DMP) method, and the quenched mean-field (QMF) method. Wei Wang et al. [9] applied the three methods in conjunction with the SIR model in 56 real-world networks. They found that the MFL method has the best performance among the three in real-world networks. The threshold predicted by the MFL method is closer to the real epidemic threshold. Shu et al. [10] used the MFL in finite-size networks and confirmed that analyzing the peak of the epidemic variability accurately determines the simulated epidemic thresholds of the SIS and SIR models.

The duration (time) of nodes or links plays an important role in the propagation process, see [11, 12]. The epidemic threshold of temporal networks is given by the interplay between the timescales of contagion [13]. In static networks, the link between two individuals indicates that the two individuals have at least one-time interaction during the sample period. The epidemic threshold of static networks is determined by the principal eigenvalue of the adjacent matrix [13].

3 Methodology

The data format in our case study is expressed as follows: (t, i, j, m_i, m_j) represents (time, identity i, identity j, status i, and status j), respectively; status: NUR = Nurses, Pat = Patients, MED = Medical doctors, and ADM = administrative staff. The mean-field approximation for the SIR model is used for simulation. The parameters are defined as follows. p is the probability of a node is infected at a specific time, p_e is the connectivity probability between nodes in the network, $\mathrm{p_r}$ is the recovery probability, p_i is the probability that an infected node transfers the disease to another node if they are connected, and $n = 75$ is the total number nodes. The comparison of the infection process between the temporal network and the static network corresponding to the SIR model is presented.

In both networks, static and temporal, the probability of recovery p_r is set at 0.8 and the probability of infection is varied from 0 to 0.3 with step 0.01. Since the experiments are stochastic, each experiment will be replicated 100 times and the average values will be calculated and used for interpretation. The result will determine at which probability of infection the disease will survive in the network. Further analysis will be performed to understand the difference between these two networks in terms of disease transmission.

4 Results

This section illustrates the main findings of the simulation using the Python language and NetworkX package. Section 4.1 shows the topological analysis of static and temporal networks. The SIR results are demonstrated in Sect. 4.2. More analysis of infection transmission in the proposed data is presented in Sect. 4.3.

4.1 The Topological Analysis

Topological analysis of the network represents the main features of the network, including the number of nodes, edges, graph type, and network degree, see Table 1.

Table 1. Topological parameters of the static network

Item	Value	Item	Value
Number of nodes	75	Number of components	1
Number of edges	1139	Clustering average	0.64
Graph type	Undirected	Betweenness centrality	‘1769’
Density	0.41	Connectivity	True
Degree (min, average, max)	(6, 30.37, 61)		

This network is small due to its few numbers of nodes, 75, compared with large-scale networks in the literature. The density is high due to many contacts compared to the number of people or nodes. We have found out that node ‘1525’ has the lowest number of contacts while ‘1098’ has the highest number of contacts. Moreover, the patient number

'1769' has the minimum length path in the network, so patient number '1769' serves as a bridge from one part of the network to another. In the temporal network, each day always contains the main component and isolated nodes. When interactions between nodes are active through a specific period, the number of isolated nodes is few as shown in day1, while isolated nodes increase when interactions are reduced such as (d) or day5 in Fig. 1.

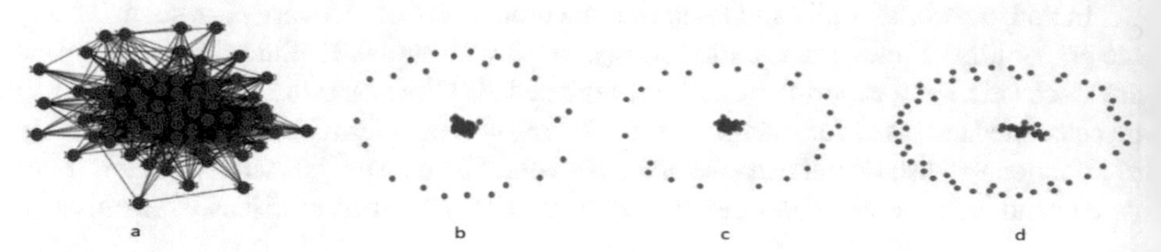

Fig. 1. (a) is the static network, and (b), (c), and (d) are the temporal network nodes interactions in day1, day3, and day5, respectively

4.2 Dynamic Simulation of the SIR Model

The patient in the SIR can recover and get immunity or die after becoming infected. Figure 2 shows the simulation of the SIR model tested on the static and temporal networks.

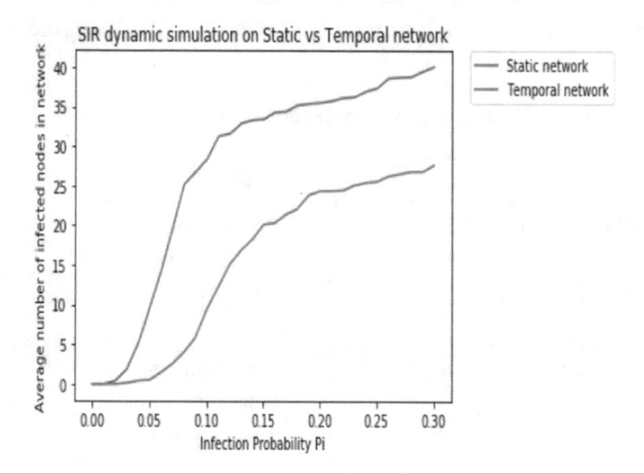

Fig. 2. SIR model for static and temporal networks

The disease propagation starts quite late for the temporal network on the SIR model ($p_i = 0.09$) and the average maximum number of infected nodes is maintained around 25/75, almost half the size of the static network.

4.3 Disease Transmission Analysis

This section concentrates on individuals to track the most infected people in this temporal network using the SIR scheme simulation. The simulation parameters are $p_i = 0.2$ and $p_r = 0.8$. The number of iterations is 100, each time we replicate the experiment 5 times, such that in each replication, the highest 5 infected nodes, maximum number of switches "either from normal to infected or the opposite way", the lowest infected nodes and eventually the nodes that never changed through the entire experiment were computed. Then, the most frequent results in all five experiments are reported.

The obtained results show that the highest infected nodes in all replications are the nurses, then the administrators. Besides, patients and physicians are less likely to become infected. It is found that the nurse ID "1295" has a dominant probability. Interestingly, most of these nurses' connections are with people who themselves have a higher probability of infections in the system. These nurses have a higher probability to transfer diseases to others, which on the other hand reflects the reality due to nurses' frequent interaction with patients and workers alike. Secondly, the nurses' number is higher than physicians or other staff as a majority that plays an important role in disease propagation.

5 Results

The obtained results show that the static network seems to be more vulnerable to the increment of infection probability. The temporal network required a much larger value of infection probability to be threatened by the epidemic. In a static network, every connection throughout the whole time will be aggregated together to form the network. In the temporal network, every connection for each node will only be considered during a specific time frame, which is dynamic and represents reality. The connection between some sets of nodes will appear on time t but might disappear in time $t + 1$ or $t + 2$. This behavior reduces the network density and makes the network more resistant to epidemic deployment.

The average maximum value of infected nodes in the static network is significantly higher than the temporal network. The explanation of this behavior may reside in the community structure of the temporal network. During a different time, the temporal network creates different community components and clusters. Those clusters contribute to isolating the spread of disease in some specific experiments and decreasing the total number of infected nodes. This result supports [6] claim, "the diffusion dynamics are affected by the network community structure and by the temporal properties of waiting times between events" [14]. Consequently, disease prevalence is lower in temporal networks than in static networks. In addition, the presented SIR model was able to capture most of the relevant information of the given data. The SIR simulation showed that the epidemic structure has an exponential form, which matches with the literature review and particularly, with the results reported in [4]. To prevent disease transmission, the transmission rate should be less than 10%.

6 Conclusion

This study elucidates the way of controlling and monitoring disease propagation in hospitals and alerts policymakers about the risk rate of the epidemic. The SIR model is used and tested on the proposed temporal network dataset and its aggregated (static) network. The temporal network represents reality due to its advantage of involving time as a main part of the data structure. The patient's interaction with staff occurs in an intermittent form, which was reflected in the topological analysis of the temporal network. It is found out that nurses and administrators have a higher probability of becoming infected compared with medical doctors or patients.

There are many limitations to our study, including the use of homogeneous assumptions. Even though this is a common method to make the results achievable; however, in real life, the medical staffs have a better awareness of the disease and well-knowledge of the prevention of infection, so that they don't have the same infection probability as patients. Future research can consider more detailed based on these different characters.

References

1. WHO: What is the global incidence of influenza? (August 2020). https://www.medscape.com/answers/219557-3459/what-is-the-global-incidence-of-influenza
2. Albrich, W.C., Harbarth, S.: Health-care workers: source, vector, or victim of MRSA? Lancet Infect. Dis. **8**(5), 289–301 (2008)
3. Barrat, A., Cattuto, C., Tozzi, A.E., Vanhems, P., Voirin, N.: Measuring contact patterns with wearable sensors: methods, data characteristics and applications to data-driven simulations of infectious diseases. Clin. Microbiol. Infect. **20**(1), 10–16 (2014)
4. Holme, P.: Epidemiologically optimal static networks from temporal network data. PLoS Comput. Biol. **9**(7), e1003142 (2013)
5. Holme, P.: Temporal network structures controlling disease spreading. Phys. Rev. E **94**(2), 022305 (2016)
6. Moinet, A., Pastor-Satorras, R., Barrat, A.: Effect of risk perception on epidemic spreading in temporal networks. Phys. Rev. E **97**(1), 012313 (2018)
7. Nadini, M., Sun, K., Ubaldi, E., Starnini, M., Rizzo, A., Perra, N.: Epidemic spreading in modular time-varying networks. Sci. Rep. **8**(1), 2352 (2018)
8. Shu, P., Wang, W., Tang, M., Do, Y.: Simulated identification of epidemic threshold on finite-size networks. arXiv preprint arXiv:1410.0459 (2014)
9. Valdano, E., Ferreri, L., Poletto, C., Colizza, V.: Analytical computation of the epidemic threshold on temporal networks. Phys. Rev. X **5**(2), 021005 (2015)
10. Vanhems, P., et al.: Estimating potential infection transmission routes in hospital wards using wearable proximity sensors. PloS one **8**(9), e73970 (2013)
11. Vanhems, P., et al.: Risk of influenza-like illness in an acute health care setting during community influenza epidemics in 2004–2005, 2005–2006, and 2006–2007: a prospective study. Arch. Intern. Med. **171**(2), 151–157 (2011)
12. Wang, W., Liu, Q.-H., Zhong, L.-F., Tang, M., Gao, H., Stanley, H.E.: Predicting the epidemic threshold of the susceptible-infected-recovered model. Sci. Rep. **6**, 24676 (2016)
13. Zhang, J., Lu, D., Yang, S.: Comparison of mean-field based theoretical analysis methods for SIS model. arXiv preprint arXiv:1704.01025 (2017)
14. Delvenne, J.C., Lambiotte, R., Rocha, L.E.: Diffusion on networked systems is a question of time or structure. Nat. Commun. **6**(1), 1–10 (2015)

Hospital Supply Chain Management and Quality of Services Within Hospitals: A Preliminary Review

Amer Alqudah[1(✉)], Hussein Mohammed Abualrejal[1,2], and Ezanee Elias[1,2]

[1] School of Technology Management and Logistics, College of Business, University Utara Malaysia, Sintok, Kedah, Malaysia
alqudahamer99@yahoo.com, abualrejal@uum.edu.my

[2] Knowledge Science Research Lab, School of Technology Management and Logistics, College of Business, University Utara Malaysia, Sintok, Kedah, Malaysia

Abstract. The most significant changes that face organizations nowadays are the growth of the globalization phenomenon and the new conditions and its development. In terms of the direction, the rapid growth work patterns and interactions between these factors prompted organizations to come up with new ways, also to deal with the suitable qualified and sudden changes affected by the changes that the economic environment has witnessed. Quality management (QM) and the supply chain (SC) are some of the significant changes facing organizations today and have been highlighted in many articles. They are management philosophies, not just simple tools or techniques. As a result, the purpose of such a study is to examine prior studies founded on this philosophy of overloading and to provide a fundamental notion in that framework for future research studies. This research will look into how improving medical care and treatment services has become urgent at the local and global levels as governments and the health care sector have begun to adopt total quality management. The study's goal is to provide a completer and more achievable model of controlling the relationship between supply chain and hospital service quality that has a significant impact on health. The study is useful for patients and health professionals to have a fundamental awareness of the relationship between supply chain and hospital service quality in Jordanian government hospitals, that aims to develop a healthier and better Jordanian generation.

Keywords: Hospital supply chain · Quality services · Government hospital Jordan

1 Introduction

The emergence of a new Coronavirus disease has impacted public health care organizations around the world. In Jordan, Coronavirus negatively affected healthcare for patients and has also forced a downturn in the production of medicines and respiratory equipment throughout the industries, and has further damaged supply chains that generally maintain

F. Saeed et al. (Eds.): IRICT 2021, LNDECT 127, pp. 775–784, 2022.
https://doi.org/10.1007/978-3-030-98741-1_66

health organizations' supplies [1]. Many organizations have adopted quality management as a key concept, and management ideology and lifestyle enable them to do so in the face of successful and rapid environmental conditions, as well as to raise customer awareness of the quality of the goods or services they supply [2]. Customer satisfaction is an important part of quality assurance, and comparable customer interactions have also been vital for improving service quality [3] To provide it, the importance of the supply chain in this field must be recognized as a major and essential area, both in the public and private sectors, and a significant contribution and focus on its effectiveness must be made through the use of the supply chain management information system, which is a part of the information system that measures, processes, and reports useful management information in making smooth decisions [4]. Consumers are encouraged to play a more active role in their own health management in today's healthcare environment. The quality of medical provided, on the other hand, is extremely variable and changing. Little is known about people's ideas and views concerning the quality of health utilized in medical car [5]. In the face of the foreign market's international competitive and totalitarian environment, enterprises must implement a "quality enhancement" strategy that caters to systems and services, allowing them to develop efficiently in international markets [6].

In general, the implementation of the concept of TQM translates into an improvement in service quality, which in turn leads to increased patient (customer) satisfaction, which is also taken into account to be among the basic tools for measuring the quality of service provided in health systems [3]. Kisuma et al. (2013) was also shown that the more successful the service quality assessment, the more significant the appealing precedents of customers enhance their relationship with them. Because health care providers give reliable information (feedback) that reflects the performance of health institutions, health care quality assessment of health care providers is a vital aspect in determining the effectiveness of these critical sectors [7].

The healthcare industry exists to serve the public by providing patients with high-quality care and safety at a low cost. As a result, having a responsive supply chain can help achieve this goal [8]. Chowdhury and others (2017) emphasized that the fundamental goal of the supply chain in service industries is to lower the costs associated with providing high-quality services [4]. Accordingly, the purpose of this study is to examine the difficulties surrounding the supply chain and quality of service' as they influence the health of government hospitals in Jordan as a first step toward proposing an academic improved model to improve health care service quality. In Jordan, there aren't enough models addressing or assessing the efficacy of the supply chain, and more models are needed to understand its utilization and its impact on health-care quality.

2 Business Model

The study aims to clarify the impact of the dimensions of supply chain management (relationship with suppliers, specifications and standards, delivery, and after-sales service) as the Independent variables on the dimensions of health service quality (suitability, responsiveness, trust, and safety) in Jordanian government hospitals (the Dependent Variables) (Fig. 1).

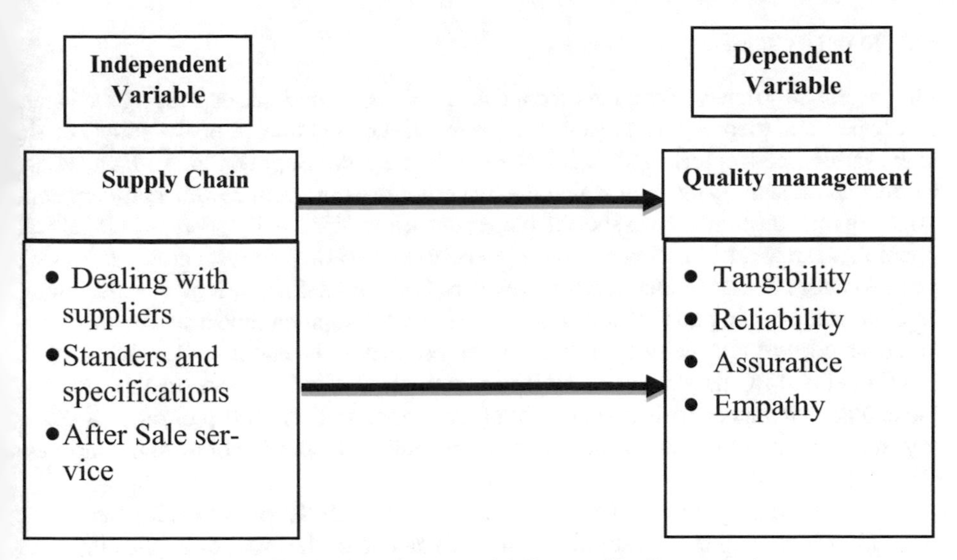

Fig. 1. Research business model (Prepared by Researcher)

3 Literature Review

The researcher reviews some previous research regarding healthcare services quality management and the supply chain of the hospital correlation of healthcare services in Jordanian government hospitals. Therefore, the researcher introduces several SC concepts, quality management, and healthcare service quality. During the discussion of the study theoretical literature previous studies, An overview of the development of supply chain management and related ideas present.

3.1 HealthCare Quality Service

Quality management is considered one of the modern management concepts that continuously improves and develops understanding by responding to client requirements continually [9]. Quality management is defined as a cooperative approach of company performance based on the shared skills of managers and employee, with the goal of continual quality and productivity development through work teams [10]. Quality of health care is described by the World Health Organization as conforming to standards and accurate performance in a safe, community-acceptable manner at a reasonable cost, resulting in a change and influence on the percentage of illness cases, deaths, disability, and malnutrition [11]. Many researches on assessing the quality of hospital services and patient satisfaction have shown numerous challenges, emphasizing the importance of continuing to pay attention to quality issues and informing hospital managers about potential problems so that they can be addressed [12].

Quality healthcare, in the classical sense, entails meeting professional standards, specifications, and norms. Medical personnel as nursing practiced and taught by leaders of the medical profession during a given period of social, cultural, and professional growth in a particular country are referred to be good medical care [13].

3.2 Supply Chain

The theoretical frameworks addressed a wide range of definitions, expressing the ideas, ideologies, and theoretical concepts of each researcher and thinker on the supply chain from various conceptual angles. SC is described by the Supply Chain Management Council as an activity chain in which raw materials are transported from a primary supplier to a final customer. Also sharing materials, information, and materials in logistical operations ranging from collecting raw materials to delivering end-user products, as well as all vendors and customer service providers [14]. SC defined a logical sequence of creative value-adding activities that commence with the procurement of raw materials and conclude with the delivery of the finished product to the end user [15]. Burns et al. (2021) defined SC as a series of facilities, activities, functions, and organizations of those organizations encompassed in manufacturing as well as service or product delivery, starting with raw material suppliers and extending in all directions to the ultimate client. [16].

The Relationship Between Supply Chain and Health Services Quality Ben Daya et al. (2020) highlighted the supply chain (SC) as one of the areas of application with considerable potential to reap the benefits of the Internet of Things in their evaluation of Internet of Things (IoT) applications in supply chain management. They proposed possible study subjects that benefit from rapid technological improvements in SC, based on the results of this literature review. [17]. In a field of knowledge on the impact of supplier investment, quality management, and supply chain information on SME performance, Zhou and Li (2020) investigated the importance of quality management and value chain practices. The research added to the literature in a number of ways [18]. Initially, it investigates the connections between supplier investment, supply chain information sharing, quality management, along with the effects on development and market share performance.

Furthermore, geographic settings such as coastal areas and interior provinces could have a considerable influence on the practices and performance of SMEs in the supply chain. Additionally, competition intensity could affect small and medium-sized enterprises' decisions regarding investing in provider investment projects. Fourth, the different stages of development (i.e., presentation, growth, and maturity) in which SME choices concerning supplier investment, quality management, and supply chain information sharing are unaffected. Al-Saa'da et al. (2013) from the standpoint of quality, the dimensions of supply chain management, namely, specifications and standards, supplier connection, after-sale service, compatibility, and delivery on health care quality and their impact on health care quality dimensions (security, response, and confidence) in Jordan's private hospitals were studied [19] according to the procurement staff. The research further seeks to explain the variation between the quality of health care and supply chain as a result of certain demographic factors. According to the research, supply chain management parameters, which include specifications and standards, after-sales support, supplier connection, and delivery, have a moral impact on health service quality. The outcomes, on the other hand, demonstrate that there are no sex, level of education, age, or knowledge disparities in health-care quality, along with supply chain management. Jordan's health-care system's quality has been evaluated (Abu-kharmeh 2012). The quality has been assessed in five dimensions, namely concrete, reliable, responsive, assured, and sympathetic. According to the findings, Jordanian hospitals provide moderate health services. With the exception of assurance factors and the high response, the service quality dimensions appeared likewise modest [20]. De Vries and Huijsman (2011) centered on the topic of whether there are any parallels seen between healthcare services, along with industrial centers concerning developments in supply chain management [21].

4 Methodology

A literature review method was used in this study depending on supply chain and healthcare service quality as well as hopes for future empirical investigations to go into the specifics of the links between supply chain and healthcare service quality. This study will consider the 'supply chain and healthcare service quality among Government hospitals in Jordan with the goal of developing a new academic-enhanced approach that would serve as a complete and achievable approach for controlling service quality that might have a considerable effect on patients. The study's exploratory approach attempts to determine the impacts of the supply chain on the quality of service. The conclusions may not be deduced from electronic sources, necessitating additional study (Table 1).

5 Discussion

Warehouses, factories, operations centers, and distribution centers are all part of supply chains. Among the responsibilities and activities addressed are forecasting, buying, stock management, data management, quality control, manufacturing, distribution, delivery, and, finally, customer service. [25]. From an administrative standpoint, El-Shoghari and Abdallah (2016) noted that supply chain management will have an impact on service quality, as it will allow institutions to monitor service quality in order to better utilize existing resources and attract new ones to satisfy demand. [26]. Ali et al. (2012) investigated the extent to which Jordanian hospitals use comprehensive quality management to improve their performance. A total of two health-related industries were investigated: Both public and private hospitals (Irbid-King Abdullah University Hospital) are available (Amman-Jordan Hospital and Medical Center) [27]. The results revealed that eight principles of comprehensive quality management were strongly linked to the hospital's performance, and that overall quality management had a very good association with the hospital's performance in Jordan. Starting with a review of existing literature, various approaches to supply chain integration might be examined. Additionally, knowledge gained from the studies presented in this special issue must be reviewed and contextualized in the context of any additional investigation that could be necessary. By outlining several important study areas that are connected to healthcare management as well as supply chain management, this book contributes to the literature in both fields. The researcher aids researchers and administrators in grasping the complexity of health-care supply chain management.

Table 1. Provides research carried out on supply chain and quality of health service.

Author	Independent variable	Mediating & moderating variable	Dependent variable	Methodology	Findings
Gentle and Arrive, 2020	SCM		Health care service quality	Qualitative analysis and questionnaire	The findings are based on a sample of students from a single Italian state institution A cross-sectional approach is provided in this study [23]
Jan, De Vries, 2011	SCM		Health services	Exploratory, qualitative approach	Starting with a classification of current studies, five major study topics affecting supply chain management in healthcare and care settings have been identified. Furthermore, in addition to studies with a monodisciplinary emphasis, a multidisciplinary attention on Supply chain issue in health services appears to be necessary
Xianghui Peng, 2017	SCM		A quality		The findings indicate the efficacy of the suggested framework. According to the findings, SCM is an important organizational construct that has a considerable beneficial direct influence on organizational performance. According to studies, SCM is also a facilitator for management, measurement, investigation, and knowledge creation, all of which impact organizational success

(*continued*)

Table 1. *(continued)*

Author	Independent variable	Mediating & moderating variable	Dependent variable	Methodology	Findings
Agyabeng-Mensah et al., 2020	Green supply chain	TQM		Qualitative analysis	The results show that GSCPs integrate with TQM and JIT to enhance OP as well as BP significantly. However, green TQM and supply chain management combination add greater value to BP and OP as opposed to the synergy between GSCPs and JIT [24]
Gutama Getele, 2020	SCM		Healthcare service quality	Questionnaire used in this study	All the variables are associated; all of the variables have a strong and substantial association. Current study results show that the quality of healthcare in Ethiopia is linked to a combination of timely delivery of health care products, specifications, the standard of healthcare product providers, and after-sale services in private health sectors
Mahmoud BakkarAbdel Tawab, 2019	Total quality management		SCM	Descriptive-analytical method	The results of the positive research of TQM in all its dimensions (support to senior management), Customer focus, continuous improvement, employee training working in the public domain The supply chain dimensions (the company, customer recovery, customer relations, information flow) Across the supply chain, internal supply chain operations (public sector industries firms

(continued)

Table 1. (*continued*)

Author	Independent variable	Mediating & moderating variable	Dependent variable	Methodology	Findings
Raghavendraand Njaguna, 2015	SCM		Service quality		Clearly indicates that there is significant relationship between the supply chain Practices and the service quality of the restaurant. Our findings are also discussed in terms of their significance for practicing managers. Our findings imply that in their strategic planning efforts, supply chain managers should consider the practices highlighted in this study when determining the optimal amount of supply chain integration in the five service quality dimensions
Alsaida, 2013	Management of the supply chain			Quality service health	In Ethiopia, the quality of healthcare is connected to a combination of timely provision of health care goods, specifications, After-Sale services in the private health sector, and the standard of healthcare product suppliers

6 Conclusion

Total Quality Management (TQM) is a method utilized by organizations that provide high-quality service. Total Quality Management (TQM) is a management method that gives organizations a competitive edge. TQM was defined as a change in the organization's structure that also entails focusing the organization's efforts on the continuous improvement of all operations and systems, as well as, most importantly, the various stages of work, because performance is nothing more than knowing the client's requirements and converting them into requirements that meet the client's requirements. In addition, healthcare SCM is a dynamic model that takes into account production and provider resources, as well as the availability of services and goods for patients and providers, which is considered as an intrinsically difficult operation, which necessitates a continuous commodities' flow, information, orders, as well as financial transactions among phases. Despite the fact that SCM considers a phased operation, the COVID-19 pandemic damaged the majority of the chain for several grounds, leading to a shortage of several personal protective devices and medical services on the medical frontlines because of insufficient data quality. The impact on daily life of a disturbance in the flow of services and medical goods from the patients' factory as well as doctors, with far-reaching implication.

References

1. J. World Health Org. (2020)
2. Al-Maamari, Q.A., Hashemi, A., Aljamrh, B.A., Al-Harasi, A.H.: The relationship between total quality management practices and individual readiness for change at petroleum exploration and production authority in Yemen. Int. J. Bus. Industr. Mark. **6**(2), 48–55 (2017)
3. Nguyen, T.L.H., Nagase, K.: The influence of total quality management on customer satisfaction. Int. J. Healthc. Manag. **12**(4), 277–285 (2019)
4. Chowdhury, A.H.M., Alam, M.Z., Habib, M.M.: Supply chain management practices in services industry: an empirical investigation on some selected services sector of Bangladesh. Int. J. Supply Chain Manag. **6**(3), 152–162 (2017)
5. Tao, D., Lerouge, C., Smith, K.J., De Leo, G.: Defining information quality into health websites: a conceptual framework of health website information quality for educated young adults. JMIR Hum. Fact. **4**(4), E6455 (2017)
6. Debattista, J., Auer, S., Lange, C.: Luzzu—a methodology and framework for linked data quality assessment. J. Data Inf. Q. JDIQ **8**(1), 4 (2016)
7. Cho, W.H., Lee, H., Kim, C., Lee, S., Choi, K.S.: The impact of visit frequency on the relationship between service quality and outpatient satisfaction: a South Korean study. Health Serv. Res. **39**(1), 13–34 (2004)
8. Srivastava, S., Garg, D., Agarwal, A.: A step towards responsive healthcare supply chain management: an overview. Adv. Manuf. Industr. Eng. 431–443 (2021)
9. Wagner, C., Groene, O., Thompson, C., et al.: Development and validation of an index to assess hospital quality management systems. Int. J. Qual. Health Care **26**, 16–26 (2014)
10. Abbas, J.: Impact of total quality management on corporate sustainability through the mediating effect of knowledge management. J. Clean. Prod. **244**, 1–11 (2020)
11. Hamed, O.: Quality of health services provided to patients in government hospitals, applying to locality and Medani Al-Kubra, Gezira State - Sudan (2020). World J. Econ. Bus. **9**(2), 318–332 (2020)
12. Parand, A., Dopson, S., Renz, A., Vincent, C.: The role of hospital managers in quality and patient safety: a systematic review. BMJ Open **4**(9), 1–15 (2014)
13. Mcglynn, E.A.: Measuring and improving quality in the US: where are we today? J. Am. Board Family Med. **33**(Supplement), S28–S35 (2020)
14. Mathur, B., Gupta, S., Meena, M. L., Dangayach, G.S.: Healthcare supply chain management: literature review and some issues. J. Adv. Manag. Res. (2018)
15. Abdel-Basset, M., Manogaran, G., Mohamed, M.: Internet of things (IoT) and its impact on supply chain: a framework for building intelligent, secure, and efficient systems. Futur. Gener. Comput. Syst. **86**, 614–628 (2018)
16. Burns, N., Minnick, K., Smith, A.H.: The role of directors with related supply chain industry experience in corporate acquisition decisions. J. Corp. Finance, 101911 (2021)
17. Ben-Daya, M., Hassini, E., Bahroun, Z., Banimfreg, B.H.: The role of internet of things in food supply chain quality management: a review. Qual. Manag. J. 1–24 (2020)
18. Zhou, H., Shou, Y., Zhai, X., Li, L., Wood, C., Wu, X.: Supply chain practice and information quality: a supply chain strategy study. Int. J. Prod. Econ. **147**, 624–633 (2014)
19. Al-Saa'da, R.J., Taleb, Y.K.A., Al Abdallat, M.E., Al-Mahasneh, R.A.A., Nimer, N.A., Al-Weshah, G.A.: Supply chain management and its effect on health care service quality: quantitative evidence from Jordanian private hospitals. J. Manag. Strategy **4**(2), 42 (2013)

20. Abu-Kharmeh, S.: Evaluating the quality of healthcare services in the hashemite of the Kingdom of Jordan. Int. J. Bus. Manag. **7**(4), 195–205 (2012)
21. De Vries, J., Huijsman, R.: Supply chain management in health services: an overview. Supply Chain Manag. Int. J. (2011)
22. Iyengar, K., Mabrouk, A., Jain, V.K., Venkatesan, A., Vaishya, R.: Learning opportunities from COVID-19 and future effects on health care system. Diabetes Metab. Syndr. **14**(5), 943–946 (2020)
23. Getele, G.K., Li, T., Arrive, J.T.: The role of supply chain management in healthcare service quality. IEEE Eng. Manag. Rev. **48**, 145–155 (2020)
24. Agyabeng-Mensah, Y., Ahenkorah, E., Afum, E., Agyemang, A.N., Agnikpe, C., Rogers, F.: Examining the influence of internal green supply chain practices, green human resource management and supply chain environmental cooperation on firm performance. Supply Chain Manag. Int. J. (2020)
25. el Shoghari, R., Abdallah, K.: The impact of supply chain management on customer service (a case study of Lebanon). Management **6**(2), 46–54 (2016)
26. Agyabeng-Mensah, Y., Afum, E., Agnikpe, C., Cai, J., Ahenkorah, E., Dacosta, E.: Exploring the mediating influences of total quality management and just in time between green supply chain practices and performance. J. Manuf. Technol. Manag. (2020)
27. Ali, J., Kumar, S.: Information and communication technologies (ICT) and farmers' decision-making across the agricultural supply chain. Int. J. Inf. Manag. **31**(2), 149–159 (2011)

Author Index

F. Saeed et al. (Eds.): IRICT 2021, LNDECT 127, pp. 785–787, 2022.
https://doi.org/10.1007/978-3-030-98741-1

Printed in the United States
by Baker & Taylor Publisher Services